The RCEM Lecture Notes: Emergency Medicine

The RCEM Lecture Notes:
Emergency Medicine

Edited by

Catherine Williams

Emergency Medicine Consultant, Royal Bolton Hospital, Bolton, UK
Health Education North West, Manchester, UK

Amy Nickson

Emergency Medicine Consultant, Royal Bolton Hospital, Bolton, UK
Sexual Offences Examiner, Lancashire SAFE Centre, Preston, UK

Fifth Edition

This Fifth Edition is edited by Catherine Williams and Amy Nickson, has been revised and updated by contributors, and is based on the Fourth Edition of *Lecture Notes: Emergency Medicine* which was authored by Chris Moulton and David Yates.

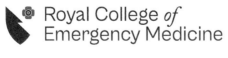
Royal College *of* Emergency Medicine

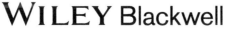
WILEY Blackwell

Registered Offices
John Wiley & Sons, Inc., 111 River Street, Hoboken, NJ 07030, USA
John Wiley & Sons Ltd, The Atrium, Southern Gate, Chichester, West Sussex, PO19 8SQ, UK

For details of our global editorial offices, customer services, and more information about Wiley products visit us at www.wiley.com.

Wiley also publishes its books in a variety of electronic formats and by print-on-demand. Some content that appears in standard print versions of this book may not be available in other formats.

Library of Congress Cataloging-in-Publication Data
Names: Williams, Catherine (Consultant in emergency medicine), editor. |
  Nickson, Amy, editor. Lecture notes. Emergency medicine. |
  Royal College of Emergency Medicine (Great Britain), issuing body.
Title: The RCEM lecture notes. Emergency medicine / edited by Catherine
  Williams, Amy Nickson.
Other titles: Royal College of Emergency Medicine lecture notes. Emergency
  medicine
Description: Fifth edition. | Hoboken, NJ : Wiley-Blackwell, 2024. |
  Preceded by Lecture notes. Emergency medicine / Chris Moulton, David
  Yates. 4th ed. 2012.
Identifiers: LCCN 2023016562 (print) | LCCN 2023016563 (ebook) | ISBN
  9781119325819 (paperback) | ISBN 9781119325840 (Adobe PDF) | ISBN
  9781119325857 (epub)
Subjects: MESH: Emergencies | Emergency Treatment–methods | Emergency
  Medicine–methods
Classification: LCC RC86.7 (print) | LCC RC86.7 (ebook) | NLM WB 105 |
  DDC 616.02/5–dc23/eng/20230912
LC record available at https://lccn.loc.gov/2023016562
LC ebook record available at https://lccn.loc.gov/2023016563

Cover Design: Wiley
Cover Image: © Christine Müller/EyeEm; Tyler Olson

Set in 8/10.5pt Utopia by Straive, Pondicherry, India
Printed and bound by CPI Group (UK) Ltd, Croydon, CR0 4YY

C9781119325819_131223

Contents

List of contributors, vi

Preface to the fifth edition, vii

Preface to the fourth edition, viii

Preface to the second edition, ix

Preface to the first edition, x

About the Companion Website, xi

1 What every Emergency Physician needs to know, 1
Catherine Williams

2 Major trauma and multiple injuries, 19
Lt Col Alan G A Weir RAMC

3 Head injuries, 34
Kate Clayton

4 The neck and the back, 48
Fiqry Fadillah and Catherine Williams

5 Facial injuries, 64
James Conroy and Abu Hassan

6 Injuries to the trunk, 73
Fiqry Fadillah

7 The lower limb, 88
Abu Hassan

8 The upper limb, 113
Katie Fulcher and Abu Hassan

9 The hand, 132
Shah Rahman and Sophie Jefferys

10 Burns, contamination and irradiation, 141
Jodie Wilkinson

11 Cardiac arrest and cardiac dysrhythmias, 157
Rob Summerhayes

12 Chest pain, 184
Vivek Chhabra and Amy Nickson

13 Respiratory distress, 205
Amy Nickson

14 Collapse and sudden illness, 233
Amy Nickson

15 Poisoning, 277
Jodie Wilkinson

16 Abdominal pain and GI problems, 310
Catherine Williams

17 Obstetric, gynaecological and genitourinary
problems, 326
Amy Nickson

18 Children's problems in the emergency
department, 341
Catherine Williams

19 The disturbed patient, 373
Antonia Hazlerigg and Laura Cottey

20 Medicolegal aspects of emergency medicine, 392
Amy Nickson

21 Small wounds and localised infections, 410
Catherine Williams

22 Ophthalmic, ENT and facial conditions, 428
Amy Nickson

23 Global health, 443
A.D. Redmond

Index, 458

List of contributors

Vivek Chhabra
York and Scarborough Teaching,
Hospitals NHS Foundation Trust,
Calderdale and Huddersfield NHS Foundation Trust, UK

Kate Clayton
Queen Elizabeth Hospital Birmingham,
Birmingham, UK

James Conroy
Leeds Teaching Hospitals, Leeds, UK

Laura Cottey
Academic Department of Military Emergency Medicine,
Royal Centre for Defence Medicine

Fiqry Fadillah
Royal Free Hospital, London, UK
Magpas Air Ambulance, Huntingdon, UK

Katie Fulcher
Bradford Teaching Hospitals NHS Foundation Trust,
Bradford, UK

Abu Hassan
Sheffield Children's Hospital and the Northern General
Hospital, Sheffield, UK

Antonia Hazlerigg
Emergency Department, Royal Infirmary of Edinburgh,
Edinburgh, UK
Academic Department of Military Emergency Medicine,
Royal Centre for Defence Medicine

Sophie Jefferys
St Mary's Hospital, Imperial College Healthcare
NHS Trust, London, UK

Amy Nickson
Royal Bolton Hospital, Bolton, UK
Lancashire SAFE Centre, Preston, UK

Shah Rahman
Oxford Deanery, Oxford, UK

A.D. Redmond
Humanitarian and Conflict Response Institute,
University of Manchester, Manchester, UK

Rob Summerhayes
University Hospital Southampton, Southampton, UK
Hampshire and Isle of Wight Air Ambulance

Alan G A Weir
UK Defence Medical Services, Lichfield, UK
Academic Department of Military Emergency Medicine,
Royal Centre for Defence Medicine, Birmingham, UK
Major Trauma Centre, University Hospital
Southampton, Southampton, UK

Jodie Wilkinson
Northern Care Alliance,
Royal Oldham Hospital, Oldham, UK

Catherine Williams
Royal Bolton Hospital, Bolton, UK
Health Education North West, Manchester, UK

Preface to the fifth edition

Emergency medicine is facing some of the greatest challenges since the specialty first began. Departments are faced with crowding, exit block and higher attendances than ever before. Our bright and talented doctors want to provide the highest standards of care but are struggling to do so. Maintaining our compassion in the face of extremely challenging working conditions is clearly essential for the patients that we care for and has also been demonstrated to reduce physician burnout and emotional fatigue.

Despite its challenges, emergency medicine remains an innovative and forward-thinking speciality, which is rising to meet these challenges and continually adapting to meet the needs of our patients. The joy and challenge of Emergency Medicine has always been the intellectual stimulus of providing high-quality emergency care for the very sickest patients and managing the broad range of undifferentiated patients attending our departments, and this remains undimmed.

We hope this book provides you with a strong foundation to begin your journey into Emergency Medicine. Most of the important skills you will need cannot be learned from a book alone. Practical skills and pattern recognition only come with thousands of hours of deliberate practice under the supervision of experienced clinicians. Amongst those, we hope you find a role model for the type of doctor you would like to be – a leader, a pioneer, a teacher. We hope you find satisfaction in working in the most challenging of careers, where each of your actions can have such a profound impact on the lives of others.

Attempting to produce a textbook for a speciality as wide ranging and rapidly evolving as Emergency Medicine is a daunting task. In updating this text, we hope that we have represented the changes in both Emergency Medicine practice, and in society, in the years since previous editions. In doing so, we are highly cognisant that we are standing on the shoulders of giants. We would like to express sincere gratitude for the mentorship and support of the previous editor of this book, Dr Chris Moulton, and for the training, challenge and constructive criticism of all the colleagues, trainers and patients who have shaped our practice.

Catherine Williams and Amy Nickson, 2023

Preface to the fourth edition

The intervals between editions of this text are getting shorter, perhaps reflecting the increasing speed of change in medicine in general and emergency medicine in particular. We have introduced new material on emerging topics and updated information on established topics and now support this with a bank of multiple-choice questions (MCQs) available online. The MCQs are supplemented by short explanations to reinforce your understanding.

The original layout has been retained – providing immediately accessible didactic advice supported by evidence-based rationale. The latter is now firmly established in the practice of the specialty, vindicating the aspiration in our first preface that 'future developments must ensure that the scientific method is woven into the fabric of the department'™.

There is an increasing tendency for more professionals to be exposed to the emergency department for shorter periods of time and, to many, the sometimes deceptive lure of the internet as a source of immediate knowledge seems to be all-satisfying. We hope that you will agree that, although search engines can reinforce a book, they can never replace it. Using both, you will gain knowledge and understanding. Your patients will then be treated by the experienced rather than be used by you to gain experience.

We are very grateful to Anne Bassett whose help improved the quality of this book.

Chris Moulton and David Yates, 2012

Preface to the second edition

Emergency physicians work in an environment where measured interrogation is a luxury, where life-saving skills can be required urgently and where the art of rapid and effective communication is essential. Add to this list the expectation that the doctor will have an encyclopaedic knowledge of the emergency aspects of every medical condition – and not a few social crises – and it is not surprising that most medical students and young doctors approach the emergency department with excitement that is tinged with anxiety.

This book is designed, in its approach, layout and content, to address these fears. Information is presented in an order that is relevant to the enquirer. It is demand led. Pathophysiology and relevant explanations follow. The reader learns how to deal with the emergency and then reads the background to the crisis and how, perhaps, it could have been avoided. This link with prevention is an increasingly emphasised part of emergency medicine, together with its concern to blur the boundaries between hospital and community care. Our primary aim has been to equip the reader with the knowledge to deal with crises, but we hope that we have shared, in these pages, our concern to ensure that doctors are also trained to try to avoid them.

Professor AD Redmond was the co-author of the first edition of this work, with Professor Yates. Although the book has been completely rewritten, we have retained all the innovations that were so successfully introduced in *Lecture Notes on Accident and Emergency Medicine* in 1985. Professor Redmond has provided valuable advice on the development of this new edition, and it is a pleasure to record our appreciation of this support and encouragement.

The authors are very grateful for the support of their families, whose accidents and emergencies were neglected during the writing of this book.

Chris Moulton and David Yates
Manchester, UK, 1999

Preface to the first edition

Our aim has been to cover all aspects of the work of a doctor in a busy accident and emergency department. Much of the text should be of interest to medical students during their clinical studies, but we hope that the book will be of special value to doctors studying for postgraduate diplomas.

Clearly, some restrictions must be placed on our definition of accident and emergency work unless we are to be overwhelmed, both here as authors and in our departments as casualty officers. These lecture notes have not been conceived as comprehensive treatises on the management of the many topics discussed – for only some aspects of most diseases and injuries are germane to the accident and emergency department. But it is precisely these aspects that are often inadequately covered in the standard texts. This book is based on our daily experience of the plethora of conditions presenting to what is inevitably an unstructured environment.

Sections devoted to 'Urgent action' are designed to facilitate the book's use during emergencies. The remaining text continues this rather didactic format but is supported by background material, which attempts to justify our dogma. It is, however, not always enough to state that the advice given here has worked in practice (but it has!). Emergency medicine, like all other branches of medicine, must be based on sound scientific principles. A significant recent development has been the acceptance that emergencies are better treated by the experienced than used to gain experience. Future developments must ensure that the scientific method is woven into the fabric of the department.

The academic base for accident and emergency medicine in Manchester has been created by the foresight and hard work of three men. We wish to record our thanks to Professor MH Irving, Dr GS Laing and Professor HB Stoner who have given so much to the specialty in its early days and who have supported us during the preparation of this book. The doctors, nurses, clerical staff and patients of Salford and Stockport have also given us invaluable help. Their encouragement has been greatly appreciated. Jackie Fortin typed some of the preparatory work and Julie Rostron exercised great skill and patience in compiling the manuscript.

Veronica Yates responded to our vague requests for pictures with precise illustrations, and our publishers displayed remarkable tolerance during a long gestation.

DW Yates and AD Redmond,
August 1984

About the Companion Website

This book is accompanied by a companion website:

www.wiley.com/go/LNEM5

This website includes:

- Case studies
- Best practices
- Test questions

What every Emergency Physician needs to know

Catherine Williams

Emergency Medicine Consultant, Royal Bolton Hospital, Bolton, UK
Health Education North West, Manchester, UK

People from many different backgrounds, of all ages and with an enormous variety of problems, present to an emergency department (ED) both by day and by night. The definition of 'what constitutes an emergency' is highly variable, and the ED often acts as a medical and societal safety net.

EMERGENCY ASSESSMENT OF THE UNDIFFERENTIATED PATIENT

All emergency physicians must be able to respond to, and manage an undifferentiated patient, presenting with a sudden emergency. A structured initial approach, following the ABCDE format discussed below, will ensure that immediately life-threatening problems are addressed in order or priority. In many cases, where multiple clinicians are involved, these elements may be undertaken in parallel, but it remains important for a team leader to maintain a structured overview.

Cardiac arrest → Chapter 11, p. 157.
Children → p. 342.

The ABCDE assessment

A rapid initial ABCDE assessment should be possible in about 30 seconds. Immediate threats should be addressed at each stage before moving on.

Special considerations of the ABCDE assessment in trauma Chapter 2, p → 22.

A – Airway

The airway may be:

- patent, partially obstructed or completely obstructed (from physical obstruction or loss of muscle tone)
- adequately protected or at risk (this depends on the protective reflexes of the airway).

Check for responsiveness

Is the patient alert and responsive to questions? A verbal reply confirms that there is:

- a maintained and protected airway
- temporarily adequate breathing and circulation
- cerebral functioning.

If responsive, then the patient will usually be able to elaborate on the cause of the sudden deterioration that has brought him or her to an ED.

Failure to respond indicates a significantly lowered level of consciousness and therefore an airway that may be obstructed and is definitely at risk. There may be a need for airway-opening manoeuvres and action to protect the airway.

> Foreign body obstruction may initially present as a distressed, very agitated, cyanosed patient – 'choking'.

The RCEM Lecture Notes: Emergency Medicine, Fifth Edition. Edited by Catherine Williams and Amy Nickson.
© 2024 John Wiley & Sons Ltd. Published 2024 by John Wiley & Sons Ltd.
Companion website: www.wiley.com/go/LNEM5

Cardiorespiratory arrest → p. 157.
Choking → p. 205.
Respiratory arrest → p. 209.

Look for signs of partial upper airway obstruction

> Complete upper airway obstruction will be silent.

- **Snoring**: the familiar sound of obstruction caused by the soft tissues of the mouth and pharynx. Often it accompanies the reduced muscle tone of a lowered level of consciousness.
- **Rattling or gurgling**: the sound of fluids in the upper airway.
- **Stridor**: a harsh, 'crowing' inspiratory (or occasionally biphasic) noise. Stridor suggests obstruction at the level of the larynx and upper trachea, which may be caused by foreign body or local infection. In cases of suspected supraglottic swelling, instrumentation of the throat (including the use of tongue depressor) should not be carried out, and examination should be undertaken very carefully as there is a risk of precipitating complete obstruction.
- **Drooling**: suggests obstruction at the posterior pharynx.
- **Hoarseness**: gross voice change suggests obstruction at the level of the larynx.
- **'See-saw' respiration (abdominal expansion with thoracic wall indrawing)**: is indicative of airway obstruction with ongoing respiratory effort.

> Cyanosis and reduced saturation readings on a pulse oximeter are very late signs of airway obstruction.

Allergic reactions → p. 306.
Laryngotracheal obstruction → p. 205.
Surgical airways → p. 23.

> Assess the need for cervical spine protection before any airway intervention.

Clearance and maintenance of the airway

There are two main ways in which the airway becomes blocked.

Depressed level of consciousness: the most common cause. When muscle tone is lost, the relaxation of soft tissues around the airway, in particular the tongue, may precipitate airway obstruction.

Physical obstruction: from a variety of causes such as direct trauma, external or intramural mass or foreign body.

Airway obstruction may be immediately relieved by:

- removing the cause of the obstruction (suction, manual removal or choking manoeuvre)
- chin lift/head tilt manoeuvre
- jaw thrust – pushing the jaw and the hyoid bone and their attached soft tissues forward
- use of an oro-pharyngeal/nasopharyngeal airway, supraglottic airway (i-gel or laryngeal mask) or endotracheal intubation
- reducing the swelling with vasoconstrictor drugs (adrenaline)
- tracheal intubation
- bypassing the cause of obstruction with a surgical airway.

Protection of the airway

Airway reflexes may be compromised by specific nerve palsies (e.g. stroke), the effect of drugs (including alcohol) and decreased conscious level. They may also be impaired at the extremes of age and in states of general debilitation. Vigilance is required in all such situations as there is a risk of aspiration of vomitus.

- The recovery position should be used whenever possible if consciousness is decreased. This allows fluid and vomitus to drain from the airway under gravity, and the airway should be positioned to ensure patency. A high-flow suction catheter must always be near the patient's head.
- The patient trolley must be capable of tilting 'head down' to drain vomitus out of the airway.

Obtunded patients require consideration of endotracheal intubation for airway protection.

> Over 10% of normal individuals have no gag reflex, and thus presence or absence of a gag reflex is not a good predictor of need for intubation.
>
> In a patient with a reduced level of consciousness, the airway must be assumed to be at risk until proved otherwise.

Protection of the cervical spine

If the patient has an injury to the cervical spine, there is a risk of damage to the spinal cord during the procedures needed to maintain the airway. Because of the potentially devastating outcomes of cervical cord injury, care must be taken to protect the cervical spine in patients who are:

- unresponsive with a history of trauma or no clear history
- suffering from multiple trauma
- difficult to assess
- showing any symptoms or signs that might be attributable to the cervical spine.

Adequate protection of the potentially unstable cervical spine conventionally consists of a rigid collar and blocks secured with tape. Cervical immobilisation makes airway management more challenging and can be distressing for the patient and so in these circumstances, manual inline stabilisation may be preferable.

Exclusion of cervical spine injury → p. 54.

B – Breathing

Look for

- **Difficulty in talking**
- **Abnormal respiratory rate**: usually fast, laboured breathing. Very slow respiratory rates may occur just before respiratory arrest or due to poisoning with respiratory depressant drugs (e.g. opiates)
- *Nasal flaring and use of shoulder and neck muscles*
- **Paradoxical respiration**: a see-sawing movement of the chest and abdomen, which indicates airway obstruction, fatigue of the diaphragm or occasionally cervical cord injury
- *Unequal, diminished or abnormal breath sounds*
- *Hyperresonance or dullness to percussion*
- *Displacement of the trachea or apex beat*
- *A flail segment*
- **In children, subcostal or intercostal recession and tracheal tug**: indrawing of the elastic tissues caused by increased respiratory effort.

All the above suggest that the patient is struggling to achieve normal respiration. Failure to oxygenate the blood adequately and hence the tissues are shown by:

- **Tachycardia:** the nervous system has detected hypoxia and is stimulating the heart
- **Pallor and sweating**: caused by sympathetic stimulation
- **Cyanosis**: a late sign
- **Irritability, confusion or reduced responsiveness**: the brain is short of oxygen. This is an extremely worrying sign
- **A low SaO$_2$ (<94%)**: pulse oximetry should be established as soon as possible

Allergic reactions → p. 306.

Chest decompression and drainage → p. 76.
Chest injuries → p. 74.
Respiratory distress → p. 205.

Oxygen therapy

The common denominator of most life-threatening illness, irrespective of cause, is the failure to deliver adequate amounts of oxygen to the tissues.

In the initial phase of assessment of the critically ill patient, high-flow oxygen (usually via a non-rebreathing mask) is an appropriate temporising measure. It is increasingly recognised that administration of high-flow oxygen carries its own risks, so once accurate oxygen saturation measurement has been obtained, the FiO$_2$ should be reduced to target oxygen saturations at 94–98% in most patients and 88–92% in those with chronic obstructive pulmonary disease. It is important to recognise that oxygen is a treatment for hypoxia and not breathlessness.

Some patients present with apparent breathlessness due to a non-respiratory cause (metabolic acidosis, DKA) – these patients will not generally benefit from oxygen in the absence of hypoxia. Conversely, pneumothoraces may reduce in size up to four times more rapidly in a patient breathing high-flow supplemental oxygen.

Ventilatory support

This should always be considered when:

- the patient cannot maintain a clear airway, often as a result of significantly reduced conscious level
- high-flow oxygen via facemask (or continuous positive pressure device if appropriate) is insufficient to maintain acceptable oxygen saturations
- spontaneous ventilation is inadequate
- there has been a return of spontaneous circulation following a prolonged cardiac arrest
- the patient is multiply injured
- the patient has a severe chest injury (particularly multiple rib fractures and/or flail segments)
- the patient is to be transferred, and there is a risk of severe deterioration en route.

The emergency induction of anaesthesia for the purpose of intubation and ventilation in a hypoxic or unstable patient is a challenging task. It should be carried out by a clinician with appropriate anaesthetic training and well-maintained skills.

> A pneumothorax is more likely to tension in a positive-pressure ventilated patient. Chest drains should be inserted before ventilating patients with chest injuries.

C – Circulation

Check for a central pulse (over 10 seconds)

The absence of a central pulse (*or a rate of <60 beats/min in infants*) indicates the need to follow procedures for cardiorespiratory arrest:

Asystole → p. 161.
Pulseless electrical activity (PEA) → p. 161.
Ventricular fibrillation (VF) → p. 158.

If a pulse *is* detected, ensure that continuous electrocardiography monitoring is applied, and arrangements are made for a 12-lead ECG.

Look for

- **Pallor and coolness of the skin:** the body diverts blood away from the skin when there are circulatory problems, and these signs are thus very useful indicators of shock
- **Pallor and sweating:** signs of gross sympathetic disturbance
- **Active bleeding or melaena**
- **A fast or slow heart rate:** fast heart rates usually mean that either there is a cardiac arrhythmia or more commonly the sympathetic nervous system is responding to another problem (such as hypoxia, hypoglycaemia, pain or fear) and is driving the heart to beat faster. A slow heart rate usually means that something is wrong with the heart itself. The worst cause of this is severe hypoxia (or hypovolaemia) and, in this case, it means that terminal bradycardia and asystole are only seconds away
- **Abnormal blood pressure:** be aware that automatic blood pressure cuffs can be inaccurate at the extremes of blood pressure and may give inaccurate results in atrial fibrillation (particularly diastolic measurement). If in doubt obtain manual readings
- **A prolonged capillary refill time:** it should be less than 2 seconds if the circulation is satisfactory. However, peripheral vasoconstriction in a cold, wet patient can easily produce a prolonged refill time
- **Absent or quiet heart sounds and raised jugular venous pulse (JVP):** classically suggestive of tamponade if accompanied by hypotension and tachycardia; these signs can be difficult to detect in a busy resuscitation room, and their absence cannot be used to rule out tamponade. JVP will not be raised if there is also hypovolaemia
- **A precordial wound**
- **An abnormal electrocardiogram (ECG) trace on the monitor**
- *Signs of left ventricular failure* (dyspnoea, gallop rhythm and crepitations)
- *Signs of abdominal, pelvic or occult bleeding* (may need per rectum examination and a nasogastric tube or ultrasound scan)
- *Signs of dehydration* (especially in children)
- *Purpura* (e.g. meningococcal sepsis)

Inadequate circulation will reduce tissue oxygenation and thus may also cause:

- a raised respiratory rate
- altered mental status.

Initial bolus resuscitation fluid should comprise 500 mL crystalloid containing sodium of 130–154 mmol/L over 15 min. In elderly patients, those of low body weight or where there are concerns about fluid tolerance (cardiac or kidney disease), smaller boluses of 250 mL with frequent reassessment are appropriate.

Abdominal bleeding → pp. 82 312 and 316.
Allergic reactions and anaphylaxis → p. 306.
Blood transfusion → p. 25.
Cardiac arrhythmias → p. 172.
Cardiac failure → pp. 219 and 251.
Cardiac tamponade → pp. 80 and 253.
Resuscitative thoracotomy → p. 83.
Pelvic bleeding → p. 86.
Renal effects of shock → p. 258.
Shock → p. 25 and 250.

Cardiac function

The stroke volume is the amount of blood ejected from the heart with each beat. It is determined by the left ventricular filling pressure, myocardial contractility and systemic vascular resistance. The product of heart rate and stroke volume is the cardiac output – the most important parameter of cardiac function. (Cardiac index is cardiac output divided by body surface area.) An increase in heart rate will directly increase the cardiac output and is the earliest cardiac response to hypoxia. However, the faster the heart beats the less time there is for it to fill and, eventually, a rise in heart rate will no longer be matched by a rise in cardiac output.

Myocardial function is compromised at high pulse rates because coronary blood flow occurs chiefly in diastole. When the heart rate rises above about 130 in an adult, the filling time is so reduced that cardiac output will actually fall.

Pulse and blood pressure

The autonomic response to hypovolaemia is complex. Rapid blood loss can produce reflex bradycardia, but when associated with tissue damage, it produces the more familiar tachycardia. Systolic blood pressure is the product of cardiac output and systemic vascular resistance. A high catecholamine response to hypoxia and hypovolaemia will produce a high systemic vascular resistance. This will maintain a 'normal', or even high, blood pressure in the presence of a falling cardiac output.

> Knowledge of systemic blood pressure provides only very limited information about cardiac function and is a very late indicator of haemodynamic instability.

Maintenance of systemic vascular resistance is a vital response to hypovolaemia and hypoxia. (Skin pallor reflects this early on but is an imprecise clinical sign.) Similar to other compensatory mechanisms to hypoxia, this vasomotor response consumes oxygen and will eventually fail.

Measurements of pulse and blood pressure are very poor indicators of haemodynamic function in critically ill patients. Central venous pressure may not reflect the functioning of the left side of the heart and is thus of limited use in the assessment of overall cardiac performance.

Point of care ultrasound (POCUS) and echocardiography can give valuable information in the assessment of cardiovascular and fluid status and should be used in parallel with clinical examination wherever the equipment and skills are available → p. 10.

Fluid replacement

Left ventricular filling pressure (and hence cardiac output) is a function of the circulating blood volume. Increases in heart rate, systemic vascular resistance and myocardial contractility can maintain cardiac output and blood pressure in the early stages of hypovolaemia. This will, however, be at the expense of increased oxygen demands by the cardiovascular system and reduced tissue perfusion in many other areas. The Bezold-Jarisch reflex, comprising sudden bradycardia, hypotension and apnoea, can result from contraction of the empty ventricle triggering vagal efferent fibres.

Older patients with deteriorating physiological reserve, those with pre-existing organ dysfunction and those on certain medications will be less able to mount and maintain the compensatory reflexes. Early restoration of circulating volume can mitigate against the harmful effects of hypovolaemia.

> Early restoration of blood pressure by transfusion does not necessarily indicate the correction of the circulatory deficit, nor normalisation of oxygen delivery to tissues.

The delivery of oxygen to the tissues depends not only on the pumping mechanism of the heart but also on the red cells in the circulating blood. A modest fall in haematocrit can reduce viscosity and increase blood flow while maintaining oxygen delivery but will still require an increase in cardiac output to be effective. Maintenance of haemoglobin levels by blood transfusion may reduce the impact of hypoxia by increasing the effectiveness of each cardiac cycle and reducing the need for an increase in cardiac output. Transfused blood will also maintain the oncotic pressure of the circulating fluid, thereby increasing the filling pressure. However, adequate levels of 2,3-diphosphoglycerate (2,3-DPG) are also necessary for satisfactory oxygen delivery, and stored blood is deplete in 2,3-DPG such that even with a restored haemoglobin concentration, oxygen delivery is likely to be substantially lower than normal → p. 25.

Maintenance of adequate tissue perfusion is not synonymous with the return of a normal blood pressure. Indeed, the latter may be contraindicated in the ED in an actively bleeding patient (e.g. with an aortic aneurysm). Resuscitation can be achieved while keeping the blood pressure relatively low. This has been shown to improve survival until definitive surgery can be undertaken ('permissive hypotension'). A similar approach is recommended in the prehospital management of injured adults and older children with presumed blood loss, in which fluid resuscitation may be titrated against the presence of peripheral pulses (or central pulses in the case of penetrating trauma).

When rapid fluid replacement is required, warmed IV fluids (40°C) delivered through a rapid infuser should ideally be used. Many clinicians believe that a balanced solution such as Plasmalyte or Hartmann's solution is preferable to 0.9% saline if large volumes are required; however, evidence of a difference in patient outcomes is lacking.

The management of massive blood loss is summarised in Figure 1.1.

D – Disability

After A, B and C (airway, breathing and circulation) have been assessed and management is in progress, it is necessary to look at the state of the brain. In this context, the

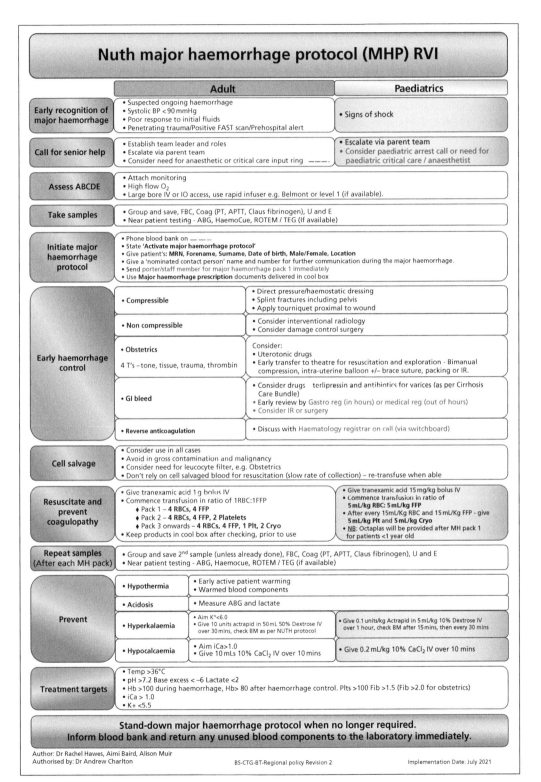

Nuth major haemorrhage protocol (MHP) RVI

	Adult	Paediatrics
Early recognition of major haemorrhage	• Suspected ongoing haemorrhage • Systolic BP < 90 mmHg • Poor response to initial fluids • Penetrating trauma/Positive FAST scan/Prehospital alert	• Signs of shock
Call for senior help	• Establish team leader and roles • Escalate via parent team • Consider need for anaesthetic or critical care input ring ————	• Escalate via parent team • Consider paediatric arrest call or need for paediatric critical care / anaesthetist
Assess ABCDE	• Attach monitoring • High flow O$_2$ • Large bore IV or IO access, use rapid infuser e.g. Belmont or level 1 (if available).	
Take samples	• Group and save, FBC, Coag (PT, APTT, Claus fibrinogen), U and E • Near patient testing - ABG, HaemoCue, ROTEM / TEG (If available)	
Initiate major haemorrhage protocol	• Phone blood bank on ——— • State **'Activate major haemorrhage protocol'** • Give patient's: **MRN, Forename, Surname, Date of birth, Male/Female, Location** • Give a 'nominated contact person' name and number for further communication during the major haemorrhage. • Send porter/staff member for major haemorrhage pack 1 immediately • Use **Major haemorrhage prescription** documents delivered in cool box	
Early haemorrhage control	• **Compressible**	• Direct pressure/haemostatic dressing • Splint fractures including pelvis • Apply tourniquet proximal to wound
	• **Non compressible**	• Consider interventional radiology • Consider damage control surgery
	• **Obstetrics** 4 T's –tone, tissue, trauma, thrombin	Consider: • Uterotonic drugs • Early transfer to theatre for resuscitation and exploration - Bimanual compression, intra-uterine balloon +/– brace suture, packing or IR.
	• **GI bleed**	• Consider drugs terlipressin and antibiotics for varices (as per Cirrhosis Care Bundle) • Early review by Gastro reg (in hours) or medical reg (out of hours) • Consider IR or surgery
	• **Reverse anticoagulation**	• Discuss with Haematology registrar on call (via switchboard)
Cell salvage	• Consider use in all cases • Avoid in gross contamination and malignancy • Consider need for leucocyte filter, e.g. Obstetrics • Don't rely on cell salvaged blood for resuscitation (slow rate of collection) – re-transfuse when able	

Resuscitate and prevent coagulopathy	• Give tranexamic acid 1g bolus IV
	• Commence transfusion in ratio of 1RBC:1FFP
	  ♦ Pack 1 – **4 RBCs, 4 FFP**
	  ♦ Pack 2 – **4 RBCs, 4 FFP, 2 Platelets**
	  ♦ Pack 3 onwards – **4 RBCs, 4 FFP, 1 Plt, 2 Cryo**
	• Keep products in cool box after checking, prior to use
		• Give tranexamic acid 15 mg/kg bolus IV
		• Commence transfusion in ratio of
		  5 mL/kg RBC: 5 mL/kg FFP
		• After every 15mL/Kg RBC and 15mL/Kg FFP - give
		  5mL/kg Plt and 5mL/kg Cryo
		• **NB:** Octaplas will be provided after MH pack 1 for patients <1 year old

Repeat samples (After each MH pack)	• Group and save 2nd sample (unless already done), FBC, Coag (PT, APTT, Claus fibrinogen), U and E • Near patient testing - ABG, Haemocue, ROTEM / TEG (if available)	
Prevent	• **Hypothermia**	• Early active patient warming • Warmed blood components
	• **Acidosis**	• Measure ABG and lactate
	• **Hyperkalaemia**	• Aim K$^+$<6.0 • Give 10 units actrapid in 50mL 50% Dextrose IV over 30 mins, check BM as per NUTH protocol	• Give 0.1 units/kg Actrapid in 5 mL/kg 10% Dextrose IV over 1 hour, check BM after 15mins, then every 30 mins
	• **Hypocalaemia**	• Aim iCa>1.0 • Give 10 mLs 10% CaCl$_2$ IV over 10 mins	• Give 0.2 mL/kg 10% CaCl$_2$ IV over 10 mins
Treatment targets	• Temp >36°C • pH >7.2 Base excess < –6 Lactate <2 • Hb >100 during haemorrhage, Hb> 80 after haemorrhage control. Plts >100 Fib >1.5 (Fib >2.0 for obstetrics) • iCa > 1.0 • K+ <5.5	

Stand-down major haemorrhage protocol when no longer required.
Inform blood bank and return any unused blood components to the laboratory immediately.

Author: Dr Rachel Hawes, Aimi Baird, Alison Muir
Authorised by: Dr Andrew Charlton

BS-CTG-BT-Regional policy Revision 2

Implementation Date: July 2021

Figure 1.1 The management of major haemorrhage. Newcastle Hospitals NHS Foundation Trust, Dr Rachel Hawes, Consultant Anaesthetist, Alison Muir, Transfusion Lab Manager, Aimi Baird, Transfusion Practitioner.

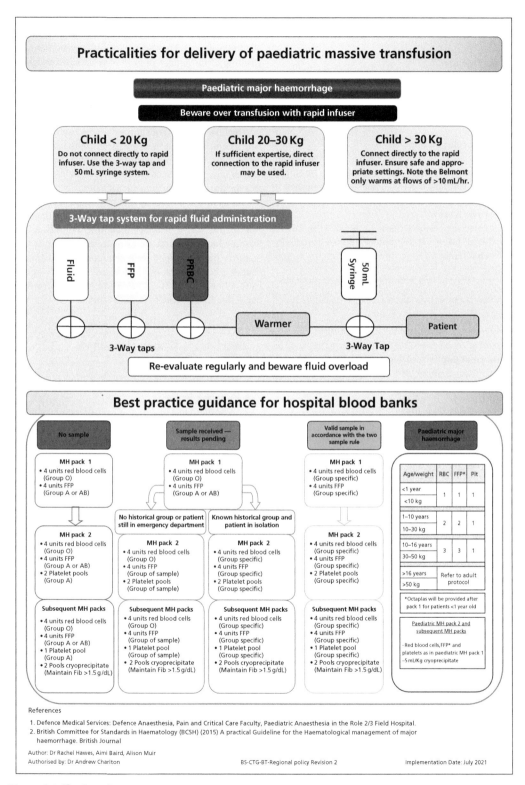

Practicalities for delivery of paediatric massive transfusion

Paediatric major haemorrhage

Beware over transfusion with rapid infuser

Child < 20 Kg
Do not connect directly to rapid infuser. Use the 3-way tap and 50 mL syringe system.

Child 20–30 Kg
If sufficient expertise, direct connection to the rapid infuser may be used.

Child > 30 Kg
Connect directly to the rapid infuser. Ensure safe and appropriate settings. Note the Belmont only warms at flows of >10 mL/hr.

3-Way tap system for rapid fluid administration

Fluid — FFP — PRBC — Warmer — Patient

50 mL Syringe

3-Way taps   3-Way Tap

Re-evaluate regularly and beware fluid overload

Best practice guidance for hospital blood banks

No sample

Sample received — results pending

Valid sample in accordance with the two sample rule

Paediatric major haemorrhage

MH pack 1
- 4 units red blood cells (Group O)
- 4 units FFP (Group A or AB)

MH pack 1
- 4 units red blood cells (Group O)
- 4 units FFP (Group A or AB)

MH pack 1
- 4 units red blood cells (Group specific)
- 4 units FFP (Group specific)

Age/weight	RBC	FFP*	Plt
<1 year <10 kg	1	1	1
1–10 years 10–30 kg	2	2	1
10–16 years 30–50 kg	3	3	1
>16 years >50 kg	Refer to adult protocol		

No historical group or patient still in emergency department

Known historical group and patient in isolation

MH pack 2
- 4 units red blood cells (Group O)
- 4 units FFP (Group A or AB)
- 2 Platelet pools (Group A)

MH pack 2
- 4 units red blood cells (Group O)
- 4 units FFP (Group of sample)
- 2 Platelet pools (Group of sample)

MH pack 2
- 4 units red blood cells (Group specific)
- 4 units FFP (Group specific)
- 2 Platelet pools (Group specific)

MH pack 2
- 4 units red blood cells (Group specific)
- 4 units FFP (Group specific)
- 2 Platelet pools (Group specific)

*Octaplas will be provided after pack 1 for patients <1 year old

Paediatric MH pack 2 and subsequent MH packs

- Red blood cells, FFP* and platelets as in paediatric MH pack 1
- 5 mL/Kg cryoprecipitate

Subsequent MH packs
- 4 units red blood cells (Group O)
- 4 units FFP (Group A or AB)
- 1 Platelet pool (Group A)
- 2 Pools cryoprecipitate (Maintain Fib >1.5 g/dL)

Subsequent MH packs
- 4 units red blood cells (Group O)
- 4 units FFP (Group of sample)
- 1 Platelet pool (Group of sample)
- 2 Pools cryoprecipitate (Maintain Fib >1.5 g/dL)

Subsequent MH packs
- 4 units red blood cells (Group specific)
- 4 units FFP (Group specific)
- 1 Platelet pool (Group specific)
- 2 Pools cryoprecipitate (Maintain Fib >1.5 g/dL)

Subsequent MH packs
- 4 units red blood cells (Group specific)
- 4 units FFP (Group specific)
- 1 Platelet pool (Group specific)
- 2 Pools cryoprecipitate (Maintain Fib >1.5 g/dL)

References

1. Defence Medical Services: Defence Anaesthesia, Pain and Critical Care Faculty, Paediatric Anaesthesia in the Role 2/3 Field Hospital.
2. British Committee for Standards in Haematology (BCSH) (2015) A practical Guideline for the Haematological management of major haemorrhage. British Journal

Author: Dr Rachel Hawes, Aimi Baird, Alison Muir
Authorised by: Dr Andrew Charlton   BS-CTG-BT-Regional policy Revision 2   Implementation Date: July 2021

Figure 1.1 (Continued)

term *disability* is now widely used to describe a brief assessment of neurological functioning.

Look for

1 **A reduced level of consciousness**: this is the most important sign of any problem affecting the brain. AVPU scoring is useful initially:

A – Alert

V – Voice elicits a response

P – Pain elicits a response. (Attending relatives are usually in a highly distressed state so be careful how you elicit this sign) Pain should be elicited in the cranial nerve territories, in case of spinal injury.

U – Unresponsive

Later, the Glasgow Coma Scale (GCS) should be used (→ *p. 35* for adults and → *p. 345* for children).

> Always consider hypoglycaemia as a cause for a reduced level of consciousness.

2 **Abnormal pupils**: look for size, equalness and reactivity. These features can be affected by both drugs and brain disease.

> Physiological anisocoria is present in up to 20% of the healthy population.

3 **Abnormal posture and limb movements**

Severe intracerebral problems may also cause:

- airway obstruction
- respiratory depression (respiration, unlike the heartbeat, requires an intact brain stem)
- bradycardia and hypertension (Cushing's response)
- neurogenic pulmonary oedema (caused by massive sympathetic vasoconstriction).

Diagnosis of death using neurological criteria → p. 405.
Head injury → p. 34.
Hypoglycaemia → p. 254.
Intracranial pathology → p. 236.
Poisoning → p. 277.

Depression of consciousness

There is a continuum of consciousness that ranges from an alert and oriented patient to one with brainstem death. Causes of impaired consciousness → *Box 1.1.* To maintain consciousness requires at least one functioning

cerebral hemisphere and a working reticular activating system (RAS) in the brainstem. The RAS may be affected by brainstem stroke or increased intracerebral pressure leading to movement of cerebellar tonsils through the foramen magnum ('coning'). For both cerebral hemispheres to be impaired suggests systemic insult such as inadequate oxygen delivery, hypoglycaemia, or the effect of toxins.

Unconsciousness is an imprecise term usually describing a condition of an unaware patient with whom verbal communication is not possible; unresponsive is thus a better description. Such patients will usually be amnesic for the duration of the unresponsiveness.

The ability to protect the airway decreases as the level of consciousness falls, and finally, the ability to maintain an open airway is also lost. Breathing indicates a functioning brain stem; in a cardiac arrest patient, it often returns quickly after cerebral circulation is restored. Sudden cerebral trauma may cause transitory apnoea and all of the causes of impaired consciousness listed in → *Box 1.1* may lead to terminal apnoea.

> **Box 1.1 Causes of impaired consciousness**
>
> - Hypoxia, hypovolaemia or cerebral ischaemia
> - Hypoglycaemia
> - Hypothermia
> - Poisoning or gross metabolic disturbance (including CO_2 narcosis)
> - Injury to the brain
> - Intracranial pathology (bleeding, thrombosis, embolism, infection, swelling, tumour, fits, etc.)
>
> If prolonged, many of the above problems (including hypoxia, ischaemia, hypoglycaemia and status epilepticus) will lead to a remarkably similar outcome – selective neuronal necrosis and permanent brain injury.

E – Environment and exposure

In cases of trauma, collapse and depressed conscious level, the whole body must be exposed – including the back – so that nothing important is missed. In major trauma, rolling the patient is best avoided prior to imaging, due to the risk of exacerbating spinal or pelvic injury → *p. 49.*

Control of body temperature is important for successful resuscitation. Remove wet clothes and, if high volumes of IV fluids are to be given, they should be warmed. Even at this early stage, avoid extrinsic factors that may harm the patient.

Look for

- Medical alert bracelets/necklaces or drug patches
- Cold extremities
- Shivering
- Wet clothing
- Pyrexia and clamminess
- The position in which the patient is most comfortable
- Uncomfortable splints (including collars and spinal boards)
- Loss of the protective reflexes of the eyes
- Areas where pressure sores might form
- The proximity of the next of kin.

Attention to these details early on can radically change the well-being (and demeanour) of a patient.

> If a patient cannot blink, then the eyes should be covered to protect them.

Hyperpyrexia and hyperthermia → p. 249.
Hypothermia → p. 247.

F – Fits

Fits or seizures deprive the brain of oxygen and make assessment almost impossible. Stopping them is as important as the ABCs.

Look for

- Frank tonic or clonic activity
- Spasmodic twitching
- Post-ictal drowsiness
- Gurgling, rattling or other signs of post-ictal airway obstruction
- Cyanosis: there is increased demand for oxygen and ventilation may be inadequate
- Signs of head injury
- Signs of other injury caused by a convulsion (e.g. a bitten tongue and intraoral bleeding)
- Hypoglycaemia
- Pyrexia or other signs of infection (especially in children).

Convulsions must be terminated before any further action can be effective.

Convulsions in adults → p. 243 and in children → p. 356
Hypoglycaemia → pp. 254 and 346.

Fitting indicates that something is wrong with the brain or its fuel supply. The list of possibilities is almost the same as that for causes of reduced consciousness

→ Box 1.2. Convulsive activity causes a dramatic increase in cerebral and muscle oxygen demand; a post-ictal acidosis is inevitable following all but the briefest of seizures. The uncoordinated muscle action that occurs during the tonic or clonic stages of a fit makes control of the airway extremely difficult; some regurgitation may also occur. Ventilation of the lungs is usually reduced for the same reason. Alveolar oxygenation is thus poor at a time of high oxygen demand. This combination explains why prolonged fitting can be associated with permanent neurological damage.

 Box 1.2 **Causes of fits**

- Hypoxia
- Shock
- Hypoglycaemia
- Poisoning
- Metabolic disturbance
- Intracranial pathology:
  - bleeding
  - trauma
  - thrombosis
  - embolism
  - infection
  - swelling
  - tumour
  - epilepsy

G – Glucose

The human body can be compared to an engine that needs an oxygen supply (airway and breathing) delivered in the bloodstream (circulation). However, we should not forget that the oxygen is required to burn fuel (glucose). Fat and protein are, of course, also important, but the brain uses glucose almost exclusively.

Look for

- Restlessness, agitation or other mental change ('jitteriness' in a neonate)
- Inappropriate lack of cooperation or aggression
- A reduced level of consciousness
- Convulsions
- Signs of insulin usage
- A low blood sugar level on testing with a reagent strip.

A reagent-strip measurement of blood glucose should be performed in all patients who have depression of consciousness. If hypoglycaemia is found, it should be immediately treated with IV/IO glucose solution (50 mL of 50% glucose for a normal adult, 0.2 g/kg for a child). If no venous access is immediately available or rapidly obtained, then glucagon 1 mg by intramuscular (IM) injection is a useful standby.

Hypoglycaemia → pp. 254 and 346.

> Hypoglycaemia is always waiting to catch you out. A comatose, or bizarrely behaving, patient with profuse sweating should always make you think of low blood sugar.

H – History

At this juncture, a brief history becomes a necessity using the mnemonic 'AMPLE':

A	Allergies
M	Medication
P	Past and present illnesses of significance
L	Last food and drink
E	Events leading up to the patient's presentation

The people who accompany the patient to the department are a vital source of this information, hence the need to collect facts before the paramedic team leaves the ED.

> **Adrenocortical suppression**
>
> Patients who are undergoing prolonged treatment with steroids (i.e. for >3 weeks) may develop adrenocortical suppression. This can also occur for up to a year after stopping long-term steroid therapy. During a medical crisis, such patients should be given supplementary corticosteroids (e.g. IV hydrocortisone 100 mg) in the ED.

I – Immediate analgesia and investigations

> This is the point (if you have not already done it) to call for help. There should be no hesitation in seeking another pair of hands or a more experienced opinion.

In many patients who are not in extremis, the above will take only a matter of seconds. Once life-threatening problems have been identified and treated, it is necessary to perform the tasks that are at the very heart of emergency medicine – to ensure the immediate relief of suffering. This will include the following:

- Administration of analgesia: *assessment of pain → Box 1.3*
- Provision of splintage and support for injuries: *lower limb → pp. 89 and 95; upper limb → p. 114*
- Further relief of dyspnoea
- Reassurance.

> **Box 1.3 Assessment of pain**
>
> Pain is a subjective experience. Clinical assessment of a patient's level of pain depends on:
>
> - the patient's description of the pain
> - the patient's behaviour
> - the known injuries or condition
> - any observed signs of pain (sweating, tachycardia, posture, etc.)
> - the use of visual pain scales – analogue or image type (pain ladders and faces, etc.)

This is not just a matter of humanity. The trust of the patient (and the relatives and friends) is more easily gained by staff who are seen to address the patient's distressing symptoms. This trust leads to the provision of better information and more easily achieved concordance with treatment. Conversely, nothing distresses relatives or friends more than the sight of a doctor or nurse asking endless questions whilst the patient continues to suffer. It is always better to overestimate pain rather than to underestimate it.

Relevant imaging and other investigations can now be requested. Twelve lead ECG and blood gas analysis are helpful early on. In the vast majority of cases, venous blood gas analysis is adequate and obviates the need for the difficulty and discomfort often associated with arterial blood gases. A low or normal pCO_2 on venous blood gas analysis rules out hypercapnia with a high degree of certainty.

Point of care ultrasound

It is not possible to learn ultrasound from a textbook, and a detailed description of the physics and techniques is beyond the scope of this text; however, Point of Care Ultrasound (POCUS) is an extremely valuable tool that has now become widely used in the evaluation of patients in the ED. In appropriately trained hands, POCUS can be used as an extension of the clinical examination. As an addition to the clinical evaluation of the critically ill patient, POCUS can facilitate the rapid identification of reversible life-threatening pathologies, such as pneumothorax, haemothorax, cardiac tamponade, pulmonary embolism and aortic aneurysm.

Analgesia

The administration of analgesia does not mask significant clinical signs. Conscious level is not greatly depressed by the judicious administration of small doses of IV opioids; abdominal signs remain unchanged. Tenderness can still be located and guarding is an involuntary mechanism, which is unaffected. The biggest change will be in the ease of examining a trusting, cooperative patient who was previously distressed and agitated.

> The immediate relief of suffering, in all its forms, is the most important function of an ED.

The needs of relatives and friends

The needs of the patient's loved ones cannot be ignored. These may vary from simple reassurance to medical treatment. As soon as practicable, and with the patient's consent if conscious, the relatives or friends must be informed of the patient's current situation and what is going to happen next. In some cases, it may be necessary to telephone people important to the patient, deliver an update or ask them to attend the department. At all times, the patient's right to confidentiality and autonomy must be respected – it may sometimes be necessary to limit the number or nature of visitors to safeguard this principle. (→ *Box 1.4*).

 Box 1.4 Summary of immediate assessment and management

Airway
Establish and maintain a clear airway
Ensure airway protection
Consider the need for cervical protection
Breathing
Give high-concentration oxygen
Ensure adequate ventilation of the lungs
Decompress pneumothoraces
Begin to correct severe respiratory problems
Circulation
Restore the circulating blood volume
Ensure adequate cardiac function
Commence monitoring
Disability
Assess cerebral functioning
Consider causes of depression of
    consciousness
Environment/exposure of the whole body
Check the body temperature and positioning
Ensure protection from further harm
Expose the whole body for examination
Fits
Control convulsive activity
Glucose
Correct hypoglycaemia
History
Take brief but AMPLE details
Immediate analgesia and investigations
Provide analgesia and splintage
Relieve remaining dyspnoea
Give reassurance
Request major investigations

FURTHER MANAGEMENT IN THE ED

How much history, how much examination?

History-taking in emergencies should be guided by the presenting complaint. The familial medical history will rarely be relevant in a patient with a dog bite; it might be vital in someone with haemophilia and a swollen joint. The art of adjusting the acquisition of information to the circumstances is a difficult one.

Most new clinicians take an over-long history first, but familiarity with common ED presentations allows this to be appropriately reduced as experience is gained. Mechanism of injury is particularly important in trauma; events that lead to the patient's presentation, the timing and speed of onset are essential in medical cases.

The examination must also be tailored to the patient. At times it can be limited, but often it must be thorough. Experience teaches the relative uselessness of some physical signs and the enormous value of others. The examination in trauma patients is usually performed from top to toe rather than in systems and is called the secondary survey. The back of the patient and the perineum are the parts that are often missed.

Investigations

Investigations should be targeted to answer a clinical question – requesting large numbers of investigations without a clear idea of how the results will alter management is rarely fruitful. Investigations should generally only be requested if the results could have an impact on immediate care or disposal.

Tests should be performed for precise indications rather than as a general screen. The possible exception to this is in elderly patients who present with non-specific events such as collapse. They can be very difficult to evaluate clinically. Consequently, before considering sending them home, it is best to carry out a brief screen including CXR, ECG, haemoglobin, white cell count and blood urea level – and a pelvic radiograph if concerned about mobility.

Definitive care

This may involve:

- accurate liaison with other specialists in the hospital or community
- safe transport to another facility
- careful follow-up arrangements
- rehabilitation

Social problems and homelessness

Socially excluded people are more likely to experience health inequality and have less access to preventative healthcare, as a result of a combination of minoritisation, low literacy, lack of trust in services, transience or poverty. Life expectancy of people in this group is substantially shortened compared to the general population, and morbidity is high. This group is consequently more likely to present to the ED. Every presentation is an opportunity to provide advice, essential healthcare and ensure that referral and signposting to other services takes place. This may sometimes mean the Emergency Physician provides management that is not strictly 'Emergency' in nature. Presentations are often complex combinations of mental and physical health problems, sometimes combined with substance use. In this vulnerable group, every opportunity should be taken to build trust, intervene and connect the patient to relevant services.

> The standardised mortality rate for homeless people is three times higher than that of the UK population as a whole.

Many patients who come to an ED have nowhere to sleep or to shelter. There is a statutory requirement in the UK to identify and refer patients who are homeless or at risk of becoming so.

People experiencing rough sleeping die on average 30 years earlier than the general population. Efforts should always be made to find temporary accommodation for these patients. The most likely sources of help are:

- Social Services
- the Salvation Army
- Shelter

Patients should be given contact details for local agencies, soup kitchens and charitable organisations. If discharge from hospital is a possibility, it is important to consider the practicality of the discharge plan – for example if your patient is advised to keep their limb elevated and return to outpatient clinic, but is sleeping rough, following this advice is likely to be impossible. Follow-up with a GP should not be recommended if the patient is not registered with a practice. In certain circumstances, therefore, a lower threshold for inpatient admission is appropriate.

> Health inequalities in the UK are increasing. The differences in life expectancy between rich and poor areas of the country are at their greatest since the Victorian era.

Major incidents

The management of major incidents is outside the scope of this book, but in essence, the following should be implemented:

- All departments should have a written policy for dealing with events that have the potential to overwhelm the standard facilities of the hospital.
- Action cards for all personnel should be available together with a special supply of equipment and drugs.
- Regular practice sessions are essential.

(Note that the last is a legal obligation in the UK under the Civil Contingencies Act 2004. The Act is divided into two parts – Civil Protection (Part I) and Emergency Powers (Part II). For the purposes of Civil Protection, local responders are divided into two categories. Category 1 responders (which include hospitals, primary care trusts and ambulance services) have a duty to make and execute effective plans for major incidents. Category 2 organisations (such as utility and transport companies) are obliged to cooperate with other responders.)

Contamination and irradiation → p. 151.

Sedation and general anaesthesia

Most ED patients are self-referred, and many will return to their homes or workplaces within a matter of hours. Some patients arrive in a state of unconsciousness, and others will require sedation. All are, by definition, unexpected. This combination of circumstances leads to special problems with the safe administration of sedative drugs:

- Most patients are not fasted.
- Painful conditions delay gastric emptying.
- Many patients will have ingested alcohol.
- There is no opportunity for pre-planned assessment of fitness or review of case notes.
- The need for sedation is invariably nearly immediate.
- The fitness of patients for discharge and the circumstances to which they depart require very careful consideration.

The safety of the patient is paramount; emergency situations do not obviate the need for standard precautions. Consideration must be given to the medical preparedness and fasting state of all patients. Senior staff should be consulted.

Preparation for sedation and selection of patients

The objective of ED sedation is to minimise discomfort for the patient during essential urgent procedures. It is, therefore, essential to ensure that alternatives to sedation are considered, and that analgesia is given appropriately before deciding on sedation. Consider the urgency of the proposed procedure, the required depth of sedation and any patient factors which may render the sedation higher risk (→ Table 1.1).

Most patients will not require investigations to assess their fitness for the procedure; those who do are generally not suitable for sedation in the ED

Patients with the following problems are generally unsuitable for sedation in the ED:

- Severely intoxicated
- Previous problems with sedation
- Chronic illnesses – which may complicate sedation or aftercare
- Other severe injuries
- Coexistent significant head injury
- At the extremes of age
- Inadequate circumstances for discharge.

Patients who are deemed unsuitable for sedation but whose condition does not allow delay (e.g. vascular compromise distal to a dislocation) must be discussed with a senior colleague immediately.

Most patients in the ED will not be fasted, and both pain and opiate analgesia delay gastric emptying. The decision to proceed with sedation should be based on a careful consideration of the urgency of the procedure and the nature of the sedation required. Senior staff with training in sedation and airway management must be present. Pain must be alleviated with parenteral analgesia (before the radiograph if indicated) and the subsequent doses of sedative drugs must be then adjusted accordingly.

> Sedation is not the same as analgesia. Pain relief is still needed.

Facilities for the administration of sedation or general anaesthesia

The minimum requirements include the following:

- Medical and nursing staff trained in the management of patients with a depressed level of consciousness

Table 1.1 American society of Anaesthesiologists classification of grades of sedation

	Minimal sedation (anxiolysis)	Moderate sedation (conscious sedation)	Deep sedation	General anaesthesia
Responsiveness	Normal response to verbal stimulation	Purposeful response to verbal or tactile stimulation	Purposeful response after repeated or painful stimulation	Unrousable even with painful stimulus
Airway	Unaffected	No intervention required	Intervention may be required	Intervention often required
Spontaneous ventilation	Unaffected	Adequate	Maybe inadequate	Frequently inadequate
Cardiovascular function	Unaffected	Usually maintained	Usually maintained	Maybe impaired

- Areas suitable for high-dependency observation
- A full range of resuscitation and monitoring equipment
- All necessary drugs for resuscitation, including specific antidotes (e.g. naloxone, flumazenil).

> When a doctor is performing a procedure on a sedated patient, a separate member of staff must be responsible for the overall care of that patient. The operator should never try to monitor the patient at the same time.

Conditions during the period of sedation

During sedation, and until recovery is complete, all patients should:

- be accompanied by a responsible member of staff
- be on a trolley with side rails, which can be tipped head-down
- have an IV cannula *in situ*
- be given a high concentration of oxygen by mask
- be monitored by pulse oximetry, end-tidal capnography, ECG and BP recording
- have a high-volume suction catheter in place under their pillow
- have equipment required for emergency airway management immediately available.

Effective sedation is greatly facilitated by pleasant, quiet surroundings and the presence of attentive, reassuring and obviously competent staff.

Assessment of the level of sedation

> The scores for measuring coma (AVPU and GCS) must be understood and practised by all ED staff. They can be used when assessing the level of sedation.

General anaesthesia and sedation are both induced states of depression of consciousness. Depth of sedation is a spectrum ranging from full consciousness with mild anxiolysis to general anaesthesia. The depth of sedation required will depend on the procedure to be undertaken and on patient factors. Patient individual response to drugs used for sedation may be highly variable, and removal of painful stimulus mid-procedure (e.g. as the joint is reduced) may lead to sudden deepening of sedation. The clinician managing sedation must be prepared to manage this if required.

Drugs for sedation in the ED

All drugs that are used for sedation are capable of inducing general anaesthesia and vice versa; the principal difference is dose administered.

Sedation should always be accompanied by adequate analgesia before, during and after the procedure. Short-acting opiates, such as fentanyl, are useful for painful procedures where the expectation is for significant pain reduction post-procedure (e.g. reduction of dislocation). Antiemetics may be given as required, but there is little evidence that their routine use reduces the risk of aspiration.

Sedation and analgesia for children → p. 366.
Sedation of the disturbed patient → p. 375.

Propofol

Propofol is a lipophilic agent thought to act on GABA receptors. It is widely used for ED sedation and is a good option in experienced hands. Propofol has a rapid onset of action and a short duration of effect.

Propofol can cause significant hypotension and respiratory depression, especially if administered rapidly, and induction of deep sedation may inadvertently occur. The sedationist must be prepared to manage these complications.

Most patients will require 0.5–1 mg/kg for induction of sedation; however, in frail and elderly patients, slow titration of 10 mg aliquots is a safer strategy. Patients who drink alcohol regularly often require higher doses than may be expected.

Intravenous benzodiazepines

Intravenous benzodiazepines such as midazolam or diazepam emulsion have been traditionally used for ED sedation although have become less popular in recent years.

- Initial adult dose of IV midazolam is approximately 1–2 mg
- Initial adult dose of IV diazepam is approximately 2.5–5.0 mg.

The correct initial dose should be adjusted according to the age, weight and general health of the patient. Elderly people may need only very small amounts. Subsequent doses, given after a delay of a few minutes, should be titrated against apparent effect. The muscle relaxation that is a feature of sedation with benzodiazepines makes these drugs appropriate for use in the reduction of dislocations.

Short-acting opioids

Short-acting opioids such as fentanyl can provide an excellent combination of sedation and analgesia:

- IV dose of fentanyl = 1–3 mcg/kg.

This should be titrated slowly at a rate of no more than 1 mcg/kg per min up to a maximum dose of 5 mcg/kg in 1 hour. The onset of action is within 3 min and the effects of a single dose wear off in less than 1 hour. Opioids may cause some muscular rigidity.

Low-dose inhaled nitrous oxide

Low-dose inhaled nitrous oxide is useful as a supplement to other drugs or to give background sedation. It is often administered, for the purpose of analgesia rather than sedation, in a fixed concentration (50%) from a cylinder premixed with oxygen (e.g. Entonox) via a demand valve. Such valves require a negative pressure to open them (which varies greatly with the make of the demand apparatus). The generation of this pressure may be beyond the ability of younger children and some adults.

Proper sedation with nitrous oxide requires a constant flow of gas, and this is best achieved with a purpose-built system such as the Quantiflex machine. Using this apparatus, nitrous oxide may be administered in subanaesthetic concentrations of 30–70% via a non-re-breathing circuit with a guaranteed minimum of 30% oxygen.

Ketamine

Ketamine is a derivative of phencyclidine and is often recommended as an anaesthetic for prehospital use. It is a dissociative anaesthetic and analgesic, which results in a trance-like state, which can be clinically recognised by the characteristic pupillary dilatation and nystagmus. Ketamine has both sedative and analgesic effects and in sedative doses does not compromise the airway or the circulation as much as other comparable drugs. It is an excellent and safe sedative for use in the ED with a success rate of more than 90%. Contraindications to sedation with ketamine include:

- Age <12 months due to an increased risk of laryngospasm and airway complications (children aged between 12 and 24 months should receive ketamine sedation only from expert staff).
- High risk of laryngospasm (active respiratory infection, active asthma)
- Unstable or abnormal airway
- Active upper or lower respiratory tract infection
- Proposed procedure within the mouth or pharynx
- Significant cardiac disease
- Recent significant head injury or reduced level of consciousness
- Intracranial hypertension with cerebrospinal fluid (CSF) obstruction
- Intraocular pathology (glaucoma, penetrating injury)
- Uncontrolled epilepsy
- Hyperthyroidism or thyroid medication
- Porphyria

- Previous psychotic illness
- Severe psychological problems such as cognitive or motor delay or severe behavioural problems
- Prior adverse reaction to ketamine.

The recommended doses are as follows:

- IV dose of ketamine for sedation = 1 mg/kg. The sedation starts within 60 seconds and lasts for 5–10 min. A further top up dose of 0.5mg/kg is sometimes required
- IM dose of ketamine for sedation = 4–5 mg/kg. The onset of sedation is around 5 min with an effective duration of up to 35 min. A top-up dose of a further 1 mg/kg can be given if either the first dose proves to be inadequate or there is a requirement to prolong the duration of the sedation. The effects of ketamine are surprisingly predictable and reliable when it is administered by the IM route.

Laryngospasm and excess salivation are uncommon side effects and prior administration of atropine is unnecessary. Emergence from sedation is usually uneventful however emergence phenomena including agitation, dysphoria and hallucination can occur. The risk of this is minimised by ensuring minimal stimulus (quiet room, dimmed lights, silenced monitors) during the recovery phase. About 5% of children will have transient clonic movements, and the same number will vomit during the recovery phase.

Discharge of patients who have received sedative drugs in the ED

The patient who is fit for discharge after sedation must fulfil all of the following criteria:

- Alert and oriented
- Able to walk steadily and unaided
- Able to drink liquids
- Not suffering from any disabling condition such as
  - vomiting
  - dizziness
  - shortness of breath
  - severe pain
- Accompanied by a responsible adult
- Suitable for the available transport
- Returning to adequate home circumstances.

Aftercare advice for patients who have received sedative or opioid (narcotic) drugs in the ED → p. 408.

End-of-life care

It is inevitable that some patients will attend the ED during the last days or hours of life. This may be as a consequence of an unexpected catastrophic event or trauma, be as a result of uncontrolled symptoms in a patient known to be approaching end of life or may be the culmination of a slow process of increasing frailty and decline.

It is often the instinctive response of emergency care staff to default to aggressive and invasive emergency treatment – in many cases this is the right thing to do. However, in a patient who is imminently or inevitably dying, burdensome and futile treatments may deny the patient, and their family, a calm and dignified death. There comes a point at which the focus of care should alter, from aiming for definitive diagnosis and curative treatment to patient and family centred, comfort focussed care. These decisions should be taken by an experienced clinician, with the skills to recognise that a patient is dying or that treatment is very likely to be futile.

Initiating end-of-life conversations in the ED can be challenging without the prior opportunity to establish a relationship of trust, often with limited information, and in a potentially pressured and hectic environment. These should not be reasons to abdicate this responsibility. Discussion should be undertaken sensitively, using clear language and avoiding the use of jargon or euphemism. Active listening, particularly around the patient's goals of care, can pave the way for discussions about management priorities, treatment that may not be appropriate and resuscitation. Using the SPIKES model can help guide this sensitive conversation (→ *Figure 1.2*). It is likely that many patients approaching the end of life will already have considered their priorities and preferences, for place of care, presence of individuals and religious requirements-these choices should be supported as far as possible.

Do not attempt Cardiopulmonary Resuscitation decisions (DNACPR)

Cardiopulmonary resuscitation was introduced as a treatment for sudden collapse due to arrythmia following cardiac arrest. It is potentially effective in a patient who deteriorates suddenly due to a cardiac arrythmia, or other reversible cause such as airway obstruction or hypoxia. It is however, at best, a bridge to definitive treatment. CPR carries risk of harm, and even the most effective cardiac arrest management will return the patient to a state of health rather worse than that experienced immediately before the arrest occurred. In situations where a slow decline has occurred and definitive treatment is not possible, or deterioration has occurred despite maximal appropriate therapy, cardiopulmonary resuscitation will not prevent death, but may prolong or increase suffering, and deny a dignified death. In these situations, cardiopulmonary resuscitation is not in the patient's best interests.

Anticipatory care planning ideally occurs before the patient arrives in the ED and before a crisis point. Where this has not happened, and it is evident that the patient is

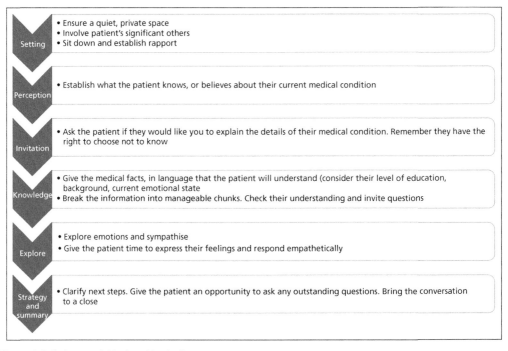

Figure 1.2 Spikes model for breaking bad news.

approaching end of life, it is important that these issues are explicitly considered and anticipatory decisions made wherever possible. There must be a presumption in favour of patient involvement in this discussion. When a DNACPR decision is made on the basis that CPR has no realistic prospect of success, this decision must be sensitively explained to the patient wherever possible. Those close to the patient should also be informed unless the patient's wish is for confidentiality. In the UK, it is accepted that consent from the patient and those close to them is not essential to implement a DNACPR decision where there is no prospect of success. Patients do not have the right to demand treatment which is clinically inappropriate, and healthcare professionals are not obliged to offer such treatment. In the occasional situation where the DNACPR decision is not accepted by the patient, a second opinion should be sought.

Risk management

The essence of emergency medicine is the assessment and management of the undifferentiated patient. This inherently carries with it a broad differential diagnosis and a high level of uncertainty.

One of the key skills of an emergency physician is effective risk management. The emergency physician needs to consider the most serious and immediately concerning diagnoses and take steps to either rule these out to an acceptable degree or expedite the next steps of emergency management.

It may not always be possible to reach a definitive diagnosis in the ED. In these cases, acknowledgement of this is often wiser than attempting to label symptoms with an inaccurate or uncertain 'diagnosis of convenience'. Where a definitive diagnosis cannot be reached, the emergency physician needs to establish

- whether immediate further investigation is required
- whether hospital admission or specialist opinion is necessary
- whether outpatient investigation and follow-up are required
- whether the risk is sufficiently low for the patient to be discharged with 'safety netting' advice to seek medical care if required. This risk is rarely truly zero and attempts to achieve this impossible goal can paradoxically increase harm by over-investigation, side effects from treatment and hospital-acquired deconditioning as a result of prolonged stay.

Safety netting

When patients are discharged from the ED, they should be advised regarding symptoms or signs that may herald a deterioration or need to return. Wherever possible these instructions should be written (an advice leaflet is often used for conditions such as head injury). Instructions should be detailed, specific and include advice on where and how to seek care if required. Provision of specific parameters requiring reassessment is likely to reduce anxiety and paradoxically reduce inappropriate reattendance.

Human factors in emergency medicine

'Human factors' refers to the complex interplay between the people and culture within a department, and the systems and processes which underpin and support practice. The ED is a complex and demanding environment and represents one of the highest risk areas in healthcare. Demand often exceeds resource, and high stakes, time critical decisions are often required on the basis of limited information. Unfamiliar multi-disciplinary teams must be assembled with little notice, and without rehearsal, to manage critically unwell patients. The emergency physician must be conscious of the impact of human factors on the delivery of care and avoidance of error. More errors and patient harms are caused by poor communication, loss of situation awareness, and the effect of cognitive biases, than result from lack of knowledge.

Some techniques that can be employed in the ED to improve safety and performance include

- Structured communication
  - Use an SBAR format to communicate the Situation, Background, Assessment and Recommendation
- Briefings and debriefings
  - Use departmental handovers, or the moments before a standby patient arrives, to ensure colleagues are aware of the current situation, team composition and experience, identify potential risks and allocate roles.
- Use of checklists
  - Certain scenarios, for example, rapid sequence induction of anaesthesia, sedation and some procedures are well suited to the use of standardised checklists
- Closed Loop Communication
  - Communicate a message or instruction to a team member using their name wherever possible. Verbal feedback from the team member confirms understanding and then completion of the task.
- Shared Mental Model
  - Verbalising the current situation, working diagnoses, priorities and plans creates more effective team working. This also enables the team to challenge or

prompt the team leader if key information has been overlooked or alternative options need consideration.

- Promoting Team wellbeing
  - Fatigue, hunger, external stressors and psychological triggers can all impair the effective functioning of team members. Ensuring team members take breaks and are appropriately supported has a direct impact on error reduction and patient safety.
- Civility
  - Incivility between members of the healthcare team has a measurable and profoundly negative impact on patient safety. Promoting civil communication reduces medical errors.

2

Major trauma and multiple injuries

Lt Col Alan G A Weir RAMC

UK Defence Medical Services, Lichfield, UK
Academic Department of Military Emergency Medicine, Royal Centre for Defence Medicine, Birmingham, UK
Major Trauma Centre, University Hospital Southampton, Southampton, UK

Epidemiology

There is a pandemic of trauma throughout the world. In high income countries, trauma is the leading cause of death in the first four decades of life and is surpassed only by cancer and atherosclerosis throughout life. Moreover, because it affects young people, trauma wastes more years of life than any other cause – an average of 36 years per trauma death. It is responsible for 8.3% of all 'life-years' lost in people under the age of 75 years in the UK. In addition, for every death from trauma, there are more than two survivors with serious or permanent disabilities.

> In the UK, accidents cause almost 2% of all deaths and account for 7% of total NHS expenditure.

The absolute number of accidental deaths is greatest in people aged 65 years and over. In this age group, more than half of all fatal trauma results from falls. However, for most of the population, road traffic is the greatest danger, being responsible for about 40% of trauma deaths and seriously injuring somebody every 20 minutes in the UK. Falls from a height and motor vehicle accidents commonly lead to multiple injuries ('polytrauma').

> People from deprived backgrounds are more likely to be injured than those from higher social classes.

Alcohol is a significant factor in about one in seven of all fatal car crashes and in over 40% of deaths from falls. (*For further information on alcohol and injury → p. 395*)

Speed also kills. A car hitting 100 pedestrians:

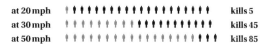

at 20 mph	kills 5
at 30 mph	kills 45
at 50 mph	kills 85

Deaths from trauma were commonly said to occur in a triphasic distribution:

1 **Immediate death, within minutes of injury**: complete airway obstruction, damage to the brain, brain stem, proximal spinal cord, heart, aorta or other large vessels
2 **Delayed deaths, within hours of injury**: intracranial bleeding or blood loss into the chest, abdomen or pelvis
3 **Late deaths, days or weeks after injury**: sepsis and organ failure.

However, in the UK, most fatalities (around 80%) actually occur at the scene of the injury, and later deaths do not

The RCEM Lecture Notes: Emergency Medicine, Fifth Edition. Edited by Catherine Williams and Amy Nickson.
© 2024 John Wiley & Sons Ltd. Published 2024 by John Wiley & Sons Ltd.
Companion website: www.wiley.com/go/LNEM5

neatly fit into this classification. Prevention is thus the best way to reduce the effect of injury, next is protection to mitigate its impact and finally, there must be timely and effective treatment.

TRAUMA CARE

The Advanced Trauma Life Support (ATLS) system, developed by the American College of Surgeons in the late 1970s, has become the standard method for the initial assessment and management of trauma victims. There are three main phases:

1 Primary survey and resuscitation
2 Secondary survey
3 Definitive care.

Senior healthcare professionals involved in managing trauma patients may wish to attend the European Trauma Course (ETC). This practical course is predominantly delivered via simulation and scenario-based training to give the technical and non-technical skills required to deliver and lead effective trauma care.

> This chapter adopts the ATLS approach but is no replacement for attendance on an ATLS course. The practical skills and team approach to trauma care cannot be learned from a book.

Preparation for reception of trauma victims

If warned of the imminent arrival of patients who are multiply injured:

- Assemble a Trauma Team in the Resuscitation Room. The trauma response initiated varies by the institution; however, the response can broadly be divided into two, the activation of which is criteria led:
  - **ED Trauma Team**: Senior EM Doctor, junior EM Doctor, ED Nurse, ED HCA
  - **Hospital Trauma Team**: ED Trauma Team plus Anaesthetist, Intensive Care Clinician, General Surgeon, and Orthopaedic Surgeon
- Warn additional appropriate inpatient specialties (such as Neurosurgery) if prehospital alert indicates they may be required
- **Allocate tasks**: the anaesthetist is usually allocated to airway and disability, doctor/nurse to breathing and circulation, nurse to apply monitoring, doctor/nurse to obtain IV access and draw blood samples, senior nurse to record findings and interventions, nurse to support relatives, senior doctor as team leader

- Check equipment and put on protective clothing
- Obtain 'Hands-off Handover' from ambulance crew, if patient status allows
- Pay particular attention to circumstances of the traumatic event as this may contain clues as to injuries sustained (→ *Box 2.1*)

> **Box 2.1 Factors associated with severe injury**
>
> Fall from a height of 5 m or more or a road traffic accident involving:
>
> - impact at high speed
> - fatality of other passenger(s)
> - ejection from vehicle
> - pedestrian struck by vehicle
> - motorcyclist with no crash helmet
> - steering wheel or windscreen damage
> - significant intrusion into passenger compartment

The primary survey and resuscitation phase (initial assessment and management)

Also → Chapter 1.

- Assess and secure the airway whilst protecting the c-spine. Manual in-line stabilisation may be needed.
- Provide high-flow oxygen.
- Ensure continued c-spine protection with blocks and tape.
- Assess the breathing; exclude/treat tension pneumothorax and other critical chest injuries. Cover 'sucking' chest wounds with a flap dressing (*Chest Injuries → Chapter 6, p. 73*)
- Stop external bleeding by direct pressure and establish venous access at two sites – large cannulae in large veins; intraosseous access may be required.
- **Draw blood for**: cross-matching, a coagulation screen, baseline glucose, electrolytes, haemoglobin, and venous blood gas.
- Take and record the pulse, BP and respiratory rate. Attach the patient to a pulse oximeter and a cardiac monitor.
- If a patient exhibits signs of shock (*Circulation → p. 4*) and requires fluid resuscitation, this should ideally be in the form of blood products (*Blood Transfusion → pp. 6 and 25*).
- Determine the level of consciousness (*AVPU → pp. 8 and 27*) and the size and reactivity of the pupils.

- Assess limb movements to confirm spinal cord integrity.
- Remove remaining clothing and expose the patient to allow further assessment.
- Obtain brief details of the patient and the trauma that he or she has suffered (*AMPLE → p. 10*).
- Consider early analgesia.
- **Request appropriate imaging**: in the severely injured patient, this is commonly a polytrauma CT that is performed to a clearly defined protocol and is applied uniformly across a trauma network.
- If life-threatening injuries (e.g. uncontrolled major haemorrhage) cannot be managed in the Resuscitation Room, the patient may need to be transferred, with ongoing resuscitation, to the Operating Theatre or Interventional Radiology Suite for definitive management.

> An understanding of the biomechanics of the trauma will suggest the likely extent of the injuries – many of which may not be obvious at this stage.

The secondary survey (further assessment)

- Once the primary survey has been completed and life-threatening injuries identified and managed, a thorough head-to-toe examination is required to identify other injuries.
- If any features in the primary survey are still giving cause for concern, return to these and address them.
- **When the front of the trunk and the limbs have been assessed, consider performing a log-roll to assess the patient's back**: frequently the back is not directly examined during the primary survey as the patient will rapidly move to the CT scanner; however, an exception to this may be in penetrating trauma when other wounds/exit-wounds need to be identified.
- During the log-roll the spine and perineum are examined, and a rectal examination is performed. The last will reveal the anal tone, presence of perineal injuries, position of the prostate and any blood.
- Document the injuries discovered.
- Consider the priorities for further investigation and treatment. Discuss the patient with doctors from other specialties and arrange timely transfer for ongoing care, i.e. Intensive Care Unit (ICU), operating theatre and inpatient ward.
- Maintain contemporary notes and repeat the ABCs and baseline observations frequently.

The chain of care

> Patients can appear deceptively stable even after significant injury – particularly blunt trauma. Inadequate assessment and treatment are commonplace, yet the consequences are not immediately evident. Complications on the ICU may be a result of inadequate resuscitation in the Emergency Department (ED) and deterioration in an ED may be caused by inadequate treatment at the scene.

Prehospital

In urban areas, with short transfer times to a definitive care centre and no delay involved in releasing the injured patient, a 'scoop and run' prehospital policy may be advocated. Pause only to secure the airway and protect the neck. In other situations (e.g. entrapment or prolonged transfer time), field resuscitation may be helpful (→ *Box 2.2*). Try to treat in transit; do not delay and play!

Emergency department

The primary concerns here are:

1. adequate oxygen delivery to vital tissues
2. treatment of critical problems as soon as they are identified
3. prevention of further deterioration.

> **Box 2.2 Prehospital management**
>
> - **Secure the airway**: jaw thrust, oropharyngeal or nasopharyngeal airway. Consider intubation
> - **Protect the cervical spine**
> - **Ensure adequate ventilation and oxygenation** (this may necessitate decompression of the chest: → *p. 77*)
> - **Cover open chest wounds**
> - **Control external haemorrhage by direct pressure**
> - **Start intravenous (IV) infusions only if this does not delay transfer**
> - **Protect thoracic and lumbar spine**: backboard or 'scoop' stretcher
> - **Provide analgesia**
> - **Record initial assessment of cardiorespiratory and neurological status**
> - **Communicate with the hospital**: assessment, management and expected time of arrival

This can be achieved by a well-rehearsed team working to agreed protocols and integrated into a comprehensive trauma care system.

PRIMARY SURVEY AND RESUSCITATION

This must be carried out in strict order of priority, although concurrent assessment is encouraged, i.e. A & D assessment by anaesthetist whilst B & C assessed by primary survey clinician. Problems are corrected as they are identified. The ATLS formula for the primary survey is:

A – Airway
B – Breathing
C – Circulation
D – Disability
E – Exposure

A to E assessment see also Chapter 1, page 1

Airway

Check for responsiveness.

> In an unresponsive patient, the airway is always at risk.

Then look for the following:

- No movement of air (complete airway obstruction or apnoea)
- Noises from the upper airway (partial airway obstruction); there may be snoring, rattles, stridor or other sounds (→ *Box 2.3*).

Box 2.3 Causes of upper airway obstruction in trauma

Oropharyngeal: tongue, teeth, dental plates, foreign bodies, blood and vomit
Facial: fractures of the maxilla or mandible
Cervical: laryngeal injury
Intracerebral: altered level of consciousness after head injury, alcohol or drugs

Any injury severe enough to compromise the airway may also have damaged the cervical spine.

Tx All severely injured patients should be commenced on high-flow oxygen, which can then be titrated appropriately as assessment and management progresses. The airway must be:

- *cleared* of foreign material with suction, Magill's forceps and fingers, if necessary
- *maintained* using a jaw-thrust manoeuvre, a Guedel oropharyngeal airway, a nasopharyngeal airway or by endotracheal intubation (the nasopharyngeal airway is safe and well tolerated in the conscious patient and is much less likely to stimulate gagging than the Guedel airway)
- *protected* by vigilance, suctioning and positioning.

When traumatic disruption of the facial or laryngeal structures prevents intubation, surgical access to the airway must be obtained. Emergency tracheostomy is difficult and dangerous and has been superseded by the technique of cricothyroidotomy. Needle puncture of the cricothyroid membrane is preferable in children aged <12 years (→ *Box 2.4*).

Box 2.4 Artificial airways in trauma

Standard orotracheal intubation: this is the route of choice in the apnoeic patient.
Nasotracheal intubation: this is a valuable technique in some special situations, such as for the non-paralysed patient. It should not be performed in the presence of a possible fracture of the base of the skull. The traditionally advocated method of 'blind' nasal intubation requires considerable skill and must not be attempted by inexperienced staff.
Surgical cricothyroidotomy: this is the method of choice in adults. It is contraindicated in children aged <12 years because of the importance of the cricoid cartilage in tracheal support and the long-term problems that result if it is damaged (→ *Box 2.5*).
Needle cricothyroidotomy: this procedure is performed using a large cannula and only allows oxygenation NOT ventilation. Bag-and-mask ventilation is ineffective via such a small opening. The patient must be oxygenated with high-flow oxygen from either a flow meter or the wall supply (at 50 lbf/in^2 [psi], or 4000 cm H_2O pressure). Intermittent flow is achieved using a Y-piece, a three-way tap or a hole in the side of the tubing. Exhalation takes place through the upper airway and not through the cannula. CO_2 retention occurs and thus this procedure should not be used for more than 20 min, i.e. buys time for a definitive airway to be established (→ *Box 2.6*).

Box 2.5 **Cricothyroidotomy**

- Extend the patient's neck while controlling the head
- Mark the skin over the centre of the cricothyroid membrane (which lies between the thyroid and cricoid cartilages → *Figure 2.1*)
- Support the larynx and tighten the overlying skin with the non-dominant hand
- Make a small transverse incision through the skin and spread the edges outwards
- Make a transverse incision through the cricothyroid membrane and open the wound with the handle of the scalpel
- Insert an appropriate size of endotracheal or tracheostomy tube
- Start ventilation and check for air entry
- Secure the tube

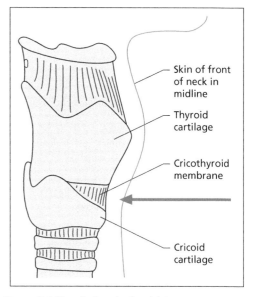

Figure 2.1 The site for cricothyroidotomy.

 Box 2.6 **Needle cricothyroid puncture**

- Extend the patient's neck while controlling the head
- Mark the skin over the centre of the cricothyroid membrane (which lies between the thyroid and cricoid cartilages → *Figure 2.1*)
- Attach a cannula and needle of an appropriate size (at least 12G for an adult) to a small syringe
- Support the larynx and tighten the overlying skin with the non-dominant hand
- Puncture the skin and cricothyroid membrane with the needle, aiming for the small of the back, aspirating as the needle is advanced
- When air is easily aspirated, advance the cannula and withdraw the needle
- Recheck the ease of aspiration of air (it is surprisingly easy to miss the trachea with a needle, especially in children)
- Attach the cannula to either the wall or the flow-meter oxygen supply via an in-line Y-connector. In a child, start with a flow meter set at a delivery rate in litres equal to the child's age in years
- Adjust the flow rate and inspiratory time until adequate chest movement is achieved. Expiration may take several seconds
- Secure the cannula

The cervical spine

Cervical spine injury must be assumed to have occurred in all patients who have sustained polytrauma until excluded by clinical examination and good-quality imaging. Patients at particular risk include those who have sustained:

- any injury above the clavicle
- head injury associated with depressed consciousness
- a high-speed injury
- a fall from a height.

A normal neurological examination does not exclude cervical spine injury. Moreover, conscious patients with other painful injuries may not always complain of neck discomfort.

Tx Movement of the cervical spine must be limited in order to protect against further spinal and/or spinal cord injury. Traditionally this has involved the application of a well-fitting hard collar plus blocks applied on either side of the head and attached to the stretcher. However, controversies exist as to the efficacies of hard collars, and there is a lack of compelling evidence either way. Collars may be uncomfortable and provoke agitation, and undoubtedly make airway management more challenging. Therefore, cervical protection should be provided in accordance with the local trauma network guidelines, which may include collar and blocks, blocks alone or manual in-line stabilisation from a healthcare professional.

Breathing

Look for

- External signs of injury
- Abnormal respiratory rate or pattern
- Unequal chest movement
- Tracheal shift and displacement of the apex beat
- Decreased breath sounds
- Increased or decreased resonance
- Low SaO_2 (arterial O_2 saturation)
- Signs of hypoxia (tachycardia, agitation or confusion and cyanosis).

Five major chest injuries require immediate recognition and treatment during the primary survey:

1 Tension pneumothorax
2 Open pneumothorax (sucking chest wound)
3 Massive haemothorax
4 Flail segment of the chest
5 Cardiac tamponade.

Other injuries, which may cause dyspnoea or shock, may become apparent in the secondary survey:

- Pulmonary contusion
- Myocardial contusion
- Aortic disruption
- Traumatic diaphragmatic hernia
- Tracheobronchial disruption
- Oesophageal disruption.

Tx

*Diagnosis and treatment of major chest injuries →
    Chapter 6.*

Upper airway patency does not ensure adequate ventilation. Assisted breathing using a bag, mask and airway or tracheal intubation may be required. Before attempted intubation, the patient must be preoxygenated using a bag, mask and airway technique, and intubation should be performed quickly by an experienced operator. Prolonged, unsuccessful attempts at intubation must be avoided.

> Attempted intubation in a patient who is not paralysed may cause a dramatic rise in intracranial pressure.

A small, uncomplicated, and possibly undiagnosed, simple pneumothorax may rapidly develop into a life-threatening tension pneumothorax if the patient is mechanically ventilated in either the operating theatre or ICU. Prophylactic chest drains should be considered in any patient with chest injury requiring ventilation.

Circulation

In the primary survey, the state of the circulation is quickly assessed by observation of:

- skin colour and temperature
- pulse rate and volume
  - Young people preferentially increase their ejection fraction initially, which can mask significant hypovolaemia
  - Tachycardia may signify significant hypovolaemia
- capillary refill time (usually 2 seconds or less)
- BP (blood pressure)
- JVP (jugular venous pressure) and heart sounds
- level of consciousness (in the patient who has not sustained a brain injury).

> Hypotension with a raised JVP and absent heart sounds suggests cardiac tamponade: → *p. 80.*

The assessment of hypovolaemia in the trauma patient is difficult because of the following:

- The interaction of autonomic reflexes, head injury, pain, drugs and blood loss is complex.
- Compensatory mechanisms may prevent a fall in systolic blood pressure until 30% of the blood volume has been lost.
- Rapid blood loss may produce reflex bradycardia.
- In elderly people, tachycardia may not be present as a result of limited cardiac response to catecholamines or treatment with β blockers.
- Haematocrit is an unreliable index of shock; a nearly normal value does not rule out significant blood loss.

> All abnormalities of colour, pulse, BP and consciousness should be regarded with suspicion.

Methods of assessing organ perfusion → Box 2.8.
Signs of shock → Box 2.7.

The blood loss potential of evident injuries should be considered (→ *Table 2.1*); the mechanism of injury may suggest occult blood loss. Hypovolaemia is seldom caused by head injury alone, except occasionally in infants. Open fractures will cause greater blood loss than similar closed injuries.

Tx

*General management of major haemorrhage → Figure 1.1
    on p. 6 and 7.*

Box 2.7 Guides to organ perfusion

- Mental state
- **Urinary output:** adequate volume replacement produces a urine output in the adult of about 50 mL/h
- **Arterial blood gases:** metabolic acidosis implies inadequate tissue oxygenation requiring increased oxygen and fluids (not bicarbonate)
- **Shock index:** calculated by dividing the pulse rate in beats/min by the systolic BP in mmHg. The normal range is 0.5–0.7. Values >0.9 suggest significant haemorrhage
- Core/periphery temperature gradient
- **Aortic flow** (measured by Doppler ultrasound probe)
- **Serum lactate:** high lactate is increasingly recognised as a good indicator of tissue hypoxia and a poor prognosis

Box 2.8 Signs of shock

- Altered mental state
- Delayed capillary refill (>2 seconds)
- Tachycardia
- Pale, cool skin

- Control external blood loss by direct pressure at the bleeding site.
- Consider the use of tourniquets
- Insert at least two large-calibre (14 G) cannulae into large veins. If percutaneous venous access is difficult, use the interosseous route. Large bore vascular access devices are available and effective when inserted by an appropriately skilled healthcare professional.

Table 2.1 Estimation of traumatic blood loss in an adult (closed injuries)

Site	Volume (L)
Pelvis	0.5–3
Shaft of femur	1–2
Tibia	0.5–1
Chest	>2
Abdomen	>2
Arm	0.5–1
Forearm	0.5–1

- Take a sample of blood for group and cross-match, and coagulation screen.
- Evidence of shock in the trauma patient requires resuscitation with blood products (→ *Figure 1.1 on pp. 6 and 7*). If blood products are not immediately available, then boluses (250 mL) of IV crystalloid may be administered, to achieve organ perfusion, until blood is available. Caution must be used as this will dilute clotting factors and the oxygen-carrying capability of the circulating blood volume. Ideally, IV fluids should be warmed to 40°C. Vasopressors must be used with caution in hypovolaemic shock as they could decrease end-organ tissue perfusion, although conflicting evidence exists in the literature.
- Consider the possibility of cavity bleeding and the need for surgical intervention.
- Consider the possibility of blood loss from a major pelvic fracture. Do not try to 'spring' the pelvis to demonstrate its instability – this may increase bleeding by either disrupting the already formed blood clot or displacing the fracture. Application of an external pelvic binder will help reduce bleeding (→ *Figure 2.2*). This should be thought of as a resuscitation manoeuvre to help control the circulation in the primary survey-have a low threshold for applying one.

The return of a normal BP after the infusion of, for example, 1000 mL does not mean that only a litre has been lost – the true amount is likely to be much higher. When blood pressure can be maintained only by continuing infusion, cardiovascular collapse is imminent; the cause of the hidden blood loss must be sought.

Failure to respond to fluids usually means inadequate transfusion or unrecognised fluid loss. However, it may also be caused by:

- tension pneumothorax → *p. 76*
- cardiac tamponade → *p. 80*
- myocardial infarction
- acute gastric distension
- neurogenic shock → *p. 54*.

Blood transfusion

Indications for blood components→ Box 14.29 on p. 270.
Overview of the management of major haemorrhage → Figure 1.1 on p. 6 and 7.

Military surgeons avoid 'old blood' and crystalloids and use large volumes of whole blood with fresh frozen plasma (FFP).

Modest haemodilution and a fall in haematocrit to 30% improve erythrocyte passage through the

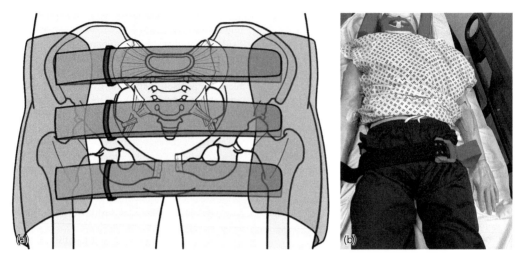

Figure 2.2 (a) Pelvic binder. Anterior view of a fractured pelvis with a pelvic binder in place. Mostafa, A. M. H. A. M., et al. 2020/SAGE Publications/Licensed under CC BY 4.0. (b) Pelvic binder applied to a manikin.

microcirculation. This allows optimal oxygen delivery to the tissues – until the haematocrit falls below 25%. However, when estimated blood loss exceeds 1.5 L in an adult, blood should be transfused to maintain the haematocrit >25% or a haemoglobin concentration >8 g/dL.

SAG-M blood (which consists of plasma-poor red blood cells in saline, adenine, glucose and mannitol) is frequently supplied by the National Blood Service in the UK. (The adenine maintains 2,3-diphosphoglycerate or 2,3-DPG activity in stored blood to allow more normal uncoupling of oxygen from oxyhaemoglobin and thus improved tissue oxygenation.) This red cell concentrate is presented in units of 300 mL, each with a packed cell volume (haematocrit) of 0.55–0.65.

If a blood sample is taken when the initial intravenous lines are established, grouped blood (type specific) should be available within 20 min. Cross-matched blood (whether by urgent or full cross-match) is seldom available within 1 hour and is therefore not normally appropriate for unstable hypovolaemic patients. These patients should receive blood that is matched only for the recipient's ABO and rhesus group. This will, of course, increase the incidence of transfusion reactions.

In situations of such urgency that delay – even for grouped blood – is unacceptable, O-negative blood should be given to women of childbearing age and O-positive blood should be given to males and females not of childbearing age (to help preserve stocks of O-negative blood).

Rapid blood transfusion may produce the following:

- **Coagulopathy:** requiring platelets and/or FFP
- **Hypocalcaemia:** as a result of calcium binding by anticoagulants in stored blood (at infusion rates

of <50 mL/min, this should not be a problem); plasma ionised calcium must not be allowed to fall <1 mmol/L
- **Hypothermia** (which may itself cause a significant reduction in coagulation).

Thus, if a large volume of blood is transfused rapidly, it should be filtered and warmed.

> Immunocompromised and pregnant patients should always receive CMV-negative blood (i.e. blood that is free of cytomegalovirus).

Control of severe bleeding

> The 'coagulopathy of trauma' is due to many factors: consumption of fibrinogen and clotting factors, dilution of plasma proteins, hypothermia, acidosis, inflammation and shock. If present on admission, it is associated with a mortality rate of almost 50%.

In the presence of intractable bleeding, deficiency of clotting factors should be considered and haematological advice sought. In particular, in the absence of any known disease, acquired haemophilia may be a possibility (→ *p. 271*). If a site for bleeding is identified, further investigation should never delay surgical attempts to 'turn off the tap'.

Tranexamic acid: tranexamic acid inhibits fibrinolysis. It has been shown to safely reduce mortality in bleeding trauma patients without increasing the risk of adverse events, provided that it is given within 3 hours of the time of injury. It is particularly useful when other treatments directed at coagulopathy (e.g. FFP, platelets and cryoprecipitate) are unavailable. A loading dose of 1 g is given intravenously over 10 min, followed by an infusion of 1 g over the next 8 hours.

Clotting factor replacement: patients who are susceptible to bleeding (e.g. congenital and acquired haemophilia, inherited factor VII deficiency, Glanzmann's thrombasthenia) may be the victims of trauma. Remember to consider clotting factor replacement in these individuals and discuss early with a Haematology Consultant.

Haemostatic substances for local application: severe bleeding from damaged tissue, blood vessels or even organs may sometimes be controlled by the local application of haemostatic substances. The most effective of these is MPH (Microporous Polysaccharide Hemospheres), a patented powder synthesised from raw materials derived from potatoes! The MPH particles dehydrate the blood and concentrate blood solids on their surfaces, thus creating a high concentration of gelled, compacted, clotting material.

Resuscitative thoracotomy

Resuscitative thoracotomy may be life-saving for some patients with penetrating injuries to the chest (→ *p. 81*). This allows cardiac tamponade to be relieved and compression of the thoracic aorta to optimise cerebral circulation during the critical period. Thoracotomy is of no value if the patient is already lifeless on arrival at the department or has sustained blunt trauma where there is no evidence of a surgical target, i.e. cardiac tamponade on bedside ultrasound.

Disability

A rapid assessment of the patient's neurological status completes the primary survey:

- Level of consciousness
- Pupil size and reaction
- Posture and spontaneous movements.

A simple classification of the level of consciousness is the AVPU system:

A – Alert
V – Responds to voice
P – Responds to pain
U – Unresponsive

Alternatively, if time allows, the Glasgow Coma Scale (GCS) can be used.

Exposure

All parts of the patient should be exposed and examined. The spine must be well controlled when clothing is disturbed. Some clothes can only be safely removed during log-rolling. The areas most often missed are the back and the perineum.

> Beware of hypothermia.

At the end of the primary survey, attention must be given to the following:

- **Glucose**: check for hypoglycaemia with a reagent stick or on VBG. Some degree of hyperglycaemia is inevitable in most trauma patients; hypoglycaemia can precipitate trauma (→ *pp. 254 and 346*)
- **History**: the AMPLE format (→ *p. 10*)
- **Immediate analgesia**: small aliquots of IV morphine carefully titrated against response
- **Investigations**: trauma CT or the three initial radiographs of multiple trauma (chest, lateral cervical spine and pelvis), trauma system dependent.

> Do not forget to communicate as frequently as possible with the patient's relatives (→ *pp. 11 and 348*).

FURTHER CARE OF THE TRAUMA PATIENT

The secondary survey

On completion of the primary survey – when the resuscitation phase is complete – remove all the patient's remaining clothing while controlling the entire spine. The detailed secondary survey can now begin. It should be carried out in a top-to-toe rather than a systems-oriented order.

> Much of the information of the secondary (and primary) survey is best recorded on a purpose-designed trauma form.

The following features must be included in the examination.

Head and neck

- GCS score
- Pupillary size and reactions
- Posture, movement and cranial nerve function – lateralising signs
- Scalp – haematomas, lacerations, depressed fractures
- Ears and nose for cerebrospinal fluid and/or bleeding. Look with an auroscope for haemotympani or ruptured tympanic membrane
- Facial skeleton
- Mouth and teeth
- Neck – swelling, wounds and tenderness.

Chest

- Respiratory rate, pattern and depth; watch and feel for the abnormal movement of a flail segment
- Clothing imprints or bruising
- Wounds – especially small penetrating injuries
- Surgical emphysema
- Rib tenderness
- Tracheal displacement
- Air entry, percussion note and breath sounds
- Heart sounds and position of the apex beat
- Trends in SaO_2
- Arterial blood gases
- ECG.

Abdomen

- Clothing imprints or bruising: which usually indicate severe compression
- Wounds
- Localised or generalised tenderness and guarding
- Bowel sounds: an unreliable guide to injury
- Buttocks, anus, genitalia and perineum
- Consider rectal and vaginal examination ($\rightarrow$ *p. 311*).

Back (will need log-roll)

- Bruising, swelling and wounds
- Gaps and swellings in the line of the spinous processes
- Tenderness: especially ribs, spine and loins
- Perineum and anus ($\rightarrow$ *p. 87*).

Limbs

- Swelling and bruising
- Tenderness
- Wounds
- Deformity and compound fractures
- Circulation, nerve and tendon function distal to injuries
- General peripheral neurological function.

At the end of the secondary survey, re-examine the ABCs.

Tx

- Summon further appropriate specialist help
- Reduce any fracture or dislocation that is threatening distal circulation or overlying skin
- Splint other fractures
- Clean and dress wounds
- Catheterise the bladder and measure the urine output
- Obtain further information from the patient, paramedics, bystanders, relatives or the GP
- Consider further investigations ($\rightarrow$ *below*).

Prophylactic antibiotics: These are indicated for:

- severe contaminated wounds with tissue destruction
- compound limb fractures
- penetrating intestinal injuries.

> Antibiotics are not indicated for simple contaminated wounds, but thorough surgical toilet is always required.

Tetanus prophylaxis: Tetanus immune status should be confirmed as soon as possible, and antitetanus toxoid and immunoglobulin should be given as appropriate ($\rightarrow$ *p. 415*). If no history is available, the patient should be treated as unimmunised.

Investigations in trauma

Blood tests

Blood should be taken for FBC, blood group and cross-match, coagulation screen and biochemistry (including glucose). When the cause of coma is in doubt, plasma osmolality can be useful ($\rightarrow$ *p. 235*).

Radiological priorities

In well-developed trauma systems, the aim is to perform a head-to-toe trauma CT within 30 min of the patient's arrival in ED. However, in less-developed trauma systems, this may not be possible and plain radiographs may be utilised. In such cases, radiological priorities are chest, pelvis and lateral cervical spine. Portable or overhead machines should be used so that the patient does not have to be moved out of the resuscitation area. Further non-critical imaging should be delayed until resuscitation is underway and the patient is stable. In this scenario, Focused Assessment with Sonography in

Trauma (FAST) whereby bedside ultrasound is utilised may be of additional benefit.

Assessment of cervical spine injury → p. 49.
Assessment of chest injury → p. 73.
Assessment of pelvic injury → p. 86.

Trauma radiograph of the chest: The ideal view of the chest is the erect posteroanterior (PA) film, which will demonstrate:

- pneumothorax
- haemothorax
- mediastinal widening
- subphrenic air
- rib fractures.

However, in the trauma patient, this is not practical due to the need to protect the spine. Therefore, a supine anteroposterior (AP) film should be obtained and interpreted in relation to clinical findings.

Trauma radiograph of the pelvis: Clinical assessment of pelvic injury by pressure on the anterosuperior iliac spines is unreliable and may restart or exacerbate pelvic bleeding. An AP radiograph of the pelvis is taken to assess the congruity of the bony pelvic ring; however, plain films underestimate a significant number of pelvic fractures. Therefore, if there is any suspicion of pelvic fracture a CT must be obtained.

Trauma radiograph of the cervical spine: A good cross-table lateral view of the cervical spine will exclude many significant injuries. Often, the body of C7 and the C7–T1 junction are not adequately visualised on the initial film, and a coned view of this area with gentle shoulder traction is needed.

If the lateral radiograph of the neck is normal and the patient is fully conscious without significant neck pain, then the cervical immobilisation may be removed to allow clinical assessment of the cervical spine. In the patient with depressed consciousness, the cervical spine must remain immobilised while awaiting AP and odontoid peg views, discussion with an Orthopaedic/Spinal surgeon and, if necessary, a CT scan.

Clearance of the cervical spine → p. 54.

CT scan: CT provides an excellent assessment of intracranial injuries and their sequelae. It is also essential for:

- assessment of the cervical spine where there remains clinical doubt after plain films
- further assessment of spinal injuries seen on plain films
- detailed examination of thoracic injuries, especially those involving the mediastinum
- assessment of abdominal injuries in relatively stable patients before laparotomy
- detailed assessment of pelvic fractures.

If CT is to be performed, all necessary images should be obtained at the same time. Routine use of 'top-to-toe' scanning is now recommended in the adult trauma patient if no indication for immediate intervention exists. A CT scan with contrast is often required.

Ultrasound scan (FAST): In experienced hands, ultrasonography can be a highly sensitive diagnostic technique. It is particularly useful for the detection of free fluid and the identification of solid organ injury. It is less valuable in the assessment of bowel damage. The ultrasound machine can be brought to the patient rather than moving an unstable patient to the CT room, and it may be useful in environments where CT cannot be obtained in a timely fashion. FAST is not sufficiently accurate to be used as a substitute for CT, where CT facilities are available, and should never delay CT.

Further assessment of the abdomen in multiple trauma

Abdominal injuries have special significance because of the following:

1 They can cause profound haemorrhage.
2 They can be difficult to diagnose clinically – especially in unresponsive patients. Signs may be poorly localised or equivocal.

Exclusion of intra-abdominal damage is particularly important in any patient who:

- is shocked or unstable
- has signs attributable to the abdomen
- has a reduced level of consciousness or is otherwise difficult to assess clinically
- is about to be anaesthetised or transferred to another department for the management of other injuries.

Methods of abdominal assessment include:

- immediate laparotomy
- ultrasound examination
- CT scan
- diagnostic peritoneal lavage (superseded by trauma CT; may have a role in less developed trauma systems).

More on assessment of abdominal injuries → p. 81.

Definitive care of the trauma patient

The trauma patient should be moved to an area for definitive care as soon as possible. This may be an operating theatre, a specialised surgical unit, an ICU or a bed in a ward. Rapid referral and transfer of a properly assessed and stabilised patient is associated with a decreased risk of complications and is (obviously) a reassurance for both patients and relatives.

> Do not forget the continuing need for analgesia.

Refer to appropriate chapters for specific injuries.

SPECIAL SITUATIONS

Choking → p. 205.
Electrocution → p. 150.
Exposure to radiation and contamination by radioactive substances → p. 151.
Gunshot wounds → pp. 30, 401 and 418.
Major burns → Chapter 10 on p. 141.

Blast injuries

Explosions have the potential to cause complex and varied polytrauma to large numbers of people. These injuries are compounded when the explosion occurs in a confined space. Blast injuries are divided into four classes – primary, secondary, tertiary and quaternary:

1 Primary injuries are caused by the effect of blast overpressure waves (shock waves) on human tissue. The degree of injury depends on the level of pressure, its duration, and the orientation of the patient to the blast. These types of injuries are especially likely when a person is close to exploding munitions, such as a landmine. Unlike water, air is easily compressible and so a primary blast injury almost always affects airfilled structures. The ears are most often injured, followed by the lungs and the hollow organs of the gastrointestinal (GI) tract. GI injuries may present after a delay of hours or even days and are very hard to diagnose. Absence of tympanic membrane injury does not rule out blast injury.
2 Secondary injuries are caused by flying shrapnel, glass, debris and other objects propelled by the explosion. These injuries may affect any part of the body and often result in penetrating trauma and bleeding.
3 Tertiary injuries are a feature of high-energy explosions. Displacement of air by the explosion creates a blast wind that can throw victims against solid objects. There may be both blunt and penetrating injuries. Fractures are common. Children are particularly vulnerable because of their low body weight.
4 Quaternary (or miscellaneous) injuries include all other injuries not included in the first three classes such as burns, crush injuries, toxic inhalations and radiation exposure.

All patients exposed to a significant explosion must be carefully examined with special attention paid to their tympanic membranes, lungs and abdomen. A chest radiograph (CXR) should be performed. Blunt injuries, fractures, crush injuries, burns and superficial injuries from flying glass should all receive standard investigation and treatment. Penetrating injuries from shrapnel and other debris are best regarded as low-velocity gunshot wounds (GSW) and should be considered to be highly contaminated, particularly with human tissue and blood-borne viruses.

Gunshot wounds

The approach to a patient with a GSW should take the same form as for any other trauma, but special attention should be taken to the following:

- The police should be informed to ensure the safety of the public, staff caring for the patient and potentially the patient themselves – if at risk of further attempts on their life.
- The pattern of internal injury depends on the type of bullet, its velocity and mass but usually represents significantly more damage than apparent from the entry wound. Cavitation, shearing and compression forces contribute to tissue and vessel damage.
- The patient must be fully exposed to look for exit wounds.
- Apparent injury to the abdomen, shoulder or neck can result in significant intrathoracic injury – have a low threshold for resuscitative thoracotomy in the peri-arrest patient. →*pp. 82 and 83*

Burns → Chapter 10 on p. 141.
Burns from white phosphorus in incendiary munitions → p. 149.
Exposure to radiation and contamination by radioactive substances → p. 151.
Gunshot wounds → pp. 401 and 418.

Drowning

Drowning is suffocation resulting from submersion or immersion in a liquid and as such causes injury by the effects of fluid in the airway and lungs and by generalised hypoxia. There may also be:

- precipitating causes, e.g. alcohol or drug intoxication, myocardial infarction, hypoglycaemia, fit
- coincidental injury, e.g. from a fall or dive into water (especially injury to the cervical spine)
- other consequences, e.g. hypothermia.

Toddlers and teenagers are the most common victims of drowning – which is the leading cause of accidental death in children worldwide.

The difference between the effects of seawater (hypertonic) and freshwater (hypotonic) drowning is probably less important than once believed. In many cases, there is immediate laryngospasm and thus little inhalation into the lungs. The patient is likely to be unresponsive and hypotensive with signs of cerebral hypoxia and perhaps also negative pressure pulmonary oedema following rapid airway obstruction from laryngeal spasm.

Tx

Cardiac arrest → p. 157.

- Clear the airway of debris and then secure it. Consider the need for cervical spine protection.
- Give high-flow oxygen with a continuous positive airway pressure (CPAP) circuit if possible. Patients in whom breathing is inadequate should be ventilated immediately – with the help of an anaesthetist if possible. These patients will usually need decompression of the stomach with a wide-bore tube.
- Establish IV access and fluid infusion.
- Monitor SaO_2, respiratory rate, pulse, BP, ECG and core temperature.
- Send blood for FBC, blood chemistry, glucose and blood gases.
- Obtain a 12-lead ECG and CXR.
- Treat hypotension, wheezing or pulmonary oedema. Severe acidosis can be corrected with bicarbonate.
- Treat hypothermia (→ *p. 247*).

All patients must be admitted – most to an ICU. Delayed exacerbations may occur up to 24 hours after injury. Patients with signs of cerebral hypoxia (usually unresponsive) should be ventilated even in the presence of satisfactory oxygenation because they are likely to have cerebral oedema.

Suffocation and asphyxiation

Suffocation is a state in which there is inadequate availability of air for inhalation – usually due to external obstruction of the mouth and nose. Asphyxiation describes oxygen deficit from a wider range of causes such as gassing and strangulation. The signs of both are those of prolonged hypoxia and developing cerebral oedema. The treatment is similar to that detailed above for drowning.

The frail injured patient

Older and frail patients have a different pattern of injury than the younger population. Minor mechanisms of injury that may be trivial in a younger patient may result in serious injury. Significant trauma is most often sustained in falls from standing height, and the head and thorax are the most common areas injured.

Frail injured patients (FRIPs) are often under triaged and the significance of their injuries overlooked or recognised late. Higher baseline systolic blood pressures, rate control medication (e.g. beta blockers) and anticoagulant medication may mean severity of haemorrhage is underestimated. Osteoporosis will increase the risk of fractures. Reduced physiological reserve, lower elasticity of tissues and comorbidity reduces the frail patient's ability to compensate for and recover from injury. Rib fracture mortality in particular increases with increasing age. There is a high risk of cervical spine injury accompanying head injury, and clinical 'clearance' is more challenging as the Canadian C-spine rule cannot be applied. Central cord syndrome is relatively common.

Patients should be assessed by a senior clinician and examined carefully. A lower threshold for imaging is often appropriate. A multidisciplinary team should be involved early in the patient's journey in the hospital. The risks of delirium and associated morbidity and mortality are significant. Management should aim to be patient-focused, rather than specific injury focused.

Paediatric trauma

The principles of trauma assessment are similar for both adults and children, with the exception of trauma imaging. Childhood covers the period from birth through adolescence to adulthood, and there is no single answer to how a child with a particular injury should be imaged. The use of adult trauma imaging protocols in children is not appropriate. Locally agreed protocols should be produced in keeping with guidance from the Royal College of Radiologists document: *Paediatric Trauma Protocols.*

Differences in anatomy, physiological parameters and equipment are dealt with in *Chapter 18*. The most important differences in managing a child when compared with an adult in trauma care are as follows:

- The airway is narrower, floppier and more difficult to maintain.
- The lungs have a very limited oxygen reserve, but the body has a higher metabolic rate.
- The circulation may suddenly decompensate, and thus shock appears with very little warning.
- The vertebrae are relatively elastic and so there may be spinal cord injury without radiological abnormality (abbreviated to the acronym SCIWORA).
- The ribs are also elastic and so underlying viscera may be injured without evidence of rib trauma.

- A child becomes hypoglycaemic and hypothermic very easily.

> A child's lungs, liver and spleen are like fresh eggs in an AMBU bag. Hit the bag with a hammer, and the eggs are smashed but the bag (the ribs) returns to its former shape. An adult's organs are like hard-boiled eggs in a tin can. Hit the can and it is damaged (there are rib fractures) but the eggs may survive intact.

Trauma in pregnancy

The relevant anatomical and physiological changes of pregnancy must be considered during assessment, along with early involvement of the Obstetric team:

- The tidal volume is increased, respiratory rate is stable and so $PaCO_2$ (arterial CO_2 partial pressure) is slightly reduced.
- The BP is normally slightly reduced, and the pulse is increased.
- Compression of the inferior vena cava in the supine patient in the last trimester of pregnancy is very significant and reduces cardiac output. The risk of sudden maternal collapse is reduced by manual displacement of the gravid uterus towards the left.
- Gastric emptying is delayed.

Systemic (maternal) hypovolaemia results in a selective reduction in placental blood flow. The fetus is very vulnerable to hypoxia, but the maternal circulation is partially protected by physiological hypervolaemia. Deterioration in oxygen supply to the fetus can occur very rapidly after a period of apparent normality.

XR Consider early ultrasound scan of the abdomen, uterus and fetus.

Tx There are, of course, two patients:

1 **The mother:** for the most part, the care of a pregnant woman is identical to that of a non-pregnant patient. Important additions are the following:
   - Hypoxia and hypovolaemia must be treated particularly quickly and vigorously. If blood is to be given, it must be CMV negative.
   - Patients in the last trimester of pregnancy should have the gravid uterus displaced to the left to prevent compression of the inferior vena cava with consequent reduction in cardiac filling and circulatory collapse. This will be either by placing the patient on a spinal board and tilting this to the left or by manual displacement of the gravid uterus.

Inserting a wedge will cause rotation of the spine and potentially result in spinal column and/or cord damage.
   - There is an increased risk of aspiration pneumonia (Mendelson's syndrome), especially if the mother has a reduced level of consciousness or needs sedation or anaesthesia. Prophylaxis is aimed at reducing the acidity of the gastric contents as quickly as possible – give at-risk patients IV ranitidine (50 mg diluted to 20 mL over 2 min) or IV omeprazole (40 mg diluted to 100 mL over 20 min).
   - Rhesus D-negative women with abdominal injury are at risk of developing antibodies against a rhesus-positive fetus. Any pregnant woman who may have had abdominal trauma should be blood grouped and, if found to be rhesus D negative, given anti-D immunoglobulin.

2 **The fetus:** the well-being of the fetus depends almost entirely on the state of the mother.

> The initial management of the fetus is the support of the maternal airway, breathing and circulation.

Methods of assessing the fetus include:

- auscultation with a Pinnard's stethoscope or Doppler fetoscope
- fetocardiotocography (FCTG)
- abdominal ultrasonography.

In late pregnancy, urgent delivery of the fetus may be required for the health of both parties. This may be by caesarean section if the situation and time allows. In cases where the pregnant patient suffers a witnessed traumatic cardiac arrest, or is so severely ill that they are at risk of cardiac arrest, performing a resuscitative hysterotomy to deliver the fetus and improve the patients cardiac output is indicated. Peri-mortem caesarean section may occasionally save the life of the baby when the mother is recently deceased. *Resuscitative hysterotomy →* *Chapter 11, Box 11.1, p.167*

Abdominal trauma in pregnancy → p. 85.

OTHER ASPECTS OF TRAUMA CARE

Bereaved relatives

As with cardiac arrest, a fatality from trauma will leave relatives in a state of sudden and unexpected bereavement. The care of these people is part of the complete spectrum of trauma management.

Outline of bereavement care → p. 171.

Trauma scores

Trauma scoring systems are useful for audit, research and planning purposes but should not be used to determine in-hospital care. They have limited use in prehospital triage. There are four main types:

1 Scores used at the site of an incident, which are based on direct observation of evident abnormalities

2 Scores that are based retrospectively on the anatomical injuries, e.g. the injury severity score (ISS)
3 Scores that are calculated from the currently observed physiology, e.g. the revised trauma score (RTS)
4 More complex scores – usually derived on the ICU – which take account of both the current status and the pre-existing health of the victim, e.g. the Acute Physiology and Chronic Health Evaluation (APACHE score).

3

Head injuries

Kate Clayton

Queen Elizabeth Hospital Birmingham, Birmingham, UK

In the UK, traumatic brain injury (TBI) results in around 900 000 emergency department (ED) visits and over 200 000 admissions to hospital every year.

> In the UK, TBI remains the most common cause of death and disability in the <40 age group, and over 1.5 million people are living with the effects of severe brain damage. Survivors of severe TBI face an increased all-cause mortality, loss of independence, social isolation, reduced employment potential and relationship breakdown. Males are twice as likely as females to experience a TBI across all age groups.

Primary damage to the brain occurs at the time of injury. Secondary damage is the result of extracranial factors such as hypoxia or hypovolaemia, which lead to impaired cerebral oxygen delivery. Reperfusion of damaged brain (with the release of oxygen free radicals and lipid peroxidation) is now recognised as an additional secondary factor that can complicate recovery from traumatic brain injury. The problems that cause secondary damage – namely hypoxia, hypoglycaemia and hypotension – can be minimised by effective systemic resuscitation. In the future, intracranial factors may be amenable to pharmacological interventions.

A decreased level of consciousness indicates that something is wrong with the brain or its fuel supply. It may be injury or:

- hypoxia or shock
- hypoglycaemia
- hypothermia
- poisoning or gross metabolic disturbance (including CO_2 narcosis)

- intracranial pathology (bleeding, thrombosis, embolism, infection, swelling, tumour, fitting).

Biomechanics and brain injury

Direct trauma may cause:

1 Focal scalp injury
2 Depressed vault fracture
3 Extradural haemorrhage
4 Focal brain injury
5 Contre-coup injury
6 Brain laceration and intracerebral haemorrhage
7 Subdural haemorrhage.

These may or may not be associated with loss of consciousness. **Sudden acceleration/deceleration** causes shearing injury to the brain and diffuse axonal injury (DAI). This is associated with loss of consciousness, but external evidence of head injury may be lacking. DAI is more common with the longer deceleration time characteristic of restrained passengers in traffic crashes. Extradural haemorrhage is more common in falls.

Cervical spine injury is more likely to be associated with a brain injury if the mobile head hits a fixed object (deceleration/acceleration) than if a mobile object hits the fixed head (assault).

THE PATIENT WITH A DEPRESSED LEVEL OF CONSCIOUSNESS

This section deals with the management of those patients who, when first assessed, have a Glasgow Coma Scale (GCS) score <15 (→ *Table 3.1* page 35). Serious brain injury must be suspected. The principal objective of

The RCEM Lecture Notes: Emergency Medicine, Fifth Edition. Edited by Catherine Williams and Amy Nickson.
© 2024 John Wiley & Sons Ltd. Published 2024 by John Wiley & Sons Ltd.
Companion website: www.wiley.com/go/LNEM5

Table 3.1 The Glasgow Coma Scale (GCS)

Response elicited	Score
Response of eyes	
Open spontaneously	4
Open to speech	3
Open to pain	2
No response	1
Best motor response	
Obeys commands	6
Localises pain	5 (supraorbital ridge pressure)
Withdraws from pain	4 (normal flexion)
Abnormal flexion	3 (decorticate response)
Extension to pain	2 (decerebrate response)
None	1
Best verbal response	
Oriented	5
Confused	4
Inappropriate words	3
Incomprehensible sounds	2
None	1

emergency management is to limit the effects of this primary insult by preventing deleterious secondary events, which could impair cerebral oxygen supply. A detailed neurological examination to determine the extent of the primary injury must be deferred until treatable secondary events have been controlled.

Immediate assessment and management

The ABC approach is vital:

- Clear and maintain the airway and give high-concentration oxygen. Have suction available.
- Ensure that the cervical spine is assessed and protected if required
- Obtain anaesthetic assistance as soon as possible if emergency induction of anaesthesia is likely to be required.

> Ensure that cardiorespiratory resuscitation is initiated and the neck is protected before assessing brain injury.

- Obtain intravenous (IV) access.
- Monitor and record pulse, BP, SpO_2, respiratory rate and ECG.
- Assess neurological status by AVPU criteria:
  A – Alert
  V – Responds to voice
  P – Responds to pain
  U – Unresponsive
  and assess the pupils for size, equality and reaction.
- Check blood glucose.
- Treat reversible conditions (and reassess after therapy):
  Hypoglycaemia: take blood for glucose estimation before giving IV dextrose (0.2–0.5 mg/kg); avoid hyperglycaemia
  Fits: give IV lorazepam 4 mg (0.1 mg/kg) or IV diazepam 10 mg (0.25 mg/kg) slowly
  Opiate toxicity: give IV naloxone 0.4 mg
  Aggression and restlessness: give 100% oxygen; check the airway and the SaO_2; catheterise the bladder; address pain and rule out hypoglycaemia. Sedation should be given only after consideration of the causes.
- Ask witnesses/paramedics if the level of consciousness has changed since the impact. Did the patient briefly recover and speak and then deteriorate? Obtain a brief history (*AMPLE → p. 10*). Try to establish the mechanism of the injury.
- Obtain a blood gas measurement.
- Tranexamic acid probably reduces head injury-associated mortality if given early (within 3 hours) to those with intracranial bleeding. Research is ongoing to establish whether or not tranexamic acid has a role in older adults with head injury (CRASH-4 trial).

> Steroids are of no benefit in the treatment of head injuries.

Further assessment and management

- Carry out a detailed secondary survey
- Seek surgical/neurosurgical advice
- Consider catheterising the bladder.

The secondary survey searches for other injuries and establishes the neurological status. It must include examination of the following:

- The scalp
- The auditory canals and tympanic membranes (caution → p. 45)

- The pupils and limbs
- The face
- The neck.

Neurological assessment

There are three groups of observations:

1 **Global**: the level of consciousness should be assessed using the GCS (→ *Table 3.1* page 35). This is a sensitive and reproducible indication of early neurological deterioration. The motor component is of more significance in detecting deterioration, and therefore the individual components of the GCS must be clearly recorded as well as the overall score.
2 **Focal**: neurological signs (e.g. variation in muscle tone, asymmetrical limb movement and reflexes, disconjugate eye movements) help to identify the site and severity of brain damage.
3 **Physiological**: the components of 'Cushing's response' (slow pulse, raised BP and dilated, sluggish pupils) are easily measured but are very late indicators of high intracranial pressure (ICP).

All of the above observations should be repeated at appropriate intervals and plotted on a chart.

> GCS maximum score = 15 (not necessarily equivalent to neurologically intact)
> GCS minimum score = 3 (even if dead!)
> GCS of 8 or less = coma

Children's Coma Score → p. 345.

Other injuries

About 50% of patients with major brain injuries have serious injuries elsewhere. The more injuries there are, the greater the risk of missing some of them.

Multiple injuries → Chapter 2 on p. 19.

Imaging

As soon as the patient with a depressed level of consciousness is stabilised, a CT scan of the brain should be obtained (→ *Boxes 3.1 for adults and 3.8 for children*). Some patients will need to be intubated and ventilated before scanning. In a patient who is aged over 65, if the only positive CT indicator from *Box 3.1* is amnesia of events for more than 30 min before the injury or a dangerous mechanism of injury, then admission for neurological observations with CT within 8 hours of injury is acceptable.

 Box 3.1 Indications for CT of the brain in adults with head injuries

Children aged <16 years → Box 3.8

(Incorporating the UK National Institute for Health and Clinical Excellence's [NICE's] head injury guideline, 2014 – updated 2023)

1 The threshold for CT examination should be lowered if there are other life-threatening injuries, particularly if these will require surgery under general anaesthetic
2 The CT examination should include the cervical spine if the head or other body areas are being scanned
3 Patients who return to the ED within 48 hours of discharge with persistent complaints that could be attributed to their head injury should be discussed with a senior clinician and considered for CT

Immediate CT scan (= imaging performed and provisional results reported within 1 hour of the scan being performed)

- GCS <12 when first assessed in the ED
- GCS <15 when assessed in the ED 2 hours after injury
- Suspected open or depressed skull fracture
- Sign of fracture of skull base (→ *p. 43*)
- Focal neurological deficit
- Post-traumatic seizure
- More than one episode of vomiting

CT scan within 8 hours (= imaging performed within 8 hours of the time of injury and provisional results reported within 1 hours of the scan being performed)

- Dangerous mechanism of injury with a history of loss of consciousness or amnesia (pedestrian or cyclist hit by motor vehicle; occupant ejected from motor vehicle; fall from a height of >1 m or five stairs; lower heights are applicable for infants and young children)
- Amnesia >30 min for events before the impact
- Age 65 years with a history of loss of consciousness or amnesia
- Coagulopathy (history of bleeding or clotting disorder)
- For people who have no other indication for CT but who are on anticoagulant or antiplatelet treatment (excluding aspirin monotherapy) consider CT within 8 hours (if return in case of deterioration may be difficult) or within 1 hour if presenting >8 hours post injury.

Table 3.2 Risk of intracranial haematoma in adults with head injuries

	No skull fracture	Skull fracture
Fully conscious	1 in 8000	1 in 45
Impaired consciousness	1 in 180	1 in 5
Comatose	1 in 27	1 in 4

Table 3.3 Risk of intracranial haematoma in children with head injuries

	No skull fracture	Skull fracture
Fully conscious	1 in 13000	1 in 157
Impaired consciousness	1 in 580	1 in 25
Comatose	1 in 65	1 in 12

For safety, logistical and resource reasons, MRI is not currently indicated as a primary investigation in patients with head injuries. Moreover, it is contraindicated in both head and cervical investigations unless there is an absolute certainty that the patient is not harbouring an incompatible device, implant or metallic foreign body.

Skull radiographs do not contribute to the management of head injury, except in resource-poor settings where CT scanning is not available (→ *Tables 3.2 and 3.3 illustrate the increased incidence of intracranial haematoma with proven skull fracture*). Therapy is concerned with brain injury rather than bone injury, and this is detected initially by neurological signs.

The indications for imaging of the cervical spine in patients with head injuries are summarised in *Boxes 3.2a and 3.2b*. In most cases of adults with a head injury, CT scan is now the preferred modality for investigation of cervical spine, especially in older patients. In children with head injury, where the risk of cervical spine injury is lower, and the risk to the thyroid gland from ionising radiation is higher, 3-view cervical spine X-rays are recommended unless indications for CT are present (→ *Box 3.2b*). In children where there is a particularly high suspicion of spinal cord or cervical spine injury, an MR scan may be preferred if available. → *Chapter 4, p. 55.*

Management of specific problems

Airway and breathing

Inadequate respiration leads to hypoxia, hypercapnia and acidosis. This results in cerebral vasodilatation and a rise in ICP. Although simple manoeuvres to clear and maintain the airway may be initially successful,

 Box 3.2a Indications for imaging of the cervical spine in adults with head injuries

(Incorporating NICE's head injury guideline, 2014 – updated 2023)

Assessment of the injured neck → p. 54.

Perform immediate CT scan if

- GCS <12 on initial assessment
- Has been intubated
- Plain films are technically inadequate, suspicious or definitely abnormal
- Continued clinical suspicion despite normal plain films
- There has been blunt polytrauma involving the head and chest, abdomen or pelvis in someone who is alert and stable
- Clinical suspicion of cervical spine injury plus any of the following:
  - Aged over 65
  - Dangerous mechanism of injury,
  - Focal peripheral neurological deficit
  - Paraesthesia in the upper or lower limbs
- Definitive diagnosis required urgently, e.g. before surgery or anaesthesia

If no indications for CT, perform immediate plain radiographs if

- Cannot actively rotate neck to 45° (left and right)
- Not safe to move neck (→ p. 54)
- There is a pre-existing condition, predisposing to higher risk of injury to the cervical spine.

intubation and ventilation are required for most patients with impaired respiration (→ *Box 3.3*).

Intubation should never be attempted without sedation, analgesia and muscle paralysis (even in apparently 'flat' head-injured patients) because the stimulus involved would result in a sudden rise in ICP.

In ventilated patients with a head injury, aim for a PaO_2 >13 kPa and a $PaCO_2$ of 4.5–5.0 kPa.

Even patients with no apparent respiratory disturbance may benefit from controlled ventilation. (→ *Box 3.4*). Hyperventilation to a $PaCO_2$ <5.3 kPa causes cerebral vasoconstriction and a consequent fall in ICP. Excessive hyperventilation can, however, be dangerous. Only the undamaged brain responds to changes in blood gas tension, and vasoconstriction in normal areas may result in redistribution of blood flow to the injured tissue. This increases the penumbra around the damaged area. Brain ischaemia leads to lactic acidosis and reflex vasodilatation.

Box 3.2b Indications for imaging of the cervical spine in children with head injuries

(Incorporating NICE's head injury guideline, 2014 – updated 2023)

Assessment of the injured neck → p. 54.

Immediate plain radiographs

- Cannot actively rotate neck to 45° (left and right)
- Not safe to move neck (→ *p. 54*)
- Neck pain or midline tenderness with:
  - dangerous mechanism of injury (fall >1 m or five stairs; axial load to head: diving injury, ejection from a motor vehicle, high-speed motor vehicle collision or roll-over, bicycle collision, crash involving motorised recreational vehicles), a condition predisposing to higher risk of cervical spine injury e.g. osteogenesis imperfecta

Immediate CT scan

- GCS <13 on initial assessment
- Has been intubated
- Focal neurological signs (including paraesthesia in the extremities)
- Plain films are technically inadequate, suspicious or definitely abnormal
- Strong clinical suspicion despite normal plain films
- Patient is being scanned for head injury or multi-region trauma
- Definitive diagnosis required urgently, e.g. before surgery

Box 3.3 Indications for intubation and ventilation after head injuries

Aiming for PaO$_2$ >13 kPa and PaCO$_2$ of >6 kPa

- Coma (GCS 8 or less), or deteriorating conscious level (one or more points on the motor score)
  - Consider the individual components of the GCS, placing greater significance on motor score deterioration.
- Apparent loss of protective airway reflexes
- Ventilatory insufficiency as judged by oximetry/blood gas measurement:
  - PaO$_2$ <10 kPa on air or <13 kPa on oxygen
  - PaCO$_2$ >6 kPa
- Spontaneous hyperventilation causing a PaCO$_2$ <4 kPa

- Irregular respiration
- Multiple fits
- Significant facial injuries
- Bleeding into the airway
- Extreme agitation

Box 3.4 Reasons for intubating and ventilating patients with brain injuries

1 To clear, maintain and protect the airway
2 To ensure normoxia and normocarbia to minimise secondary neurological injury
3 To facilitate CT
4 To allow safe patient transport

Circulation

In a healthy person, changes in arterial BP between 80 and 200 mmHg do not influence cerebral blood flow. Brain injury impairs this autoregulatory function, and hence cerebral blood supply in damaged areas is less well protected from changes in systemic circulation. Hypotension, even transiently, in a patient with a serious brain injury may have a significant impact on survival and morbidity. A single systolic blood pressure below 90 mmHg has been associated with a 150% increase in mortality.

Hypotension is only very rarely caused by brain injury. Trauma to the trunk and neck must be considered together with the biomechanics of the impact.

Cushing's response (bradycardia and hypertension) is a late sign and indicates rising ICP.

Neurogenic pulmonary oedema is occasionally seen, usually beginning within minutes to hours of insult. It is thought to be caused by vasoconstriction resulting from sympathetic overactivity (an alpha effect). It should be treated aggressively with standard drugs and almost always necessitates ventilation to ensure normoxia and normocarbia (→*p. 219*).

Raised intracranial pressure

Hyperglycaemia increases brain swelling and must be avoided. Hyperosmolar agents such as IV mannitol 1 g/kg are sometimes used as a temporising agent to reduce brain swelling before clot evacuation, although the evidence of benefit is weak; IV 5% sodium chloride (6 mL/kg) is an alternative. Neither drug should be used for the long-term management of cerebral oedema.

Seizures

Both ICP and metabolic demand for oxygen rise dramatically during a fit, and this may increase the extent of the brain damage. Intravenous lorazepam or diazepam is usually effective in terminating seizures, but be aware of the possibility of respiratory depression. Head-injured patients who suffer a seizure should be loaded on Levetiracetam 20 mg/kg as a first-line anticonvulsant; phenytoin is now considered the second-line agent.

Suspected alcohol intoxication

Alcohol intoxication increases the risk of sustaining a head injury and of that injury causing brain damage. Nevertheless, changes in conscious level must not be attributed to alcohol or other drugs except after the exclusion of all other possible causes – and in retrospect.

> Unconscious patients suspected of simple alcohol intoxication should have regular neurological observations for up to 2 hours – if by then the GCS is not improving they should have a CT scan of the brain.

Urine output

Catheterisation of the bladder is mandatory in an unresponsive, brain-injured patient. A full bladder leads to increasing restlessness. In addition, the urine output is a good indicator of adequate tissue perfusion – it should be at least 1 mL/kg per hour.

Pain

Analgesia may be needed if the patient is not deeply unconscious and has other painful injuries. Early fracture splintage is helpful in this regard. Once baseline observations are established, give small doses of opiates intravenously.

Bleeding from the scalp

Examination of the scalp must be meticulous; the hair may be trimmed off to a distance of 1 cm around the wound edges. Lacerations should be palpated with a gloved finger to detect fracture lines and foreign bodies. Severe bleeding can be controlled by direct pressure, followed by staples or a single layer of deep sutures, using 2/0 silk on a hand-held needle; proprietary haemorrhage control devices are also available. A pressure dressing should then be applied.

Deterioration

Early, rapid, neurological deterioration may result from:

- rapidly expanding intracranial haemorrhage (typically extradural)
- severe primary brain injury
- hypoxaemia
- hypovolaemia.

Guidelines for neurosurgical consultation

> Before telephoning a neurosurgeon, ensure that resuscitation has been initiated and that life-threatening or serious extracranial injuries have been identified and addressed.

Regional neuroscience centres should collaborate with their linked EDs and ambulance service to provide clear written guidance on consultation and referral practices. In particular, the definition of 'surgically significant' must be agreed by both parties. There is increasing evidence that all seriously brain-injured patients will benefit from care at a neuroscience centre, whether or not neurosurgical intervention is required, but clearly, it is imperative that all those requiring surgery should be transferred as soon as possible. Seek neurosurgical/neurointensive care advice in any of the following instances:

- Positive intracranial findings on CT scan including cerebral oedema
- Penetrating injury (definite or suspected)
- Depressed skull fracture
- Basal skull fracture
- Skull fracture with any depression of consciousness, seizures, severe headache, persistent vomiting or acute focal neurology
- CSF leak
- GCS persistently <8 after initial resuscitation
- Unexplained confusion persisting after >4 hours
- Deterioration of GCS (especially one or more points on the motor score)
- Progressive focal neurological signs.

Transfer from an ED to a neuroscience centre should be well-planned, well-resourced, speedy and documented. In all circumstances, complete initial resuscitation and patient stabilisation and establish comprehensive monitoring before transfer to avoid complications during the journey. If the patient is persistently hypotensive despite resuscitation, do not transport until the cause has been identified and the patient stabilised.

A doctor with appropriate training should accompany the patient. Child or infant transfers are ideally performed by clinicians with relevant paediatric critical care expertise, but time-sensitive injuries should not be delayed awaiting a specialist transfer service.

THE AMBULANT PATIENT WITH A HEAD INJURY

These patients will mostly have a GCS score of 15. This score does not necessarily imply normal mental functioning because the GCS score is not sensitive to changes in alertness or higher intellectual function. Some ambulant patients may be confused (GCS score = 14).

The diagnosis of a minor head injury can be made only in retrospect. The following points should help to distinguish between those with no significant brain injury and those at risk of serious complications.

History

The history of the incident is important because it often influences management. When the history is unknown or unreliable, there should be a lower threshold for admission to hospital.

- Establish the speed of impact and the nature of the object struck by the head. The part of the head involved and the area of contact are also important (e.g. occiput hitting a carpeted floor is less serious than temple hitting the corner of a radiator).
- Establish the pattern of subsequent behaviour and ask about any period of unconsciousness, confusion, amnesia or fitting. Ask about the occurrence of headache and vomiting. Changes to hearing and vision, including diplopia, must also be noted.

Post-traumatic amnesia

The duration of post-traumatic amnesia (PTA) correlates fairly well with the degree of primary brain injury. Under 1 hour usually denotes mild injury, whereas over 24 hours is associated with severe injury, although PTA is difficult to estimate reliably. It should be measured up to the time when the memory of consecutive events returns. This usually corresponds with the duration of spatial disorientation and is much longer than the period during which the patient did not speak.

Retrograde amnesia

Retrograde amnesia (for events before the accident) can be very unreliable and extremely variable, especially in patients who have been drinking alcohol. However, in others, it is a useful indicator of injury severity.

Drugs and alcohol

These are often implicated in the aetiology of head injury, but deterioration in a patient should not be attributed to their effects. Very high blood alcohol levels (>6000 mg/L) have been recorded in ambulant patients, therefore direct measurement of alcohol levels is rarely, if ever, helpful. Put alcohol at the bottom of the list of causes of altered consciousness.

Medical history

A medical history is usually obtained from relatives, neighbours, a phone call to the GP or by searching clothing. It is valuable in two respects:

1 Factors relevant to present management (e.g. diabetes, steroid treatment)
2 Factors relevant to the prevention of a further incident (e.g. transient ischaemic attack, alcohol misuse).
3 Social circumstances, including the risk of accidental falls and interpersonal violence.

> Always enquire about any bleeding diathesis or anticoagulant therapy – such as DOACs, warfarin or clopidogrel.

Assessment

- **Behaviour**: it is common for a patient to appear 'normal' on casual assessment, whereas enquiry a few days later reveals no recollection of the first interview.
- **Cognition**: assess for confusion, orientation, recall and amnesia.
- **Movement**: look especially for loss of coordination and ataxia. Examine limb movement, sensation and reflexes.
- **GCS** (→ Table 3.1).
- **Pupil size and reactivity**: pupil changes and the other classic signs of raised ICP are very late indicators of deterioration. Eighty per cent of the rise in pressure required to cause brain-stem coning occurs without any change in these indicators.
- BP, pulse, respiratory rate, SpO_2, temperature.
- Examine the head, noting any wounds, swellings or depressions. Palpate, as well as inspect, with gloved hand. Interpretation of imaging is facilitated by being able to link common areas of radiological and clinical abnormality.
- Examine the neck.
- Exclude injuries elsewhere.
- Imaging.

Imaging

CT allows visualisation of the brain and almost all pathology that may require operative treatment. Fractures of the base and vault of the skull may be seen on 'bony windows'. Depressed fractures may be identified and the depth of depressions calculated.

Indications for CT of the brain in patients with head injuries → Boxes 3.1 and 3.8.

Skull radiographs have now been replaced by CT and observation on short-stay wards. However, they still have a place in the assessment of potential non-accidental injury and occasionally the assessment of some complicated patients. In resource-poor settings, skull radiography can be used to give an indication of the risk of intracranial haematoma → *Table 3.2.*

Patients at risk of developing complications after a head injury

Patients with one or more of the following features have a significant risk of developing intracranial complications:

- Impaired level of consciousness at the time of presentation (including those who are showing GCS = 15 but not fully alert)
- Post-traumatic amnesia of over 15 min duration
- Abnormal neurological signs
- Seizures
- Symptoms of raised ICP (severe headache, persistent vomiting)
- Vault fracture on radiograph (→ *Tables 3.2 and 3.3*)
- Clinical evidence of base of skull fracture (→ *p. 45*).

Indications for observation in hospital following a head injury → Box 3.5.

Tx *Indications for CT imaging →Box 3.1 and 3.8*

All patients with a significant risk of developing complications must be admitted and observed carefully by professionals who understand the GCS and are trained in the early detection of changes in neurological status. The following observations should be made:

- Best eye-opening response
- Best motor response (noting lateralising signs)
- Best verbal response
- Pupil size and reaction to light
- Respiratory rate
- Pulse and BP
- Temperature.

Perform and record these observations at 30-min intervals until the GCS = 15. Thereafter, continue at 30 min for 2 hour, then hourly for 4 hour and then 2-hourly.

Changes requiring urgent review in patients admitted to hospital with head injuries → Box 3.6.

Box 3.5 Indications for observation in hospital after head injuries

(Adapted from NICE's head injury guideline, 2014 – updated 2023)

Patients with head injuries who have any of the following features should be admitted to hospital for observation

- New clinically significant abnormalities on imaging
- Failure to return to GCS of 15 (or baseline GCS) regardless of any imaging results
- Fulfil the criteria for CT imaging (→ *Boxes 3.1 and 3.8*) but cannot be scanned because of patient state or equipment failure
- Continuing symptoms or signs for concern (e.g. persistent vomiting, severe headache)
- Other coexisting problems (e.g. drug or alcohol intoxication, other injuries, CSF fluid leak, suspected non-accidental injury, meningism)

In patients who are fully alert on examination, a history of an altered level of consciousness before arrival at hospital increases the risk of intracranial haematoma by a factor of 4.

Box 3.6 Changes requiring urgent review in patients admitted to hospital with head injuries

(Adapted from NICE's head injury guideline, 2014 – updated 2023)

Consider immediate CT scan if

- Development of agitation or abnormal behaviour
- Drop of 1 point in GCS score for 30 min or more (especially in motor score)
- Drop of ≥2 points in GCS motor score
- Drop of ≥3 in eye-opening or verbal GCS component affected
- Development of persistent severe headache or persistent vomiting
- New or evolving focal neurological symptoms or signs (e.g. pupil inequality or asymmetry of limb or facial movements)

Ambulant patients with head injuries who are not obviously at risk

There is a remote possibility that intracranial complications will occur after apparently trivial head injury. The highest risk period for clinically important deterioration is in the first 6–8 hours after injury. A culture of risk aversion might suggest that all patients should be admitted; this would not only result in a vast number of people being admitted to make an uneventful recovery but could also have significant economic and social implications. Only those patients who have histories, symptoms or signs that put them at risk should remain in hospital for observation. However, if social circumstances appear inadequate or there is no one able to accompany and supervise the patient at home, admission may be required.

Advice to discharged patients ('head injury instructions')

Discharge criteria for patients with head injuries → Box 3.7.

1 Insist on the presence of a relative or a friend and never discharge a head-injured patient unless a third party is aware of the injury and will accompany the patient home.
2 Ensure that the patient's household has access to a phone and encourage the relatives to bring the patient back for assessment if they have any concerns.

> **Box 3.7 Discharge criteria for patients with head injuries**
>
> *Patients who fulfil all of the following criteria may be discharged home to a caring relative or friend:*
>
> - Fully conscious on presentation
> - No abnormal neurological signs
> - Loss of consciousness or PTA of <5 min
> - No severe headache or vomiting
> - No suspicion of skull fracture
> - No bleeding disorder
> - Appropriate social circumstances, adult supervision arranged
> - Reliable relative or friend available to take patient home from the ED (in appropriate transport)

3 Provide verbal and written advice. The following points should be made:
- Nausea and mild headache are common, but the patient should seek review if these symptoms persist or increase. Persistent vomiting must be taken seriously.
- Alterations in the level of consciousness are an important early sign of the development of complications and necessitate urgent referral back to hospital. Changes should not be attributed to drugs or alcohol.
- Any other unusual change in vision, hearing or movement should prompt a discussion with the hospital.
- Recovery from a mild traumatic brain injury often takes much longer than commonly expected. A period of rest and time off work is usually appropriate. Alcohol may delay recovery.
4 If concussive symptoms persist, the GP should arrange a referral back to an outpatient clinic for specialist assessment.

Head injuries in children

In a school-age child, the most common cause of death is a brain injury from a road traffic incident. Minor head injuries are also important, even if they do not produce immediate major complications; repeated minor head trauma in children has been linked to lowered IQ. Young children are less likely to lose consciousness than adults. Significant brain injury may thus occur without a history of unconsciousness.

Risk of intracranial haematoma in children after head injuries → Table 3.3.

Assessment can be difficult. The Children's Coma Scale (a modified GCS) should be used for children aged <5 years (→p. 345). In the evening, children may be sleepy but, nevertheless, a normal child is easily woken. Parents are in the best position to judge minor alterations in their children's level of consciousness.

Children are more prone to head injury when fractious, feverish or in the prodromal stage of an acute illness. A cause for unsteadiness should always be sought and the temperature recorded. All head injuries in a non-ambulant child should be reviewed by a senior clinician with experience in the assessment of safeguarding concerns and non-accidental injury.

Non-accidental head injury: Unexplained or atypical head injuries may be a result of non-accidental injury, especially if bilateral. Non-accidental head injury (NAHI) is most frequently seen in infants aged <6 months. It has a mortality rate of 20–30% and is the most common cause of death in the case of non-accidental trauma. The triad of injuries sometimes called the 'shaken baby syndrome' is subdural haematoma, hypoxic cerebral injury and retinal haemorrhage, usually without skull fracture. It is thought to be caused by either violent shaking alone or shaking with head impact. The presentation of NAHI may be very variable – fits, coma, drowsiness, irritability, apnoeic attacks, poor feeding or general malaise.

Non-accidental injury and safeguarding → p. 369.

> Most serious head injuries in the first year of life result from non-accidental injuries.

IMAGING

Imaging of the cervical spine is summarised in → Boxes 3.2a and 3.2b.
Indications for CT of the head in children aged <16 years are summarised in Box 3.8.

- Skull radiographs still have a valuable part to play in the assessment of children aged <12 years with suspected non-accidental injuries. The most common cause of skull fractures in children aged <18 months is NAHI. There may be multiple, branching fractures that involve more than one skull bone. Occipital fracture is characteristic, and underlying brain injury is relatively common.
- Early cerebral oedema may not be visible on the CT scan of a child's brain
- Separation of the suture lines of the skull (diastasis) may sometimes be seen after injury. This can fail to close, resulting in a 'growing fracture'.

Tx Most aspects of the management of a child's head injury are identical to that in the adult. Children are unique in invariably having a carer with them. This means that most can go home with their carer and written head injury instructions. They often sleep after trauma and do not need to be kept awake. Instead, they should be checked on by their carers two or three times during the night. All that is required is for the carers to be confident that the child has a normal response to a mild stimulation (verbal or tactile). It is not necessary to wake the child completely or to examine the pupils. Parents and carers are much better judges of their children's night-time behaviour than healthcare professionals.

Some injuries, especially those to the occiput, may cause severe and prolonged vomiting. Isolated vomiting in head injury has a low correlation with clinically important brain injury (0.2%). Deterioration is most likely to occur in the first 6–8 hours after head injury. Therefore in children with isolated vomiting, it is appropriate to initially manage them with observation. If the vomiting is

persistent, CT imaging will be required to rule out intracranial injury. Children in this situation may occasionally require observation in hospital for symptom control, even in the context of a normal scan. (Indications for CT imaging → *Box 3.8.*)

> Pituitary damage occurs in around 30% of moderate-to-severe head injuries. It may lead to endocrine failure (e.g. short stature or delayed puberty) that is only discovered several years after the injury.

Box 3.8 Selection of children (aged <16) for CT of the head

(Adapted from NICE's head injury guideline, 2014 – updated 2023)

Immediate CT scan

- Suspicion of non-accidental injury
- Post-traumatic seizure without history of epilepsy
- On initial ED assessment GCS <14 (or in children <1 year, GCS <15)
- GCS <15 at 2 hours after injury
- Suspected open or depressed skull fracture or tense fontanelle
- Any sign of basal skull fracture (haemotympanum, 'panda' eyes, cerebrospinal fluid leakage from the ear or nose, Battle's sign).
- Focal neurological deficit.
- For infants <1 year, the presence of bruise, swelling or laceration of more than 5 cm on the head.

CT scan within 1 hour if **more than one** of the following risk factors are present:

- Loss of consciousness >5 min
- Abnormal drowsiness
- Three or more discrete episodes of vomiting
- Amnesia (anterograde/retrograde) >5 min
- Dangerous mechanism of injury (→ *Box 3.1*)
- Any current bleeding or clotting disorder

Children who have only 1 of these risk factors should be observed for at least 4 hours from time of injury, and CT scan performed if they have:

- Further vomiting
- Further episode of abnormal drowsiness
- GCS <15

Delayed presentations

Occasionally, young children are brought to the ED by their parents with a large fluctuant of swelling over the parietal area (cephalohaematoma). There is a history of an injury a few days before but the child is otherwise well. CT scan usually shows a long, linear fracture that may extend over most of the side of the skull. It is normal for the swelling to be delayed and for a relatively late presentation. Although unlikely, the possibility of non-accidental injury must still be considered and excluded. Most of these children will need observation over a period of 24 hours and assessment by paediatricians.

SPECIFIC INJURIES

Fracture of the vault of the skull

Fracture of the skull vault most commonly results from a fall onto a hard surface. The lateral parts of the skull are the most vulnerable; intoxication is a predisposing factor.

IMAGING A CT scan of the cranium will detect most fractures of the vault of the skull.

IMAGING A skull radiograph is indicated only when CT is not available (except in suspected non-accidental injury page 42).

Indications for skull radiographs → Box 3.9

TX All patients with a new skull fracture should be admitted for observation. In the same way that a broken egg box may contain smashed eggs, a fractured skull may contain traumatised brain. Expressed more scientifically, the presence of a skull fracture greatly increases the risk of a patient developing an intracranial haematoma (→ *Tables 3.2 and 3.3*).

> Around 70% of intracranial haematomas occur in the presence of a skull fracture.

Box 3.9 Indications for skull radiographs

In the absence of facilities for CT or other problems in adhering to the NICE guidelines, skull radiographs are indicated if any of the following is present:

- Altered consciousness or amnesia at any time
- History unknown or unreliable
- Significant mechanism of injury (e.g. high-speed incident, injuring agent heavy/sharp, fall on hard surface)
- Abnormal neurological signs
- Swelling or bruising to temporal or parietal areas
- Extreme headache
- Vomiting (even once)
- Clinical suspicion of depressed vault fracture (e.g. trauma with hammer, golf club, etc.)
- Clinical suspicion of penetrating injury
- Clinical suspicion of basal skull fracture
- 'Drunk' patient with uncertain history of any event

Skull radiographs are unnecessary if all of the following apply:

- No loss of consciousness
- Occipital or frontal injury
- Low-speed impact or injuring agent flat/soft
- Normal neurological status at time of examination
- No scalp damage (or, if laceration, no associated swelling)

> Non-accidental injury is the most common cause of a skull fracture in an infant (→ p. 42).

Compound fracture of the skull

Antibiotics are not routinely indicated for compound linear fractures of the skull. Lacerations over fractures that are not depressed can be closed in the normal way and the injury then treated in the same way as a simple vault fracture.

Depressed fracture of the skull

Depressed fractures are often missed. The history is the key to diagnosis – direct force will usually have been applied over a small area of the head, e.g. a blow from a hammer or a golf club. The injury is usually associated with lacerations and soft tissue damage. Cerebral irritation may manifest itself as fitting.

IMAGING A CT scan is required when there is a suspicion of a depressed skull fracture (→ *Boxes 3.1 and 3.8*). In the absence of a CT scan, a plain film tangential view can be used to assess the amount of depression but will give no indication as to the extent of any underlying damage.

Tx Treat the brain injury first. Discuss the management of all depressed fractures with a neurosurgeon. Surgical elevation of the fragments is usually indicated.

Fracture of the base of the skull

This is usually the result of indirect violence. It often occurs in a drunken patient and may follow uncontrolled 'rag doll'-type falls.

The patient may sometimes feel unwell and vomit. A complaint of reduced hearing in one ear points to a haemotympanum. There will be one or more signs:

- Bleeding from the ear canal
- Haemotympanum (causes reduced hearing)
- Bleeding from the nose in the absence of direct injury
- Nasopharyngeal bleeding (may be torrential and compromise the airway)
- Cerebrospinal fluid leakage from the nose or ear
- Subconjunctival haemorrhage without a posterior edge
- Retro-orbital haematoma (*for emergency treatment → p. 431*)
- Bilateral periorbital haematomas ('raccoon' or 'panda eyes')
- Bruising around the mastoid area (Battle's sign) (occurs late).

Blood in the external auditory meatus after trauma is usually caused by basal fracture but is occasionally secondary to temporomandibular joint injury.

> Deep auroscopic examination of the canal should be avoided because it may introduce infection via torn meninges.

IMAGING A CT scan of the cranium will detect most fractures of the base of the skull. High-resolution sections may be required.

There is usually no evidence of a basal skull fracture on plain radiographs. However, there may be:

1 Blood in the sphenoid sinus (look for a fluid level)
2 A vault fracture line that appears to continue towards the base of the skull.

Tx
- Admission for observation for 48 hours or until any discharge has ceased for at least 24 hours
- Discussion with a neurosurgeon, ophthalmologist or ENT surgeon as appropriate
- Antibiotics are no longer recommended for base of skull fractures however fractures through any air-filled spaces will require antibiotic cover.
- If CSF leak is present, administration of pneumococcal vaccine is indicated.

Aerocele

A fracture involving a bony sinus may result in intracranial air. The presence of this aerocele is suggested by periorbital surgical emphysema.

IMAGING An aerocele is usually an incidental finding on a CT scan of the brain or a plain skull radiograph. Look for a fluid level (under the vault or in the sphenoid fossa) but be aware of the orientation of the head when the film/scan was taken – it could appear as a 'vertical' line if the patient was supine.

Tx The aerocele may expand if the pressure in the sinuses is increased, so the patient should be warned not to blow his or her nose. Such injuries require antibiotic cover to avoid the risk of osteomyelitis or brain abscess. Discuss with a neurosurgeon; early decompression is sometimes necessary.

Extradural haematoma

A blood clot in the extradural space results from direct trauma and, in adults, is usually associated with a skull fracture (of the squamous temporal bone). A lucid interval between initial trauma and the onset or return of depressed consciousness is said to be characteristic but is by no means inevitable.

The signs are those of increasing ICP. An impaired level of consciousness is the first feature. The classic, unilateral, fixed, dilated pupil is a very late sign; it occurs as the result of an ipsilateral third nerve palsy that is caused by cerebral herniation through the foramen magnum. Limb weakness, from direct pressure on the motor cortex, is usually found on the contralateral side. Lateralising signs may be preterminal.

IMAGING CT will detect almost all extradural bleeds. In the very early stages, the blood may have the same density as the brain tissue and thus be difficult to identify. Extradural collections usually appear biconvex on CT scan, whereas subdural collections have inner concave borders (→ *Figure 3.1*). On plain skull radiographs, a fracture that overlies the vascular markings of the middle meningeal artery may be associated with an extradural bleed.

Tx Resuscitation and stabilisation (→ *p. 34*) should precede transfer to a neurosurgical centre. Major coincidental extracranial injuries must always be identified before transport is initiated.

> Outcome in a patient with an extradural haematoma is compromised if the time to decompression is more than 2 hours from the point of deterioration.

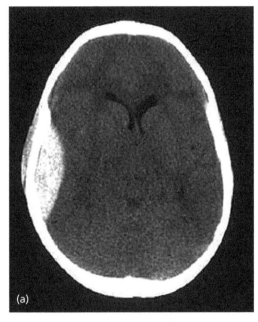 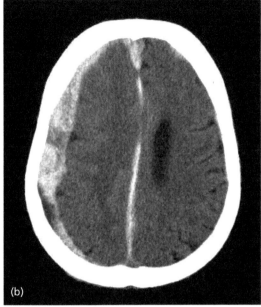

(a)   (b)

Figure 3.1 Comparison of (a) extradural. Springer Nature. (b) Subdural haemorrhages. **Extradural:** There is an injury to the middle meningeal artery or to one of its branches. The expanding haematoma strips the strongly-attached dura from the skull to form a characteristic biconvex shape with a well-defined inner margin. **Subdural:** There are often ruptured veins in the subdural space. The bleeding spreads between the dura and the arachnoid to make a crescentic appearance with an irregular inner margin.

Acute subdural haematoma

Bleeding from the veins that traverse the subdural space results in a more insidious clinical picture than extradural haemorrhage. Alteration in conscious level is the cardinal feature; lateralising signs may be absent or minimal. A unilateral increase in limb tone is sometimes apparent.

Acute subdural haematomas are most commonly seen in those:

1 Who are intoxicated with alcohol. There may be no apparent injury. The first sign may be a failure to wake up after an episode of heavy drinking. A CT scan should be obtained in all patients with head injuries who do not recover to GCS score of 15 within 2 hours of injury (→ *Box 3.1*). Intoxication may make this difficult. In such cases, consider general anaesthesia. Even in patients with confirmed alcohol intoxication and no clear evidence of head injury, a CT scan is prudent if their GCS does not start to improve within 2–3 hours of arrival.
2 Who are on anticoagulant or anti-platelet therapy (e.g. warfarin or clopidogrel). The trauma may be minimal.
3 Who have coexisting extensive brain injury from major trauma (lacerations and contusions).

IMAGING A CT scan is diagnostic, showing a collection with an irregular, inner concave border (compare extradural → *Figure 3.1*).

TX Patients with subdural haematomas must be discussed with a neurosurgeon immediately.

> Outcome in a patient with an acute subdural haematoma is compromised if the time to decompression is more than 4 hours from the accident.

Chronic subdural haematoma

This is usually seen in elderly patients with a history of a trivial head injury, or no injury at all. The symptoms and signs develop after a latent period of days or even months and, characteristically, fluctuate in severity as a result of alternating bleeding and resorption of clot. There is headache, memory loss, confusion and drowsiness. Localising signs are rare.

A CT scan should be performed if the diagnosis is suspected. Neurosurgical intervention is sometimes required.

Subarachnoid haemorrhage

A subarachnoid haemorrhage (SAH) may sometimes occur after trauma. In a conscious patient, there may be a severe headache, neck stiffness and photophobia (→*p. 238*). Diagnosis is confirmed by CT scan and then neurosurgical advice must be sought. IV nimodipine is not indicated in the treatment of traumatic SAH.

Cerebral contusions

Bruising to the brain may result in a similar clinical picture to subdural haematoma, with delayed recovery from trauma or alcohol intoxication. Frontal contusions cause disinhibition.

IMAGING CT scan is diagnostic.

Tx All patients with contusions should be discussed with a neurosurgeon. Spontaneous resolution may take several weeks.

Transient complications after minor head injury

Cortical blindness

Sudden visual loss after a head injury is uncommon but very frightening. The loss of vision can be confirmed by testing for the absence of the blink reflex (i.e. an object rapidly approaching the eye will not cause blinking). A CT scan of the brain is required to exclude serious pathology. The patient should be admitted and examined by an ophthalmologist. Vision usually returns spontaneously within a few hours.

Impact brain apnoea

Impact to the head may induce a period of apnoea and/or irregular respirations, even after an apparently minor head injury. This phenomena is most commonly observed in the prehospital setting. A CT scan should be obtained to exclude significant intracranial pathology. Total recovery is to be expected. The mechanism is presumably similar to that of cortical blindness and temporary abducens palsy.

Abducens palsy

Unilateral sixth nerve palsy is occasionally seen after an otherwise uncomplicated minor head injury. CT scan should be obtained to exclude significant intracranial pathology. The condition resolves spontaneously.

Concussion

Many patients with a minor traumatic brain injury, who do not have demonstrable intracranial lesions or abnormal signs, will have persisting symptoms for an extended period of time. These complaints include the following:

- Minor lapses in concentration and memory
- Inability to undertake complex tasks
- Fatigue
- Occipitofrontal headache
- Emotional lability (or behavioural disturbance in children).

In 90% of cases, concussion occurs without loss of consciousness at the time of initial insult. Children and adolescents are more susceptible to concussion and tend to take a longer period to fully recover. It is probable that some patients will have subtle structural brain damage – a minor form of diffuse axonal injury. This is unlikely to be seen on CT scan but has been demonstrated on MRI.

There is increasing recognition that the effects of sequential 'minor' head injuries can have significant long-term effects such as chronic traumatic encephalopathy (a dementia-like syndrome).

IMAGING A CT scan may be undertaken in some cases (as a delayed procedure) to exclude treatable causes and to give a more reliable prognosis.

Tx The patient should be reassured that recovery will occur but may take several weeks. Advise against alcohol and recreational drug use.

Patients should be counselled on a step-wise return to activity. A relative rest period of 24–48 hours is recommended, during which physical activity, reading and screentime are minimised and kept to short periods. Once completely asymptomatic at rest, a return to sedentary normal activity can occur (reading, school, work, socialising) as tolerated. Return to sport should be delayed until the patient has been asymptomatic for at least 24–48 hours of normal activity (48 hours is recommended for patients <19 years). A graduated return to sport and exercise can then begin, starting with light exercise before building up slowly in a step-wise fashion. If at any stage in return to activity, the patient experiences a recurrence of symptoms, they should reduce their activity until asymptomatic for 24–48 hours before gradually building up again. For contact sports, this will mean a minimum of 12 days before return to play for an adult and a minimum of 23 days for a patient <19 years. Young patients (<13 years) may require even longer.

Follow-up by the GP or specific neurorehabilitation follow-up may be valuable in some cases.

4

The neck and the back

Fiqry Fadillah[1,2] and Catherine Williams[3,4]

[1] Royal Free Hospital, London, UK
[2] Magpas Air Ambulance, Huntingdon, UK
[3] Emergency Medicine Consultant, Royal Bolton Hospital, Bolton, UK
[4] Health Education North West, Manchester, UK

The possibility of spinal injury should always be considered in:

- major trauma
- multiple injuries
- high-speed injuries
- falls
- sports injuries (especially in diving, trampolining, riding and rugby accidents)
- head injuries
- all unresponsive patients.

Complications can arise if there is excessive movement to the spine, but also secondary to low spinal perfusion, oedema and ischaemia. Injury most commonly occurs at the junction of a fixed and mobile portion of the spinal column (lower cervical and thoracolumbar junction). 10–15% of patients with one identified spinal fracture will be found to have another.

Anatomy

The vertebral column consists of 33 vertebrae; 7 cervical, 12 thoracic, 5 lumbar, 5 sacral and 4 coccyx. It provides the base support for the body and allows movements while protecting the spinal cord. The spinal cord runs from the foramen magnum down to the T12 to L3 region. Below this, a bundle of spinal nerves forms the cauda equina. The spinal cord gives rise to the sympathetic fibres (T1–L3) as well as parasympathetic fibres (S2–S4).

Initial management of the patient with possible spinal injury

It is important to note that the following actions are applicable for major trauma patients who are at high risk of a spinal injury. This may include a dangerous mechanism, concerning clinical signs or more minor mechanism in the elderly population.
    ABCDE assessment → Chapter 1 page 1 and Chapter 2 Page 20

- Ensure an adequate airway and give high-concentration oxygen. The jaw-thrust manoeuvre is safer than the chin-lift technique in this situation. Suctioning may stimulate the vagus nerve, triggering a vagal reaction that can result in bradycardia and hypoxia and thus should be performed with caution.
- The neck should be protected by manual in-line stabilisation if more extensive airway intervention is needed.
- Ensure appropriate spinal immobilisation, ensuring minimal movement to the spine. → *page 49 and Box 4.1*
- Assess respiratory function and rate, and measure oxygen saturation with a pulse oximeter.
- Set up an intravenous (IV) infusion and monitor BP and pulse.
- Record the Glasgow Coma Scale (GCS) score.
- Screen for →
  - Neck or back pain
  - Loss of sensation to limbs

The RCEM Lecture Notes: Emergency Medicine, Fifth Edition. Edited by Catherine Williams and Amy Nickson.
© 2024 John Wiley & Sons Ltd. Published 2024 by John Wiley & Sons Ltd.
Companion website: www.wiley.com/go/LNEM5

Box 4.1 **Log roll**

A 'log roll' is a way of moving a patient with suspected spinal trauma to minimise movement of the spine and reduce further damage to the spine. It is useful to examine the patient's back, or if the patient needs to vomit, use the bedpan or have a change of wet sheets. In the polytrauma patient, tilting should be kept to an absolute minimum (e.g. 20°) to prevent disruption of any clots that may be keeping the patient from exsanguinating. Trauma mattresses are used to move the patient easily from trolley to CT scan to prevent repeated log rolls.

Log roll is a skill best learned the practical way, but here are the basic steps:

- One team member takes control of the patient's head and neck with manual inline stabilisation and acts as 'leader' of the log roll. The blocks (and collar if being used) are removed.
- Three other team members control the body and legs, standing along the side the patient will be

rolled towards. Team members should be ordered by height, with the tallest at the head end. Consider which direction will be more comfortable for the patient to be rolled, considering their other injuries, and make sure they have had adequate analgesia and explanation of the procedure.

- The patient crosses their arms across their chest (if able). One team member has a hand on the contralateral shoulder and elbow of the patient. The next on the pelvis and under the knee. The third person has a hand under the contralateral thigh (crossing arms with the second person) and one under the ankle.
- On 'ready, steady, roll', all team members follow the 'head and neck' person. The fifth team member can then perform the examination and whatever else is needed.
- The return to supine position if performed with the same, steady control and then blocks are repositioned.

- Loss of movement to limbs
- Burning or electric shock type pain in the limbs or trunk.
- Minimise unnecessary log-rolling, especially if it will not change the immediate management.
- Pay special attention to pressure points (sores develop rapidly) and core temperature (the patient may be thermolabile).
- Consider the need for early analgesia.
- Complete the primary survey and continue resuscitation.

Spinal immobilisation

Traditionally, standard cervical spine immobilisation has been by means of collar, head blocks and tape. It is increasingly recognised that rigid collars have potential to cause harm in certain circumstances.

A rigid collar may:

- impede venous return, cause unnecessary pain and discomfort and result in pressure sores.
- make airway management more difficult.
- increase intracranial pressure.
- be difficult to fit in patients with large body habitus, spinal deformity, short or wide necks.
- increase agitation (and therefore movement) in confused, distressed or intoxicated patients.

- occasionally worsen neurological symptoms or signs in patients with spinal injury.

Method of immobilisation should be tailored to the patient and specific clinical circumstances:

- Rigid collars are contraindicated if the airway is compromised and should be replaced with manual inline stabilisation.
- Patients with spinal deformities, e.g. ankylosing spondylitis or kyphosis, may not be able to tolerate a standard rigid collar. In these instances, padding or bolsters may be used to support the neck and a position of comfort should be applied.
- Consider allowing an uncooperative, agitated or distressed patient to find their own position of comfort.
- The conscious cooperative patient may not always require formal cervical spine immobilisation.

If not using a rigid collar, it may be helpful to place blocks either side of the patient's head as a 'reminder' to both patient and staff that spinal injury has not yet been excluded.

Extrication devices such as a 'spinal board' or scoop stretcher may cause pressure area damage and thus should be removed as soon as practicable after extrication.

In a patient with suspected spinal injury, movement should be kept to a minimum and a 'log-roll' technique used when repositioning is necessary. → *Box 4.1*

Steroid therapy

Steroids are not currently recommended in the acute phase following spinal cord injury. Steroids given within the first 8 hours following an acute spinal cord injury failed to show a statistically significant short-term or long-term improvement in patients' overall motor or neurological scores compared to controls who were not administered steroids. For the same comparison, there was an increased risk of pneumonia and hyperglycaemia compared to controls.

INJURY TO THE SPINAL CORD

In the fully conscious adult, the presence of paralysis and anaesthesia after trauma immediately points to spinal cord injury. However, in the obtunded patient, the diagnosis may be difficult. Similarly, incomplete cord damage is often misdiagnosed. Paralysis may mask multiple injuries. Pain may be absent as may the signs of intra-abdominal trauma.

Localisation of spinal cord damage

Primary spinal cord injuries arise from mechanical disruption, transection, or distraction of neural elements. Twisting forces are most likely to cause fractures at the junction of mobile and fixed parts of the column, i.e. at C7-T1 and T12-L1. Upper thoracic spine injury may be associated with sternal fractures – massive forces may buckle the thoracic cage. Direct blows are commonly associated with injuries elsewhere.

Partial transection of the cord may be inflicted by a knife or a bullet, but complete separation is unusual. A twisting or bending movement resulting from indirect blunt violence is more common. This causes a combination of crushing and tearing which produces a mixed picture of neuronal damage. There is often total loss of neural continuity with complete distal motor and sensory loss.

Distal reflex activity may not be clearly related to the extent of cord section in the immediate post-injury phase. Complete section usually causes immediate flaccid paralysis with later return of reflex activity. Rarely, some reflexes are preserved throughout.

The level of cord injury may be difficult to determine because of the following:

1 Most muscles receive efferent fibres from more than one level.
2 Dermatomes have imprecise boundaries.
3 Closed cord lesions usually extend over several centimetres, involving more than one level.

Table 4.1 Nerve roots supplying tendon and superficial reflexes

Tendon reflexes		Superficial reflexes	
Biceps	C5	Abdominal	T8–12
Supinator	C5–6	Cremasteric	L1–2
Triceps	C7	Plantar	S1
Knee	L3–4	Anal	S3–4
Ankle	S1–2		

It is important to detect change in neurological status over time. Identify and document the lowest functional muscle groups and the extent of skin anaesthesia (→ *Table 4.1 and Figure 4.1*). The Standard Neurological Classification of Spinal Cord Injury proforma produced by the American Spinal Injury Association (ASIA) is a useful tool to document neurological findings in suspected spinal cord injury.

Particular considerations in spinal injury in children

Spinal cord injury is rare in children overall in comparison to adults. Less than 2% of children involved in major trauma will sustain a spinal injury. Spinal immobilisation is particularly distressing for children and challenging for clinicians. Manual inline stabilisation of the neck is better tolerated.

The spinal column is anatomically different in children than adults, which results in a different pattern of injury. The relatively large head, flexible ligaments and muscles, and (until about age 7 of years) anteriorly wedged vertebrae, generates a high fulcrum of movement. High spinal injury is therefore relatively more common (80% of injuries). Children are also prone to *SCIWORA* → *page 58*.

Children who have been involved in a road traffic collision, particularly who have been restrained with a lap belt, may have sustained a sudden hyperflexion injury of the thoracolumbar spine. Look for abdominal bruising – 50% of children with seatbelt bruising from this mechanism will have sustained a spinal injury. This hyperflexion injury can cause an unstable transverse fracture extending through the vertebral body, pedicles and spinous process, known as a Chance fracture. This typically occurs at the thoracolumbar junction.

Cord syndromes

Incomplete cord damage produces several discrete syndromes. Some degree of recovery is more likely than in complete lesions in which there is no sign of any spinal

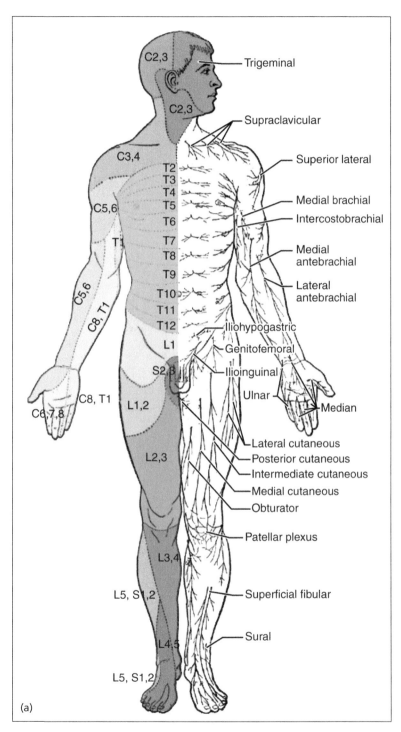

Figure 4.1 (a and b) Sensory dermatomes of the body. Mikael Häggström, Public domain, via Wikimedia Commons.

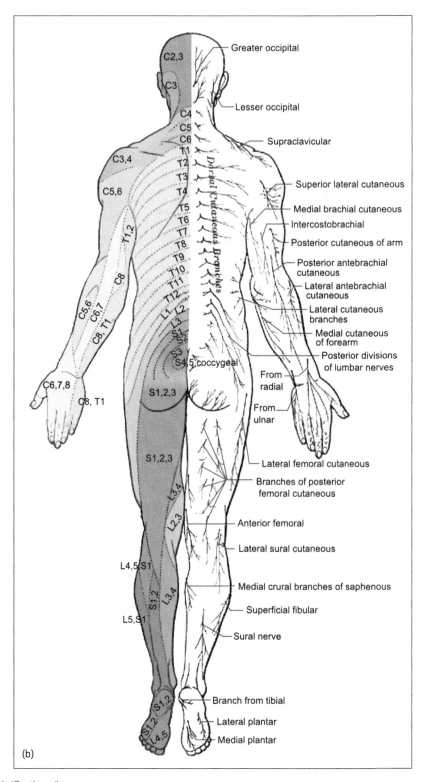

Figure 4.1 (Continued)

cord function below the level of the injury. The mixed nature of the signs can lead to misdiagnosis.

Lesser degrees of damage produce spinal cord contusions. There may be non-specific weakness, poor mobility and myoclonus. The diagnosis is usually only made on an MR scan. Recovery is usually slow but complete.

Central cord syndrome

This usually occurs in older patients with spondylitic spines following a relatively minor hyperextension injury. The spinal cord is compressed between the osteophytic vertebral body anteriorly and the stiff ligamentum flavum posteriorly. The more centrally situated parts of the corticospinal and spinothalamic tracts are the worst injured. These fibres supply the arms where the damage results in a flaccid (lower motor neuron) paresis – typically distal function is worse affected than proximal. The legs are less affected with a spastic (upper motor neuron) type of weakness. Varying levels of pain or sensory deficit may be present below the level of injury. The sacral fibres are often spared, so perineal sensation and bladder and bowel function may be normal.

> Central cord syndrome should be suspected in the elderly patient with a forehead injury who can walk but complains of altered function in the upper limbs.

Anterior cord syndrome

The anterior part of the spinal cord is usually injured by a mixture of bony encroachment and ischaemia. Typically, a flexion–rotation force causes a dislocation or a compression fracture of the vertebral body with accompanying anterior spinal artery compression. The anterior spinal artery supplies both the spinothalamic and corticospinal tracts, and so there is loss of power as well as reduced pain and temperature sensation below the level of injury.

Traumatic herniation of a cervical vertebral disc

This may occur during an acute flexion injury and cause extensive injury to the anterior part of the spinal cord. There is impaired motor function with reduced pain and temperature sensation. The posterior horns and posterior columns are usually undamaged so that touch and proprioception remain intact. *Also → p. 59.*

Posterior cord syndrome

Hyperextension injuries with fractures of the posterior elements of the vertebrae may injure the posterior columns.

Loss of proprioception may cause profound ataxia in the presence of normal power and pain and temperature sensation.

Brown–Séquard syndrome

This lateral cord syndrome can be precisely produced only by a knife or gun, although closed injuries (lateral mass fractures) may also give rise to some of its classic features. These are the signs of a hemisection of the cord. On the injured side there is reduced power, but relatively normal pain and temperature sensation because the spinothalamic tract crosses over to the opposite side. The uninjured side has normal power, but reduced sensation for pain and temperature.

Special problems that may accompany injury to the spinal cord

Spinal shock

This is rare. After a cord injury, spinal concussion causes a generalised flaccidity below the level of the lesion. Reflex activity may initially be present but later disappears.

This diagnosis can be made only in retrospect. An initial finding of proximal paralysis with sparing of distal neurological function (e.g. sphincter tone) is likely to be associated with cord concussion and carries a more favourable prognosis. Reflex activity and neurological signs may begin to improve in the first 24–48 hours, and the mean overall duration of spinal shock is several weeks. Concussion and permanent cord damage may coexist.

Respiratory failure

Intercostal muscle paralysis occurs with most cervical cord lesions. High lesions transect the phrenic nerve nucleus (C3–5) and are usually fatal. Even when the diaphragm is spared, vital capacity is greatly reduced and a compensatory tachypnoea occurs. The tidal volume and vital capacity should be measured if possible.

Paradoxical ('see-saw') respiration is an important sign. As the diaphragm descends during inspiration to create a negative intrathoracic pressure, intercostal muscle paralysis allows rib retraction rather than the normal expansion. Deteriorating respiratory function is an indication for the need for ventilation. Specific to spinal cord injury, the following patients should be assessed for intubation:

- Hypoventilation
- Persistent hypoxemia (SaO_2 ≤90%) despite supplemental oxygen
- Neck injury with the potential for airway obstruction from oedema or haemorrhage

- Persisting agitation (and associated movement) with ongoing concerns for spinal injury
- Injuries to C5 and above

Neurogenic shock

Neurogenic shock is usually associated with a cervical or high thoracic spinal injury. Impairment of descending sympathetic pathways in the spinal cord (i.e. cord damage at T6 or above) leads to a loss of sympathetic tone and thus unopposed parasympathetic response driven by the vagus nerve. This results in vasodilatation, relative bradycardia and distributive shock. Paralytic ileus often occurs in addition with a risk of vomiting and aspiration. Other injuries may have been sustained and can cause true hypovolaemia and either a bradycardia or a tachycardia. Any reduction of blood supply to the damaged cord will further impair its function.

Hypotension from loss of sympathetic tone should first be treated with adequate intravenous fluid resuscitation, to allow appropriate compensation for the vasogenic dilatation that occurs. Persistent hypotension once the patient is euvolaemic is an indication to starting vasopressor agents, aiming a mean arterial pressure of 85–90 mmHg to improve spinal cord perfusion. Bradycardia usually responds to atropine or glycopyrrolate. Symptoms last from several hours to several weeks depending on the level and the severity of the cord damage.

Retention of urine

Bladder tone is lost immediately after spinal transection. Distension leads to ureteric reflux and renal damage. Intermittent catheterisation may be the treatment of choice in the spinal unit, but it is preferable to insert and retain a catheter during the initial period of resuscitation and interhospital transfer.

Impaired thermoregulation

The patient is unable to sweat and thereby lose heat at high ambient temperatures. More commonly, too much heat is lost at low temperatures because of a failure of cutaneous vasoconstriction. The environmental temperature should be near to normal body temperature if the patient has to be exposed for long periods (e.g. for the diagnosis and treatment of other injuries). At other times, insulation is used to prevent heat loss to a cooler environment. Core temperature must be measured regularly.

Associated injuries

The signs of abdominal, pelvic and major limb injury may be masked by the motor and sensory loss. Apply a low threshold for CT scans to assess for abdominal trauma even in the absence of external signs or haemodynamic instability. Abdominal swelling may occur with a full bladder or from a paralytic ileus. Severe swelling from any cause may splint the diaphragm. Multiple fractures are present in around 5% of patients with spinal injuries.

Late-onset paralysis

Secondary cord injury can occur after spinal injuries in a similar way to the much more common complications of brain injury. Paralysis that develops hours after the incident is rare and is usually a result of cord ischaemia or oedema (causing infarction or vascular occlusion, respectively). An extradural haemorrhage may cause cord compression. Delayed signs are very unlikely to result from direct injury. Gentle handling, as described above, will not further damage a spine that has been subjected to forces sufficient to render it unstable.

IMAGING AND CLEARANCE OF THE SPINE IN TRAUMA

Often the need for radiographic imaging of the spine is obvious, e.g. penetrating trauma or marked neurological deficit. In the vast majority of patients presenting with blunt trauma, e.g. following motor vehicle collisions, a validated clinical decision rule should be used to aid decision-making.

Indications for CT cervical spine imaging in patients with head injuries → Chapter 3 pp. 37 and 38 Boxes 3.2a and 3.2b

Suspected cervical spine injury

It is often possible to clinically 'clear' the cervical spine of a conscious, cooperative patient using the Canadian C-Spine Rule.

Canadian C-Spine Rule

The Canadian C-Spine Rule was developed by Stiell and colleagues in 2001 and validated for use in the emergency department (→ *Figure 4.2*).

A person is classified as **high risk** if they have one of the following risk factors and should get imaging:

- age ≥65 years old
- dangerous mechanism (fall from a height of greater than 1 m or 5 steps, axial load to the head – for example diving, high-speed motor vehicle collision, rollover motor accident, ejection from a motor vehicle, accident involving motorised recreational vehicles, bicycle collision and horse riding accidents)
- paraesthesia in extremities.

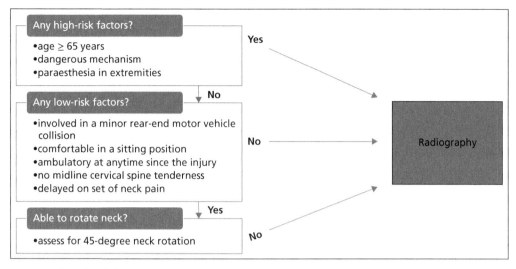

Figure 4.2 Canadian C-Spine Rule.

In the absence of any high-risk factors, patients should be evaluated for **low-risk** factors:

- involved in a minor rear-end motor vehicle collision
- comfortable in a sitting position
- ambulatory at any time since the injury
- no midline cervical spine tenderness
- delayed onset of neck pain.

In the **absence** of any low-risk factors, patients should be referred for imaging. In the **presence** of any low-risk factors, patients should be assessed for 45-degree neck rotation. If the patient fails to perform lateral rotation of the neck, he/she should be referred for imaging.

The following exclusions apply:

- Glasgow Coma Scale <15
- Critically unwell patients
- Old injury >48 hours
- Penetrating trauma
- Acute paralysis
- Known vertebral disease (ankylosing spondylitis, rheumatoid arthritis, spinal stenosis and previous spinal surgery)
- Return visit for reassessment of the same injury
- Pregnancy
- Although not formally validated in the paediatric population, it has been widely adopted and included in national guidelines. A child's developmental stage must be taken into account when deciding whether this rule can be used in an individual patient.

In the case of pregnancy, trauma remains one of the leading causes of non-obstetric maternal mortality and fetal loss. In trauma, when there is concern for the mechanism of injury, CT remains the mainstay of imaging. The risks of radiation are small compared with the risk of missed or delayed diagnosis of trauma.

If the patient is thought to be at high risk of cervical injury, proceed immediately to CT scan of the neck. In lower risk cases, particularly in young patients and children, plain radiographs may be appropriate initially.

Negative plain radiographic imaging of the spine does not exclude spinal injury, so have a low threshold to proceed to CT if ongoing concerns either of the mechanism or the examination findings. *Interpretation of Cervical Spine radiographs Page → 56*

Cervical spine imaging in children

In children with head injury and suspicion of cervical spine injury, indications for CT are as in *Chapter 3 → Box 3.2b.*

In children with isolated injury of the neck in whom there is a high level of clinical suspicion of spinal injury, indicated by abnormal neurological signs or symptoms, or by application of the Canadian C-spine rule, an MR scan is the preferred modality of imaging. The risk of ionising radiation to the thyroid is higher in this group, and they have a significantly higher risk of SCIWORA, which will be missed on CT (→ *p. 58*).

In children without high-risk factors, who do not meet criteria for MR scan, but in whom the cervical spine cannot be 'cleared' clinically, perform plain radiographs. Cervical spine radiographs can be difficult to interpret in children and should be discussed with a radiologist.

Suspected thoracic or lumbosacral spine injury

(*Adapted from NICE guideline 41: Spinal Injury: assessment and initial management 2016*)

Consider the possibility of spinal injury in patients who:

- are over 65 years and complaining of thoracolumbar back pain
- have pre-existing spinal pathology or osteoporosis
- had a dangerous mechanism of injury (fall >3 m, axial loading, high-speed RTC, ejection from vehicle, rollover RTC, lap belt only restraint, accident involving motorised recreational vehicles, bicycle collision and horse riding accident)
- have suspected spinal fracture in another region of the spine
- have new neurological symptoms (weakness, paraesthesia and numbness)
- have new neurological signs (motor or sensory)
- have new deformity or midline tenderness on palpation or percussion
- have midline spinal pain on coughing
- on attempted mobilisation have significant pain or abnormal neurological symptoms.

In patients requiring CT imaging for the cervical spine, or if there is high suspicion of thoracic or lumbosacral spinal injury with abnormal neurological symptoms or signs, arrange a CT of the whole spine.

If the CT is normal, but neurological symptoms or signs attributable to spinal cord injury are present, an MR scan of the spine will be required.

If there are no neurological symptoms or signs, and the injury is restricted to the thoracic or lumbosacral spine only, perform plain radiography as the initial investigation. If fracture is detected on plain radiography, CT imaging should follow.

Use and interpretation of cervical spine radiographs

For plain radiographic imaging,

1 request a coned view of the lower cervical spine with the shoulders pulled down OR
2 request a swimmer's view of the lower cervical spine (the swimmer's view is better at demonstrating the previously obscured vertebrae but is much harder to interpret).

If one of the above views does not allow visualisation of the C7–T1 junction, proceed to a CT scan of the neck.

There are three standard views of the cervical spine in UK practice:

1 Lateral
2 Upper anteroposterior (AP) ('open-mouth' or 'peg')
3 Lower AP.

Lateral view (→ *Figure 4.3a*)

Look for steps. Normal slight lordosis is lost when there is painful muscle spasm. C2 may appear to be subluxed forward on C3 in young children; the same appearance is less frequently seen of C3 on C4. These are normal variants that occur in up to 10% of children aged <7 years and disappear on extension of the neck.

Bones: Compare the height and shape of each vertebral body, looking for wedging and fractures.

Examine each apophyseal joint and spinous process for malalignment and fractures.

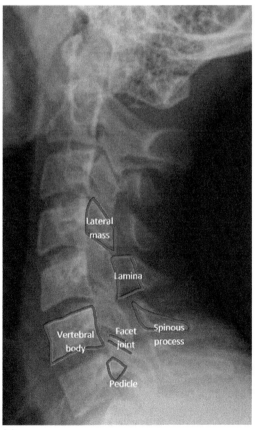

(a)

Figure 4.3 (a) Lateral view. (b) Upper AP (odontoid peg) view. Hellerhoff/Wikimedia Commons/CC BY-SA 3.0. (c) Anteroposterior view.

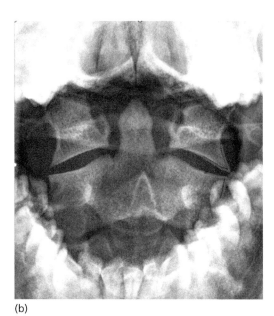

(b)

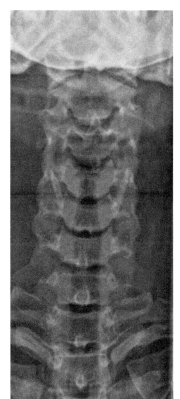

(c)

Figure 4.3 (Continued)

Look at the integrity of the odontoid peg and for increased space between the peg and the anterior arch of C1. Look for fracture of the posterior arch of C1 and for 'hangman's fracture' of the pedicles of C2.

Cartilages: Examine each intervertebral joint looking for osteophytes and narrow disc spaces.

Soft tissue: The soft-tissue shadow, anterior to the vertebral bodies, is increased if there is a fracture, haematoma or anterior ligament injury. Air is trapped in this area if there is damage to the posterior pharyngeal wall. Above the larynx, the width of the prevertebral soft-tissue space should be less than a third of the diameter of the vertebral body. Below this level, the space is accepted as normal if it is no wider than a whole vertebral body.

Look for widening of the space between the spinous processes (torn interspinous ligaments).

Alignment: Confirm the continuity of the curve along the following four lines:

1 Anterior borders of the vertebral bodies
2 Posterior borders of the vertebral bodies (the anterior edge of the vertebral canal)
3 Posterior edge of the vertebral canal
4 Tips of the spinous processes.

Upper AP (odontoid peg) view
(→ *Figure 4.3b*)

Alignment: Look at the lateral masses of C1, on either side of the odontoid peg. They should line up with the equivalent parts of C2. Spread suggests a burst (Jefferson's) fracture.

Bones: Look at the integrity of the odontoid peg.

Anteroposterior view (→ *Figure 4.3c*)

Alignment: Look for symmetry of the apophyseal joints.

Bones: Examine the transverse processes for fracture, or buttressing of C7 or a cervical rib. Thyroid cartilage wings are often misinterpreted as calcified vertebral arteries.

Cartilages: Confirm that the disc spaces are equal. Spaces above and below the centre of the X-ray beam appear narrower but should be bilaterally symmetrical.

Soft tissue: Confirm the central shadow of tracheal air.

Radiographs of the thoracolumbar spine

Similar to radiographic imaging of the cervical spine, have a low threshold for performing a CT scan to evaluate the thoracolumbar spine, especially when the history suggests violent impact and there are significant injuries above and below the diaphragm.

Spinal cord injury without radiographic abnormality (SCIWORA)

This is often seen in children, although very rarely can present in adults. The term had traditionally been used to describe an acute traumatic neuropathy in the absence of spinal column findings on plain radiographs, flexion–extension radiographs and/or computed tomography.

With the growing use of MRI, demonstrable injury to the spinal cord, soft tissue or vertebral body endplates are increasingly being described in patients who have had a normal CT finding.

If there are ongoing concerns with the neurological examination, patients should remain under spinal precautions until an MRI is performed. It is important to remember that the clinical presentation may be transient and delayed by a few hours or days; thus, there should be a low threshold to performing an MRI if SCIWORA is suspected.

'Clearing the C spine' → *p. 54*

X-ray is generally not indicated, however if performed radiographic findings may reveal the following:

- **Evident recent bony injury**: exercise spinal precautions and seek orthopaedic or neurosurgical advice. MRI may be warranted to exclude ligamentous injuries.
- **Loss of the normal lordosis with no bony injury**: this is caused by muscle spasm and usually indicates a more severe injury. Recovery may take longer than average but treatment remains as described below.
- **Pre-existing osteoarthritis**: the patient may have been asymptomatic previously. Some clinicians believe that spondylosis is associated with prolonged symptoms.
- **No radiographic abnormality**: this is the most common finding. This does not mean there is nothing wrong – there is a soft-tissue injury and symptoms are likely to get worse during the next 24–48 hours.

> The prognosis is difficult to determine on initial presentation to the ED. Symptoms are usually worse and more protracted than most clinicians anticipate.

NECK AND BACK INJURIES

'Whiplash' injury (strain injury to the neck)

'Whiplash' strain injury to the neck is poorly understood and is usually the result of a motor vehicle accident. It is much more common than similar injuries to other spinal regions for all vehicle occupants in all crash configurations. Drivers, females and younger people seem to be most at risk. The strain injury appears to be caused by sudden hyperextension and hyperflexion of the cervical spine. The circumstances of the incident will help assessment of the forces applied to the neck and so aid prognosis. The most common story is of a stationary vehicle being hit from behind.

Mobility may be good initially, with little pain, and then symptoms typically increase over the first 24 hours. There may be an associated headache, and pain may radiate to the shoulders. Sometimes, there is slight paraesthesia in one or both hands, but there are no long tract signs. Occasionally, the patient complains of difficulty in swallowing as a result of inflammation of the adjacent muscles.

On examination, there is usually tenderness of the paravertebral areas. Movements are restricted, particularly lateral flexion (in the direction of tenderness), and flexion and extension of the lower cervical spine. Movement at the atlanto-occipital joint is normal and will allow the head to flex forward without movement of the rest of the cervical spine. Rotation is variably restricted; forward flexion against resistance is almost always painful.

Tx

- Reassure the patient that symptoms will gradually settle over the next few weeks but warn him or her that they may increase over the first 24 hours.
- Prescribe an oral non-steroidal anti-inflammatory drug (NSAID).
- Encourage gentle range of movement exercises.
- Do not prescribe a cervical collar. The use of these devices has been shown to prolong symptoms without short-term benefit.
- Consider physiotherapy (heat lamp and massage at home may suffice). Early treatment probably reduces the incidence of chronic symptoms.

Clay shoveller's fracture

The muscular effort associated with strenuous digging – classically in clay – may avulse the spinous process of C7. There is localised pain over this vertebra prominens, which worsens on attempted flexion and extension.

Tx Fracture clinic referral is indicated for all spinous process fractures, although they heal spontaneously with conservative treatment.

Torticollis

Pain and spasm of one of the sternomastoid muscles may occur spontaneously (wry neck) or reflect local or generalised pathology. Most commonly, the symptoms occur on waking or after a sudden neck movement. The head is turned to the opposite side and cannot be rotated, but slight flexion and extension are usually possible. The muscle may be locally tender.

Local causes include pharyngitis, adenitis, retropharyngeal or parapharyngeal abscesses or rarely, spinal injury, spinal epidural haematoma following trauma or neurosurgical procedures and central nervous system tumours. Athetoid movements because of extrapyramidal excitation may present as atypical torticollis.

Imaging: When there are no other positive findings and there is no history of trauma, radiographs are unnecessary. Plain radiographic imaging may be unhelpful. A CT scan is warranted if infection, tumour or trauma is suspected.

Tx Idiopathic torticollis may be extremely painful but usually responds to reassurance and oral analgesia. Consider referral for physiotherapy.

Atlantoaxial rotary subluxation is one of the most common structural neck injuries of childhood. A rotational displacement of C1 on C2 is thought to be caused by retropharyngeal oedema, leading to laxity of the ligaments and capsular structures.

It may present with torticollis after trauma and is very difficult to identify on plain radiographs. If suspected, a CT scan of the neck is indicated.

Cervical spondylosis

Degenerative disease of the cervical spine is very common and often asymptomatic. The condition is usually diagnosed incidentally in the ED, on radiographs taken to exclude bony injury after trauma. Neurological function should be assessed and recorded.

If symptoms are long-standing and attributable to the cervical spondylosis, referral to the orthopaedic department or the patient's GP is appropriate.

Diffuse neck pain

The history is important:

- Mode of onset
- Site and character of pain and any radiation
- Associated headache and systemic symptoms.

The temperature must be taken and the mouth, ears and neck examined. A brief neurological examination should also be performed. Consider:

- Meningeal irritation (meningitis or subarachnoid haemorrhage)
- Spinal disease (infection, degenerative disease or rheumatoid arthritis)
- Intervertebral disc herniation
- Herpes zoster
- Pathology in the chest (e.g. myocardial infarction or pneumomediastinum)
- ENT pathology (e.g. Ludwig's angina, Lemierre's syndrome).
- **Cervical nerve root pain:** cervical nerve entrapment can be caused by degenerative disease, prolapsed intervertebral disc or in a relatively normal neck for reasons that are unclear.
- **Cervical spondylosis:** degeneration often affects the C7 distribution and causes pain and paraesthesia in the upper arm, dorsal forearm and dorsum of the hand, extending to the index and middle fingers. There may be weakness of triceps and the extensors of the wrist and fingers. The triceps reflex may be absent. Treatment is difficult. Adequate analgesia is essential and physiotherapy may be helpful. Specialist review may be indicated for patients whose symptoms or signs fail to resolve.
- **Cervical intervertebral disc prolapse:** this may arise spontaneously or after a sudden lifting or twisting movement. There is acute pain and spasm of the neck muscles with pain and paraesthesia radiating down the arm. In severe cases, there is anaesthesia, weakness and loss of reflexes in the arm. An MRI scan is diagnostic. Treatment consists of analgesia and physiotherapy. Patients with prolonged symptoms (more than 2 weeks) or any neurological signs require specialist referral.

Fractures of the thoracolumbar spine

> Injuries to the thoracolumbar spine are easily overlooked in patients with polytrauma.

- Knowledge of the mechanism of the injury will help in the assessment of the forces involved. As part of the secondary survey, ensure a thorough neurological examination is performed. This should include the anus (tone) and rectum (blood and swelling).
- In the presence of a normal CT and normal neurological examination, log-roll the patient carefully. Look for swelling, bruising, tenderness and steps in the vertebral column. Examine the bony spines, paravertebral structures and perineum.

- Consider the possibility of renal injury; test the urine for blood.
- Chest or abdominal injuries may coexist → *Chapter 2 Major Trauma*

Severe soft-tissue injury to the back

Patients with severe bruising to the back are often unable to walk. Many such patients require admission for analgesia and mobilisation. The possibility of renal injury must always be considered; the urine should be tested for blood.

Fractures of the transverse processes

These fractures, which are often multiple, are caused by either direct trauma – usually a fall from a height – or psoas muscle avulsion. Significant force is required and so other concomitant injuries are common. The retroperitoneal structures are particularly vulnerable; the urine must always be examined for the presence of blood. Over 10% of patients with a fractured transverse process also have a further lumbar spine fracture.

X̲ʀ The bisected transverse process is often missed on a plain AP radiograph. A CT scan is usually indicated to detect both retroperitoneal and more severe spinal injuries.

T̲x Admission is required for observation, bed rest and especially for analgesia.

Acute back pain

Back pain of sudden onset is a common presentation in young or middle-aged patients and affects 60% of the population to a significant degree at some point in their lives. It usually occurs while lifting. The clinician should enquire about the following:

- Onset of the pain/relation to lifting or injury
- Site and character of the pain
- Aggravating and relieving factors
- Radiation and referral of the pain, especially sciatica
- Neurological symptoms, including bladder and bowel function
- Previous episodes
- Coexisting diseases and drug therapy (especially steroids).

The clinician should then:

- Observe the patient's degree of mobility.
- Examine the spine and paravertebral areas for tenderness.

- Check the mobility of the lumbar spine with the patient erect and supine.
- Determine the extent of sciatic nerve sheath tethering by measuring straight-leg raising bilaterally. Perform the sciatic stretch test:
  - Raise one leg until back/thigh/calf pain is felt
  - Record this angle. Normal would be 80°–90°
  - Dorsiflex foot. Test is positive if pain is reproduced
  - Flex the knee. This should relieve the pain.
- Record subjective or objective sensory loss in the lower limbs.
- Look for muscle weakness (commonly at ankle or toe) and reflex loss.
- Examine the perineum for sensory loss and sphincter laxity.
- Measure pre- and post-void bladder volumes.

Detailed in Box 4.2 → *Cauda Equina Syndrome p. 62*

> Mechanical low back pain is usually exacerbated by movement in specific directions. Global pain (with all movements) is either more sinister or associated with psychological overlay.

X̲ʀ Urgent plain radiography is unhelpful in most younger patients. Older men (>55 years) and postmenopausal women may have osteoporotic collapse of the vertebrae or other diseases. The differentiation between new and old collapse of the bone can be very difficult on plain films. Indications for radiography see Box 4.3.

T̲x Negative neurological findings in the presence of low back pain suggest minor ligamentous injury in the

Box 4.2 Atypical ('red flag') features in a patient with back pain

- Age <20 years or >55 years
- Recent onset of pain without trauma or lifting
- Severe pain at rest or progressively worsening pain
- Bilateral sciatic pain
- Thoracic pain
- Obvious structural deformity
- Neurological symptoms or signs
- Urinary or bowel symptoms
- Malaise or weight loss
- History of carcinoma, HIV infection, IV drug use or recent steroid therapy

Box 4.3 Indications for radiography of the lumbar spine in patients with atraumatic back pain

- History suggestive of non-mechanical back pain (i.e. the pain is constant, progressive, worse at night and unrelated to activity)
- History of coexisting condition that may give rise to non-mechanical back pain (i.e. malignancy or inflammation)
- Patient at risk of spontaneous vertebral collapse (on steroids, elderly)
- Neurological symptoms or signs
- Pain persisting for more than 4–6 weeks

young or degeneration in the older patient. Most patients will be helped by the following:

- Analgesia to take home (to be taken on a regular basis)
- Written instructions on the care of the injured back
- Review by the GP after this time if there is no improvement. A letter should accompany the patient.

Physiotherapy should also be considered. Regular exercise is important, and patients should be advised to return to work as soon as possible. Some patients may be confined to bed as a consequence of their pain, but this should be limited to 2 days as a maximum and should not be considered as a primary treatment. It is important to reassure patients that early mobilisation will not cause harm.

Over 95% of patients with simple mechanical low back pain will recover spontaneously within 6 weeks. There is an 85% chance of recurrence, with around 8% of affected patients becoming chronically disabled.

Collapsed vertebral bodies are an indication for an orthopaedic or neurosurgical opinion. Nursing care and analgesia are usually required before mobilisation. Patients with osteoporotic collapse who are referred back to their GP should be considered for bone protection treatment. This may include hormone replacement therapy (dependent on age and gender), calcium, vitamin D and bisphosphonates.

Atypical back pain

If back pain is not related to direct trauma and did not come on while the patient was lifting or twisting, the insidious onset of a more sinister disease should be considered. This could include the following:

- Secondary deposit (breast, bronchus, prostate, thyroid and kidney)
- Myeloma

- Pelvic neoplasm or infection
- Epidural abscess or other spinal infection
- Aortic aneurysm
- Renal or pancreatic disease or peptic ulceration
- Ankylosing spondylitis
- Paget's disease
- Herpes zoster.

A leaking aortic aneurysm commonly presents with pain experienced in the back and myocardial infarction may cause isolated back pain.

The examination should be tailored to the history but may need to include:

- abdominal palpation and rectal examination
- urinalysis
- breast examination
- a search for causes of weight loss.

Investigations: Full blood count (FBC), blood chemistry, C-reactive protein (CRP) and erythrocyte sedimentation rate (ESR) may be helpful as screening tests. CT and MR scans are often of more diagnostic value than plain films. Point of care ultrasound (POCUS) can look for abdominal aortic aneurysm.

Tx Assess the patient and ask for advice. Older people with backache tend to be under-investigated.

Spinal epidural abscess

Infection of the spinal epidural space is easily overlooked; the diagnosis is delayed in around half of all cases. During this time, damage to the spinal cord by direct infection, compression or vascular compromise may occur. Epidural abscess may be found at all ages but is more common in males and in high-risk groups such as intravenous drug users. Haematogenous spread from almost any site can infect the epidural space but, often, no source is identified. The most common pathogen is *Staphylococcus aureus.*

Back pain – often of disproportionate severity – is the main symptom, although irritation of nerve roots may cause the patient to complain of chest or abdominal pain. Unlike mechanical and sciatic back pain, symptoms get progressively worse rather than better. Only a third of patients have a raised temperature; some have neck stiffness. Neurological features may initially be absent and, when present, can be very variable and atypical. There may be motor and sensory deficits in isolation or findings suggestive of incomplete cord syndromes. Reflexes may be absent or increased and sphincter disturbance can occur.

Investigations: Only half of patients with an epidural abscess have a raised white cell count. ESR and CRP are more sensitive. Lumbar puncture is relatively contraindicated. An MR scan (or CT myelography) is diagnostic. Oedema of the paraspinal muscles may be seen in addition to the epidural infection.

Tx The patient should be discussed with a spinal surgeon. Antibiotics are required for 3–4 weeks ± surgical decompression. Anti-staphylococcal therapy (such as IV flucloxacillin and vancomycin) may be given initially until cultures are available (following CT-guided aspiration of the abscess).

Discitis

Discitis may present in either adults or children. Risk factors include immunocompromise and intravenous drug use. Infection of the intravertebral disc generally results from haematogenous spread. It usually presents with insidious back pain, low-grade pyrexia, malaise and sometimes abdominal pain. The patient may have difficulty walking, tenderness to spinal percussion and worsening of pain with forward flexion. Neurological examination is usually unremarkable.

Investigations: Plain X-rays are generally unremarkable. Blood tests (WBC and CRP) may show some elevation but are often normal. MRI scan will be diagnostic.

Tx Discussion with the spinal team and admission for intravenous antibiotics is required.

Other spinal infections: subdural abscess, vertebral osteomyelitis and paraspinal infections may all occur. Diagnosis and treatment is similar to that for epidural abscess. Tuberculosis of the spine may also cause severe, intractable back pain.

Sciatica

Pain in the distribution of the sciatic nerve is most commonly caused by the lateral prolapse of an intervertebral disc. The pain, which may be severe, radiates across the buttock, down the back of the thigh and along the medial aspect of the leg to the foot. Backache may be absent, especially when the sciatic pain is of more gradual onset.

The examination should be the same as that detailed above for low back pain. Consider alternative, particularly vascular, causes of the pain. Bilateral sciatica/radiculopathy is suggestive of a central disc prolapse, which is high risk for cord compression and cauda equina syndrome. These patients should usually have same-day MRI scan imaging.

XR Plain films are not helpful. An MRI scan will demonstrate the prolapsed disc(s), the degree of protrusion and any impingement on the cauda equina.

Tx The initial management of sciatica is similar to that for back pain. Initial conservative treatment should be employed, with analgesia and early mobilisation.

The patient should be warned that sciatica can be slow to settle. Fortunately, the majority of sufferers will be better in 6 weeks, and many of the remainder will have resolved before 6 months have elapsed.

Cauda equina syndrome (CES)

Central prolapse of the L4–5 or L5–S1 intervertebral disc may cause compression of the terminal branches of the spinal cord. In the absence of prompt treatment, cauda equina syndrome results in severe and permanent neurological damage. Consequently, the presenting symptoms and signs must not be missed:

- Acute low back pain (which may be superimposed upon a chronic history of recurrent pain)
- Radiation of pain to the legs – usually but not always bilateral
- Bilateral sciatica should prompt urgent MR scan
- Weakness or sensory disturbance in the legs – often present but not invariable; this may cause an abnormal gait
- Alteration of perineal sensation ('saddle anaesthesia') – usually but not exclusively bilateral
- Sphincter dysfunction presenting as urgency, frequency or incontinence
- Alteration of bladder and bowel habit (leading to retention and constipation).

It is worth noting that absence of any of the above symptoms does not rule out cauda equina syndrome. Alteration of bladder and bowel habit is often a late sign, and the aim is to identify and treat cauda equina before permanent neurological damage and loss of sphincter control occurs. Unfortunately, none of the clinical symptoms or signs are sufficiently accurate in isolation to rule in or rule out cauda equina syndrome. Abnormal ankle jerks bilaterally, dermatomal sensory loss and bilateral leg pain have been suggested to be most predictive. Normal digital rectal examination and normal perianal sensation are not sufficiently sensitive to rule out CES with sensitivities of 35% and 50%, respectively.

Investigations: Plain films are not helpful. An MRI scan will demonstrate the prolapsed disc(s), the degree of protrusion and compression of the cauda equina. MRI should be performed urgently, and pathways should exist to ensure local access to a centre with 24-hour MRI capability.

Post-void residual volume is a useful adjunct to conventional clinical assessment and allows risk stratification in managing suspected cauda equina syndrome. A post-void residual volume ≥200 mL is suggestive of CES.

Tx Immediate admission and referral for urgent decompression is essential. Surgery undertaken more than 48 hours after presentation is rarely successful.

Injury to the coccyx and coccydynia

The coccyx may be injured by a fall on to the buttocks. There is local pain and extreme tenderness. Dyschezia (pain on defecation) may also occur. A haematoma can sometimes be felt between the coccyx and rectum, but pain usually prevents a rectal examination. Prolonged symptoms are inevitable; sitting is likely to be uncomfortable for months.

Pain in this region (coccydynia) can also be caused by prolapse of an intervertebral disc, pelvic inflammatory disease, and tumours of the spine and sacrum.

XR Radiographs of the sacrum and coccyx are often of poor quality, especially in obese patients. Moreover, management is rarely changed by an initial radiograph. If imaged, a fractured coccyx is often seen to be anteverted or displaced. Anterior subluxation of the entire coccyx can also occur, with or without an accompanying fracture of the distal sacrum.

Tx Analgesia is the mainstay of treatment, and the patient should be advised to sit on an inflatable rubber ring cushion. A swimming ring is a cheap and easily available alternative. Constipation must be avoided. The patient should be warned that pain will persist for several months. Physiotherapy (ultrasound treatment) can sometimes be helpful. For severe, prolonged coccydynia, excision of the coccyx may be necessary.

WOUNDS TO THE NECK AND BODY

Major wounds to the neck

A major neck wound is defined as any injury in which the platysma muscle is thought to be divided. Look for further wounds if the patient has been stabbed.

Neck wounds are often deeper than a casual examination might suggest, and wounds near the base of the skull and the root of the neck are particularly dangerous.

The neck is divided into three zones when considering penetrating neck traumas:

- **Zone 1**: extends from the clavicle to the cricoid cartilage
- **Zone 2**: extends form the cricoid cartilage to the angle of the mandible
- **Zone 3**: extends form the angle of the mandible to the skull base.

Major vascular injury may remain occult for many hours or even days. A normal carotid pulse does not exclude arterial damage. Look for any direct airway injury, suggested by hoarseness, stridor, tachypnoea, subcutaneous emphysema or laryngeal crepitus.

Air embolisation may follow venous injury.

Emergency exploration may be indicated if there is persistent haemorrhage especially within Zone 2, associated with haemodynamic instability.

Tx Position the patient with a slight head-down tilt to lessen the risk of air embolism. Gain venous access and ensure anti-tetanus cover.

Major neck wounds should not be explored under local anaesthesia in the ED. Patients with such wounds must be referred urgently for specialist assessment, observation and surgical exploration. CT angiography is likely to be required in most cases.

Stab wounds to the back

Stab wounds to the back should be treated as for penetrating trauma of the chest and abdomen. The vast majority will require CT imaging and management as major trauma.

Major trauma → Chapter 2
Injuries to the trunk → Chapter 6

5

Facial injuries

James Conroy[1] and Abu Hassan[2]

[1] Leeds Teaching Hospitals, Leeds, UK
[2] Sheffield Children's Hospital, Sheffield, UK

Facial injuries are commonly seen following assaults in adults and falls in children. They need special consideration because:

- the airway may be compromised
- the eyes, nose, mouth and ears are functionally and cosmetically important
- the skin is closely bound to underlying tissue, which complicates wound care and local anaesthesia
- deep tissue injuries may be masked; delay in their treatment can lead to major disability.

FRACTURES OF THE FACIAL BONES

Management of fractures in the emergency department (ED) involves:

- airway care (may be difficult)
- control of profuse bleeding
- pain relief
- initial clinical and radiographic assessment
- administration of antibiotics for compound fractures
- tetanus prophylaxis
- consideration of other injuries.

The airway

Airway patency may be threatened by profuse bleeding and distortion of the skeleton and soft tissues. The airway may be maintainable in a fully conscious patient, but in the unresponsive patient with major facial injury endotracheal intubation becomes essential. Rarely, very extensive facial injuries may make this technically difficult or impossible and warrant urgent cricothyroidotomy or tracheostomy (→ *pp. 22 and 23*).

Neck injuries

These must be considered when facial injury is sustained by the moving head striking a fixed object (e.g. in a car). Although neck damage is less likely if the immobile head is struck by a mobile object (e.g. in an assault), it is essential to examine the cervical spine of all patients with facial injuries.

> An elderly patient with a bruise on the forehead and weak arms should be assumed to have sustained a central cord injury (→ *p. 53*).

The facial skeleton is designed to withstand the vertical forces associated with mastication, but it collapses readily when struck from the front. Injuries can be divided into lower third (mandible), middle third and upper third (frontal). The last type is considered in Chapter 3.

Facial fractures are not always obvious. Examination begins with an assessment of facial contours, often best achieved by looking at the face from above and behind. Bony tenderness may be difficult to detect if soft-tissue bruising and swelling are already present. However, pressure for a few seconds over bony points (e.g. the infraorbital margin) will usually displace sufficient interstitial fluid to allow assessment of bony contours and orbital contents.

Facial radiography

For initial investigation of most facial injuries, 'facial views' consisting of two occipitomental views are appropriate. The head position required to obtain occipitomental views can however be dangerous in the presence

The RCEM Lecture Notes: Emergency Medicine, Fifth Edition. Edited by Catherine Williams and Amy Nickson.
© 2024 John Wiley & Sons Ltd. Published 2024 by John Wiley & Sons Ltd.
Companion website: www.wiley.com/go/LNEM5

of cervical spine injuries. These can never be excluded immediately in the severely injured or obtunded patient and so it is unwise to request facial views in such patients. The usual brow-up, lateral view has two advantages: (1) minimal patient movement and (2) easier demonstration of paranasal sinuses. In some circumstances such as co-existing significant head or spinal injury, suspicion of basal skull fracture, or very severe facial injury, it may be appropriate to proceed directly to CT. A CT scan overcomes issues of positioning but should not be undertaken at the expense of treating more immediately important injuries.

Antibiotics for compound fractures

Fractures of the facial bones, which communicate either with skin wounds, sinuses or buccal mucosa carry a similar theoretical risk of infection as an open fracture to a limb or elsewhere. Antibiotics may be indicated and are usually recommended for mandibular fractures and those associated with skin wounds. Evidence is less clear for other facial fractures. Consult local guidance with regard to indications and recommended targeted antibiotic prophylaxis – the usual recommendation is co-amoxiclav (or clindamycin in penicillin allergic patients).

Special features associated with facial fractures

Surgical emphysema of the face

This indicates the presence of a fracture into an air-containing sinus. Antibiotics and referral for maxillofacial surgical review are required. Advise the patient to avoid blowing their nose as this will increase volume of surgical emphysema.

Facial sensory loss

Anaesthesia in the area of distribution of the infraorbital nerve (terminal branches of V2) is often associated with:

- fractures of the malar complex
- fractures of the floor of the orbit
- Le Fort II and III fractures
- severe soft-tissue injuries to the cheek.

The area of numbness may include the ipsilateral upper lip and also the anterior gums and teeth (anterior superior alveolar nerve). Oedema in the infraorbital canal is the usual cause. This is where the dental nerve separates off, leaving the terminal part of the maxillary nerve to exit from the infraorbital foramen as the infraorbital nerve. Oral surgical follow-up is indicated.

Intraoral damage

Examination inside the mouth is very important. Malocclusion of teeth, or displacement of dentures in the absence of primary dental damage, is strongly associated with injury to bone or to the temporomandibular joint (TMJ). Palatal irregularities suggest a Le Fort fracture. Buccal mucosal lacerations may be associated with mandibular fractures. The inability to open the mouth fully is an indication for imaging.

Injuries affecting the eye

Assessment of visual acuity, conjunctival sac, cornea, anterior chamber and fundus is an essential part of facial assessment. The weakest point of the orbit is the floor, and so increased intraorbital pressure due to a blow, often leads to fracture of the orbital floor. Displacement of the eye, inwards or downwards, is associated with injury to the infraorbital plate. Extraocular muscle damage or distortion may complicate any damage to the bony wall of the orbit and is clearly demonstrated on testing the full range of eye movements. The presence of a subconjunctival haemorrhage without evidence of direct trauma to the eye is a strong indication of the presence of a facial fracture, usually in the infraorbital region.

Other causes of subconjunctival haemorrhage → *pp. 45 and 431.*

Wounds associated with major fractures

Closure of major wounds associated with displaced facial fractures must await reduction of the fractures and should usually be carried out by the maxillofacial surgery team. The wounds may offer surgical access to bone and facilitate reduction. Until this has been carried out, it may not be possible to achieve cosmetically acceptable reconstruction of the soft tissues.

Mandibular fractures

The most common mandibular fracture, through the extracapsular part of the neck of the condyle, is usually sustained by a blow on the chin. It can be unilateral or bilateral. Examination reveals dental malocclusion, often a lateral cross-bite, and absence of forward movement of the condylar head on opening the mouth. The force may have been sufficient to drive the head of the condyle backwards and cause a fracture of the squamous temporal bone. This produces bleeding and a cerebrospinal fluid (CSF) leak into the external auditory meatus.

Fractures of the ramus, angle and body will be revealed by local tenderness of the cheek and difficulty in opening the mouth. There may be surprisingly little swelling. The presence of mucosal lacerations and irregular dentition helps confirmation. Displacement is determined by the configuration of the fracture line in relation to the pull of the masticatory muscles. Anaesthesia to the lower may reflect damage to the inferior dental nerve.

> The ability to open the mouth fully and to clench the teeth normally makes the presence of a fracture of the jaw very unlikely. In the 'tongue blade test', a patient is asked to bite down on a wooden tongue depressor which the clinician then twists medially until it breaks. In the presence of significant injury, the patient will be unable to hold on. This test has a reported sensitivity of 95% for a mandibular fracture.

XR An orthopantomogram (OPT or OPG), a rotational tomogram that gives a circumferential view of the face, is especially helpful and easy to interpret. If this cannot be obtained, the best plain radiographs are lateral oblique, posteroanterior (PA) and Townes' views (for the condyles).

Tx No immediate treatment is required in the ED for any of these fractures themselves. Unstable and painful fractures will require early repair; specific management of mandibular fractures is complex, and it is therefore recommended that all patients are discussed with a maxillofacial surgeon. Some displaced condylar fractures can be managed conservatively with good functional results, but there is an increasing trend towards internal fixation. All patients will need analgesia and a soft diet. Patients with an open mandibular fracture should be given a broad-spectrum antibiotic whilst in the ED. A systematic review of antibiotic prophylaxis in the treatment of open mandibular fracture found that short-term antibiotic therapy (<48 hours) reduces infection rates threefold.

Temporomandibular joint dislocation

This may occur spontaneously (as the inability to close the mouth after yawning) or result from a blow to the open mouth. It is often recurrent and is particularly common in elderly people.

XR An OPG of the jaw is usually diagnostic. TMJ views may be requested but can be difficult to interpret. Fractures of the condyles must be excluded but are unlikely in the absence of trauma.

Tx Reduction can usually be achieved without general anaesthetic but must be carried out by an experienced clinician using appropriate analgesia or sedation. The jaw is held by putting both (gauze wrapped) thumbs inside the mouth along the line of the lower teeth on each side, while the forefingers grasp the bone from outside. Pressure is then applied downwards and backwards by the thumbs intraorally pressing bilaterally against the angle of the jaw. Post-reduction radiographs are taken to confirm relocation, although the patient is usually in no doubt. Specialist follow-up on an outpatient basis is appropriate.

Malar fractures

The malar complex provides the bony prominence on the cheek and is commonly fractured in isolation by a blow to that area. The strong central part of the bone usually remains intact, the force being transmitted to the three buttresses. These bones then fracture or dislocate either individually or, more frequently, simultaneously (a 'tripod fracture'):

1 **Infraorbital fracture:** fracture in the infraorbital region usually causes neuropraxia of the infraorbital nerve. Subconjunctival haemorrhage may occur.

> Sensory loss after a facial injury merits specialist follow-up. It may involve the upper lip, gum and front teeth on the affected side (→ p. 65).

2 **Displacement of the zygomaticofrontal suture:** this may be associated with injury to the suspensory ligament of the eye.
3 **Fracture of the zygomatic arch (zygoma):** this may be sufficiently displaced to impinge on the coronoid process of the mandible and prevent normal jaw movement. Even if this does not occur at the time of injury, exuberant callus formation may cause problems later.

Examination will reveal tenderness over one or more malar processes. Bony irregularity can be assessed by intraoral examination behind and above the upper molars, and by careful palpation along the inferior and lateral borders of the orbit and along the line of the zygomatic arch. Diplopia may occur because of injury to the suspensory ligament or displacement and damage to the extraocular muscles. The latter is usually transient.

> Surgical emphysema in the area of a malar injury indicates a (compound) fracture into an air sinus. Antibiotics and follow-up are indicated.

X_R Facial radiographs confirm the diagnosis. The most common pair of views are occipitomental projections at 10° and 30°.

T_X Once the diagnosis has been made, the patient should be referred for specialist care. If reduction and elevation of the displaced malar are required, this can be achieved relatively simply, under a short general anaesthetic on a day-case basis within the following week.

Retrobulbar haemorrhage

This may occasionally occur after a fracture of the zygomatic complex. It causes:

- retrobulbar pain
- very marked proptosis
- diminished vision (which may quickly become permanent)
- massive facial swelling.

> Severe retrobulbar bleeding with orbital displacement is a surgical emergency. The area must be decompressed by lateral canthotomy.

Lateral canthotomy →Chapter 22 p. 431

Middle third fractures

When the face is struck directly from the front, the delicate bony skeleton formed by the maxilla, palatine, nasal and ethmoid bones may be crushed and forced backwards and downwards. The nasal bones may be broken in isolation (→ *below*), but the other bones tend to collapse en masse. Le Fort first described the three fracture complexes that are commonly seen (→ *Figure 5.1 and Box 5.1*).

Examination may reveal a dished-in face if the middle third has moved backwards and downwards. The nose appears flattened and widened. This appearance is best confirmed from the side and from above. Swelling and bruising are usually marked. By holding the vault of the skull with one hand and the maxilla complex with the other (between gloved index finger on the hard palate and thumb over the upper incisors), instability may be elicited with surprising ease and without too much pain.

There may be diplopia on upward gaze and damage to the lacrimal system. Damage to the cribriform plate may produce anosmia, but this can be difficult to confirm in the ED because blood is usually present in the nasal cavity which will seriously impair the sense of smell even in the absence of damage to the olfactory apparatus. Any minor occlusion deformity is readily appreciated by the patient

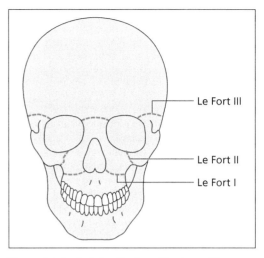

Figure 5.1 Le Fort classification of fractures of the middle third of the face.

> Box 5.1 **Le Fort fractures (→ *see Figure 5.1*)**
>
> *Le Fort I* fracture runs across the lower face, including the hard palate and alveolus.
> *Le Fort II* is pyramidal, extending variably upwards in the midline to involve the ethmoids. An associated leak of CSF may occur.
> *Le Fort III* is more transverse but at a uniformly higher level than Le Fort I. Essentially, it separates the face from the skull and has been described as craniofacial disjunction.

and is a reliable indicator of bony injury. The backward displacement of the middle third of the face will produce a reverse overbite (upper incisors behind lower incisors). The associated tilting results in an anterior open bite.

X_R Le Fort fractures can be difficult to spot on facial views, so CT may be required.

T_X Immediate specialist inpatient care is required. Significant bleeding and airway compromise may occur, and in this case an anaesthetist should be called.

Nasal fractures

The nasal bones may be dislocated from their normal relationship with the maxilla or fractured. The nasal cartilages usually deform to accommodate violence and do not break. The nasal septum may be deformed, deviated laterally and fractured.

> Trauma to the nose may produce a large septal haematoma that can obstruct the nostril and damage the nutrient vessels to the septum. This can result in avascular necrosis of the bone and septal collapse.

The nose has a good blood supply, and all these injuries are associated with epistaxis.

Examination should first exclude more serious facial injuries. Local tenderness over the nasal bones will be present, but the appearance of swelling may be delayed. The tip of the nose may be upturned. Lateral deviation may not be obvious to the examiner. The patient should be given a mirror and asked to compare present and previous facial appearance. An obvious deformity may relate to a previous injury.

More extensive fractures involving the ethmoids are associated with widening of the intracanthal distance, a transverse cleft across the glabella and CSF rhinorrhoea. Intranasal examination should be carried out with a speculum and good light; it is essential to exclude a septal haematoma.

Xʀ Radiological confirmation of nasal fractures is of no immediate value. Indeed, an undisplaced fracture may be difficult to distinguish from a vascular marking.

Tx Bleeding usually settles with alar pressure (→ p. 436). Septal haematoma or uncontrolled bleeding is an indication for immediate referral. Patients with clearly deformed noses should be referred to ENT clinic. There is a large group of patients who have marked swellings but an uncertain amount of deformity. They should be told to let the swelling settle over 5–7 days and then return for reassessment (according to local agreement) if they are unhappy with their appearance. Reduction under anaesthesia should usually be carried out within the first 14 days.

FACIAL WOUNDS

Minor wounds to the face → Chapter 21 on p. 410.

Facial skin is unusual. It is an integral part of the deep structures, bound to them by the facial muscles that arise from and insert into the subcutaneous tissues. Consequently, it is difficult to undermine and close quite small defects without causing deformity. Wounds near the circular muscle around the eyes or mouth may influence their function. The importance of cosmesis and the psychological impact of facial scarring should not be underestimated. The threshold for referral onwards for wound closure under theatre conditions should be significantly lower for facial wounds than for those elsewhere.

Initial assessment should include the following:

- Mechanism and direction of injury
- Wounding agent (especially glass)
- Contamination
- Delay to presentation
- Sensation and function (before anaesthetising the wound)
- Involvement of specialised areas.

Record details of wound site, size and configuration. When making notes, annotation of a diagram of a facial outline may be helpful. Many such injuries are the result of assaults and you may be called to describe the wound in court.

> Wounds to the chin may be associated with fractures of the condyles of the jaw.

Prerequisites for definitive care in the ED are:

- patience (and time)
- good operating conditions
- adequate anaesthesia
- a compliant and cooperative patient
- a knowledge of facial anatomy
- a knowledge of the general principles of wound management.
- technical skill.

Standard suture sets, provided in EDs, often contain large and unreliable instruments. Finer, good quality instruments for face and hand use may be useful if available.

Anaesthesia

This is essential to permit adequate exploration and cleaning. In children, a general anaesthetic may be required for a relatively small wound; this may warrant admission.

Exploration

Deep wounds may damage the facial or infraorbital nerves, or the parotid, submandibular or lacrimal ducts. The suspicion of damage to any of these structures requires expert assessment by the appropriate specialist. Early referral is essential.

Cleaning

This must be very thorough. Dirt and foreign bodies such as windscreen glass may be driven deep into facial wounds. An appreciation of the direction and force of the injuring agent will facilitate exploration. Remove dirt from grazes as soon as possible because residual dirt is taken up by inflammatory cells and may produce a tattoo effect. It may be necessary to use a scrubbing brush or toothbrush to remove ingrained dirt, and this will require adequate anaesthesia. A second operation to retrieve a foreign body is always more difficult and produces a more pronounced scar.

Special areas

Wounds involving the eyelid margins should always be referred to an ophthalmic surgeon. Incorrect apposition of the various layers may produce entropion or ectropion. Extreme care is also required when repairing wounds that involve the margin of the lips (vermillion border). A slight malalignment will produce a major cosmetic defect. In most cases (other than very minor wounds, or where the patient does not wish it), lacerations crossing the vermillion border should be referred to maxillofacial or plastic surgery.

Similarly, the line of the eyebrows must be carefully preserved. Adequate local anaesthesia can be difficult to achieve around the nose and ears.

Tissue loss

Large wounds and those with tissue loss should be referred for specialist plastic surgery or maxillofacial assessment. Undermining facial wound edges is technically difficult and can increase rather than decrease the deformity associated with tissue loss. An experienced plastic surgeon should be involved in the management of such wounds from the outset. The excellent blood supply of the face allows even the most tenuous flap to survive with appropriate management. Trimming of wound edges should be left to a senior doctor with plastic surgery experience.

Closure with sutures

Two layers are usually adequate. Troublesome bleeding may require the occasional ligature, but haemostasis is usually achieved on wound closure. Haematoma formation is rarely a problem. Subcutaneous closure with interrupted, plain absorbable sutures (about 4/0) is advisable in larger wounds. The skin is then apposed with interrupted sutures. Tension must be avoided. Correct alignment is best achieved by initial insertion of a few sutures at intervals along the wound.

Fine-diameter sutures are generally recommended for use on the face, but the contused wounds often seen in an ED do not lend themselves to very fine sutures. Placing adhesive tapes on top of a sutured wound may reduce the tension on the sutures and improve the final result.

Suture removal

Facial wounds heal rapidly. Those not subject to undue stress (e.g. on the forehead or cheek) will be sufficiently strong to allow suture removal at 4–5 days. Wounds over convex surfaces may open up at this stage and can be protected by adhesive tapes. The early replacement of sutures by tapes has the advantages of reducing scarring around the needle puncture marks. This is not recommended under the chin and other areas where saliva or excessive movement may impair their adhesion.

Closure with adhesive tapes

Some facial wounds can be closed with adhesive tapes. Cleaning before the application of these tapes must be just as thorough as cleaning before the insertion of sutures. This often requires local anaesthesia. Wounds on convex surfaces will tend to open up in the early stages of healing, as a result of a combination of reduced tissue strength and oedema. Tapes should not be used if the wounds cannot be kept dry and immobile (e.g. the chin or eyebrows of children) but are ideal for small wounds of the forehead and cheek.

Closure with tissue glue

This can also be considered for some small wounds. The same precautions apply as for adhesive tapes.

Bites

This type of wound is considered in detail on p. 418.

The practice of leaving bites open, to heal by secondary intention, has no benefit and should not be applied to the face. Primary closure usually gives good cosmetic results. The wounds must be cleaned meticulously and then a broad-spectrum antibiotic (e.g. co-amoxiclav) prescribed. Follow-up wound review is advisable.

INJURIES INSIDE THE MOUTH

> Wounds associated with dental damage should be explored for tooth fragments, which may lead to a severe infection if not removed. The possibility of tooth aspiration should also be considered.

Injuries to the tongue

Isolated or small lacerations rarely require any specific treatment, especially if centrally located. Healing is rapid and the cosmetic result good, despite initial deformity caused by the pull of the intrinsic muscles. Large flap lacerations, bisecting wounds or uncontrolled bleeding should be discussed with the maxillofacial specialists. An antiseptic, analgesic, oral rinse (benzydamine hydrochloride) may be valuable. This is particularly important in patients who are reluctant to drink and in whom a dry mouth may predispose to secondary infection.

Injuries to the buccal mucosa and gingiva

Simple lacerations are treated in the same way as injuries to the tongue; if more extensive then look for a fracture.

Full thickness wounds

Full thickness, or 'through and through' wounds are often caused by a tooth biting through the lip or cheek when a patient falls onto the face. This type of wound require meticulous cleaning and irrigation and closure in three layers, which requires experience – often best left to the maxillofacial surgeon.

> The patient (or the parents) should be warned that a yellow exudate will form over the wound. This is caused by the normal commensal bacteria of the mouth and is not harmful. It will last a few days and may give rise to slight halitosis.

Injuries to permanent teeth

Teeth may be chipped (fractured), displaced (forwards, backwards or intruded) or avulsed. Occasionally, they can be bruised (concussed), making the tooth tender and slightly discoloured, which settles over time. The site of injury should be described using the dental formula shown in → Box 5.2.

Tx
Conditions that require immediate dental advice → Box 5.3.

A chip confined to enamel or dentine (→ *Figure 5.2*) will be very sensitive but does not pose any immediate threat to the viability of the tooth. Varnish may be applied to reduce thermal pain and the patient referred to his or her own dentist the next day.

If the pulp is exposed (→ *Figure 5.2*), there is a risk of infection and immediate dental referral is necessary. The pulp is recognised by its red colour.

- Incisor teeth may be displaced (subluxed) but otherwise apparently undamaged. Immediate specialist advice should be obtained in the case of permanent teeth because there is only a 4-hours window of opportunity for easy repositioning. Manipulation of

Box 5.2 Dental formula

1 Determine the quadrant (as if you are looking into the mouth):

upper right	upper left
lower right	lower left

2 Count out from the midline:

1, 2 incisors	3 canines
4, 5 premolars	6, 7, 8 molars

e.g. outer upper right incisor 2⌋
    lower left canine ⌊3

Box 5.3 Dental injuries for which immediate specialist advice is needed

- Exposed pulp of any tooth
- Avulsed permanent tooth
- Subluxed permanent tooth
- Mobile segment of alveolar bone
- Severe soft-tissue injury with dental damage

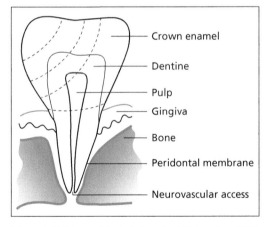

- Crown enamel
- Dentine
- Pulp
- Gingiva
- Bone
- Peridontal membrane
- Neurovascular access

Figure 5.2 Types of dental injury in relation to the dental anatomy.

the tooth in the ED may loosen it further, with subsequent risk of inhalation.

- Sometimes, several incisor teeth are loosened together with a segment of the underlying alveolar bone (alveolar plate fracture). Again, this needs immediate specialist treatment including splintage and antibiotics.
- Avulsed (permanent) teeth should immediately be:
  - washed very gently with saline
  - kept in saline

- handled as little as possible
- reimplanted and splinted in place.

Reimplantation is often successful, but the chances of a good outcome are directly related to the speed of reimplantation – within 30 min is ideal. If definitive dental care is delayed, the socket can be cleaned with saline, local anaesthetic gel instilled and the tooth replaced in ED. Temporary stabilisation is obtained by using tissue glue and wire or metal strips to bridge the tooth to the one either side. Aftercare includes consideration of tetanus prophylaxis and antibiotics.

Injuries to deciduous (milk) teeth

For the purposes of treatment, it is important to differentiate the permanent dentition from the deciduous teeth. Permanent teeth are bigger and have a different shape from milk teeth. They usually appear after the age of 6 years in the lower jaw and after the age of 7 years in the upper jaw. The 32 permanent teeth replace 20 deciduous teeth. The first milk tooth erupts at about 6 months of age, and thereafter one or more appears every month. They are all shed by the age of 13 years. For children, the dental formula is written in the usual way (→ *Box 5.2*), but the letters A–E are used to designate the deciduous teeth.

Avulsed milk teeth are common and require no immediate treatment. However, there are two possible long-term effects on the permanent teeth:

1 The gap may affect their positioning.
2 The trauma may impair their development. This risk is increased by attempts at reimplantation.

The child should see his or her own dentist on the following day.

Deciduous teeth that are subluxed or intruded (pushed into the jaw) should also be seen by the dentist on the following day.

Very loose deciduous teeth may be removed, but other loose milk teeth can be safely left to the patient's dentist. We all have 20 loose milk teeth at some time in our lives and survive without aspiration.

Chipped deciduous teeth are dealt with in the same way as the permanent dentition.

INJURIES TO THE EAR

Injuries involving the cartilage of the ear

The elastic cartilage of the ear receives its blood supply from the overlying skin. If the cartilage is exposed on both sides by skin avulsion or is separated from the skin by haematoma, it will necrose and collapse, resulting in a 'cauliflower' ear.

Lacerations

Most lacerations of the pinna involving cartilage require specialist care. Small pieces of cartilage exposed at the edge of the pinna may be trimmed, before skin closure, without causing significant cosmetic problems.

Auricular haematoma

If left undrained, these can cause necrosis of ear cartilage and the 'cauliflower ear' appearance which is seen in some boxers and rugby players.

Acute auricular haematoma presents as a tender, tense, fluctuant collection of blood, typically on the anterior aspect of the pinna. The overlying skin can be erythematous or ecchymotic. If the haematoma has begun to clot and organise (approximately 24 hours after injury), it may become firmer.

Tx Drainage is performed under auricular nerve block (see p. 436). Patients with auricular haematomas that are <2 cm in diameter and present within 24 hours can undergo needle aspiration rather than incision and drainage. All others with require opening with a scalpel to evacuate clots.

The incision wound should be irrigated and sutured, and patients followed up to check for re-accumulation and infection in ENT clinic. Although evidence is lacking, patients are usually given 7 days of antibiotics with pseudomonas cover, such as levofloxacin or co-amoxiclav.

A bolster made of gauze tucked and taped in the antihelix with a firm bandage over can help prevent re-accumulation.

Bites to the ear

Bites to the ear may result in extensive mixed flora infection and cartilage destruction. They are usually caused by humans.

Tx Most such injuries should not be closed. Clean the area thoroughly, give antibiotics (e.g. coamoxiclav) and ensure protection against tetanus. The advice of an ENT or plastic surgeon will usually be required.

Bites (general considerations) → *p. 418.*

INJURIES AROUND THE EYE

Assessment of the eye → *p. 428.*
Corneal and other ocular injuries → *p. 428.*

Blow-out fractures of the orbit

These injuries result because the eyeball is stronger than the floor of the orbit. A direct blow on the eye by a fairly large object (e.g. a squash ball) may cause little damage to the eye – acuity may not be impaired – but push it backward and downward through the infraorbital plate. Surprisingly, the condition may go unrecognised. Suspicion is aroused by the mechanism of injury and sometimes by restriction of the extraocular muscles, resulting in double vision. Patients will be much more aware of subtle eye movement restriction (causing diplopia) than may be obvious to the clinician.

XR There may be a fluid level (blood) in the maxillary antrum on the AP radiograph and sometimes a 'teardrop' soft-tissue shadow at the top of the antrum. 'Eye brow' sign is a lucency under the superior orbital ridge, representing air from maxillary sinus in the orbit.

An associated fracture of the malar may occur, but the infraorbital plate fracture is often difficult to identify.

A CT scan shows the 'tear drop' to be orbital contents herniating into the antrum through the fracture.

Tx Elevation and reconstruction of the orbital floor may be necessary; early referral is essential. Blow-out fractures in children often cause severe vomiting and need early repair for this reason.

Eyelid lacerations

These wounds require expert assessment and repair and so must be referred to an ophthalmic surgeon immediately. Injuries below the medial canthus may involve the lacrimal apparatus; this damage is easily overlooked.

6

Injuries to the trunk

Fiqry Fadillah

Royal Free Hospital, London, UK
Magpas Air Ambulance, Huntingdon, UK

Injuries to the trunk can be difficult to diagnose and are easily overlooked, especially when associated with:

- a depressed level of consciousness
- painful skeletal injuries.

They may be immediately life-threatening but can also cause delayed deterioration. A careful and repeated systematic review of the chest, abdomen, pelvis and thoracolumbar spine should be undertaken in all patients who may have sustained multiple injuries.

> If blunt trauma results in injuries both above and below the trunk (e.g. to the head and femur), then the trunk itself is also likely to be injured.

Bruises, clothing imprints and friction burns, together with any history available from the patient or witnesses, can help to determine the direction and severity of the injuring agent.

> Stab wounds must be assumed to involve vital organs until proven otherwise.

Repeated physical examination is essential.

> Always examine the back and the perineum – they are often forgotten.

CHEST INJURIES

Chest injuries are commonly caused by major trauma such as assaults, road traffic accidents and falls. They vary in severity from minor bruising or an isolated rib fracture to severe chest wall, pulmonary and cardiac injuries that may:

- disrupt the mechanism of respiration
- impair gas exchange
- produce hypovolaemia
- cause cardiogenic shock.

Immediate assessment and management

- Initial assessment should follow the ABCDE format as described in *Chapter 1 and Chapter 2*.
- Provide supplementary oxygen as needed.
- Consider tension pneumothorax.
- Cover open (sucking) wounds of the chest wall with firm, waterproof dressings. For open pneumothoraces, use a three-sided dressing, or purpose-made seals with unidirectional valves.
- Obtain intravenous (IV) access.
- Connect the patient to appropriate monitors (arterial O_2 saturation [SaO_2], ECG and blood pressure [BP]) and measure the respiratory rate.
- Consider need for urgent imaging (→ page 28).
- Obtain a 12-lead ECG.
- Consider early analgesia.
- Consider blood gas analysis.

The RCEM Lecture Notes: Emergency Medicine, Fifth Edition. Edited by Catherine Williams and Amy Nickson.
© 2024 John Wiley & Sons Ltd. Published 2024 by John Wiley & Sons Ltd.
Companion website: www.wiley.com/go/LNEM5

Further assessment and management

Ask about

- Site and character of pain
- Dyspnoea
- Mechanism of injury
- Past medical history.

Look for

- Sweating, pallor and cyanosis
- Increased respiratory rate and work of breathing
- Uneven or abnormal chest movements
- Areas of tenderness, bruising, abrasions or crepitus
- Dullness or hyperresonance on percussion
- Reduced air entry and abnormal breath sounds
- Abnormal position of apex beat or trachea
- Increased pulse rate or paradoxical pulse
- Inaudible heart sounds (tamponade)
- Distended neck veins
- Abdominal tenderness
- SaO_2, BP and ECG abnormalities.

It is important that the back is appropriately exposed and examined – this is likely to require log rolling in multiply injured patients. The timing of this will depend on stability and need for urgent cross-sectional imaging. Minimise unnecessary log-rolling, especially if it will not change the immediate management.

Radiographs of the chest

In major trauma, when there is concern for the mechanism of injury, CT is the preferred modality of imaging. In patients with severe respiratory compromise, or if there is a delay in access to or unavailability of CT, a portable chest radiograph may be beneficial to help identify any immediate life-threating injuries that may necessitate intervention.

These may include:

A – Airway obstruction or disruption
T - Tension pneumothorax
O – Open pneumothorax
M – Massive haemothorax
F – Flail chest
C – Cardiac tamponade

> In stable patients, without concerns for spinal injury, the chest X-ray should be performed with the patient erect to permit fluid-level detection. With the patient supine, fluid present in the pleural cavity will lie behind the lung and produce a diffusely opaque lung field (→ Figure 6.1). Radiography must not precede or prevent careful initial clinical assessment.

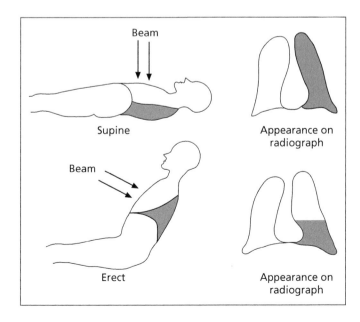

Figure 6.1 Appearance on fluid on supine and erect chest radiographs.

Wounds to the chest wall

Sucking wounds, although unusual, attract immediate attention. In contrast, small stab wounds may be underestimated. They must be assumed to penetrate the parietal pleura until proved otherwise. Confirmation of the mechanism of wounding is essential. Establish, wherever possible, the details of the weapon involved. These patients will require CT imaging followed by observation of progress (if necessary, with repeated CXRs or CT scan) and careful examination of the anaesthetised wound by an experienced surgeon in an operating theatre (but not in the ED). A long, incised wound at right angles to the line of the ribs is usually superficial.

Tx The presence of surgical emphysema, pneumothorax or haemothorax is strongly suggestive of pleural penetration. A chest drain will usually be required. This should not be inserted through the wound, but via a new incision. Most cases resolve without surgical management; thoracotomy is indicated only if bleeding is severe or if a large air leak persists.

Anti-tetanus cover must be established (→ *Chapter 21 p. 415*) and the wound covered with an antiseptic dressing. Be aware that an open wound may effectively prevent the development of a tension pneumothorax. Stab wounds should be examined, explored and closed in theatres.

Pneumothorax and haemothorax

Traumatic pneumothorax may follow rib injury, stab wounds or barotrauma. The degree of pleuritic pain and dyspnoea is very variable. Clinical suspicion should be followed by radiographic confirmation except in the case of tension pneumothorax, which should be immediately decompressed.

> A simple pneumothorax may develop into a tension pneumothorax – particularly when the patient receives positive-pressure ventilation. In the positive-pressure ventilated patients, any increase in peak airway pressures or resistance in hand-ventilation should raise the suspicion on an evolving tension pneumothorax.

An open pneumothorax occurs when the wound is equal to or bigger in size compared to the tracheal diameter. This results in preferential flow of air through the wound rather than the upper airway.

A tension pneumothorax is a life-threatening emergency; the rapid increase in intrapleural pressure compresses and shifts the mediastinum, compressing the opposite lung and impairing venous return. The patient has:

- dyspnoea
- unilaterally reduced breath sounds
- distended neck veins
- tracheal deviation (late sign)
- impaired cardiac output
- cyanosis (a late sign)
- hyperresonance to percussion over the affected side.

Haemothorax may also follow multiple rib fractures as a result of intercostal vessel damage. The bleeding is often brisk and continuous from the high systolic pressure of the intercostal arteries. In contrast, bleeding from the low-pressure pulmonary vessels usually stops with the collapse of the lung. A stab wound may cause profound bleeding from the internal thoracic artery or other intrathoracic structures. Symptoms and signs usually reflect the initial injury.

Imaging If a chest radiograph is performed, look carefully for small pneumothoraces – especially apically, laterally and medially (close to the heart border). If there is clinical suspicion of a tension pneumothorax, imaging is likely to delay treatment, and decompression should be undertaken promptly on clinical suspicion. This is especially important if the patient is intubated and receiving positive-pressure ventilation. Point of care ultrasound can help with the diagnosis, especially when there is clinical uncertainty. This will show absent lung sliding and a barcode/stratosphere sign on M-mode.

If taken, radiographs will show a hyper-expanded lung field that is displacing the mediastinum, depressing the diaphragm and compressing the opposite lung. Haemothorax may appear as blunting of the costophrenic angles. A large quantity of blood lying parallel to the diaphragm is often missed (a subpulmonary haemothorax). Depending on the patient's clinical state, haemodynamics, mechanism and suspected injuries, it may be appropriate to proceed immediately with a CT scan, thoracostomy/thoracotomy and/or surgical intervention.

Tx

- Provide supplementary oxygen as needed, including intubation and mechanical ventilation if needed. Beware of positive-pressure ventilation and monitor for signs of deterioration
- Monitor SaO_2, BP and ECG
- Consider early analgesia
- For open pneumothoraces, consider using a three-sided dressing, or purpose-made seals with unidirectional valves
- Decompression and/or drainage of pneumothorax/haemothorax.

Identification of a tension pneumothorax warrants immediate decompression → *Box 6.1*. Due to the possibility of the catheter kinking/blocking, and the variation in thickness of the chest wall, a finger thoracostomy may be more appropriate in some circumstances, followed by a tube thoracostomy.

Choice of chest drain

In general, placement of a chest drain in traumatic chest injury is via blunt dissection of the subcutaneous tissue and muscle into the pleural cavity. Blunt dissection followed by a finger sweep (technique explained below) ensures muscle fibres are separated and that there are no underlying organs that might be damaged on insertion. It also allows the individual performing the procedure to evaluate whether the lung is collapsed or expanded. These factors are less important when injuries have been identified on cross-sectional imaging before drain insertion.

Large chest drains (>24°F) are normally used for drainage of haemothoraces, which in principle allows faster flow of fluid and lesser risk of clot formation. In practice, this has not been sufficiently proven in randomised controlled trials. For stable patients with a pneumothorax, a smaller drain inserted via seldinger technique can be effective and better tolerated than an open drain.

Some small haemopneumothoraces can be managed conservatively, if the patient is stable and there are no plans to institute IPPV. Large haemothoraces, defined as >1500 mL per hemithorax or 1/3 of the patient's blood volume in the chest cavity, will necessitate simultaneous restoration of blood volume and chest drain insertion (→ *Figure 6.2 and Box 6.1*). Small, minimally symptomatic pneumothoraces do not usually require drainage, although if positive pressure ventilation is required careful monitoring (for signs of increasing size or evolving tension) is important.

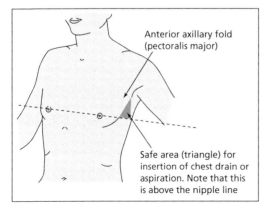

Anterior axillary fold (pectoralis major)

Safe area (triangle) for insertion of chest drain or aspiration. Note that this is above the nipple line

Figure 6.2 The triangle of safety for insertion of a chest drain.

Surgical emphysema

Gas under the skin can arise in three main ways:

1 As a complication of injury to gas-containing structures (usually lung or oesophagus – rib fracture is the most common cause)
2 After assault or injury with a high-pressure hose
3 As a result of infection with gas-forming organisms.

Subcutaneous gas in the chest or neck can usually be felt as crepitus. Other symptoms and signs result from the original insult.

Surgical emphysema after blunt trauma is usually a direct result of damage to the lung, but clinical and radiological examination may not initially confirm this. Stab and gunshot wounds may injure the pharynx or oesophagus. Infection spreading from such wounds into the mediastinum is a major, life-threatening complication.
Imaging Subcutaneous or mediastinal gas may easily be seen on a plain CXR (and CT scan) as lucent areas in the soft tissues.

Tx Look for the injury that has caused the air leak. In the case of suspected oesophageal or pharyngeal injury, prophylactic antibiotics should be started and surgical advice sought.

Rib fractures

Fractured ribs are common and result from direct blows or falls. There is local tenderness, pain on inspiration and coughing, and difficulty with trunk movements. The patient must be asked about shortness of breath and previous cardiorespiratory problems. Careful observation should reveal any significant dyspnoea. The chest should be examined thoroughly to exclude underlying pneumohaemothorax and contusion. Pain from fractures limits the patient's ability to expand their chest wall and therefore limits tidal volume. Pain reduces the ability to cough effectively. In combination, this results in atelectasis and sputum retention. This increases the risk of pneumonia, which is the commonest reason for delayed morbidity and mortality after chest trauma.

Risk factors for morbidity after rib fractures include:

Anatomical
• Number of ribs involved and degree of displacement
• Involvement of first rib
• Bilateral rib fractures
• Presence of flail segment
• Associated pulmonary contusions
Physiological
• Reduced physiological reserve:
  ○ Increasing age
  ○ Known respiratory disease e.g. COPD, asthma, obstructive sleep apnoea

Box 6.1 **Needle thoracocentesis and chest drain insertion**

Treatment of tension pneumothorax (needle thoracocentesis)

- On the affected side, identify the second intercostal space in the midclavicular line
- Insert a cannula with a syringe attached just above the rib, until air is aspirated (a cannula of at least 4.5 cm in length will be required)
- Remove the syringe and needle. There should be a hissing decompression followed by an immediate clinical improvement
- Tape the cannula in place
- Proceed to chest tube drainage
- Once the chest drain is working, remove the cannula and dress the site
- Obtain a CXR

Insertion of a chest drain

In a dire emergency, the need for a chest drain should be determined clinically, without waiting for radiographic confirmation. However, this is the exception rather than the rule. Bilateral drains may sometimes be needed. The preferred site in emergency practice is the fifth intercostal space in the midaxillary line. There are three equally important phases to the procedure:

1 Analgesia and preparation
- Position the patient in a semi-recumbent position with the affected side uppermost
- Provide supplementary oxygen as needed, attach a pulse oximeter and obtain venous access
- Consider analgesia and/or sedation depending on the patient's clinical status. Intravenous ketamine titrated to effect gives good analgesic effect without significant respiratory depression at low doses
- Perform intercostal blocks posterior to the anticipated site of drain insertion. This is done by injecting 2 mL of 1% lidocaine around the neurovascular bundle (just below the inferior border of the rib). About three intercostal nerves should be blocked to include a space above and a space below

- Infiltrate local anaesthetic down to the parietal pleura at the site of insertion. Aspiration of air bubbles into a syringe containing residual local anaesthetic is a useful confirmatory sign

2 Insertion technique
- Clean the skin and use surgical gloves and drapes
- Make an incision to the skin. Aim for the upper border of the lower rib, to avoid the neurovascular bundle
- Open the incision with forceps. Perform blunt dissection through the intercostal muscles with forceps or a curved clamp
- Pierce the parietal pleura with clamp or forceps
- Insert a gloved finger and perform a 360° sweep in the cavity to establish lung collapse
- Mount the chest drain on a clamp or pair of curved artery forceps and insert while removing finger from the incision
- Attach the drain to an underwater seal or a double Heimlich ('flutter') valve. In the case of the former, check for movements with respiration
- Advance the drain up to 15–20 cm

3 Fixation of the tube
- Secure the tube using a horizontal mattress suture wrapping both ends of the suture firmly around the drain
- Cover the site with a waterproof dressing
- Cover the dressing completely with strips of tape
- Secure the drain with a 'mesentery' of adhesive tape
- Confirm the position of the chest drain on chest X-ray
- Traditional teaching states that drains for haemothoraces should be directed downwards, and those for pneumothoraces toward the apices – in practice this is not important. A functioning chest drain should not be repositioned solely due to direction on X-ray

o Smoking history
o Overweight (BMI >25)
o Premorbid cardiovascular disease
- Reduced oxygen saturation at presentation
- Reduced vital capacity
- Post injury pneumonia

Other
- Premorbid use of anticoagulants
- Treated in low volume ('non-trauma') centres

Imaging The sensitivity for rib fractures on plain films is low, and a CT should be sought even in the presence of a

Variable	Score
Age	+1 per additional 10-year increase starting at 10 years of age
Number of rib fractures	+3 per rib fractured
Chronic lung disease	+5 if present
Pre-injury anti-coagulant use	+4
Peripheral oxygen saturation levels (SpO$_2$)	+2 per 5% decrease SpO2 starting at 94% at time of assessment

Final risk score	Probability of complications mean ± SD
0–10	13% ± 6
11–15	29% ± 8
16–20	52% ± 8
21–25	70% ± 6
26–30	80% ± 6
31+	88% ± 7

Figure 6.3 Battle score.

'normal' X-ray if the suspicion of injury remains high. It should be noted that isolated, non-complicated rib fractures may only require conservative management, and thus imaging may not always be necessary.

Scoring systems are available to predict the risk of complications after blunt chest trauma and hence influence the choice of imaging and analgesia administered. Battle score is one such tool, utilising age, number of rib fractures, chronic lung disease, pre-injury anti-coagulant use and peripheral oxygen saturation levels (SpO$_2$). A high score, together with a suspicious mechanism of injury, should prompt a CT scan → Figure 6.3.

Management of rib fractures

- Provide supplementary oxygen as needed
- Monitor SpO$_2$, BP and ECG and measure the respiratory rate
- Consider blood gases.
- Early and effective analgesia is essential
  Non-invasive
  o Paracetamol
  o Ibuprofen
  o Regular oral morphine or opioid PCA (patient-controlled analgesia)
  o Consider 5% lidocaine patches

Invasive (regional anaesthesia)
Consider invasive pathway in those >65 years of age, ≥3 rib fractures, presence of flail segments/underlying lung contusions, the presence of a chest drain, worsening pain score/oxygen saturations despite using the non-invasive pathway and a Battle score >15.

All regional anaesthetic techniques for rib fracture analgesia impair impulse transmission at various points along the intercostal nerve. Thoracic epidural analgesia remains the gold standard analgesic modality. They are the most widely studied mode of analgesia, and their use in rib fractures is endorsed by several systematic reviews and international bodies. Alternatives include serratus anterior, erector spinae and paravertebral blocks.

- Consider an urgent intensive care opinion if the patient has evidence of underlying contusion resulting in severe hypoxaemia.
- Surgical stabilisation with metal rib reinforcements may be required, especially with underlying lung injury and presence of a flail segment. This aims to allow earlier weaning from ventilator support, reduce acute complications and avoid chronic pain sometimes associated with permanent deformity of the chest wall. Consider discussion with the cardiothoracic team.

Uncomplicated rib fractures

Patients with uncomplicated rib fractures may be discharged home with adequate advice on conservative management.

- Prior to discharge ensure that the patient is able to take deep inspirations and cough adequately.
- Provision of adequate analgesia is essential and the patient should be encouraged to take this regularly.
- Breathing exercises should be recommended. Advise the patient to perform these hourly while awake:
  o Take a deep breath in through the nose to fully expand the lungs and hold for 5–10 seconds before exhaling through the mouth. Repeat 5–10 times per hour.
- Encourage patients to remain mobile to improve ventilation and reduce atelectasis
- Providing support to the chest wall by winding a scarf or similar around the chest and pulling on the crossed-over ends while coughing provides a surprising amount of pain relief. Strapping of the ribs, however, is contraindicated.
- Patients should be encouraged to stop smoking.
- Patients with large breasts may benefit from using a supportive bra, including while sleeping. The fascia and ligamentous structure of the breast is in parts directly continuous with pectoral fascia and rib periosteum and so gravitational movement of breast tissue can exacerbate pain.
- Advise the patient of the need to return in case of increasing breathlessness, signs of a chest infection, or development of surgical emphysema.

Flail segment

> When a rib is broken at two points, the middle section is not mechanically linked to the rest of the rib cage and tends to move in the opposite direction during breathing.

A flail chest occurs when a part of the thoracic cage moves independently from the rest of the chest wall. There is paradoxical movement of this free segment – it is drawn inwards on inspiration and moves outwards on expiration – and thus impedes ventilation. Flail chest has been defined in a variety of ways, but at least two fractures per rib in at least two ribs are needed to produce a flail segment. Large flail segments may extend bilaterally or even involve the sternum. This injury is best detected clinically but is often overlooked. A large area of crepitus is usually apparent on palpation. Respiratory movements are best observed from the bottom of the trolley, looking for an area of the chest wall that moves out in expiration. Even apparently minor degrees of 'paradoxical respiration' are associated with significant hypoxaemia, because there is usually a large underlying pulmonary contusion. Patients with flail segment will require positive pressure ventilation and consideration of rib fixation surgery.

Tracheobronchial tree injuries

These are potentially fatal and may occur due to direct penetrating trauma, hanging, direct blunt trauma to the neck, rapid deceleration and blast injuries. Advanced airway skills (e.g. fibre-optic insertion of an endotracheal tube past the injured site or selective intubation of the unaffected bronchus) may be required.

Larynx

There may be localised pain and tenderness, hoarseness, subcutaneous emphysema and local crepitus. An urgent ENT opinion is indicated, and a surgical airway may be required.

Trachea

The signs may be subtle and easily overlooked. If suspected, obtain anaesthetic and surgical advice. Perform CT scan and bronchoscopy.

Bronchus

This is rare, difficult to detect on physical examination and often fatal. A large air leak after a thoracostomy is suspicious. Bronchoscopy is diagnostic. Ventilation of patients with tracheobronchial injuries may be difficult and indeed hazardous.

Fracture of the sternum

Sternal fractures are not usually associated with instability of the rib cage and may be overlooked in patients with multiple injuries. Local examination reveals tenderness and sometimes swelling. Respiratory movements may not be affected. Sternal fractures may be associated with injury to the heart and great vessels.

Investigations Sternal fractures are best detected on lateral sternal radiographs and are easily overlooked on plain chest X-ray. If there are ongoing concerns, proceed to CT, especially if there is suspected underlying injury to thoracic contents. Perform a 12-lead ECG if a fracture is identified. The use of cardiac biomarkers such as troponin remains unclear. There is level 2 evidence to suggest that an underlying blunt cardiac injury can be ruled out in patients with a normal ECG and a negative troponin I with 100% negative predictive value, although the optimal timing of troponin measurement remains unclear. If troponin is elevated, it does little to characterise or prognosticate the cardiac injury.

Tx This consists of observation, exclusion of associated injuries to thoracic contents and symptomatic pain relief. Reduction or internal fixation is not usually indicated, although fractures with a large amount of depression of the inner table should be discussed with a cardiothoracic surgeon.

Traumatic asphyxia syndrome

Diffuse crushing of the chest (e.g. by a trench collapse) will cause transient venous engorgement and petechial haemorrhages over the upper chest and face. There may also be subconjunctival haemorrhages. Maximal barotrauma occurs in the presence of airway obstruction.

The prognosis is good if the patient is rescued promptly. If crushing is not quickly relieved, hypoxia is severe with lung contusion and alveolar collapse. Some patients may initially appear deceptively well after extrication. Pulmonary oedema gradually develops and gas exchange is impaired – a form of acute respiratory distress syndrome.

Tx Provide supplementary oxygen. Steroids are of no benefit. If there is associated bronchospasm in the early stages, nebulised salbutamol will be useful.

Injury to the heart

Damage may be inflicted by a gunshot, a stabbing or blunt decelerating forces. Contrary to popular belief, these injuries may not be instantly fatal and may remain undetected in the patient who is slowly dying from multiple injuries. The paucity of specific signs may frustrate early and precise diagnosis

Penetrating injury

Stab wounds anywhere between the midclavicular lines, from the lower third of the neck to the epigastrium and around the flank, have the potential to involve mediastinal structures. Beware of small entry wounds, especially in the back or axillae.

Laceration of the thick left ventricular wall may not be as catastrophic as damage to less muscular structures. Pump failure may occur because of valve damage, hypovolaemia or tamponade.

Haemopericardium may produce a life-threatening cardiac tamponade at any time, with high venous pressure, muffled heart sounds and falling BP (Beck's triad), which may be difficult to detect clinically, especially if there are other confounding injuries (very low sensitivity). There may be distended neck veins. Classically, the systolic BP is lower during inspiration (pulsus paradoxus - 98% sensitivity and 83% specificity). Tamponade may also cause a paradoxical rise in venous pressure during inspiration (Kussmaul's sign - 26% sensitivity, 96% specificity). Profound shock and IPPV may invalidate these signs.

Point of care focused ultrasound can be used to identify pericardial effusion and tamponade:

- The absence of a dilated IVC (>2.1 cm diameter) excludes the diagnosis with 97% sensitivity.
- Right ventricular collapse is 50% sensitive and 80% specific.
- Absence of right atrial collapse has a 90% negative predictive value for tamponade.

Blunt injury

Blunt injuries are more common. Most minor cardiac contusions probably resolve without detection. At the other extreme, fatal dysrhythmias may not be associated with structural damage *post mortem*. A few patients, in between, present with symptoms and signs typical of myocardial ischaemia, including ECG changes.

Direct damage to coronary arteries is rare but septal rupture, damage to papillary muscle and chordae tendineae, and tears of the atria or right ventricle do occur. Rupture of the sturdy left ventricle is rare.

It is useful to distinguish between cardiac contusion and concussion. The latter is defined as the occurrence of a dysrhythmia without ECG or biochemical evidence of muscle necrosis. Most of these dysrhythmias are transient, but sudden death has been reported after relatively minor blows to the sternum (commotio cordis).

Tx

- Provide supplementary oxygen as needed.
- Obtain IV access.
- Consider aspiration of the pericardium.
- In cases of witnessed cardiac arrest following penetrating injury, consider resuscitative thoracotomy (*Box 6.2*).
- Seek cardiothoracic advice.
- Perform routine blood tests and cross-match blood.
- Obtain an ECG.
- In less urgent cases, the problem is always the initial paucity of physical signs. Admit the patient to a high-dependency area and monitor carefully.

Injuries to the great vessels

Immediate survival depends on the formation of an acute false aneurysm. Stab wounds may inflict injury at any site, but the more common deceleration injury usually produces a lesion at the level of the aortic isthmus. The intima and media rupture, but the adventitia and adjacent mediastinal structures may provide a sufficiently strong sheath to contain the arterial pressure for a few hours, or indeed many years. The expanding haematoma may occlude the origin of one or more of the vessels arising from the aortic arch. Patients may develop neurological symptoms presenting as confusion or weakness. Blood pressure and pulse may differ in the two arms, although this is neither sensitive nor specific. Pain radiating to the back is common.

These injuries can be overlooked, even at thoracotomy. The history is important. Most are associated with injuries elsewhere after high-speed road traffic accidents or falls.

Investigations: A plain CXR, if performed, may show haemorrhage into the mediastinum and other indirect signs of blood vessel injury:

- Widened mediastinum (mediastinum/chest width >25%; may be obscured by lung injury and not present in 10% of cases)
- Trachea displaced to the right
- Left main-stem bronchus depressed
- Aortic knuckle absent
- Left apical pleural cap (the left paraspinal line is displaced laterally and extends up and over the apex of the left lung)
- Broad right paratracheal stripe
- Separation of calcium deposits in the aortic wall
- Other signs of severe chest trauma (rib fractures, pulmonary contusion, haemopneumothorax and ruptured diaphragm).

High-resolution CT (HRCT) provides much more information, especially with contrast angiography, and is the definitive investigation once the diagnosis is suspected. Focused bedside echo may reveal blood within the pericardial sac.

Oesophageal injury

This may be caused by penetrating trauma. Blunt rupture may follow vomiting (Boerhaave's syndrome → Chapter 16, page 312) or a direct blow to the epigastrium; it may also complicate endoscopy. Consider oesophageal injury if there is:

- gas in the mediastinum on radiograph
- unexplained shock after trunk injury
- left pneumothorax without rib fracture
- gastric contents in a chest drain.

Mediastinitis develops insidiously and is often fatal.
Imaging There is mediastinal gas on plain radiographs and CT scan.

Resuscitative thoracotomy

Tx Early diagnosis, antibiotics and surgery are essential.

Emergency resuscitative thoracotomy may be performed in the emergency department or in the pre-hospital environment (→ Box 6.2 and Figures 6.5 and 6.6). The main indication for resuscitative thoracotomy is in a patient with penetrating chest trauma in a peri-arrest state or established cardiac arrest for a short period of time. Consideration should be given to abdominal wounds that may breach the thoracic cavity. After more than 10 min of cardiac arrest, outcome from resuscitative thoracotomy is likely to be poor, and it is generally not recommended, although this should be determined on a case-by-case basis.

Survival after thoracotomy in blunt trauma is poor, especially when presenting with no signs of life. In blunt polytrauma patients, survival rates after resuscitative thoracotomy are in the region of 1–2%.

The European Resuscitation Council (ERC) published a guidance in 2015 on traumatic cardiac arrest and when to consider resuscitative thoracotomy (→ Figure 6.4). Relative contraindications to performing resuscitative thoracotomy include:

- Blunt polytrauma
- CPR >5 min with no return of spontaneous circulation
- Severe head injury
- Inadequate training, equipment, assistance or system resources to support ongoing care.

The clamshell thoractomy allows rapid access to the pericardium, myocardium, lungs and descending aorta.
The potential aims of the procedure are:

- to relieve a pericardial tamponade
- to gain direct control of intra-thoracic haemorrhage by suturing a myocardial wound or by using hilar compression/rotation to arrest pulmonary bleeding
- to allow internal cardiac massage
- to compress the descending aorta so that blood flow is prioritised to the brain and heart, while limiting blood loss from haemorrhage below the diaphragm.

The best prospects for success are for stab wounds in which the patient arrests in the presence of clinicians; where pericardial tamponade can be relieved, the cardiac wound repaired, and internal cardiac massage performed.

ABDOMINAL INJURIES

Around 20% of major trauma cases involve injuries to the abdomen. However, they may not be initially apparent on clinical examination, especially if patients are unconscious. Even in awake patients, the extent of the injuries may not be immediately apparent, e.g. handlebar injuries.

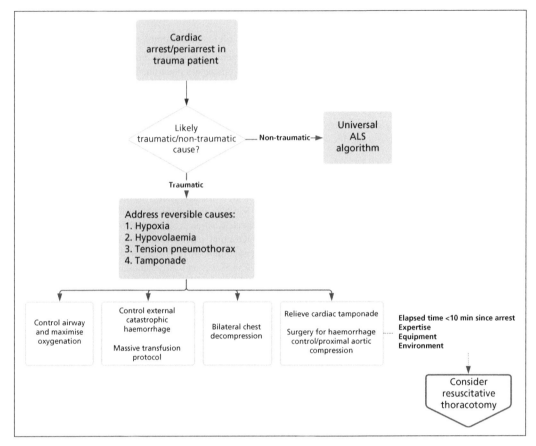

Figure 6.4 Traumatic cardiac arrest algorithm. Adapted from European Resuscitation Council guidelines 2015.

Abdominal injuries can occur following blunt and penetrating trauma. Blunt abdominal trauma often occurs secondary to compressive forces or decelerations. Assault (including kicking, punching and using a blunt weapon), falls, road traffic collisions (including injuries secondary to seat belts) and sporting accidents may inflict compressive forces.

In decelerating injuries, stretching and shearing can occur at the points where mobile contents in the abdomen are anchored. This may cause tearing of the mesentery of the bowel, injury to the blood vessels within the mesentery and shearing of organs off their vascular pedicle leading to bleeding and organ ischaemia.

Be cautious when examining patients with a history suggestive of penetrating trauma secondary to weapons, e.g. knife injury, gunshot, etc. The entry point may appear rather innocuous but is poorly predictive of the depth and extent of the underlying damage.

The initial approach to a patient with suspected abdominal injury should follow the same principles as outlined in *Chapter 2 Major Trauma*. Look in particular for:

- Bruising, abrasions or wounds suggest penetrating trauma.
- Abdominal distension in a patient with signs of hypovolaemia is suggestive of intra-abdominal haemorrhage.
- Tenderness and rigidity due to a peritoneal irritation secondary to a hollow viscus perforation may initially be absent - serial examinations are important.

Stab wounds to the abdomen

Small external wounds are poor predictors of depth and extent of the injury. Injury to the intestine and mesentery may not be accompanied by the rapid clinical deterioration usually associated with stab wounds to the liver, spleen and major vessels.

Obtain surgical advice. Laparotomy has an associated morbidity. This can be reduced if a selective approach is used.

Box 6.2 **How to perform resuscitative thoracotomy (see *Figures 6.5 and 6.6*)**

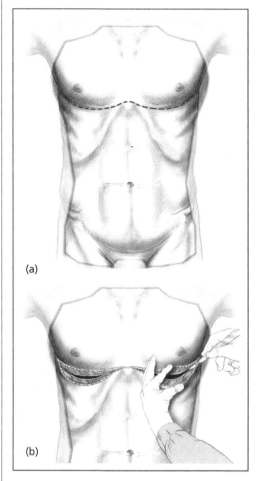

(a)

(b)

Figure 6.5 Thoracotomy incision. Journal of Visceral Surgery, Volume 154, Supplement 1, December 2017, Pages S61–S67.

1 Intubate and ventilate the patient
2 Have two operators performing the procedure. Each operator performs a finger thoracostomy on their side using a scalpel and finger (±blunt dissecting forceps) in the fifth intercostal space, triangle of safety
3 Each operator to declare if the lung feels inflated. Check if the patient has ROSC.
4 Join the skin incisions to the midline
5 Use trauma shears ('tuff cuts') to cut through the layers of intercostal muscle
6 Cut the sternum with trauma shears or a Gigli saw
7 Open the 'clam shell' using rib spreaders

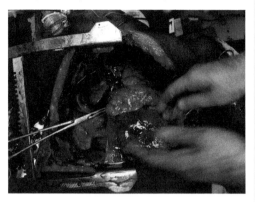

Figure 6.6 'Clamshell' thoracotomy incision follows the fourth or fifth intercostal space, joining bilateral thoracostomies in the mid axillary line. The sternum can then be divided with scissors. International Journal of Surgery, Volume 33, Part B, September 2016, Pages 202–208.

8 Tent the pericardium with forceps and open with a longitudinal midline incision. 'Deliver' the heart out of the pericardium and remove clots

Procedures after an emergency thoracotomy
• Open cardiac massage – one hand in front and one behind. The blood is 'milked' from the apex upwards at 80 bpm
• Internal defibrillation with internal paddles (up to 10 J energy)
• Cardiac haemostasis
  ○ Closure of cardiac wound with sutures/staples/pledgets fashioned from the pericardium
  ○ An 18-G French Foley catheter may be inserted through a wound in the heart and the balloon inflated inside. Gentle traction on the distal catheter then achieves temporary haemostasis. If the catheter is connected to an IV infusion, fluids and drugs can be given by the intracardiac route.
• Clamping of major lacerations of the lung or perform a pulmonary hilum twist (cut the inferior pulmonary ligament and twist the lung on the hilum – pulling the lower lobe towards you and up)
• Packing apices with towels if bleeding from this area
• Manual compression of the descending aorta (a hand behind the left lung) to optimise cerebral circulation and reduce major abdominal blood loss

Patients with immediate evidence of an intra-abdominal catastrophe may need to be taken straight to theatre for surgical exploration and repair. Most patients will require CT imaging to assess the extent of injury.

The wound should be covered with an antiseptic dressing. Antitetanus prophylaxis is required.

Blunt abdominal trauma

Blunt abdominal injury should be considered if any of the following apply:

- Localising symptoms or signs
- Marks on the abdominal wall, e.g. seatbelt sign
- Suspicious mechanism of injury, e.g. handlebar injuries, fractures to the lower ribs, etc.
- Injuries both above and below the abdomen
- Unexplained hypovolaemia
- Abnormally pale patient
- Reduced conscious level, so patient difficult to assess.

Intra-abdominal injuries in the absence of external bleeding are much slower to present and more difficult to diagnose. Handlebar injuries, for example, may lead to a perforation of the duodenum which may present with delayed onset of pain and guarding. Compression of the pancreas against the lumbar spine may result in pancreatic injury, which may present with symptoms of pancreatitis a number of hours after the injury. These injuries are not easily visualised on CT.

Stable patients with a normal initial CT scan may therefore require close observation and consideration of an explorative laparoscopy/laparotomy at the first indication of significant problems.

Abdominal pain may be caused by acute gastric dilatation or paralytic ileus associated with an injury elsewhere. Gastric dilatation is a well-recognised complication of head injury, particularly in children. Gastric stasis can also be caused by pain or secondary to medications, e.g. opiates. Insertion of a nasogastric tube may resolve distension and pain. If the tube is wide-bore, it will also remove partially digested food and thus reduce the risk of aspiration into the lungs.

Splenic injuries are common. They may occur with very little in the way of external signs. Very careful monitoring under the care of the surgical team with consideration of repeat CT scan is required. Options include conservative management, splenic artery embolisation and surgical repair or splenectomy. Post-splenectomy prophylactic antibiotics and immunisations will be required.

In patients with **microscopic** haematuria following a blunt trauma, the incidence of renal parenchymal/tract injuries requiring intervention are extremely low. In most cases, no further imaging is needed and a repeat urinalysis (e.g. in a week's time) and follow-up by a GP are all that are required. Fifty per cent of patients with **macroscopic** haematuria have renal injuries; these patients warrant a CT scan.

Children are more vulnerable to significant renal injury, and a lower threshold for considering imaging in asymptomatic haematuria following blunt abdominal trauma is reasonable.

Immediate action

- Attend to ABCs and the principles of assessment of major trauma as per Chapter 2.
- Cover eviscerated gut with warm saline packs – do not try to push it back. Manipulating the mesentery potentiates shock.
- Obtain IV access.

> Fluid loss into the abdomen is usually underestimated.

- Examine the abdomen, noting areas of tenderness, guarding and lacerations, and clothing imprints and grazes. Listen for bowel sounds.
- Administer analgesia if required.
- The back and perineum must be examined, but the timing may need to be deferred especially if unstable. Stab wounds and bullet entry and exit points may be missed if these areas are overlooked.
- Consider performing a rectal examination (noting injuries, sphincter tone, presence of blood, the wall and contents, and prostate gland).
- Obtain details of the incident, past medical history, medication and time of last food and drink.
- Consider inserting a urinary catheter if there is no urethral injury.
- Consider passing a large-bore nasogastric tube if there is no basal skull fracture.

Imaging in abdominal trauma

Computed tomography: CT is the imaging modality of choice in most cases. Any delay that it may cause must be balanced against a corresponding delay in definitive care. CT performs well for the detection of retroperitoneal pathology but may miss gastrointestinal injury such as perforation.

Point of Care Ultrasound (FAST scan): this is widely used in the ED. In experienced hands, it is good for solid organ assessment and detection of free fluid. A negative

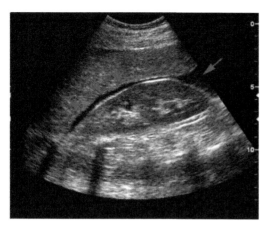

Figure 6.7 Fluid within Morrison's pouch – red arrows. Image reproduced from Public domain, via Wikimedia Commons.

scan does not rule out abdominal injury, as free fluid in excess of 200 mL is required before it can be detected by ultrasonography. Presence or absence of free fluid on ultrasound should not be used to determine need for CT.

Ultrasound should not delay CT scanning or transfer for definitive care but may be useful in resource-poor settings or if there is a delay to CT. Free fluid seen within the abdomen in an unstable patient may help with the decision to transfer to theatre instead of CT.

Three views are of interest: right upper quadrant, left upper quadrant and suprapubic. The right upper quadrant is examined by placing the curvilinear probe down the mid-axillary line starting at the right 8th rib to 11th rib.

The hepatorenal interface (Morrison's pouch) is first identified, with subsequent assessment of the sub-phrenic and pleural spaces, down to the inferior pole of the kidney.

Free fluid is shown as a black hypoechoic structure, as indicated by red arrows in the image above, sitting within Morison's pouch (→ Figure 6.7). This is repeated on the patient's left, examining the perisplenic region and the splenorenal interface.

The suprapubic view examines the most dependant peritoneal space in the supine trauma patient. The probe is held in the transverse and longitudinal views, using the bladder as a sonographic window, to examine the pouch of Douglas (in women) and rectovesical space.

Damage control resuscitation

Often severely injured patients may be too unwell physiologically to tolerate a long operation. 'Damage control' surgery is thus performed to treat life-threatening

injuries, minimise contamination and ensure adequate perfusion to vital organs. Resuscitation then continues on the intensive care unit, before considering further exploration and repair in theatres at a later date.

This aims to ensure that patients are adequately resuscitated, warmed, and any biochemical disturbance or coagulopathy are stabilised prior to definitive treatment.

Abdominal trauma in pregnancy

Changes in pregnancy

A – pregnant patients are at particular risk of aspiration due to delayed gastric emptying, elevated gastric pressures and gastro-oesophageal incompetence. The nasal mucosa is engorged and oedematous, resulting in greater resistance to air flow. Weight gain and breast enlargement can make direct laryngoscopy more difficult.

B – there is an increase in oxygen consumption. Compensatory rises in respiratory rate and tidal volume occur at the expense of a reduced functional residual capacity. This means that there is a shortened apnoeic desaturation time. Anatomically, the gravid uterus pushes on the diaphragm and decreases the expiratory reserve volume by 10–20%.

C – cardiac output increases from 5 to 7 L/min, with an increase in both stroke volume (from 65 to 80–90 mL) and heart rate (from 75 to 85–90 beats per minute). Blood pressure decreases (and is lowest in the second trimester) but steadily increases to pre-pregnancy values by the third trimester.

Signs of intra-abdominal bleeding tend to be reduced or modified in pregnancy as by the third trimester, plasma volume increases by up to 45%. Systemic vascular resistance decreases (down by as much as 40%) – in fact, the vascular system becomes fairly refractory to the effects of vasoconstrictors such as angiotensin and vasopressin. The inferior vena cava is compressed by the gravid uterus in the supine position, decreasing the preload. Pregnant women are at particular risk of postural hypotension during rapid postural changes.

Tx The treatment of an injured pregnant patient follows the usual ABCDE format, but in addition there should be consideration of the following:

• Early involvement of the obstetrics team if ≥23 weeks and/or suspected uterine contractions, placental abruption or traumatic uterine rupture.
• Manual displacement of the uterus to avoid inferior vena cava compression. This is normally required

from mid-way through the second trimester. At term, the vena cava is completely occluded in 90% of supine pregnant women.

- Extra vigilance in treating early hypovolaemia. Signs of shock are delayed because of maternal hyperaemia.
- Consider early ultrasound scan of the abdomen, uterus and fetus.
- Confirmation of the normal fetal heartbeat. A Doppler ultrasound probe is better for this purpose than a fetal stethoscope. Consider early monitoring of the fetal heart rate by fetocardiotocograph (FCTG) in seriously injured patients.
- Administration of anti-RhD immunoglobulin to rhesus D-negative women.

Pelvic injuries

Bony injury to the pelvis

There are two distinct types of pelvic fracture:

1. After violent injury, the fracture is:
    - unstable
    - crushed or displaced at more than one point
    - associated with major blood loss and visceral injury.
2. After a fall in an osteoporotic patient, the injury is:
    - stable
    - anterior and minimally displaced
    - associated with pre-existing frailty and other medical problems.

Tenderness is usually apparent. Testing stability by attempting to move the iliac wings is unreliable and contraindicated – it provokes bleeding. Straight-leg raising is usually reduced or impossible.

Imaging An AP radiograph may be useful as part of the primary survey but should not delay CT scanning, especially in patients suspected of having pelvic fractures.

Tx Initial management of major pelvic fractures includes:

- resuscitation
- pain control
- pelvic binder (*Chapter 2 Page 26*).

In a haemodynamically compromised patient with mechanism suggestive of a pelvic injury, a pelvic binder should be applied. This provides stability, allows for clot formation and may prevent ongoing haemorrhage. A pelvic binder is a treatment intervention rather than a

packaging device. Pelvic binders should be applied next to the skin, paying extra caution to the external genitalia in the male population. Appropriate application is at the level of the greater trochanter.

Single fractures of the pubic rami are rarely associated with visceral injury or significant blood loss. They are, however, painful and restrict the mobility of the elderly patients in whom they most commonly occur. Hospital admission may be required for a few days before gentle mobilisation. Look for the cause of the fall. Also consider fracture of the neck of the femur.

Injury to the pelvic viscera

Injury within the pelvis may cause profound blood loss. The pelvic venous plexus is often involved. Massive blood loss usually occurs from injury to superior gluteal artery or anterior branches of the internal iliac artery.

Imaging A CT scan is essential if visceral injury is suspected.

Tx Transfuse and refer. Apply a pelvic binder. Discuss early with interventional radiology and the surgical team.

Urogenital injuries

Perineal injury is easily missed. There may be:

- a painful desire to micturate
- local swelling or bruising
- blood at the external meatus.

Suspect damage to urogenital area if the patient has had a straddle injury. In a male patient, there may be cranial migration of the prostate (the 'missing prostate' sign). This is associated with rupture of the membranous urethra and is diagnosed by rectal examination. The corresponding sign in a female patient is bogginess of the anterior vaginal wall on pelvic examination.

Extravasation of urine into the perineal tissues is unusual immediately after injury, more commonly developing after 1 or 2 hours. It suggests injury to the extraperitoneal part of the bladder or urethra. Intraperitoneal rupture of the bladder produces the earlier abdominal signs of pain and shock.

Imaging A CT cystogram may be performed at the time of trauma CT, if there is high suspicion of a urogenital injury and the patient is otherwise stable.

A retrograde urethrogram and/or a voiding cystourethrogram may be indicated to identify urethral and bladder injury. Discuss with urology and radiology colleagues.

Tx Intraperitoneal bladder rupture will require surgical repair, whereas extraperitoneal bladder rupture may be managed conservatively. The majority of urethral injuries are incomplete transections. The maintenance of urothelial continuity will reduce the severity of late stricture formation. It is therefore important that these injuries are diagnosed early and treated gently by an experienced surgeon.

Other perineal injuries

Lacerations of the perineal body or the anal or vaginal margins should be assumed to penetrate deeply until proven otherwise. This will entail careful and skilled examination under good operating conditions. If there is any suggestion of intraperitoneal extension, laparotomy will be required – possibly with faecal diversion. Early referral is essential.

7

The lower limb

Abu Hassan

Sheffield Children's Hospital and the Northern General Hospital, Sheffield, UK

GENERAL APPROACH TO LIMB PROBLEMS

This section should be read before turning to the relevant anatomical site.

Crush injuries and myoglobinuria → p. 262.
Hand → p. 131.
Small wounds and localised infections → p. 410.
Upper limb → p. 114.

> Four four-letter words describe a structured approach to examination of the limbs: LOOK, FEEL, MOVE, X-RAY.

Immediate assessment and management

- Start with the ABCDE approach as discussed in *Chapters 1 and 2.*
- Apply direct pressure to stop any bleeding.
- Expose the affected part; cut off clothes as necessary.
- Take a brief history.
- Confirm that the presenting problem is confined to the limb.
- Confirm the presence of distal pulses and the integrity of the nerve supply.
- Splint fractures.
- Give analgesia early on; this may be systemic or local.
- Finally undertake a detailed local examination including a comparison with the opposite limb.

If there is a clear history of trauma, it is useful to reconstruct the incident to appreciate the forces applied and to consider the biomechanics of the injury:

- Healthy young bones will undergo considerable elastic deformation (e.g. the femoral shaft will bend over 10° before breaking). At breaking point, stored energy is released and the limb suddenly deforms further, inflicting secondary soft-tissue injury. Often, this is more important than the underlying fracture.
- Twisting tends to produce spiral fractures.
- Direct blows cause transverse fractures, which may be compound.
- Sheering forces raise contused skin flaps.
- Forces applied to the heel of the falling body and causing a fracture of the calcaneum will be transmitted cranially and may produce a fracture of the knee, hips or lumbar spine.
- An evident knee injury, sustained by a front-seat car passenger, may draw attention away from an occult hip dislocation.

> **Do not consider the limb in isolation as:**
>
> - Injuries around the shoulder and thigh may cause hypovolaemia.
> - Painful limb injuries may be associated with life-threatening, but less painful, trunk trauma.
> - Limb infection may have systemic effects.
> - Limb pain may be symptomatic of trunk pathology (e.g. cardiac pain, sciatica and herpes zoster infection).

Wounds

Wounds should not be explored at this stage. Sterile dressings or iodine soaks are the only necessary treatment. A photograph of the injury will prevent the need for frequent re-examination by attending clinicians. Foreign bodies must be left alone, even if they are grossly protruding, until resuscitation has begun and the environment and staff are prepared for a careful, controlled assessment. Patients with grossly contaminated wounds and compound fractures should receive intravenous (IV) antibiotics (e.g. flucloxacillin or co-amoxiclav as per local guidelines) and anti-tetanus prophylaxis as soon as possible.

Pain

Splintage and reassurance are very important. Application of a splint can provide excellent pain relief in many cases. Pain may be controlled by nitrous oxide or methoxyflurane while a splint is applied. Parenteral analgesia, often opiates, is frequently required. In some situations, a local anaesthetic block may be preferable.

Radiographs

Radiographs complement but do not replace a full clinical examination. Good radiographs demand good viewing facilities. The doctor should have a high-quality screen and charts showing the times of appearance and fusion of primary and secondary ossification centres.

> Do not attempt to interpret radiographs without first examining the patient.

Vascular problems related to injury

Specific vascular problems → p. 110.

> All urgent limb problems are related to blood supply.

Occlusion

Displaced fractures around the elbow and the knee are commonly associated with vascular occlusion. Do not assume that distal ischaemia has been caused by transient vascular spasm. Urgent specialist referral is necessary. Limb viability is threatened if a major occlusion persists for 4 hours or more.

> Healthy young limbs are more at risk from vascular occlusion of main vessels than are old ischaemic limbs because the latter have had time to develop a collateral circulation.

Bleeding

Elevation is an effective first-aid measure for major venous haemorrhage but is often impossible to achieve because of associated bony injury. Applying artery clips to spurting vessels in the emergency department (ED) will usually inflict further injury, especially as most major limb vessels run alongside peripheral nerves. Instead, local pressure should be applied. Bleeding into damaged muscle is a much more common problem.

Applying a pressure dressing

When faced with a bleeding wound to a limb, manual pressure and elevation of the limb is the first measure. Then a pressure dressing can be applied for 30–60 min prior to closure of the wound. Applying a flat dressing to the wound and wrapping with a bandage will apply pressure circumferentially to the limb, whereas a rolled bolster applied over the wound will direct the pressure onto the bleeding vessels (→ *Figure 7.1*).

Compartment syndrome

The closed fascial compartments of the limbs prevent contused muscles and haematomas from expanding indefinitely. Interstitial pressure rises causing pain and ischaemia (→ *p. 112*).

Plaster casts

Application of a cast is the most common way of immobilising an injured area of a limb, be it an injury to the bone or to the soft tissue. However, acute injuries may swell considerably in the first 48 hours and restriction of that expansion by a cast can cause severe ischaemia. The inelasticity of fascial compartments, particularly in the lower leg, can have a similar effect.

Utilising a 'backslab' (an incomplete plaster secured with bandages) or splitting a cast longitudinally reduces this risk but does not necessarily completely protect the limb from the underlying ischaemia. All plasters must be well padded, especially over bony protuberances, and the patient must have:

- instructions to elevate the limb and crutches or a sling if needed

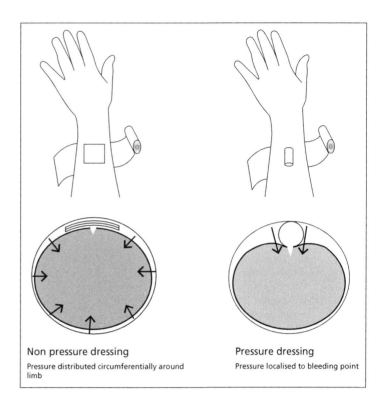

Non pressure dressing
Pressure distributed circumferentially around limb

Pressure dressing
Pressure localised to bleeding point

Figure 7.1 Pressure dressing application.

- advice on the care of the cast and written advice regarding the symptoms of compartment syndrome and ischaemia (plaster instructions)
- appropriate follow-up.

All staff who deal with patients in casts must be aware of the need to look out for the signs of compartment syndrome (→ p. 112) as well as the more widely appreciated changes to the warmth, colour and capillary refill of the digits.

The National Institute for Health and Clinical Excellence (NICE) recommends that all patients who are being treated with a plaster cast or other immobilisation of the lower limb should be risk assessed for venous thromboembolism (VTE). If they are found to be at significant risk of VTE, they should be offered thromboprophylaxis for the duration of the treatment.

Phlegmasia cerulea dolens

This is an uncommon but serious complication of DVT where complete obstruction of the deep vein causes massive fluid stasis and oedema, leading to obstruction of arterial supply, and ultimately ischaemic injury. It is characterised by severe pain, swelling and cyanosis of the affected limb. Compartment syndrome can also occur. Initial treatment is with elevation and IV heparin. In severe cases, surgical thrombectomy or catheter directed thrombolysis may be needed. The risk of concurrent pulmonary embolism in these patients is high.

Diagnosis and management of suspected deep vein thrombosis (DVT) → *p. 110.*
Risk factors for VTE → Box 13.13 on p. 228.

Physiotherapy

The help of a physiotherapist can be invaluable in treating a wide range of soft-tissue injuries and other conditions. Particular benefits are seen with early physiotherapy and include the following:

- Reduction in pain, bruising and swelling
- Maintenance of muscle fibre length and range of movements
- Early mobilisation and restoration of function.

Physiotherapy also offers:

- Re-examination of the injury and the level of function
- Assessment for and training with walking aids
- Restoration of the patient's confidence
- Skilled follow-up.

Crutches

Crutches are required for emergency patients with a large variety of differing problems. They may be utilised to enable a limb to be:

- non-weight-bearing
- partial weight-bearing

All patients given crutches must be instructed about their safe care and usage and should also be observed in action.

Local injection of steroids

The injection of a long-acting steroid-type drug into a joint, tendon sheath, bursa or other suitable area can bring long-lasting relief to a large number of inflammatory soft-tissue conditions. This is best undertaken as a pre-planned procedure in an outpatient setting (e.g. rheumatology outpatients).

Sports injuries

Soft-tissue and bony injuries, secondary to trauma sustained during sport, are common presentations. Many such injuries can also occur during non-sporting activities. There are three specific needs of the sportsperson:

1 A quick return to normal training and activity
2 Maintenance of muscle fibre length
3 Protection from re-injury when the activity is resumed.

Accurate diagnosis is essential. A good general recipe for treating sports injuries is:

- 3 days of complete rest (crutches/sling if required)
- appropriate analgesia
- early physiotherapy.

Ice and elevation are useful in the early stages to reduce discomfort and swelling. There should be a return to about 50% training levels as soon as possible and then a gradual build-up to full activity.

See also the appropriate anatomical sections of this chapter and Chapters 8 and 9.

THE HIP AND THIGH

> The hip joint capsule is innervated from the L2–4 level. These dermatomes extend to the knee, hence the common complaint of hip pathology apparently arising in the knee. The hip must be examined whenever a patient complains of a knee problem.

Dislocation of the hip

Dislocation of a native (as opposed to prosthetic) hip is a high energy injury. This is caused by axial trauma such as a force applied to the flexed knee. The dislocation is usually posterior with a fracture of the acetabular rim. Sometimes, the sciatic nerve is injured – most frequently that part destined to be the common peroneal nerve. Pain is usually severe, and the hip is held partially flexed and adducted. Central dislocation into the pelvis is associated with major (concealed) blood loss.

Dislocation of an arthroplasty of the hip is often seen after relatively minor trauma, or a contraindicated movement (e.g. hip flexion greater than 90°, or internal rotation).

Xᴿ When resuscitation has been established and analgesia given, radiographs are obtained. Later, a CT scan will aid identification of complex acetabular rim fractures.

Tx Resuscitate and provide analgesia; support the limb but do not attempt reduction of a native hip dislocation in the ED. The distal neurovascular function must be assessed, and the secondary survey completed, looking for other injuries. The patient needs an urgent referral to the orthopaedic department. Traumatic dislocation can be difficult to reduce by closed manipulation. Posterior dislocation may be treated more appropriately by open reduction and internal fixation of the bone fragments.

Reduction of a dislocated prosthetic hip may sometimes be appropriate in the ED, dependent on facility for safe sedation, patient factors, and local policy. Reduction may be more challenging than other joint dislocations, and approximately 25% of attempts are unsuccessful.

The Allis technique involves the patient being placed in the supine position, while an assistant firmly holds the pelvis down by applying pressure to both anterior iliac crests. The clinician flexes both the hip and knee to 90°. Axial traction is then applied to the distal femur and gradually increased, while the femur is slowly externally rotated. Joint stability must be assessed following reduction, and involvement of the orthopaedic team is recommended.

Fracture of the hip (fracture of the proximal femur)

There are three circumstances in which this may occur:

1 At any age – associated with major violence and multiple injuries
2 In elderly people – after a simple fall
3 Spontaneously – as a result of osteoporosis or bony metastatic deposits.

Hip fracture is a major public health issue in countries with an ever-increasing ageing population. In the UK, these fractures account for 90% of the enormous cost of osteoporosis to the NHS. The human cost is equally high – around 10% of people with a hip fracture die within 1 month and almost a third within 12 months of the injury. Most of these deaths are due to associated co-morbidities.

A detailed history must be taken and other injuries excluded. Consider the reason for an unexplained fall (medication, syncope, sarcopenia and requirement for walking aids) and assess general health. Patients presenting with fractured neck of femur typically have multiple co-morbidities which will require careful multidisciplinary management in the perioperative period and whilst in hospital. There is a high risk of other associated injuries. The following notes assume that systemic examination has been undertaken and relate to the care of the typical elderly patient with an isolated injury.

The patient typically presents unable to weight-bear after a relatively minor fall. Some patients may be able to walk, albeit with a painful limp and so the ability to weight bear should not be assumed to 'rule out' fractured neck of femur. There is pain in the hip, thigh or knee but usually no visible swelling, bruising or deformity. The affected leg may be shortened and externally rotated, but this classic appearance is dependent on the grade of the fracture. A more valuable sign is pain on gentle passive rotation (rolling) of the extended leg and pain on axial loading of the hip. If the fracture is impacted, other movements may be good, with minimal pain including on straight leg raising. Tenderness is most marked posteriorly. Significant blood loss is unusual and associated vascular and tendon damage is rare.

Fractured neck of femur in a younger patient with preserved bone density (typically <60 years) is usually a high-energy injury. In such patients, prompt surgical fixation is required, with the intent to avoid osteonecrosis and preserve the native femoral head.

Examination of the hip joint → Box 7.1.

 Radiological examination must include an anteroposterior (AP) view of the hips and pelvis, and a lateral radiograph of the affected hip. In the AP view, look for a break in the normal apparent continuity of trabeculae across the joint and disruption to Shenton line (→ *Figure 7.2*).

Osteoarthrosis is associated with intertrochanteric rather than subcapital fractures, so it is relatively unlikely that an undisplaced subcapital fracture will be hidden in the disorganised radiological pattern around a significantly arthritic joint.

The lateral view may be difficult to obtain and interpret but is nevertheless the best film on which to see a minimally displaced fracture.

Box 7.1 How to examine the hip joint

- Assess gait and continue inspection of mobility and pain as clothes are removed and the patient gets on to the couch
- Look for shortening or rotation of the leg. True shortening is caused by collapse or angulation of bone (distance between anterosuperior iliac spine and medial joint line of knee – both legs in the same position). Apparent shortening is the difference between the two sides when the patient is lying supine (distance from umbilicus to medial malleoli). It is usually caused by pelvic tilt or fixed deformity at the hip joint
- Look at the groin, perineum, buttock and lateral bony prominences, and feel for tenderness in these areas. A sinus or old scar may point to established disease, but there are usually no surface signs of acute inflammation or of joint effusion
- Assess flexion, abduction, adduction and rotation in each leg (active before passive). Keep one hand under the lumbar spine when testing flexion and one hand on the opposite iliac crest when testing abduction and adduction. Rotation is most accurately measured with the knee at right angles (lower leg over the end of the couch or patient prone). With the patient lying on his or her side attempt to extend the hip joint backwards; 5°–10° is often possible
- Examine the relationship between hip movement and lumbar spine and pelvic movement. Fixed flexion of the hip can be camouflaged by excessive lumbar lordosis. Fixed adduction is usually compensated for by pelvic tilt. The easiest way to abolish the lordosis is to fully flex the leg that is not being measured. Any passive movement off the bed of the leg under assessment is fixed flexion. Similarly, setting the pelvis square may cause fixed adduction of one leg
- Finally, ask the patient to stand on one leg. The pelvis should rise on the non-weight-bearing side. Failure to do this is a positive Trendelenburg sign and indicates disease in the weight-bearing hip or its associated abductor muscles

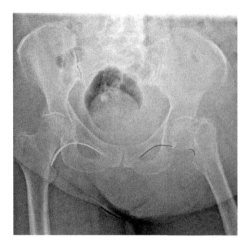

Figure 7.2 Intact Shenton line (green) and disrupted Shenton line (red) due to hip fracture.

Up to 5% of fractures in osteoporotic bone are not immediately visible on plain radiographs – this is particularly the case in lower-grade fractures. An MR scan should be performed if a hip fracture is suspected but initial radiographs are normal. A CT scan is an alternative if MRI is not available within 24 hours of admission. *For different types of proximal femoral fractures → Box 7.2.*

Tx Analgesia should be given immediately (and the effect of these measures assessed after 30 min). Regional nerve blocks, e.g. fascia iliaca block, are recommended for effective analgesia. Use of a fascia iliaca block reduces opiate requirements, which may reduce lower respiratory tract infections, promote earlier mobilisation and possibly reduce mortality. For Fascia Iliaca block technique see Box 7.3.

Long waits on hard trolleys must be avoided because these patients acquire pressure sores very quickly. Internal fixation, hemiarthroplasty or total arthroplasty is usually performed on the day of admission or ideally at least within 24 hours of injury.

Fracture of the pubic rami

The anterior pelvis should be carefully examined in all cases. Fracture of the pubic rami occurs in the same group of patients as those with fracture of the hip and gives a very similar clinical picture. The pain may be felt in the buttock or groin, but otherwise symptoms are localised to one leg and may divert attention away from the pelvis. Patients with this injury need initial bed rest and analgesia and then gradual mobilisation (*also → p. 86*).

 Box 7.2 **Hip fractures (or proximal femoral fractures)**

Fractures occurring between the edge of the femoral head and 5 cm below the lesser trochanter.

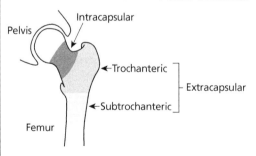

Extracapsular fractures
Fractures between the insertion of the capsule of the hip joint and a line 5 cm below the lesser trochanter. There are two subgroups:

1 **Trochanteric fractures**: including intertrochanteric (pertrochanteric) and reverse oblique trochanteric fractures
2 **Subtrochanteric fractures**: fractures up to 5 cm below the lesser trochanter

Intracapsular fractures
Fractures between the edge of the femoral head and the insertion of the capsule of the hip joint. Also known as femoral neck fractures. There are three types:

1 Subcapital
2 Transcervical
3 Basal cervical

Garden classification of subcapital (intracapsular) hip fractures
The classification relies only on the appearance of the hip on an AP radiograph:

Grade 1: incomplete (impacted) fracture
Grade 2: complete fracture without displacement
Grade 3: complete fracture with partial displacement
Grade 4: complete fracture with full displacement

Box 7.3 Fascia iliaca block

- Calculate the dose of local anaesthetic – e.g. 2 mL/kg bupivacaine, and draw up to 40 mL with saline
- Consent the patient and apply monitoring
- Confirm the side with the patient and with another staff member looking at the X-ray
- Clean the area with chlorhexidine
- Using a linear ultrasound probe with a sterile cover, identify the femoral artery and vein at the level of the inguinal crease. Moving laterally, identify the iliacus muscle with sartorius overlying like a 'beak' coming over from the lateral side
- Infiltrate 1 mL of 1% lidocaine to the skin at the lateral end of the ultrasound probe
- Using a needle with a short bevel insert through skin with the needle visualised in the long axis. Feel as the needle 'pops' through the fascia of iliacus, aspirate to check no blood is withdrawn and infiltrate a couple of mL of anaesthetic. The fluid should be seen expanding linearly along the plain of the muscle
- When satisfied with the position, continue to infiltrate the full 40 mL
- Ensure the patient is monitored carefully for 30 min afterwards for local anaesthetic toxicity and also the much more common complication of opiate toxicity (when the pain stimulus is removed by the FIB, any opiates given earlier can have a profoundly sedating effect)

The elderly patient with failure to weight-bear after a fall

All such patients must be admitted for reassessment and mobilisation. A considerable number prove to have a fracture that was not evident on the initial radiograph. An MR scan should be performed if a hip fracture is thought to be a possibility (i.e. in most elderly patients), but initial radiographs are normal. Patients with soft-tissue injuries may require prolonged rehabilitation before they are ready for discharge. Local policy dictates whether care for these patients is provided by the geriatric or orthopaedic department.

Degenerative disease of the hip

The patient presents with pain and stiffness and may relate this to a recent injury. The hip joint has a restricted range of movement. Fixed flexion may be obscured by compensatory lumbar lordosis. Fixed adduction causes pelvic tilt and an apparently short leg. Pain is usually most marked at the extremes of the range, and there is little muscle spasm. A general examination is always indicated to exclude systemic disease and injury.

XR Radiographs show reduced joint space, irregular articular surface, osteophytes, sclerosis and bone cysts. Such changes, however, are common and may not be related to the patient's symptoms.

TX In the absence of other pathology, symptomatic treatment with analgesia and a walking aid should be offered. The patient should be advised to consult their GP. Physiotherapy may help with initial mobilisation.

Extra-articular problems around the hip

Spinal and abdominal lesions may present with hip symptoms:

- Infection of the lumbar spine may produce a psoas abscess, which points just below the inguinal ligament. This may be tuberculous or as a result of a variety of infectious agents in the immunocompromised.
- A femoral hernia may be overlooked, especially in an obese, elderly patient.
- A high lumbar disc lesion may present with anterior thigh pain and limitation of hip extension (the femoral stretch test).
- Constriction of the lateral cutaneous nerve of the thigh as it passes through the inguinal ligament may cause persistent pain over the thigh (meralgia paresthetica).
- A child with haemophilia may present with hip joint spasm caused by haemorrhage into the psoas muscle.

Avulsion fractures of the pelvis

Apophyseal avulsion fractures of the pelvis are quite common in adolescents and young adults during physical activity due to the relative weakness of the apophysis compared to the tendon and muscle. There will be a sudden onset of pain during a forceful muscle contraction, e.g. kicking a ball, sometimes associated with a 'cracking' sensation. There will be tenderness at the site of avulsion and pain on moving the associated muscle group.

The avulsion can normally be seen on AP X-ray of the pelvis, remember to always compare left to right.

The common sites of avulsion include:

- Anterior superior iliac spine – sartorius
- Anterior inferior iliac spine – rectus femoris
- Ischial tuberosity – hamstrings
- Lesser trochanter – iliopsoas

Treatment is usually conservative, with rest and analgesia in the first instance and follow-up with orthopaedics.

Return to sport can take 8–10 weeks, which can be extremely upsetting for young sportspeople.

Fracture of the femoral shaft

This is associated with extensive soft-tissue injury and internal bleeding but is not usually compound. The level of trauma required to fracture the femur should suggest the possibility of serious injuries elsewhere.

XR The diagnosis is usually clinically evident without immediate resort to radiographs, which are mainly used to exclude other injuries and to check the position of the bone after the application of a splint.

Tx Priorities are as follows:

- Complete ABCs
- Give effective analgesia, initially nitrous oxide mixture and then IV opiates and/or a femoral nerve block (→ *Box 7.4*)
- Apply Thomas' or other traction splint (→ *Box 7.5*)
- Check distal pulses; vascular damage can occur with supracondylar fractures
- Perform blood tests for baseline values and cross-match
- Complete the secondary survey
- Take radiographs as appropriate
- Involve the orthopaedic team early in management

 Box 7.4 Femoral nerve block

Indications: fractures at any level of the femur
Contraindications: hypersensitivity to local anaesthetics; neurovascular complications of the injury
Method: clean and drape the skin. Insert a short needle lateral to the femoral artery just below the inguinal ligament. Advance it perpendicularly to the skin. Feel for loss of resistance when the fascia is penetrated. Inject up to 10 mL 0.5% bupivacaine. The patient may experience paraesthesia during the injection
Onset: within 15 min
Duration: variable, but often over 5 hours

 Box 7.5 Splinting a femoral shaft fracture

Traction splints and Thomas' splints are commonly available. Consider applying the splint before the radiograph if the fracture is clinically obvious. It will give immediate pain relief and reduce blood loss.

- If Thomas' splint is to be used, obtain the appropriate size and cover it with tubular bandage or webbing slings. If a traction splint is to be used much of the following can be omitted, but ensure that you know how it works before trying to apply it
- Apply the strapping from the skin traction kit to the leg. Adhesive strapping must not be used on elderly or fragile skin because its removal later may damage the skin. Instead, use a non-adhesive traction kit
- Protect the malleoli by padding
- Secure the strapping with crepe bandages
- Ensure adequate analgesia. Intravenous analgesia can be supplemented with nitrous oxide while applying the splint
- Grip the heel and forefoot of the injured leg and apply firm continuous traction. Muscle spasm will gradually disappear and angulation of the thigh will decrease. Transient increase in pain is usually reduced by continuous traction
- Instruct an assistant to manoeuvre the splint over the foot and ankle
- Maintain constant traction while the assistant pushes the splint towards the pelvis
- Protect the genitalia
- Fasten the strapping by its ropes to the end of the splint
- Tighten the traction by inserting a wooden spatula between the two ropes and twisting it until the required tension is achieved (Chinese windlass method)
- Check the foot pulses and toe movements
- Request a radiograph to check the position of the splint

The limping child

Children are commonly brought to the emergency department with a primary complaint of limp. The differential diagnosis is strongly influenced by age (→ *Box 7.6*). Observe the child moving and attempting to walk from a distance if possible. All children should have a full set of observations recorded (including temperature) and be fully examined, including examination of

> ### ⚷ Box 7.6 Causes of limp in children
>
> | Age <3 years | Age 3–10 years | 10–19 years | All ages |
> |---|---|---|---|
> | Toddler's fracture | Transient synovitis (irritable hip) | Fracture or soft tissue injury | Septic arthritis |
> | Fracture or soft tissue injury | Fracture or soft tissue injury | Slipped upper femoral epiphysis | Osteomyelitis |
> | Developmental dysplasia of the hip | Perthes' disease | Osgood Schlatter's disease | Discitis |
> | | | Sever's disease | Malignancy (primary bone tumours, soft tissue sarcoma, leukaemia and lymphoma) |
> | | | Chondromalacia patellae | Haematological disease (sickle cell and haemophilia) |
> | | | Osteochondritis dissecans | Inflammatory joint disease (e.g. Juvenile idiopathic arthritis) |
> | | | | Non-musculoskeletal conditions (intra-abdominal problems like appendicitis, testicular torsion and hernia) |

abdomen, back, testicles and skin for rashes as well as a comprehensive examination of the affected limb. A range of systemic problems may present as a limp (→ *Box 7.6*).

Take a careful history of any trauma – remember toddler's fracture may result from a fairly trivial mechanism of injury – usually a fall from standing.

Transient synovitis (irritable hip)

Common in children aged 3–10 years. There may be a history of a mild upper respiratory illness in the preceding days or weeks, but this is absent in many cases. Severity can vary, and sometimes the hip may appear to give way and raise concern of traumatic injury. Examination findings are limited. There is no erythema or clinically evident inflammation, and passive hip movements are usually normal; however, there may be discomfort on hip abduction and external rotation.

XR Radiographs are not usually required. Focused radiography guided by a thorough physical examination is all that is necessary during the initial work-up phase. The differential diagnosis may include a toddler's fracture or a foot injury (→ *p. 107*).

Ultrasound examination can demonstrate an effusion in the hip joint but cannot differentiate synovial fluid, blood and pus. A difference of >3 mm of effusion between the normal and the affected hip is considered to be pathological.

TX Complete refusal to weight bear, concurrent systemic illness or fever should raise concern for possible septic arthritis. In such cases, take blood tests and refer for orthopaedic assessment.

A child who is apyrexial with no hip spasm and no evidence of bony injury can be discharged with analgesia and instructions to rest but should be advised to return if not resolved within 72 hours (or follow-up arranged in a review clinic).

Perthes' disease

Perthes' disease is an idiopathic avascular necrosis of the proximal femoral epiphysis. It is often called an 'osteochondritis' and belongs to a group of similar diseases of epiphyseal growth (→ *p. 366*). In the UK, it affects 1 in 10 000 children and is four times more common in boys than in girls. In 10% of cases, it is bilateral. Children aged between 3 and 15 years may be affected, although it is most common in children between 5 and 8 years of age. It presents with a painful or painless limp or sometimes with hip or knee pain after exercise. Pain may be mild and is often of several months' duration. There is restriction of hip movements with muscle spasm, especially

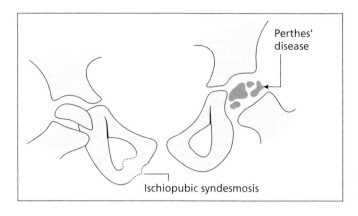

Perthes'
disease

Ischiopubic syndesmosis

Figure 7.3 Perthes' disease, with incidental normal enlargement of the ischiopubic syndesmosis.

internal rotation and abduction. Flexion is usually unaffected.

XR Radiographs may be normal in very early disease. However, they often show remarkably advanced changes in contrast to the short clinical history. The femoral neck may be widened, bone density reduced, joint space increased and the femoral head fragmented (→ *Figure 7.3*). An ultrasound scan reveals an effusion, and bone scanning shows reduced uptake in the affected epiphysis. Blood tests are all normal.

TX The child should be referred to the orthopaedic department for admission. Bed rest until the muscle spasm has resolved is now the mainstay of treatment for this condition.

Slipped upper femoral epiphysis

The capital (or proximal femoral) epiphysis may slip suddenly or gradually, usually in a teenager who is having a pubertal growth spurt. The onset may be linked to minor

trauma. There is limping and pain, which may be localised to the distal thigh or knee. Hip abduction is restricted, but adduction is often increased. Flexion and internal rotation may increase the pain, because these movements stretch the joint capsule. An acute slip is more likely to lead to ischaemia and avascular necrosis of the epiphysis than the more common chronic slip.

XR Radiographs may be difficult to interpret and should include AP and 'frog leg' lateral views of both hips. Posterior movement of the epiphysis is sometimes the first radiographic sign and is best seen on the lateral view. Slight medial displacement of the epiphysis is usually the initial change and is sometimes likened to 'an ice-cream sliding off its cone' (→ *Figure 7.4*). More specifically, a line drawn parallel to the femoral neck (Klein's line) will normally intersect with the lateral portion of the femoral epiphysis (Trethowan's sign).

TX Immediate referral to the orthopaedic department is essential. Surgical reduction of an acute slip followed by prophylactic pinning is usually recommended.

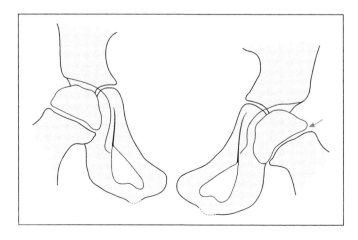

Figure 7.4 Slipped left proximal femoral epiphysis (arrowed) (anteroposterior view).

THE KNEE

Assessment of the knee joint

The knee can be very difficult to assess acutely. A detailed history will help to distinguish between the many types of injury and symptoms that may occur:

- Ask about the relationship between the onset of symptoms (especially pain and swelling) and the time of injury.
- Ask about and observe the ability to weight-bear.
- Look, feel and move the joint (→ Box 7.7).
- Confirm the presence of distal pulses.
- Exclude referred pain, especially from the hip and spine.

Vascular problems are relatively common in fractures around the knee. There are of two types:

1 Direct trauma to a major vessel by a bone fragment or by the interosseous ligament at the trifurcation of the popliteal artery.
2 Raised interstitial pressure within a closed fascial compartment of the lower leg (→ p. 112).

Damage to the distal part of the popliteal artery is particularly serious in young people, because here it is an 'end'-artery. Elderly patients may have developed a collateral circulation around the knee in response to the main vessel disease.

Examination of the knee joint → *Box 7.7.*
Indications for radiography of the knee after injury → *Box 7.8.*

Wounds around the knee

Even apparently trivial wounds around the knee may involve the joint capsule and synovium.

XR Intra-articular air may be seen on the radiograph as a radiolucent area.

Tx Suspicion of joint involvement warrants orthopaedic referral, thorough assessment, usually under general anaesthesia and prophylactic antibiotics (e.g. flucloxacillin, started before surgery).

Soft-tissue injuries to the knee

Ligamentous and meniscal injuries to the knee are often difficult to diagnose precisely on first presentation. The patient generally has variable degrees of:

- pain
- difficulty weight-bearing

Box 7.7 A method of examining the knee joint

- Watch the patient climb on to the couch
- Look for scars, sinuses, muscle wasting and joint swelling
- Ask patient to point to the site of the pain
- Test for the presence of an effusion or haemarthrosis (→ *p. 99*)
- Palpate bony landmarks for irregularities and tenderness
- Confirm the ability of the quadriceps mechanism to extend the joint
- Check for the ability to hyperextend the knee so that the heel lifts off the couch, while the back of the knee remains in contact with it. This usually signifies that the joint is not severely injured
- Determine the range of true extension and flexion and compare this with the normal side
- At 90° flexion (or as near as the pain allows), rotate the tibia on the femur by twisting the foot. Pain at the joint line suggests meniscal injury. Repeat this test with the patient prone, applying compression along the tibia. This increases pain of meniscal origin and lessens the pain of a collateral ligament lesion
- Keeping the joint at 90°, sit on the foot and attempt to pull and push the upper tibia on the femur to test the cruciate ligaments. The hamstrings must be flaccid; assess this by having the index fingers up against them while pulling forward. There is considerable variation in cruciate laxity between patients, but not between their two knees
- Test collateral ligament integrity at 10° flexion. Stand facing the supine patient, put the foot in your axilla and hold the leg just below the knee in both hands. All muscles must be flaccid while you attempt to shake the knee sideways. Normally, there will be painless – if alarming – clunks at the limits of valgus and varus stressing. A 'rubbery', painful end point suggests collateral ligament injury. Complete rupture may be less painful than partial rupture
- Move the patella sideways on the femur with the knee fully extended. If lateral pressure causes anxiety and pain, consider potential dislocation. If downward pressure is painful consider chondromalacia

Box 7.8 Indications for radiography of the knee after injury

Any of the following:

- History of fall, blunt trauma or penetrating injury
- Age >55 years
- Obvious deformity
- Severe swelling of rapid onset
- Tenderness at the head of the fibula
- Isolated tenderness of the patella
- Inability to flex to 90°
- Inability to straight leg raise
- Inability to walk four weight-bearing steps unaided in the ED
- Atypical features
- Return visit with no improvement
- Modest effusions can be detected by balloting the patella against the femur (patellar tap).
- Large effusions will prevent bony contact but are obvious
- Small effusions are best detected by emptying the suprapatellar pouch with one hand and testing for lateral fluid shift with the other. The normal concavity on either side of the patella is obliterated by quite small amounts of fluid. Pressure on the one side of the patella will push fluid to the opposite side and increase the parapatellar convexity there

- swelling
- reduction of the range of movements – due to restriction by fluid, pain and sometimes by mechanical blocks.

Serious intra-articular problems are probable in the presence of any of the following:

- A large, rapidly developing effusion
- Complete inability to weight-bear
- Demonstrable collateral or cruciate laxity.

If the patient can lie with the joint fully extended so that the back of knee is on the couch while the heel is a few centimetres off it, and also squat down with the knee fully flexed, then serious injury is extremely unlikely.

Effusions in the knee joint: the speed of onset of an effusion is as important as the size. Rapid collection suggests the presence of blood and thus damages to vascular structures such as the bone or ligament. The most common cause of a haemarthrosis is a partial tear of the anterior cruciate ligament. Fractures of the lower femur and upper tibia may extend into the joint and produce a haemarthrosis. Onset of swelling over 24 hours is typical of a synovial response, commonly associated with

damage to the avascular menisci or trauma to an osteoarthritic knee.

Meniscal injury: injury to the medial or lateral meniscus of the knee is suggested by the ability to walk immediately after the incident followed by a gradual onset of swelling with increasing pain. Tenderness is maximal at the joint line. The knee may lock or give way days later. Damage will have been inflicted by tibial rotation on the partially flexed joint, and pain at the joint line can be reproduced by recreating these stresses. The medial meniscus is the more commonly injured of the two because it has more restricting peripheral attachments than the lateral meniscus and is therefore subjected to greater shearing forces.

Collateral ligament injury: spraining of a collateral ligament in the knee is common and usually results in a very similar picture to meniscal injury. There may be pain on valgus or varus stressing but no demonstrable laxity. More significant tears or complete rupture of a collateral ligament may, paradoxically, leave the patient with very little pain. There will, however, be obvious laxity on valgus or varus stressing. The consequent instability of the knee may necessitate surgical repair.

Cruciate ligament injury: this is a major injury with long-term consequences. The anterior and posterior cruciate ligaments are very strong; their rupture is usually caused by significant trauma and is associated with damage to other structures, particularly the collateral ligaments and the menisci. Swelling is immediate, and pain and loss of function are evident. If pain permits, excessive movement will be found on attempting to move the upper tibia back and forth on the femur when the joint is at right angles. Radiographs may show an avulsed tibial spine. Referral to the orthopaedic team is essential.

Xᴿ Radiological examination is usually unrewarding but must be carried out to exclude intra-articular fracture. There may be an avulsion injury at the site of attachment of collateral or cruciate ligaments. An MR scan (or arthroscopy) is the definitive investigation.

Tx
Knee problems that require immediate referral → Box 7.9.

Early arthroscopy is increasingly used to aid diagnosis and to give appropriate treatment. Minor meniscal and collateral ligament injuries can be treated on an outpatient basis. A support bandage should be applied and crutches and analgesia given as necessary. Follow-up must be arranged, and physiotherapy may be helpful.

Withdrawal of fluid from the knee may relieve the pain caused by a tense swelling, facilitate examination, and distinguish between blood and serous effusion. However, aspiration of an effusion should only be attempted in a suitable environment by an experienced clinician.

> ### Box 7.9 Knee problems that need immediate referral
>
> - Haemarthrosis
> - Ligamentous instability
> - Locked knee
> - Complete failure to straight leg raise
> - Fracture on radiograph
> - Possibility of septic arthritis
> - Penetration of the joint

Fractures of the tibial condyles

Fractures of the proximal tibia may occur after a forcible valgus or varus strain (e.g. knee hit by a car bumper). The patient is typically in pain, unable to walk and has an obvious haemarthrosis. However, the tibial plateau may be depressed to a lesser degree in elderly patients after relatively minor trauma, in which case the knee is not very swollen and the patient is able to walk. There is:

- localised pain and tenderness at the joint line
- a modest effusion
- a reasonable amount of movement of the knee
- pain on valgus/varus stressing.

XR Minor degrees of depression of the tibial plateau are often overlooked on a radiograph (→ *Figure 7.5*). The AP radiograph requires, especially careful scrutiny. Osteoporotic bone is often present as a causative factor. The radiological appearance of osteoarthrosis may obscure the fracture.

TX Patients with tibial condyle fractures generally require referral for surgical fixation. Some minor crush fractures of the tibial plateau may be treated on an outpatient basis in a plaster cast, but most patients will need to be admitted.

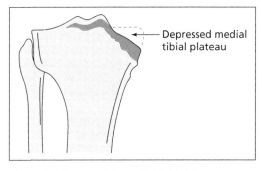

Figure 7.5 Fracture of the medial tibial plateau.

Fracture of the neck of the fibula

This injury may be associated with damage to the common peroneal nerve (causing drop-foot, paralysis of ankle everters and loss of sensation over the lateral aspect of the lower leg). It may be an isolated injury or accompany rotational injuries of the ankle (Maisonneuve's fracture).

XR Radiographs of this area are indicated when there is direct injury or tenderness accompanying an obvious ankle injury.

TX The uncomplicated injury may be treated with analgesia, crutches and fracture clinic follow-up. Other variants require immediate referral.

Diffuse inflammation of the knee

Also → p. 422 in Chapter 21.

Septic arthritis may be florid, with acute joint pain, fever and systemic illness, or more insidious with only modest pain and some joint movement. Be alert to this possibility in elderly patients and those with rheumatoid disease. Also consider the diagnosis of gonorrhoea.

Crystal arthropathy may present with exquisite local pain and joint stiffness.

Deformity secondary to osteoarthrosis and bone destruction decreases locomotor efficiency. Muscle work is increased and the patient complains of fatigue as well as joint pain. The joint line is prominent and irregular as a result of osteophytes, and there are usually a few degrees of fixed flexion. Collateral ligament instability follows tibial condyle collapse and instability predisposes to trauma. Osteoarthrosis extends recovery time after injury.

XR Radiographs may show calcified menisci or non-specific changes.

TX Referral to an orthopaedic surgeon or rheumatologist should be decided by the most likely diagnosis. Diagnostic tap may be indicated.

Loose bodies in the knee joint

Intra-articular fragments may arise from an area of osteochondritis dissecans (→ *Figure 7.6*), degenerate menisci, osteophytes or the synovium. The patient complains of intermittent locking of the knee, typically in a different position each time. There may be a small effusion.

XR The loose fragments are usually easily seen on a radiograph.

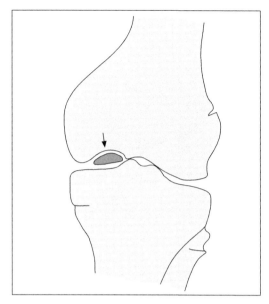

Figure 7.6 Osteochondritis dissecans (arrow).

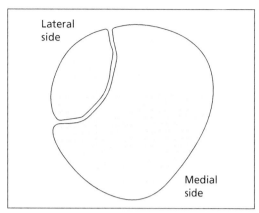

Figure 7.7 Bipartite patella.

Tx If the knee is locked, no attempt should be made to manipulate it, but orthopaedic advice should be sought. In other cases, the patient may be referred for follow up in the orthopaedic outpatients clinic.

Fracture of the patella/quadriceps injury

The patella may be fractured by a direct blow or fall or by sudden quadriceps contraction. Indirect traction force can break the quadriceps mechanism at different levels. The older the patient, the higher the lesion:

- **Young**: patellar tendon
- **Middle-aged**: across the patella
- **Older**: rectus femoris muscle.

The action of the quadriceps muscle should be assessed by active knee extension; failure to straight-leg raise suggests a significant injury.

XR Occasionally, the patella is bipartite. The upper lateral part is separated from the rest of the patella by a curved line mimicking a fracture (→ *Figure 7.7*). This is a normal variant but may not be present in both knees.

Tx Refer for specialist care. Comminuted fractures are excised. Minimally displaced fractures may be wired together. Undisplaced fractures are treated in a plaster cylinder. Transverse fractures of the patella, which extend laterally to involve the quadriceps expansion, require surgical repair, as do serious injuries of quadriceps.

Dislocation of the patella

The patella may dislocate laterally during active quadriceps action. Teenage girls are most often affected. All knee movements are painful, and the deformity is obvious. If spontaneous reduction has occurred, the diagnosis can be confirmed by a positive patellar apprehension test: pushing the patella laterally (usually in either knee) causes pain and a feeling of imminent dislocation.

XR Radiographs should be taken to exclude bony injury.

Tx Reduction should be undertaken promptly in the ED and may be facilitated by nitrous oxide, or methoxyflurane analgesia. Reduction entails a gentle straightening of the leg by the application of distal traction with firm medial pressure applied to the lateral border of the patella. A straight-leg splint is then applied in the short term, the patient given crutches and referred to fracture clinic. Patients with a clear history of dislocation of the patella in whom spontaneous relocation has occurred should be treated in the same way. Prolonged immobilisation may be counterproductive as resulting quadriceps wasting may increase the risk of further dislocation. Physiotherapy is helpful.

Patellofemoral osteochondritis

Pain behind the patella is a common cause of knee pain in young women. Trivial direct trauma may be implicated. Symptoms are exacerbated by exercise, especially going down steps. Pain is reproduced by pressing on the patella. There may be a small effusion, but the knee joint is otherwise normal.

XR Radiographs are usually normal.

Tx Analgesia and physiotherapy (to prevent wasting of the quadriceps muscles) are indicated. The condition is self-limiting and rarely requires surgical intervention. Initial referral to the patient's GP is usually appropriate.

Peripatellar bursitis

Both the prepatellar and infrapatellar bursae may become inflamed and then secondarily infected after repeated minor trauma. Colloquial names for these conditions, namely housemaid's and clergyman's knee, respectively, were derived from the most commonly affected professions and their differing kneeling positions. Nowadays – because of changing priorities in society – carpet fitters, electricians and plumbers are the people most prone to these conditions. The affected area is red, swollen and tender. Pain may limit full movements, but there is no communication between the bursa and the knee joint.

Acute traumatic bursitis may follow a direct blow or fall. In this case, the prepatellar area is very tender and swollen. There often appears to be a fluid-filled area that could be aspirated, but attempts to do this are usually unsuccessful and risk-introducing infection.

XR After severe direct trauma, the knee should have a radiograph taken to exclude an underlying fracture of the patella.

TX When there is no clinical evidence of infection (as indicated by body temperature), the patient can be treated with non-steroidal anti-inflammatory drugs (NSAIDs) and follow-up. The condition usually resolves spontaneously, but occasionally the bursa requires removal. Any suspicion of knee joint involvement demands immediate orthopaedic referral. If there is an acute localised infection of the bursa alone, incision and drainage under a general anaesthetic should be carried out by the orthopaedic team.

Rupture of a Baker's cyst

Bursae in the popliteal fossa may be connected to the knee joint. An enlarged and isolated popliteal bursa (Baker's cyst) is associated with rheumatoid involvement of the knee. If it ruptures, there is sudden pain in the upper calf as the synovial fluid is squeezed between the calf muscles. The condition is often misdiagnosed as either a tear of the calf muscles or a DVT (→ *pp. 102 and 110*).

> Exclude a popliteal aneurysm before considering other extra-articular swellings.

XR Arthrography is diagnostic.

TX Advice should be sought from the orthopaedic or rheumatology departments.

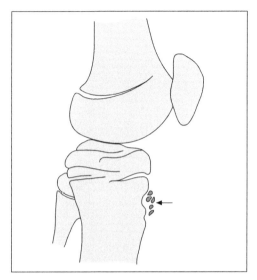

Figure 7.8 Osgood–Schlatter disease (arrowed).

Osgood–Schlatter disease

A common cause of anterior knee pain in adolescents. Most typically around the insertion of the patellar tendon and occurs generally after exercise. This is caused by an apophysitis of the tibial tuberosity. Knee movements are normal, but resisted extension is painful, along with point tenderness on palpation of the tibial tuberosity.

XR Radiographs are diagnostic but not necessary, as the diagnosis is usually made from clinical findings. The knee X-ray may show fragmentation of the tibial epiphysis (→ *Figure 7.8*).

TX Simple analgesia with reassurance that symptoms will settle with time. Ice packs over the affected area may help. Sporting activity may continue as symptoms allow. The condition always resolves when the epiphysis fuses just after puberty.

Sindig–Laarson disease: This is of similar aetiology and involves the lower pole of the patella. Treatment is as for Osgood–Schlatter disease.

> Tumours and sepsis may occasionally present with knee pain, especially in children.

THE LOWER LEG

Two anatomical features provide potential complications for injuries to the lower leg:

1 The skin, thinly stretched over the tibia anteriorly, has a poor blood supply.
2 The muscles are enclosed in a rigid fascial envelope.

Consequently:

- Many fractures of the tibia and fibula are compound.
- Wounds of the skin in this area are slow to heal.
- Muscle contusion or vascular damage in the calf may raise interstitial pressure sufficiently to occlude the circulation.

Fracture of the shaft of the tibia

Tibial shaft fractures follow a considerable amount of direct or indirect force. They are generally extremely painful injuries and render walking impossible. The fibula is usually also fractured, although a direct blow may break the tibia only. In the latter case, there will be minimal deformity and occasionally the patient is able to weight-bear with difficulty. Vascular damage should be suspected in all lower limb injuries, especially if there is either a crush or high-speed mechanism of injury. If present, early recognition and referral are essential.

XR The diagnosis is usually evident clinically. Radiographs follow splintage and will show the fracture in adults but can be difficult to interpret in young children.

Tx
Initial splintage → Box 7.10.

Most patients with a fractured tibia need admission, observation and internal fixation. Compound fractures must be debrided in theatre as soon as possible.

Some closed fractures can be managed on an outpatient basis, but the decision should be left to the orthopaedic department. The application of a well-padded, above-knee plaster cast should not be delegated to inexperienced staff. 'Check radiographs' in plaster are

---

Box 7.10 Splinting the lower leg

- Apply splintage under appropriate analgesia after removal of clothing and footwear but before radiography
- Confirm the presence of foot pulses and toe movements
- If there is gross ankle deformity, give morphine and nitrous oxide and quickly reduce the dislocation. This prevents pressure necrosis of overlying skin
- If there is a compound fracture, remove gross contaminants and take an instant photograph before applying sterile iodine-soaked pads. Do not allow repeated examination – show the photograph instead. Start antibiotics
- Apply an L-shaped splint or box splint
- Check the pulses again and review the analgesia
- Arrange for radiographs

---

essential, even if the fracture initially appeared stable and undisplaced. Displacement can occur during application of plaster. Crutches and analgesia will be required as will early orthopaedic follow-up.

Tibial fractures in children

Children with these injuries present with a limp or failure to weight-bear. A history of trauma is by no means inevitable. There may be no swelling or deformity and tenderness, although present may be difficult to localise. Knee and ankle flexion are usually unaffected, although ankle rotation may be painful. The diagnosis is thus elusive and if there is any doubt follow the procedure for the limping child as described in → Box 7.6.

XR Radiographs may not show an obvious fracture. Look at both films for a faint, long, oblique and lucent line. In the 'toddlers' fracture', radiographs are often initially normal, and the characteristic periosteal elevation is not seen for several days. Where toddler's fracture is suspected but not confirmed on radiograph, re-imaging in 7–10 days can demonstrate periosteal reaction and more easily identified fracture.

Tx Obvious fractures should be immobilised in an above-knee cast. The child will need analgesia and fracture clinic follow-up. Toddlers' fractures can be treated with rest and just analgesia, a bandage or a below-knee plaster cast depending on the degree of pain and discomfort.

Fracture of the shaft of the fibula

The shaft of the fibula may be broken by direct trauma. Although there is localised pain and tenderness, there is little swelling and the patient can weight-bear. Consequently, the injury is often missed.

XR The radiograph is diagnostic.

Tx The shaft of the fibula functions as a muscle anchor rather than a weight bearer, so a plaster cast is unnecessary. The patient requires an elastic bandage, analgesia, crutches and a fracture clinic follow-up.

Pretibial pain

Shin pain may develop acutely in athletes. The patient complains of intermittent discomfort over the front of the lower leg. There may be local tenderness, but the diagnosis is made chiefly from the history of gradually increasing pain associated with exercise. 'Shin splints', as the condition is known, is probably caused by oedema within the anterior compartment.

Other possible diagnoses are chronic or acute osteomyelitis, bone tumour or hyperplasia of the anterior tibial cortex. This last condition occurs in footballers subjected to repeated shin injury and subperiosteal haematoma.

XR Radiographs may show cortical thickening in some cases. A bone scan or MRI may be more helpful in distinguishing between soft tissue pain or a tibial stress fracture.

TX Management of these patients depends on symptoms and diagnosis. A referral to a physiotherapist or a sports injury clinic may be appropriate. Stress fractures should be immobilised in a cast. All patients should have follow-up arranged.

Calf muscle strain or tear

Disruption within the calf muscles or at the junction with the tendon may be caused by overuse or sudden stretching. There is acute localised pain, usually towards the medial side of the gastrocnemius muscle. Weight-bearing is painful as is passive ankle dorsiflexion. It is important to exclude rupture of the Achilles tendon, which gives a similar clinical picture. DVT and ruptured Baker's cyst must also be considered (→ pp. 102 and 110).

TX Patients require analgesia and crutches. Follow-up should be arranged, as should early physiotherapy.

Achilles tendonitis (tendonosis)

The Achilles tendon is the largest tendon in the human body but is prone to injury, inflammation and degeneration. Problems are usually due to a combination of repetitive stress injury and age-related degeneration, the exact proportions of each depending on the individual patient. Sudden increases in exercise, tight calf muscles, fluoroquinolone antibiotics and congenital or acquired calcaneal spurs are also implicated in the pathogenesis of the condition. Two main types are described:

1 **Non-insertional Achilles tendonitis**: fibres in the middle portion of the tendon develop tiny tears and then become swollen and thickened. This is more common in younger, active people including distance runners.
2 **Insertional Achilles tendonitis**: calcified fibres in the lower part of the Achilles tendon (at the junction with the calcaneum) become oedematous and inflamed. A bony spur may form on the heel and rub against the tendon. This type of tendonitis usually occurs in older, less active people.

Features of Achilles tendonitis include:

- Pain behind or above the back of the heel that gets worse during or after activity (sometimes on the following day)
- Pain in the region of the tendon that is worse in the morning
- Pain with ankle flexion (relatively unusual)
- Tenderness and thickening of part of the tendon.

XR Plain radiographs may show calcification of part of the tendon or a calcaneal spur. An MR scan can demonstrate degeneration and inflammation of the tendon.

TX Initial treatment includes NSAIDs and rest, including abstinence from high-impact exercises and strenuous work. Crutches or even a below-knee cast may be required. Early physiotherapy and graduated stretching exercises are helpful and heel pads often give considerable relief. Steroid injections may precipitate rupture of the tendon. Cases that fail to resolve after a few months may be referred for possible surgery. There are several recommended procedures, but there is a high incidence of postoperative pain and infection after all of them.

Rupture of the Achilles tendon

Surprisingly, acute rupture may at first be dismissed by the patient as a trivial injury. The usual history is of sudden calf pain thought to have been caused by an object hitting the back of the leg. The acute pain subsides, and the patient is able to walk flat-footed with difficulty but cannot run. On examination there is a palpable gap in the tendon, although this may be filled with inflammatory exudate. Plantar flexion is possible using the toe flexors, but it is weak. Squeezing the calf fails to cause plantar flexion of the foot and is painful. This test is most accurately performed with the feet of the prone patient extending over the end of the couch and is always compared with the normal side.

TX Refer the patient to the orthopaedic department immediately. Most patients will undergo early primary tendon repair, although immobilisation in equinus in a cast is another option. Recovery is often delayed because of pre-existing degenerative changes.

Rupture of the musculotendinous junction of the Achilles tendon: injuries that are in this area also require an immediate orthopaedic opinion.

Partial rupture of the Achilles tendon: sometimes, patients present with the hallmarks of acute rupture and a normal, but painful, calf-squeeze test. This may be caused by partial rupture of a degenerate tendon. Ultrasonography or MRI may be required to confirm the diagnosis. Management is similar to that described for a complete rupture of the Achilles tendon.

THE ANKLE

Inversion sprains

Sprained ankles are the most common injuries seen in an ED, resulting in the attendance of around 2.5% of the UK population every year! They result from stretching and tearing of the lateral ligament and tendon complex of the ankle, and so are seen in a number of different varieties, depending on the particular structures torn and the severity of the damage (→ *Figure 7.9*):

- Grade 1 sprain = stretching of the ligament complex
- Grade 2 sprain = partial tearing of the ligament complex
- Grade 3 sprain = complete rupture of the ligament complex.

Some sprains will resolve quickly without treatment, many will heal more slowly and need routine outpatient care, and a few require specialised management from the outset. It is important, but not always easy, to assign the patient to the appropriate treatment category as soon as possible.

Ask the patient about:

- history and mechanism of injury
- extent and speed of appearance of pain and swelling
- mobility
- occupational and recreational demands.

The usual history is of ankle inversion while running, playing sports or slipping down a step. A crack may have been heard, but this does not inevitably indicate bone injury. The initial pain settles and then gets worse again over the next few hours, causing difficulty in weight-bearing. This sequence is typical – but not diagnostic – of a soft-tissue injury.

Swelling and pain are often focused just anterior to the lateral malleolus – caused by injury to the anterior talofibular ligament – or over the side of the foot. Exclude ankle mortise instability by gripping the heel with one hand and the lower leg with the other. There should be no pain or movement when a sideways force is applied to the heel. In contrast, the patient will have acute pain on attempted inversion of the foot.

After examining the lateral side of the ankle, there are six other places to feel for related injuries:

1 The medial malleolus and medial ligament complex
2 The base of the little (fifth) metatarsal bone
3 The calcaneum
4 The Achilles tendon
5 The neck of the fibula
6 The midtarsal region.

The ankle must be palpated all around for bony tenderness, not just the swollen lateral side. Pain over the styloid process of the fifth metatarsal base may be caused by ligament or bone avulsion – a variation of ankle inversion injury. Fracture of the calcaneum and rupture of the Achilles tendon are injuries that are often wrongly diagnosed as ankle sprains on first presentation. The neck of the fibula should be examined because of its involvement in rotational injuries of the ankle (→ *p. 100*). Fracture dislocation at the tarsometatarsal junction (Lisfranc's fracture) causes significant pain over the dorsum of the foot, especially medially.

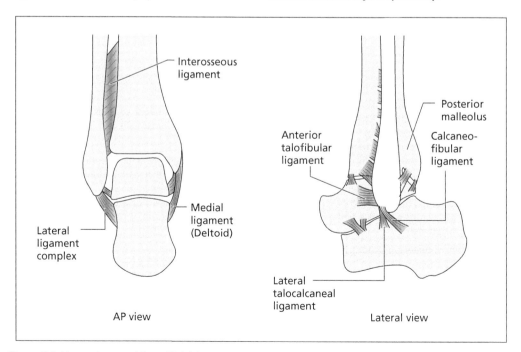

Figure 7.9 Ligaments around the ankle joint.

X$_R$ If indicated, plain radiographs of the ankle are taken to exclude significant fractures of the malleoli. They should be supplemented with other films (e.g. knee, heel and foot) if there are atypical findings on clinical examination.

Indications for ankle radiographs → Box 7.11.

Ankle sprains may be associated with an avulsed flake from the lateral malleolus or the dorsum of the talus. New flake fractures have a sharp, irregular outline without a complete marginal cortex. Do not forget to look at the calcaneum. Lisfranc's fracture may be difficult to diagnose on standard radiographs.

Some patients continue to have severe symptoms and signs despite normal initial radiographs. These patients should be reviewed by a senior doctor after 7–10 days; further radiographs may be required. Stress views or an MR scan may be indicated to help choose optimum treatment.

T$_X$ If the patient has a classic mild inversion sprain and is able to weight-bear, then treat with:

- ice and analgesia
- initial rest and elevation, leading to graduated exercise

Box 7.11 Indications for radiology of the ankle after injury

Any of the following:

- History suggesting severe injury
- Severe pain
- Age >55 years
- Inability to walk four steps unaided
- Obvious deformity
- Severe swelling of rapid onset
- Bony tenderness of the posterior border of the lateral malleolus (lower 6 cm)
- Bony tenderness of the posterior border of the medial malleolus (lower 6 cam)
- Atypical features
- Return visit with no improvement
- Foot X-ray should be requested if there is tenderness over the navicular, or the base of the fifth metatarsal

The corollary of these indications is that a radiograph is not needed in:

- a younger patient
- with a history of a simple inversion injury
- who can partially weight-bear, and
- who has no tenderness over the base of fifth metatarsal, navicular, or posterior borders of medial or lateral malleoli

---

However, if the patient is unable to weight-bear or has an obviously more severe injury, add:

- crutches (partial weight-bearing)
- early physiotherapy
- review after about 2 weeks to ensure satisfactory progress (physiotherapist or clinic).

In these patients, consideration should be given to offering immobilisation of the injured ankle in a below-knee walking cast or walking boot for between 10 and 14 days. This has been shown to be associated with less pain and discomfort during the 4 weeks after the injury, and better ankle function, activity and quality of life after 3 months. The cast should be applied after the initial swelling has subsided; this will necessitate a clinic appointment after 3–7 days. A purpose-made ankle brace is less effective than a cast but better than an elastic support bandage in effecting a speedy recovery and a cost-effective return to work. After 9 months, patients receiving any of these three methods of ankle support have similar symptoms and the same level of functioning.

Flake fractures represent variants of ligament injuries and should be treated in the same way as a sprain. However, their detection is useful because they often indicate that a more severe injury has occurred. The patient should be told of their presence to prevent a later misunderstanding.

Most patients with mild ankle sprains can expect a marked improvement after 10–14 days and to be weight-bearing almost normally within 2–3 weeks.

Eversion sprains

These injuries produce pain and swelling below the medial malleolus. They are uncommon but may produce an unstable ankle joint.

X$_R$ Radiographs should be taken unless the patient can bear full weight without pain and has very little local swelling.

T$_X$ Evidence of fracture or incongruity of the ankle joint is an indication for orthopaedic referral. Less severe injuries usually resolve with a support bandage and a short course of physiotherapy or a below-knee walking cast (→ *above*). Analgesia and crutches may be necessary.

Ankle fractures

A fracture of the ankle may follow a mechanism of injury similar to a sprain. There is usually significant pain and swelling, although some patients may be able to weight-bear. Examination must again include the knee, calf, ankle, heel and foot.

Two or more separate lesions, whether of bone or ligament, will produce a potentially unstable joint and require specialist attention. Isolated fracture of the lateral malleolus, for example, may render the ankle mortise unstable if there is concurrent rupture of the deltoid ligament (between the medial malleolus and the calcaneum). Fracture of the medial malleolus may be associated with a spiral fracture of the neck of the fibula (Maisonneuve's fracture).

XR Radiographs of the ankle are usually diagnostic but should be supplemented with views of the knee, leg, heel and foot, as clinically indicated. Vertical fractures of the posterior part of the tibia (seen on the lateral view and extending down to the ankle joint) are conveniently (but inaccurately) termed fractures of the posterior malleolus. Thus, a fracture may be described as bimalleolar or even trimalleolar.

TX Stable, undisplaced fractures of the lateral malleolus may be treated on an outpatient basis in a below-knee plaster cast. The patient should be seen at the next fracture clinic.

Unstable and displaced bimalleolar and trimalleolar fractures should be reduced under conscious sedation and a backslab applied. Post reduction X-rays must be taken. Admission under the orthopaedic team will be necessary.

Posterior displacement of the lower tibial epiphysis

This may occur in children. Reduction under general anaesthesia is straightforward, but overnight admission is usually required.

Fracture of the distal tibial epiphysis

This is also known as the Tillaux fracture. This is a type of transitional ankle fracture that occurs exclusively in the adolescent population due to the unique closure pattern of the distal tibial epiphysis. This is a Salter Harris III fracture of the antero-lateral distal tibial epiphysis. Clinical examination often reveals localised tenderness over the anterior joint line, as opposed to a sprain where the tenderness is generally below the joint line. This injury will require referral to orthopaedics.

Dislocation of the ankle

The talus, and with it the foot, may be completely dislocated after severe local trauma. Usually, the skin remains intact but is stretched tightly over the bone. An accompanying fracture is common.

XR Radiographs should be delayed until after reduction if there is evidence of skin or vascular compromise. Despite traditional teaching, if perfusion is adequate, imaging prior to reduction (if achievable rapidly) is appropriate and useful.

TX Prompt reduction is important to reduce pain and minimise the risk of tissue necrosis.

- Give IV analgesia and supplement it with nitrous oxide/ methoxyflurane or IV sedation during the procedure.
- Reduce the ankle with axial traction.
- Check the skin circulation and foot pulses.
- Apply a splint or cast.
- Obtain radiographs.
- Refer the patient to the orthopaedic team.

THE FOOT

Relative positions of the bones of the foot → Figure 7.10.

Fracture of the talus

Talar fractures present in a similar way to ankle injuries. They often produce long-term disability because of disruption of the subtalar joint; sometimes avascular necrosis occurs.

XR These fractures can be missed on radiographs unless the area is carefully inspected.

TX The patient should have analgesia and orthopaedic referral.

Fracture of the calcaneum

Calcaneal fracture is usually caused by a direct fall on to the heel from a height such as a roof or a ladder. There is:

- pain and difficulty in weight-bearing
- local tenderness and sometimes bruising
- a possibility of associated, and perhaps masked, injuries elsewhere (e.g. lumbar spine).

A fracture of this region may also occur in osteoporotic bone, following relatively minor trauma. In this case, it may superficially mimic a soft-tissue injury of the ankle.

XR Radiographs should be obtained of the ankle, heel and foot. The radiograph shows a normal ankle mortise. Single or multiple fracture lines through the cancellous os calcis are often missed. The flattening of Böhler's angle is an important radiographic sign (→ *Figure 7.11*). A CT scan may be required to assess the degree of injury and the consequent need for internal fixation.

> The calcaneum is like an egg – it can be cracked, dented or completely smashed!

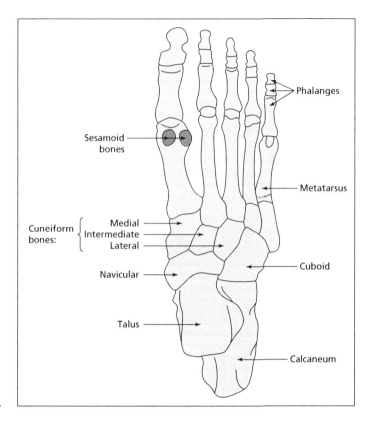

Figure 7.10 The bones of the foot.

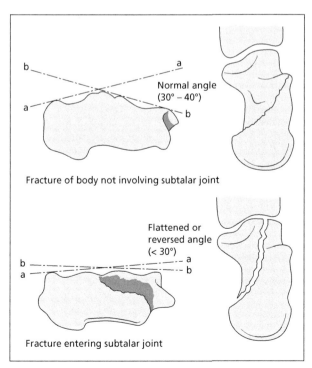

Figure 7.11 Loss of Böhler's angle.

Tx Exclude associated injuries. Patients with this fracture require strong analgesia and orthopaedic referral. Weight-bearing is usually impossible; a thick wool and crepe bandage with crutches, or a walking splint allows temporary mobility.

Tarsal fracture and tarsometatarsal dislocation

Fractures of the tarsus may be produced by crushing and twisting forces. Pain and swelling are usually prominent. The term 'Lisfranc's fracture' covers a variety of ligament and bone injuries at the junction of the mid- and forefoot. Trapping the foot in a stirrup when thrown from a horse is a typical cause. Although rare, it is difficult to diagnose and inadequate management leads to significant disability. There is usually a dislocation at the tarsometatarsal junction with associated fractures, commonly at the second metatarsal base but also at the metatarsal neck.

XR Tarsometatarsal dislocation with fracture of the second metatarsal base (Lisfranc's fracture) is important to recognise but may be overlooked on standard radiological views. A true lateral view of the area will reveal dorsal displacement.

Tx Open reduction may be necessary. Specialist advice should always be sought.

Pain in the foot

Plantar fasciitis

The patient complains of pain on the sole of the foot, often worst in the morning and after exercise. Pain is exacerbated by the heel striking the ground. There is tenderness localised to the anteromedial part of the calcaneum about 5 cm below and 1 cm in front of the medial malleolus. The condition is caused by degenerative changes in or overuse of the plantar fascia, as with jogging and military training. This results in partial avulsion of the fascia from the os calcis. Chronic symptoms may be associated with a calcaneal spur. Radiographs may be taken to exclude a fracture and identify a spur, although diagnosis is clinical in most cases. Most cases of plantar fasciitis can be effectively treated by prescribing an excavated heel cushion or a pad composed of an energy-absorbing hydrogel. NSAIDs, physiotherapy or orthotic review may be helpful. Local infiltration with a steroid is often effective but should be left to the discretion of the orthopaedic department. The presence of a calcaneal spur is not an indication for surgery, although its removal is occasionally necessary.

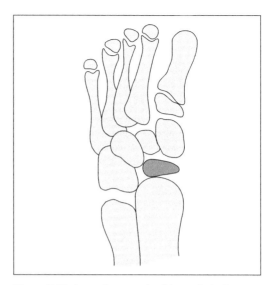

Figure 7.12 Avascular necrosis of the navicular bone.

Köhler's disease

Osteochondritis of the navicular bone occurs mostly in teenage boys. They present with chronic pain on exercise. There may be a history of minor trauma. Midtarsal and subtalar joint movements are restricted. Radiographs show a collapsed sclerotic bone (→ *Figure 7.12*). The patient should be given analgesia and referred to the next orthopaedic clinic.

Prominent navicular bone

Teenagers (most often girls) may complain of pain over the inner aspect of the foot and relate the symptoms to exercise or injury. Anxious parents point to the prominent medial end of the navicular bone as the cause of the pain. If examination of the foot is otherwise normal, they should be reassured. Periosteal inflammation may indeed make the bone appear prominent, but most cases settle spontaneously. Attention should be directed to appropriate footwear.

Metatarsalgia

Pain under the metatarsal heads is often chronic and degenerative in origin. It may be relieved by providing a metatarsal gel pad. This should extend almost up to, but not under, the prominent bone.

Fractures of the forefoot

Metatarsal fractures are common but are only of importance when there is gross disruption or the bones of the first ray are involved. Most forces through the forefoot are transmitted along the first metatarsus. A stress fracture (March fracture) is most commonly seen in the index (second) metatarsal neck.

XR Stress fractures may not be visible on a radiograph until callus formation has occurred. A bone scan may be diagnostic.

TX Multiple fractures of the metatarsal bones may require internal fixation. Patients with significant fractures of the first metatarsus should also be referred for an orthopaedic opinion. For most other metatarsal fractures, a below-knee plaster cast can be applied on an outpatient basis. The patient will require analgesia, crutches and follow-up in the fracture clinic.

Fractures of the toes

Fractures of the toes are common and usually result from a kicking or stubbing injury.

XR A radiograph is usually not necessary except where there is clinical deformity or the proximal phalanx of the big toe is involved.

TX Fractures of the proximal phalanx of the big toe may need a walking splint/boot and fracture clinic follow-up.

Angulated toes should be straightened under ring block and then neighbour strapped. Check radiographs should be obtained and follow-up arranged.

Other toe injuries are treated symptomatically irrespective of the presence of a minor undisplaced fracture. Neighbour strapping is helpful. Pain around the metatarsophalangeal joints may be helped by the application of a metatarsal pad. Bulky dressings prevent the use of normal footwear and should be avoided. Follow-up is not necessary if the patient is advised on care of the strapping and told that symptoms will abate over the ensuing month.

VASCULAR CONDITIONS OF THE LOWER LIMB

Arterial embolism

Thrombi, which embolise to peripheral arteries, may arise from several sites:

1 The left atrial appendage (usually in the presence of atrial fibrillation)
2 The left ventricle (invariably on an area damaged by a recent myocardial infarction)
3 An atheromatous plaque
4 An aortic aneurysm
5 A thrombosis in a deep vein in a patient with a patent foramen ovale (paradoxical embolism).

All of these possibilities should be considered, although the first two are by far the most common.

Emboli tend to lodge at the sites of bifurcation of arteries. Their effects depend on the extent of the occlusion of the circulation and the degree of collateral circulation that exists. The following are common sites that involve the lower limb:

- The aortic bifurcation (bilateral ischaemia to the level of the knees)
- The origin of the deep femoral artery (ischaemia to the midcalf)
- The bifurcation of the popliteal artery (ischaemia of the foot).

Sudden occlusion of the femoral artery causes the six 'Ps':

1 Pain
2 Pallor
3 Pulselessness
4 Paraesthesia
5 Paralysis
6 Perishing cold.

TX Embolism must be treated within 6 hours of the onset of symptoms or else propagation of thrombus distal to the embolus will greatly worsen prognosis. Treatment includes:

- Oxygen
- IV analgesia
- IV fluids
- IV unfractionated heparin
- referral to a vascular surgeon. Embolectomy or thrombolysis may be required.

Intra-arterial injection

Irritant substances may cause critical ischaemia if injected into an artery. IV drug users are the most common sufferers from this problem. The ischaemia results from a mixture of vasospasm and multiple small emboli. Severe pain is the prominent symptom, but the other signs described above (the six 'Ps') may be absent.

TX This is similar to the treatment described above for arterial embolism. Drugs that cause arterial dilatation may be considered.

Venous thrombosis

Thrombosis of the deep veins of the lower limb or pelvis (DVT) may be caused by changes in any of the following:

1 Blood coagulation (smoking, hormonal contraception, malignancy, recent surgery or major illness)

2 Blood vessels (pregnancy)
3 Blood flow (immobility, long-haul air or road travel and plaster casts).

> Thrombosis of veins distal to the popliteal vein ('below-knee DVT') is particularly common because of the venous sinuses present in the soleus muscle of the calf. At least 5% of below-knee DVTs spread to the proximal veins and half of all above-knee venous thromboses embolise to the lungs.

The classic clinical features of DVT are:

- swelling and oedema distal to the occlusion
- warmth, redness and deep tenderness of the thigh or calf.

These signs depend on venous occlusion. In contrast, there may be no signs in the presence of an extensive, non-occlusive thrombus.

> Homan's sign cannot be relied on – it is positive in less than 20% of patients with DVT of the leg.

- The following conditions may be mistaken for DVT:
- Chronic venous obstruction
- Superficial phlebitis (→ next)
- Post-thrombotic syndrome
- Acute or subacute arterial ischaemia (→ 110)
- Cellulitis of the leg (→ p. 423)
- Calf muscle tear (→ p. 104) or other soft-tissue injury
- Ruptured Baker's cyst (→ p. 102)
- Fracture of the lower limb
- Lymphoedema
- Hypoproteinaemia.

Investigations: The Well's scoring system for clinical DVT may be used to stratify patients into low-, moderate- or high-risk groups (→ Table 7.1). Those patients with a low risk may be further subdivided by requesting a D-dimer blood test. (This protein is a cross-linked fibrin degradation product that is released into the bloodstream from active blood clots and sites of wound healing.) A negative D-dimer has >95% negative predictive value for DVT, whereas a positive result has <70% positive predictive value. D-dimer is therefore a good test to rule out DVT in low-risk patients but is not a useful method of diagnosis. D-dimer is not useful in high-risk patients.

Proximal leg compression ultrasound is the investigation modality of choice.

Table 7.1 Well's scoring system for clinical deep vein thrombosis (DVT)

Clinical feature	Score
Cancer treatment ongoing or within last 6 months	+1
Immobilisation of lower limb	+1
Bedridden for more than 3 days	+1
Major surgery in last 4 weeks	+1
Entire leg swollen	+1
Calf swelling >3 cm in diameter	+1
Increased pitting oedema in symptomatic leg	+1
Superficial collateral veins visible	+1
Alternative diagnosis as likely or more likely	−2
Total score ≤0	Low probability of DVT
Total score = 1–2	Moderate probability of DVT
Total score ≥3	High probability of DVT

Tx Once the diagnosis has been confirmed or provisionally suspected, most patients will be treated by rapid anticoagulation (usually as an outpatient). This is usually with either a low-molecular-weight heparin (LMWH) given subcutaneously or direct acting oral anticoagulants (DOACs). If parenteral anticoagulation is used, it will be required for at least 5 days and consequently effective community liaison is essential for outpatients. Follow-up in a clinic should be arranged. Oral anticoagulants are substituted for the heparin as soon as possible and are usually continued for about 3 months. In occasional cases of rapidly progressing or life-threatening DVT, thrombolysis may be considered.

Diagnosis and management of suspected PE → pp. 227.
Risk factors for venous thromboembolism → Box 13.13 on p. 228.

Phlebitis

Inflammation of the long or short saphenous vein usually occurs in patients with varicose veins or those who have had IV therapy. The vein is red, hot and tender.

Tx Phlebitis usually settles with topical therapy and oral NSAIDs. It has however been recognised that more symptomatic cases respond better with anticoagulation treatment. If there is a systemic pyrexia, an antibiotic (e.g. co-amoxiclav) can be added.

Venous disease in IV drug users

Repeated injection into the femoral vein causes chronic venous obstruction. There is swelling and oedema of the whole lower limb and dilatation of the superficial vessels; injection sinuses are often found in the groin. Femoral vessel aneurysm, pseudoaneurysm and abscess formation may occur – hence, CT angiography should be performed prior to incision of a groin abscess. Thrombosis may result in the limb becoming hot, red and painful. This type of widespread DVT is potentially life-threatening.

Acute compartment syndrome

> A compartment is defined as a closed tissue space where muscle, neural or other soft tissue are surrounded by a layer of inelastic fascia (or bone). There are 46 such compartments in the human body, 38 of which are found in the upper and lower extremities.

Closed compartment syndrome of the limbs is caused by swollen, contused muscle or bleeding inside a rigid fascial envelope. As the intra-compartmental pressure rises, there is venous obstruction and further swelling. When capillary perfusion pressure is exceeded, ischaemia and tissue necrosis begin to occur. Eventually, there is irreversible injury to both nerves and muscles (e.g. Volkmann's ischaemic contracture). The most common cause is trauma, usually with a fracture, and male patients aged <35 years are the most frequently affected. Anticoagulant drugs increase the likelihood of developing compartment syndrome.

Compartment syndrome can easily develop unseen under a plaster cast or below an eschar from a burn. The most common site to be affected is the lower leg (which has four anatomical compartments), but the syndrome is also seen in the forearm (three fascial compartments), the foot and the hand. The anterior compartment is the most commonly affected area of the leg, whereas, in the forearm, it is the flexor compartment. Compartment syndrome is reported to occur in between 2% and 5% of patients with tibial fractures, often after comparatively low-energy mechanisms of injury.

The onset of compartment syndrome may be delayed after injury and insidious. Early symptoms are severe pain – aggravated by muscle stretching – and paraesthesia. The affected part may also, but not inevitably, be pale and cool with a slow capillary refill, although this is a later sign. Ischaemia results from compression of small blood vessels and so the presence of distal pulses are of no help in excluding the diagnosis. Venous outflow from the compartment is usually obstructed long before the entry of arterial blood is impeded.

> In compartment syndrome, the limb may not be broken, distal pulses may be present and pulse oximetry may be normal. Worsening pain, especially on passive stretch, is an important sign.

XR Arteriography will reveal arterial lesions but will not demonstrate compartment syndrome.

TX Suspicion of compartment syndrome is an indication for an immediate orthopaedic referral. Manometry is useful, particularly in patients with a depressed level of consciousness. Compartment pressures of over 40 mmHg or within 30 mmHg of diastolic blood pressure are highly suggestive of compartment syndrome. (The normal intracompartmental pressure is 10–12 mmHg.) There are four compartments in the lower leg, and all may require extensive decompressive fasciotomy. This will produce significant fluid loss, and blood transfusion may be necessary.

> Elevation of the affected limb may increase ischaemia.

8

The upper limb

Katie Fulcher[1] and Abu Hassan[2]

[1] Bradford Teaching Hospitals NHS Foundation Trust, Bradford, UK
[2] Sheffield Children's Hospital, Sheffield, UK

General principles of the management of limb injuries → p. 88.

Think about analgesia, support and splintage (→ *Box 8.1*) before starting your assessment.

THE SHOULDER AND UPPER ARM

> If the patient can put his or her hand behind the head and into the small of the back without pain, then the shoulder on that side is unlikely to be significantly injured.

Fracture of the clavicle

The clavicle provides the only skeletal continuity between the upper limb and trunk. Clavicle fractures usually result from a direct blow to the shoulder, it is a common injury, e.g. in cycling accidents. Most fractures occur at the junction between the middle and outer third of the clavicle, as this is the thinnest part of the bone and the only part not reinforced by attached musculature and ligaments.

Damage to adjacent neurovascular structures is very rare except with posterior sternoclavicular dislocation. In adults, fractures cause well-localised symptoms with obvious deformity and tenderness.

Children: greenstick fractures are common after childhood falls. There may be little deformity and remarkably good movement of the arm and shoulder girdle. Alternatively, the child may refuse to use the whole arm on the affected side and thus mimic a pulled elbow (→ *p. 119*). In children, if it looks clinically like a clavicle fracture, it may not always be necessary to perform radiographs as this will often not change the management. Follow up is not essential for minimally displaced fractures in children.

XR An anteroposterior (AP) radiograph confirms the diagnosis.

TX The weight of the arm should be supported in a broad arm sling. Figure-of-eight bandages are no longer widely used. Most displaced fractures settle to produce an acceptable cosmetic result. Prescribe appropriate analgesia and refer the patient to the next fracture clinic. Non-union is rare and usually occur in outer third fractures. In cases where there is significant displacement, skin tenting, >2 cm shortening or comminution surgical management may be indicated.

Sternoclavicular joint disruption

This is rare and usually the result of considerable indirect violence applied to the shoulder, so there should be a high index of suspicion for additional injuries. Sternoclavicular dislocation can be anterior or posterior. Anterior is more common, and there is usually a bony prominence on examination. Posterior displacement is rare but potentially very serious as it may involve damage to, or compression of, major blood vessels, the trachea or the oesophagus.

XR Radiological confirmation is difficult, especially if bilateral. Specific sternoclavicular joint X-rays can be helpful. A CT scan may be helpful to diagnose sternoclavicular dislocation and look for associated injuries

TX This can be a major injury with potentially serious consequences. Orthopaedic advice should be sought.

The RCEM Lecture Notes: Emergency Medicine, Fifth Edition. Edited by Catherine Williams and Amy Nickson.
© 2024 John Wiley & Sons Ltd. Published 2024 by John Wiley & Sons Ltd.
Companion website: www.wiley.com/go/LNEM5

Box 8.1 Upper limb support and splintage

Broad arm or triangular sling
Used to support the weight of the arm and restrict its movement. Useful for:

- fractures, dislocations and other painful conditions of the shoulder and clavicle
- fractures and other injuries of the forearm, wrist and hand including support of plaster casts
- painful conditions of the elbow and support of casts on the elbow

The high arm sling
This is a variant of the triangular sling used to decrease swelling of the hand. It is of doubtful effectiveness because flexion of the elbow above 90° may decrease venous drainage of the distal parts.

Collar and cuff
Usually made in the emergency department (ED) by securing a length of covered foam with a plastic clip, although commercial alternatives are available. It uses gravity to restrict movement while applying slight traction at the elbow and is useful for injuries of the elbow and humerus. Flexion of the elbow of more than 20° above the right angle is painful and should be avoided. Check the radial pulse.

Polysling
Various types on the market but all follow the same broad principle. Indications are the same as for a broad arm sling, but polysling may have advantages in terms of comfort and flexibility of positioning. Some can be used with a body belt to additionally restrict shoulder movement.

Advice to patients
- Wear the sling outside clothes
- Remove the sling at night and support the injured part on pillows
- Remember the importance of maintaining shoulder and hand mobility

Acromioclavicular joint disruption

This is much more common than the sternoclavicular joint disruption. The outer end of the clavicle is elevated at its articulation with the acromion. The weak fibres of the acromioclavicular joint are readily ruptured. The joint's normal stability is maintained by the conoid and trapezoid ligaments, binding the outer fifth of the clavicle down to the coracoid process of the scapula. It is the complete or partial rupture of these strong ligaments that results in an acromioclavicular dislocation or subluxation. Direct downward pressure will reduce the deformity rather painfully and only transiently. Acromioclavicular joint disruption is graded using the Rockwood classification.

Patients usually present with non-specific shoulder pain and reduced shoulder movements.

X<small>R</small> An acromioclavicular joint radiograph series can be used to evaluate the AC joint and lateral clavicle. An AP view will show widening of the joint and elevation of the distal end of the clavicle relative to the acromion process – the inferior border of the acromion should be level with the inferior border of the clavicle. If there is diagnostic uncertainty, and AC disruption is suspected but not confirmed, consider an AP film with the patient holding weights in the hands. Slight subluxation may occur normally. Grade of injury is determined by the degree of displacement of the clavicle relative to the acromion – in mild injuries there is little or no displacement of the joint (grade 1 or 2), but the clavicle in elevated above the superior border of acromion in more severe injuries (grade 3 and 5). Grade 4 refers to posterior displacement.

T<small>X</small> The raised outer end of the clavicle is accepted as a minor disability by most patients. Reduction is very difficult to maintain by closed methods and internal fixation, although successful, may leave a prominent scar. A sling and analgesia are provided until the pain has settled. The shoulder may remain weak for some months, and there may be a very slight permanent loss of power in the affected limb.

Supraspinatus tendonitis/subacromial bursitis

These two conditions are very difficult to separate. Both are caused by a combination of soft-tissue degeneration and a modest increase in activity. The patient presents with an injured shoulder often following an event such as lifting. Symptoms may occur suddenly or be more gradual in onset. Movements are restricted, particularly abduction and forward flexion. Classically, there is a painful arc from about 20° to 90° of abduction, but initially the pain may be intense and affect all movements. There may be specific tenderness in the supraspinatus fossa laterally.

X<small>R</small> Radiographs sometimes show calcification within the tendon, near its attachment to the joint capsule.

Tx A sling and non-steroidal anti-inflammatory drugs (NSAIDS) should be prescribed. In severe cases, a short course of oral steroids can give dramatic relief. Patients should be reviewed by physiotherapy, and orthopaedic referral may be considered. Surgical decompression may help in chronic cases.

Rotator cuff injury

The glenohumeral joint is stabilised by four muscles that surround it – the rotator cuff:

1 **Subscapularis**: a medial rotator
2 **Supraspinatus**: which initiates abduction
3 **Infraspinatus**: a lateral rotator
4 **Teres minor**: another lateral rotator.

The rotator cuff muscles may be acutely injured or chronically inflamed or both. This causes pain with shoulder movements, sometimes of the painful arc type. There may be a tender area anteriorly. The tendons of all the rotator cuff muscles may rupture or degenerate in a similar manner to the supraspinatus tendon (→ *above*).

Frozen shoulder → p. 117.

Tx Analgesia, together with rest in a sling, is required for a few days. Early physiotherapy is essential. The condition can be very slow to settle (up to 2 years), especially in older patients and in those with an acute onset.

Rupture of the long head of biceps

This is caused by a combination of tendon degeneration and powerful elbow flexion. The patient often gives a history of hearing a snap whilst lifting, bruising down the anterior upper arm and the sudden appearance of a painless lump reminiscent of Popeye's biceps.

Tx This is usually conservative, but a specialist opinion should be sought via fracture clinic.

Dislocation of the shoulder joint

The shoulder is the most commonly dislocated joint. This involves dislocation of the humeral head from the glenoid. This may occur after trivial injury in a predisposed individual or follow major energy transfer to the shoulder girdle and be associated with other bone and soft-tissue injuries.

Patients present with pain and an inability to move the joint. A full examination is essential to exclude associated injuries and neurovascular complications, particularly checking for loss of sensation in the regimental badge distribution supplied by the axillary nerve.

95% of dislocations are anterior and easily detected clinically and radiologically (→ *Figure 8.1*). Posterior dislocation is rarer and associated with the muscle contraction that occurs during fits and electric shocks. Inferior dislocation ('*luxatio erecta*') is very rare – the patient presents with the arm erect. A fracture of the greater tuberosity or neck of the humerus may accompany a dislocation.

Xʀ In first dislocations or those associated with significant energy transfer, radiographs must be taken before reduction is attempted. In patients with recurrent dislocation due to minor provocation, this is not always necessary. Lateral radiographs are difficult to interpret; modified axial views are more useful. → *Figures 8.2* and *8.3* demonstrate the normal appearances of the shoulder joint on lateral and apical radiographs.

> Posterior dislocation of the shoulder may not be obvious clinically and can easily be missed on the AP radiograph (→ *Figure 8.4*).

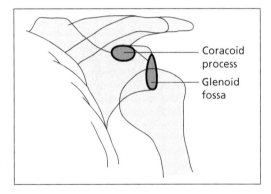

Figure 8.1 Anterior dislocation of the shoulder joint.

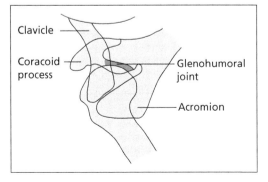

Figure 8.2 The normal appearance of the shoulder joint (apical view).

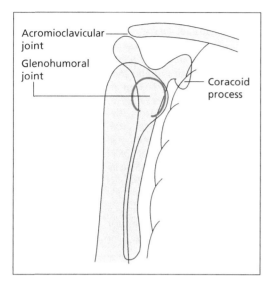

Acromioclavicular joint

Glenohumoral joint

Coracoid process

Figure 8.3 The normal appearance of the shoulder joint (lateral view).

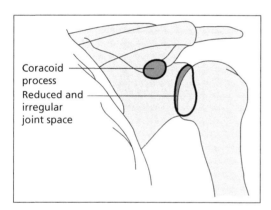

Coracoid process

Reduced and irregular joint space

Figure 8.4 Posterior dislocation of the shoulder joint.

Tx The patient will need early analgesia. In many cases, reduction can be achieved without sedation by using one of a number of techniques to overcome muscle spasm. Gentle downward traction with massage to the deltoid and biceps (Cunningham technique) is often effective. Prior analgesia helps but large amounts should not be necessary if the technique is good. The method of sedation will depend largely on the experience of the staff involved (→ p. 13). Many methods of reduction can be equally successful; a technique for anterior dislocations is described in Box 8.2. The emergency physician should be familiar with a range of techniques for shoulder reduction as no single method will be successful in all patients.

 Box 8.2 Reduction of a dislocated shoulder

- Explain the procedure to the patient and obtain consent
- Ensure that adequate sedation and analgesia are achieved and appropriate resuscitation facilities are available
- Gently hold the wrist on the dislocated side in both hands. Countertraction, if required, may be applied by a second person supporting the patient with a towel sling around the shoulder
- Slowly (over a minute or two) abduct the arm out to 90°, keeping the elbow extended. As the arm is abducting, rotate it externally (i.e. so that the palm is facing upwards)
- Apply firm, constant traction along the patient's abducted, rotated arm. The shoulder joint is approaching its most unstable position. Gentle, uninterrupted traction with reassurance to maintain muscle relaxation is the key to success. Do not use excessive force because it may damage the axillary neurovascular structures. By slightly varying the angle of pull and the axial rotation of the arm, the joint will usually relocate within about 5 min with minimal patient discomfort

The ease of reduction is dependent on a number of factors, including the build of the patient and the amount of time the shoulder has been dislocated. Shoulders which have been dislocated for some time are in most cases more difficult to reduce and may be more likely to result in complications. Inferior dislocations usually reduce easily; the arm is gently brought down to a partially abducted position and then treated as an anterior dislocation.

Fracture of the greater tuberosity may accompany a dislocated shoulder. It will usually relocate easily as the shoulder dislocation is reduced. Patients with a dislocation and a coexisting fracture of the neck of the humerus need immediate orthopaedic referral as do patients with a dislocation that is more than 24 hours old.

After reduction, the arm is immobilised in a collar and cuff or polysling. Radiographs are then repeated to confirm reduction, and the arm is again examined to exclude neurovascular damage. The patient is then referred to the next fracture clinic with instructions to keep the wrist and hand mobile. Physiotherapy and gradual mobilisation will be necessary at a later date, possibly followed by surgical repair of the lax shoulder joint capsule if there has been recurrent dislocation.

Hill-Sachs fracture and Bankart lesion are common sequelae of recurrent anterior shoulder dislocation. Hill-Sachs fracture is due to compression of the posterolateral humeral head against the glenoid. Bankart lesion results from detachment of the anterior labrum from the glenoid. Although no acute management is needed, the associated glenohumeral instability sometimes requires operative repair at a later date.

Brachial plexus injury

These injuries are caused by sudden traction on the arm (e.g. a window cleaner grasping the window ledge as the ladder slips) or by direct impact to the shoulder region (e.g. a motor cyclist struck from in front by an oncoming vehicle). They may also be seen in patients who have sustained prolonged pressure on the axilla while under the influence of alcohol or other intoxicants. Injury can involve the upper two or three nerve roots (partial injury) or all five nerve roots (complete injury). Injuries can be ruptures, where the root is still connected to the spinal cord, or avulsions where the root detaches from the spinal cord.

There may be any of the following:

- **Complete section**: neuroptmesis
- **Axonal damage**: axonoptmesis
- **Failure of transmission only**: neuropraxia
- *A combination of the above.*

Neurological examination determines the areas involved. The clinical presentation will depend on which root is involved and the degree of damage. The presence of Horner's syndrome indicates preganglionic damage.

XR Radiological examination should include the shoulder, cervical spine and thoracic outlet. Look for a first rib injury and a raised hemidiaphragm.

Tx Early specialist referral will be required. Axonal regeneration down intact sheaths occurs at a rate of about 1 mm/day (or 1 in./month). Surgical repair is rarely attempted and then mainly for distal lesions. No regeneration or repair is possible if part of the plexus has been avulsed from the spinal cord.

Fracture of the scapula

Fractures of the scapula are relatively uncommon and usually the result of direct trauma. Significant force is required to fracture the scapula and so the possibility of accompanying injuries must be strongly considered. Any part of the bone may be fractured, including the body, spine, neck, acromion process and coracoid process. Local pain and tenderness are the main clinical features; shoulder movements may be relatively intact.

XR Fractures of the scapula are often missed on radiographs. An oblique view of the shoulder (to show the scapula more clearly) may be requested in cases of doubt. CT is usually required to evaluate the extent of the fracture and assess for other injuries.

Tx Displacement of a fracture of the spine or blade is rarely significant and management is conservative. The patient should be given a broad arm sling and analgesia and then referred to the next fracture clinic. A floating shoulder is a fracture of the scapula neck and ipsilateral clavicle, and this requires surgical fixation. The scapula has an excellent blood supply and usually heals very well.

Fracture of the humeral neck

This can occur at all ages but is particularly common in elderly people. It is usually an isolated injury, caused by a low-speed impact such as fall onto outstretched hand at home. Displacement is common and may be gross but is usually unimportant and will reduce over time under gravity without needing manipulation.

A full examination should be made to exclude other injury, particularly at the wrist. The axillary nerve may be damaged, causing deltoid paralysis and an area of anaesthesia over the outer aspect of the shoulder (regimental badge patch). The joint may subluxate inferiorly because of this deltoid paralysis. The nerve will recover spontaneously over a period of a few weeks. Bruising is often very extensive and may extend down to the mid-forearm over the first few days. The patient should be warned that this rather frightening, but harmless phenomenon might occur.

XR An AP radiograph may be sufficient, but if shoulder dislocation is suspected an axial view will be required. In children, take care to distinguish a greenstick fracture, with buckled cortex, from the normal epiphyseal line.

Tx A collar and cuff, analgesia and reassurance are all that are required initially. Fracture clinic referral is arranged; physiotherapy should follow.

Frozen shoulder

Adhesive capsulitis of the shoulder joint is most commonly seen in older patients. It is a chronic fibrosing condition resulting in a reduced passive and active range of movement in the shoulder. It may be spontaneous or follow the disuse associated with any type of upper limb injury. Early mobilisation after injury will help to prevent its development (e.g. for patients with Colles' fractures remove the sling every few hours so that the arm can be moved behind the back and the neck). Patients with established disease and no recent history of trauma may present to the ED. Cervical and thoracic outlet problems must be excluded. The patient often complains of pain at the deltoid insertion but is actually tender over the anterior capsule. Abduction and internal rotation are particularly restricted.

> When assessing glenohumeral movement, always put one hand on the scapula to exclude the scapulothoracic contribution to shoulder mobility.

XR Radiographs are not generally indicated but may show an area of calcification in the shoulder joint capsule.

TX This condition may be very slow (up to 2 years) to resolve spontaneously. The other shoulder may be affected just as the first is recovering. Physiotherapy is the mainstay of treatment. Steroid injection, particularly into calcified areas of the capsule, and NSAIDs may be helpful. Manipulation under anaesthesia may sometimes be needed.

Thoracic outlet obstruction

The neurovascular outflow from the thorax and spine to the upper limb is constrained by a narrow-based triangle above the first rib. The lower parts of the brachial plexus and the subclavian artery may be compressed here if the shoulders are depressed by heavy backpacks or unaccustomed lifting. Symptoms are more likely if the brachial plexus is post-fixed (i.e. arises from the spinal cord more caudally than usual) or if there is a cervical rib. A tumour at the apex of the lung can spread upwards to involve the lower part of the brachial plexus.

The patient complains of a gradual onset of diffuse shoulder girdle pain, made worse by carrying shopping bags, etc. Symptoms can be reproduced by pulling down on the arm with the patient standing. Depending which structure is being compressed, there may be signs and symptoms of paraesthesia, weakness or circulatory changes to the upper limb. The radial pulse may be obliterated if the arm is abducted to 90°, and the patient turns their head to the opposite side. There may be weakness of the small muscles of the hand and paraesthesia in the hand extending up the inner border of the arm. The most important form of thoracic outlet obstruction not to miss is compression of the subclavian artery as this can result in limb ischaemia.

XR Radiographs are taken of the cervical spine, thoracic inlet and chest.

TX Always seek advice about management. If more sinister causes have been excluded, slow recovery usually occurs if traction on the shoulder can be avoided. Physiotherapy may help. Patients with vascular compromise may require thrombolysis and surgical intervention with resection of the first rib.

Referred pain at the shoulder

When no obvious localised cause of shoulder pain can be found on history or examination, referred pain at the shoulder must be considered. Any cause of diaphragmatic irritation may produce shoulder-tip pain, and this includes any cause of free fluid in the abdomen, cholecystitis, splenic injury, subphrenic abscess and pleurisy. Cardiac pain may present initially with a generalised ache in the shoulder joint.

Fracture of the humeral shaft

This fracture is unstable and painful and thus requires immediate splintage. These usually occur from direct blow to the upper arm or twisting action. If little force was involved, pathological fracture is a possibility. The radial nerve is often damaged, but rarely divided, as it winds around the humeral shaft in the spiral groove; check the patient's ability to extend the wrist and fingers. The radial pulse should also be checked because brachial artery injury may sometimes occur.

XR Radiographs should include the shoulder and elbow joints.

TX Provide support and analgesia. Orthopaedic referral is indicated. Internal fixation is often undertaken but external splintage with a U-slab of plaster or a humeral brace, and a collar and cuff is an alternative.

THE ELBOW

The elbow may be injured by a direct blow or by transmitted forces. In children, the constantly changing epiphyses make the interpretation of radiographs challenging (→ *Box 8.3* and *Figure 8.5*).

> Full extension of the elbow (to a bony block) without pain makes the presence of a fracture very unlikely.

Box 8.3 **Elbow radiographs**

If a fracture is not clearly demonstrated on an elbow radiograph when you are clinically suspecting one, you must look for the indirect signs of a fracture. These are:

- **Fat pads:** a visible anterior fat pad is normal but if displaced anteriorly this is abnormal (called the sail sign). A visible posterior fat pad is almost always abnormal and suggests a large elbow effusion. In the context of trauma, a posterior fat pad and/or sail sign should make one look closely for an elbow fracture, e.g. radial head or supracondylar fracture. A lack of an elevated fat pad does not exclude a fracture
- **Radiocapitellar line:** a line drawn along the longitudinal axis of the radial head and neck should pass through the capitellum, if it does not then suspect dislocation of the radial head
- **Anterior humeral line:** on a true lateral X-ray, a line drawn down the anterior humerus should intersect the middle third of the capitellum, if it does not then there is likely to be a supracondylar fracture

Interpretation may be difficult in children but is aided by a knowledge of the times of appearance and fusion of secondary ossification centres (also → Figure 8.5):

C 2: Capitellum – present by age 2 years
R 4: Radial head – appears at 3–5 years of age
I 6: Internal or medial epicondyle – present by age 6 years
T 8: Trochlea – appears at age 7–9 years
O 10: Olecranon – appears at age 9–11 years
L 12: Lateral or external epicondyle – present by age 11–14 years

- The epiphyses of the capitellum, trochlea and lateral epicondyle become one centre in the early teenage years
- All the epiphyses fuse in the teenage years, usually a year or two later in boys than in girls
- Comparative views of the other elbow, taken at the same angle, are occasionally helpful but should not be requested unless absolutely necessary (and then usually after discussion with a radiologist)

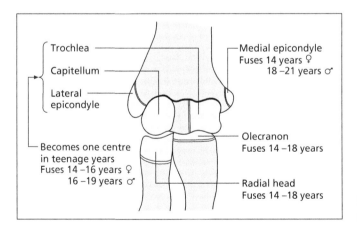

Figure 8.5 Secondary ossification centres around the elbow.

Pulled elbow

Sudden traction on a young child's arm may partially sub-luxate the radial head through the soft annular ligament which becomes stretched and entrapped. The classical history of pull on the arm is absent in about half of cases. The diagnosis should be suspected in a child who:

- is between 1 and 4 years old (rare > 6 years).
- has no history of significant trauma.
- is unwilling to use one arm.
- holds that arm limply by his or her side with the elbow semi-flexed in mid-pronation.
- has no obvious swelling, bruising or tenderness.
- cries at attempts to elevate the arm.

Xʀ Radiographs are unnecessary if you are confident in the diagnosis of a pulled elbow.

Tx There are two main methods of reduction for a pulled elbow. The most effective is hyper-pronation of the extended forearm. An alternative is gentle but determined supination of the forearm with the elbow at 90° and a thumb over the radial head, followed by full flexion of the elbow. A palpable click indicates success but is not always felt. The child should then be given some analgesia and observed playing for a while to satisfy the clinician and parents that the injury is resolved. This may take some time. Arms that have been immobile for several hours can be slightly swollen and more difficult to reduce. In older children, partial tears can occur in the annular ligament resulting in pain for a few days after reduction.

> Do not attempt to reduce a pulled elbow if you are in any doubt about the diagnosis. You will probably not do any harm, but the child's parents may be upset if you discover a fracture sometime later!

If the above procedure is unsuccessful at any stage, the whole arm should be re-examined and radiographed. If nothing abnormal is found, a collar and cuff should be supplied and the child reviewed within 48 hours. Most cases settle spontaneously in a few days.

The parents can be reassured that, although the condition may recur (in either arm), the ligaments will stiffen up after the age of 5 years and resolve the problem (*also → Box 8.4*).

 Box 8.4 The management of the child who is not using an arm

- Get a clear history and ensure the child has been given analgesia
- Watch the child playing with toys and the interaction with the parents
- Look for bruising, swelling or tenderness. Do not forget to examine the clavicle and wrist
- Decide where the problem areas are. If there are no immediately obvious areas and the arm is held limply by the side, consider pulled elbow or fractured clavicle
- If impossible to localise the area of injury, it may sometimes be necessary to obtain radiographs of the whole arm, including the clavicle. If they seem normal, look again for buckle fractures of the wrist or clavicle and effusions of the elbow. Consider plastic bowing fractures (→ *p. 125*)
- In all other cases, prescribe analgesia and a collar and cuff, reassure the parents and arrange for the child to be reviewed within 2 or 3 days

Supracondylar fracture

This injury occurs in older children (peak incidence at age 8 years) who fall on the outstretched arm. Severity varies from a hairline fracture to gross displacement, usually of the distal fragment posteriorly. These fractures are classified using the Gartland classification (→ *Figure 8.6*). All displaced fractures are associated with the risk of brachial artery injury; check distal pulses.

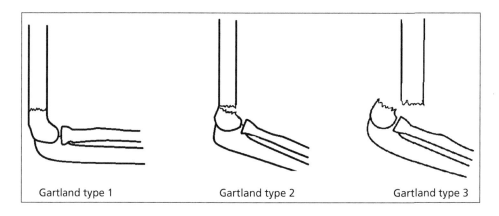

Gartland type 1   Gartland type 2   Gartland type 3

Figure 8.6 Gartland classification of supracondylar fractures.

Fractures of this area in adults are often comminuted and involve the articular surface. The elbow is swollen and movement very restricted. Neurovascular damage may occur.

Tx For displaced supracondylar fracture (Gartland classification 3 and 4), reduction under general anaesthesia by the orthopaedic team and subsequent monitoring of distal neurovascular function is essential. Failure to do this may result in Volkmann's ischaemic contracture of the forearm muscles, with permanent disability in the hand. Internal fixation is often required, especially if the articular surface is implicated. Undisplaced fractures (Gartland Type 1) can often be treated as an outpatient with an above elbow backslab and orthopaedic follow-up.

Fractures of the medial and lateral epicondyles

These fractures are caused by a varus or valgus strain at the elbow. Fracture of the medial epicondyle is more common than lateral epicondyle. Swelling may not be a major feature, but there is always a restriction of elbow extension and local bony tenderness. The medial epicondyle may be trapped in the joint; ulnar or median nerve injury may occur.

XR Radiographs may show little more than an effusion (→ *Figure 8.7*). Avulsion of an epicondyle in a child involves much more of the joint than the radiographs suggest, because most of the structure is cartilaginous.

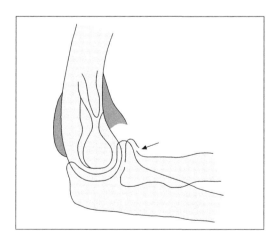

Figure 8.7 Lateral radiograph of the elbow joint showing anterior and posterior effusions (shaded) and fracture of the radial head (arrowed).

Tx An orthopaedic opinion is essential. Medial epicondyle fractures can often be managed with splinting and physiotherapy, but lateral epicondyle fractures almost always need operative management.

Fracture of the olecranon

This is sustained by falling on the point of the flexed elbow. Triceps action will distract the bone ends, and a gap can usually be felt beneath the rapidly developing haematoma and oedema. Active elbow extension is impossible. In the absence of an associated elbow dislocation, other movements, particularly supination and pronation, are often quite good and pain-free.

Tx The patient should be given a sling while awaiting specialist advice. Inpatient care and internal fixation will be necessary.

Fracture of the head or neck of the radius

This common fracture is usually sustained by a fall on the outstretched arm. Elbow flexion may be full, but extension is restricted. There is pain on palpation of the radial head, which is exacerbated during forearm rotation. Injury to the posterior interosseous nerve – which winds around the neck of the radius – is rare. There may be associated injuries, in particular fracture of the coronoid process of the ulnar and collateral ligament tears.

XR Radiographs usually show an effusion (→ *Figure 8.7*), but the fracture may be elusive. Further oblique views may be necessary.

Dislocation of the elbow joint

This requires considerable force. Consequently, there are usually associated fractures of the coronoid process, olecranon, capitellum or trochlea. There may also be damage to the brachial artery, or ulnar, median or radial nerves. The most common type of dislocation is posterolateral.

Tx Analgesia and splintage should be provided before taking a radiograph, and the radial pulse must be monitored. Reduction may be carried out in the ED by suitably experienced staff. Under sedation, axial traction is applied to the elbow while it is in about 30° of extension, with supination to allow the coronoid to pass under the trochlea, and direct pressure over the olecranon. A palpable clunk is usually felt on reduction. Place in an above elbow backslab in at least 90° of flexion, prior to obtaining post reduction imaging. Subsequent care is carried out by the orthopaedic department.

Box 8.5 Management of an injured elbow with a radiograph showing effusion but no fracture

A joint effusion seen on the lateral radiograph (→ *Figure 8.7*) usually indicates a significant injury – most commonly radial head fracture in an adult or supracondylar fracture in a child. If there is an effusion but no visible fracture then:

- re-examine the injured limb
- reconsider the possibility of a fracture of the head of the radius
- discuss the problem with a senior colleague and consider the need for further (oblique) radiographs
- explain the situation to the patient
- support the elbow in a collar and cuff
- prescribe analgesia
- arrange for follow up in 5–10 days

Radial head fracture is one of the most commonly missed limb injuries. It should be diagnosed clinically when there is:

- an appropriate history
- local tenderness
- reduced extension and supination
- a positive 'fat pad sign' on radiograph (anterior effusion)

Tx Minor undisplaced fractures are treated conservatively with early mobilisation. The patient will need analgesia, a collar and cuff, and referral to the next fracture clinic. More significant injuries may require internal fixation or excision of the radial head and should be referred immediately for specialist advice (*also* → *Box 8.5*).

Epicondylitis: Tennis elbow and golfer's elbow

Epicondylitis is most common between the ages of 40 and 60 years. There is usually a history of repetitive hand and wrist movements contributing to overuse of the forearm muscles that originate at the elbow.

'**Tennis elbow**' causes pain around the lateral epicondyle of the humerus. There is inflammation and sometimes partial avulsion of the common extensor origin, which may be tender. Nerve entrapment is occasionally responsible for the symptoms. Movements of the elbow joint are not usually reduced, although there may be slight restriction of pronation. Sudden passive flexion of the wrist, especially from the extended position, may reproduce the pain, as may gripping and twisting movements.

'**Golfer's elbow**' refers to a similar inflammation of the common flexor origin at the medial epicondyle of the humerus. There is chronic pain, which is worse on gripping, resisted wrist flexion and resisted forearm pronation.

XR Diagnosis is clinical. Radiographs are usually not necessary except where there is a history of trauma or clinical suspicion of bone disease.

Tx The inflammation is usually self-limiting, although symptoms may persist for many months. In mild cases, an oral NSAID together with advice to modify activity at work or sport may be sufficient. A wrist brace may provide some symptomatic relief. Physiotherapy is of some value and local injection of steroid often helps. Surgical division of part of the extensor (or flexor) origin is occasionally necessary.

Degenerative disease of the elbow joint

Chronic osteoarthrosis of the elbow is usually secondary to imperfectly reduced fractures involving the articular surfaces. Symptoms may begin spontaneously or be triggered by further minor trauma. The main complaint is of an inability to extend the elbow fully with some restriction of forearm rotation. Loose bodies may cause locking. If the fracture occurred during childhood, inequalities of growth may have resulted in marked deformity. A traction injury to the ulnar nerve may develop if cubitus valgus occurs after a lateral epicondyle fracture.

XR Radiographs may reveal more joint destruction than might be expected from clinical examination but are not usually indicated acutely unless there is a coexisting injury.

Tx The elbow may be rested in a sling for a few days to allow any inflammation to settle, but prolonged immobilisation may exacerbate stiffness. NSAIDs may be helpful. The patient should be referred for orthopaedic follow-up either directly or via the GP.

Olecranon bursitis

The patient presents with a large swelling over the olecranon, often after minor trauma or from repetitive injury. The elbow joint is not affected and is clinically normal except for discomfort on movement. The lump may be soft and fluctuant or tense and very painful if secondarily infected. Occasionally, the cause will be a crystal arthropathy.

Box 8.6 **Median and ulnar nerve supply to the muscles that are involved in movements of the hand**

Performing the 'Rock, Paper, Scissors, Ok?' test is an effective screening tool → *Figure 8.8*.

Muscles of the anterior forearm
Ulnar nerve flexor carpi ulnaris
  → medial half of flexor digitorum profundus
Median nerve supplies all the rest.

Intrinsic muscles of the hand
Median nerve → lateral two lumbricals
        → opponens pollicis
        → abductor pollicis brevis
        → flexor pollicis brevis
Ulnar nerve supplies all the rest.

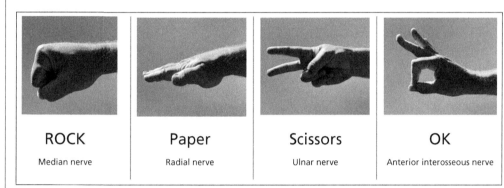

ROCK	Paper	Scissors	OK
Median nerve	Radial nerve	Ulnar nerve	Anterior interosseous nerve

Figure 8.8 Aide memoire for testing motor nerve function in the hand.

X_R Radiographs are not necessary, but if performed may reveal an underlying bony spur.

T_X The inflammation usually settles with rest and NSAIDs. Antibiotics should be prescribed if there is evidence of spreading infection or if the patient is pyrexial. If there is no sign of infection and the patient is systemically well, aspiration should be avoided as there is the risk of introducing infection. Rarely, incision and drainage will be required under anaesthesia. If the episode is non-resolving after 1–2 months, the patient may benefit from a steroid injection. If the episodes are recurrent, consideration should be given to referring the patient for formal excision of the bursa and underlying spur. If crystal arthropathy is thought to be a possibility, then the patient should be discussed with a rheumatologist.

THE FOREARM AND WRIST

Wounds to the forearm and wrist

Lacerations in this area frequently involve deep structures, and accurate diagnosis is essential. The history is usually helpful, although many injuries are either self-inflicted or sustained while intoxicated, so the patient's account may be misleading. Penetrating injuries (e.g. from glass) can cause nerve and tendon damage at a distance from the puncture wound.

A full assessment of distal neurovascular function is essential. Test all tendons and nerves individually (→ *Box 8.6*). Any positive finding of deep structure involvement must be discussed with a senior colleague. Further exploration must be carried out:

- in an operating theatre
- under adequate anaesthesia (usually general)
- with a bloodless field
- by an experienced surgeon

A divided nerve may continue to conduct some sensation for several hours if the nerve ends are touching.

Abductor pollicis brevis is paralysed in T1 root lesions but not in ulnar nerve lesions. To test this muscle, the thumb is moved vertically upwards against resistance with the hand in a supine position.

Fractures of the midshafts of the radius and ulna

The radius and ulna are bound together at the proximal and distal radioulnar joints forming a ring. Because of this ring, if the radius or ulna is fractured, it is likely there is another fracture or one of the radioulnar joints has been damaged.

There are three common patterns of injury:

1 A direct blow to the forearm produces a transverse fracture of either the ulna or both bones at the same level ('Nightstick fracture').
2 Rotational or transmitted forces produce a spiral fracture of each bone at different levels.
3 Rotational forces produce a fracture of one bone and a dislocation of the other at either of the radioulnar joints (→ *Figure 8.9*). In children a displacement of the epiphysis may occur (→ *Figure 8.10*).

Clinical and radiological examination must thus include the elbow and wrist joints, and neurovascular status must be carefully assessed. All of these forearm fractures are potentially unstable.

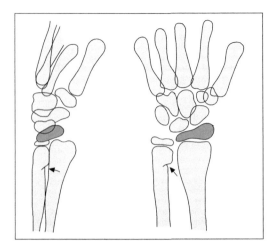

Figure 8.10 Posterior displacement of distal radial epiphysis (shaded) with buckle fracture of the ulna (arrowed).

XR One long X-ray plate, including both joints with the forearm bones, is inadequate because it produces oblique, atypical views of the joints, which are difficult to interpret. Standard films of adjacent joints should be obtained. If you see one fracture, it is important to look for another.

TX Analgesia and splintage should precede orthopaedic advice. Closed manipulation of some fractures under general anaesthetic may be successful, but this should be carried out in a fully equipped operating theatre so that failure can be quickly followed by open reduction and internal fixation under the same anaesthetic.

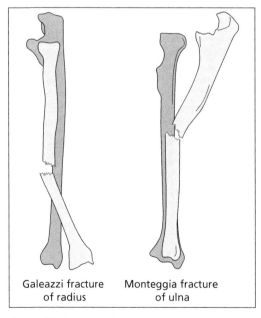

Galeazzi fracture
of radius

Monteggia fracture
of ulna

Figure 8.9 Fracture dislocations of the radius and ulna. *Galeazzi fracture dislocation*: fracture of the radial shaft with dorsal dislocation of the lower ulna from the inferior radioulnar joint. *Monteggia fracture dislocation:* fracture of the ulnar shaft with volar dislocation of the radial head into the antecubital fossa.

FOREARM FRACTURES IN CHILDREN

Children's bones are immature and more elastic than those of an adult. Because of this when a force is applied, it is possible for the bone to bend causing an incomplete fracture which is not seen in adults. This can occur to the upper or lower limb. In the upper limb, this most commonly causes a torus fracture (→ see *Figure 8.11*), plastic bowing fracture or greenstick fracture.

Torus fractures

These common 'buckle' fractures represent an incomplete fracture in the growing bone. They are inherently stable as the periosteum remains intact on both sides of

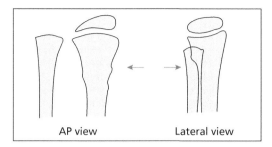

Figure 8.11 Buckle fracture of the distal radius (arrowed).

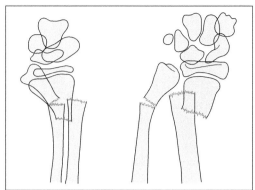

Figure 8.12 Metaphyseal (pronator quadratus) fracture of the distal radius and ulna.

the injury. Symptoms are usually mild, and examination findings may be very subtle pain on wrist pronation, and supination is often the most marked clinical finding (→ Figure 8.11).

Tx Buckle fractures are often managed in a rigid wrist splint for support. Plaster cast is unnecessary and cumbersome. Newer evidence suggests that a simple bandage or no splintage at all give similar results. Decisions can be made on a case-by-case basis depending on patient and parental preference and degree of discomfort. These fractures heal uneventfully, and no follow-up is required. Pain typically settles within 2–3 weeks.

Greenstick fractures

These result from an angulated force which causes bending of the bone and a cortical breach on only one side of the bone, the opposite cortex remains intact. In contrast to torus fractures, greenstick fracture involves damage to the periosteum on one side of the bone and therefore has potential to become unstable. They are usually mid-diaphyseal and can affect the radius, ulnar or both. A complete fracture, with breach of periosteum on both sides of the bone, and often significant displacement of the distal fragment may occur with higher energy transfer (→ Figure 8.12).

These fractures are usually mid-diaphyseal:

- there may be very little angulation.
- there is usually only a modest amount of pain.
- forearm rotation is always restricted.
- elbow and wrist movements may be full.
- neurovascular complications are unlikely.
- For these reasons, the fracture may be overlooked.

Tx A backslab with a sling, oral analgesics and outpatient follow-up is usually appropriate. Significant displacement may require manipulation under general anaesthesia.

Plastic bowing fractures of the radius and ulna

These relatively uncommon injuries are seen only in children between the ages of 2 and 5 years. The bending deformation is caused by a continuously applied longitudinal force, usually a fall on an outstretched arm. The most common variety occurs with the forearm pronated and involves bowing of the ulna with an angulated greenstick fracture of the radius. Conversely, a fall on a supinated forearm may fracture the ulna and bow the radius. Plastic bowing of both bones is the easiest variety to miss: although the child complains of pain and inability to use the arm, tenderness is difficult to localise and deformity may not be immediately obvious. Narrowing of the intraosseous space may cause pain on pronation and supination.

XR The affected bone appears bowed but with no actual fracture visible. (Microscopically, there is a series of microfractures on the concave aspect of the bone with intact cortex on the convex side.) Bowing is best seen on the lateral view. Ulnar bowing is usually convex posteriorly, whereas bowing of the radius causes an anterior angulation.

Tx Orthopaedic referral is required. In children aged <4 years, angulations of less than 20° that are not restricting movements can be left to remodel. Other plastic bowing fractures should be manipulated under general anaesthesia.

Plastic bowing fractures may also occur in the fibula, femur and clavicle.

Fracture of the distal radius

Fractures of the distal radius mostly occur in osteoporotic bone and so are most common in older women. These fractures are usually sustained by falling on the outstretched hand, and consequently injuries higher up the arm should always be excluded. In adults, impaction of cancellous bone imparts some stability compared with the obvious instability of midshaft fractures. However, pain and deformity are usually obvious, and supination is always restricted.

Colles' fracture is actually defined as any fracture of the radius within 2.5 cm of the wrist joint, but the term is usually taken to mean a wrist fracture with either dorsal displacement or anterior angulation.

Management of fractures of the distal radius with volar displacement of the distal fragment (Smith's fracture) → *p. 127.*
The six characteristic features of a Colles' fracture → *Box 8.7.*

 The degree of displacement or angulation, and therefore the need for reduction, can be estimated from the radiographs. The malposition is significant if either of the following occurs:

1 The articular surface of the distal radius on the lateral radiograph is not angulated in a volar direction, i.e. if angle ABC, as seen in → *Figure 8.13*, is <90°.
2 Radial shortening is seen on the AP view such that the ulnar articular surface is >2 mm distal to the radial articular surface.

Tx For the purposes of management in the ED, there are three main types of Colles' fracture of the distal radius:

1 **Fracture with minimal or acceptable displacement in an older patient with osteoporotic bone:**
 – confirm acceptable position (→ *Figure 8.13*).
 – exclude other injuries.
 – exclude medical cause of fall.
 – apply padded forearm backslab.
 – provide sling and analgesia.
 – encourage shoulder and hand mobility.
 – ensure adequate domestic support.
 – refer to fracture clinic.
2 **Displaced/angulated fracture in an osteoporotic wrist:** Treatment is as described in (1) above, but the fracture must be reduced under appropriate local (haematoma block), regional (Bier's block) or general-anaesthesia. (*Haematoma block* → *Box 8.8*). In some hospitals, this will take place in the ED. Satisfactory home circumstances are then of even greater importance if postoperative discharge is anticipated.
 Reduction is achieved by traction and slight hyperextension (to disimpact the fracture) and then flexion and ulnar deviation. Countertraction is applied by a colleague holding the upper arm. Unfortunately, the poor-quality dorsal cortex often allows the fracture to redisplace over the next 2 weeks. Re-manipulation may then be necessary. Good function is more important than good

---

> **Box 8.7 The six characteristic features of displaced Colles' fracture**
>
> 1 Dorsal displacement
> 2 Anterior angulation
> 3 Impaction
> 4 Lateral (radial) displacement
> 5 Ulnar angulation
> 6 Rotational deformity
>
> Avulsion of the ulnar styloid is a common accompanying feature

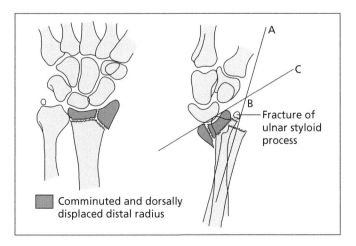

Figure 8.13 Comminuted Colles' fracture (with angle ABC identified).

A

C

B

Fracture of ulnar styloid process

Comminuted and dorsally displaced distal radius

> **Box 8.8 Haematoma block for reduction of Colles' fracture**
>
> - Use an aseptic technique; clean the skin thoroughly
> - Inject 5–15 mL 1% lidocaine into the fracture haematoma. Approach from the dorsal aspect; the fracture site lies more proximally than you might expect
> - Also inject some local anaesthetic around the ulnar styloid

anatomical and radiological reduction, but this fact should not influence initial attempts to obtain perfection. The manipulated fracture is held in its reduced position by a plaster backslab, which extends from the metacarpal heads to the antecubital fossa, over the dorsoradial aspect of the forearm. Radiographs should be taken after reduction but (if possible) before ending the anaesthetic so that an inadequate manipulation can be corrected immediately (→ *Figure 8.13*). As a result of the difficulty in maintaining a good position after reduction, many orthopaedic surgeons prefer to manipulate these fractures in theatre and then fix the bones in position with wires.

3 **Fracture in a younger patient**: After providing temporary splintage and analgesia, refer the patient to the orthopaedic team for reduction and plating of the fracture under general anaesthesia.

Smith's fracture: A 'reversed Colles' fracture' in which the distal radial fragment is displaced in a volar direction and tilted anteriorly (i.e. there is posterior angulation). It usually results from a fall onto the back of the hand. All such fractures should be discussed with the orthopaedic department.

Barton's fracture: A type of Smith's fracture in which only the anterior portion of the distal radius is involved. It should be referred to the orthopaedic team for fixation.

> Significant injury to the wrist is unlikely if:
> 1. full supination is possible without pain
> 2. there is no tenderness in the anatomical snuff box

Fracture of the radial styloid

This injury may mimic an undisplaced Colles' fracture or a scaphoid injury.

Tx A Colles-type plaster should be applied and the patient followed up in the fracture clinic.

Small chip fractures of the carpus

These are commonly seen after hyperextension or flexion injuries of the wrist.

XR The bone of origin is not always obvious. MR scan may be required to demonstrate ligamentous injuries.

Tx The wrist usually needs support in a cast or splint for 3 or 4 weeks.

Relative positions of the carpal bones → Figure 8.14.

Fracture of the scaphoid bone

The carpal bones lie in two rows, but the scaphoid bone straddles both rows on the radial side. During trauma, considerable force may be transmitted through it, thus making it the most commonly fractured carpal bone (70% of all carpal fractures).

Sites of fracture in the scaphoid bone → Figure 8.15.

Fracture of the scaphoid bone is most common in men aged between 20 and 50 years. The relative compressibility of the bone in children makes fracture uncommon under the age of 14 years, although it can occur in children as young as 8 years. Early and accurate diagnosis of fractures of the scaphoid bone is essential to avoid the complications of avascular necrosis, non-union and

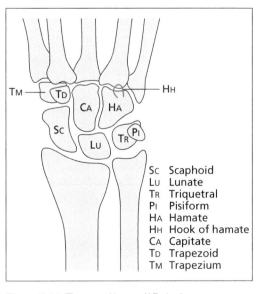

Sc Scaphoid
Lu Lunate
Tr Triquetral
Pi Pisiform
Ha Hamate
Hh Hook of hamate
Ca Capitate
Td Trapezoid
Tm Trapezium

Figure 8.14 The carpal bones (AP view).

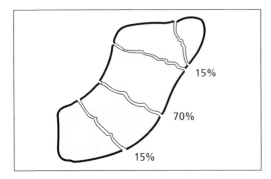

Figure 8.15 Sites of fracture in the scaphoid bone.

radiocarpal arthrosis. The diagnosis should be suspected if there is a combination of the following:

1 An appropriate mechanism of injury – usually a fall on to the outstretched hand.
2 Tenderness in the anatomical snuffbox between the long and short extensors of the thumb, and also on the dorsal and volar aspects of the scaphoid bone. In particular, the scaphoid tubercle may be tender when palpated on the palmar aspect of the wrist in radial deviation. Accompanying swelling is usually minimal. (However, the route of the cutaneous branch of the radial nerve across the snuffbox means this area is often tender even in the absence of injury – consider comparing with the other wrist)
3 A well-preserved range of movements. Forced thumb abduction and extension are usually painful as are pronation and ulnar deviation of the wrist.
4 A positive compression test (hold the thumb and apply axial pressure along the thumb metacarpal; a positive test causes wrist pain).

Unfortunately, many soft-tissue injuries, fracture of the radial styloid process and osteoarthritis of the carpometacarpal joint may present a similar clinical picture.

> The extensive articular surface of the scaphoid bone restricts the sites of vascular supply. Consequently, avascular necrosis – and long-term disability – may follow a missed fracture. This can cause more long-term morbidity than many major trunk injuries.

XR Two special radiographs of the wrist (i.e. scaphoid views = oblique and AP in ulnar deviation) should be obtained in addition to the standard two films. Even so, radiological evidence of the fracture may be elusive until bone resorption at 10–14 days has widened the fracture line. (The sensitivity of the first series of radiographs is only 65%.) Displacement of the fragments is uncommon. MRI is now replacing technetium bone scanning (scintigraphy) as the definitive diagnostic modality for carpal pathology.

TX Patients with definite fractures should have their wrists immobilised in a cast – there is no longer thought to be any benefit of a thumb extension 'scaphoid cast' over a standard 'Colle's cast' for minimally or undisplaced fractures. Early operative intervention for minimally displaced fractures has not been shown to be beneficial. It is usually accepted that proximal pole fractures should be treated operatively due to high non-union rate. Orthopaedic follow-up is required. Prolonged immobilisation (up to 3 months) will be required until there is both clinical and radiological proof of union.

If the fracture has not been confirmed on radiograph, patients may be treated in a wrist splint. After 2 weeks, the wrist should be re-examined and further imaging obtained if symptoms and examination findings remain concerning. Common practice has been to repeat plain 'scaphoid' radiographs; however, plain films are still inadequate to rule out a fracture, and therefore MR scan is now the recommended imaging modality where available.

Carpal dislocation

This uncommon problem is often missed on radiographs, although clinically there is obviously something wrong because swelling and pain are usually considerable. The lunate may be dislocated into the palm (anterior dislocation of the lunate) or the entire distal carpal row may dislocate dorsally (perilunate dislocation). In the latter, there is often an associated fracture of the scaphoid. Other variations are also described. Median nerve signs may occur as a result of direct compression in the carpal tunnel.

XR The lateral radiograph is diagnostic (→ *Figure 8.16*).

TX Immediate specialist referral is essential. Closed reduction under general anaesthesia may be successful. The injured part must be elevated and distal neurovascular function assessed.

Wrist sprain

Diffuse pain may follow either a fall on to the outstretched hand or a hyperflexion injury. Tenderness is usually maximal over the dorsum of the carpus or at the inferior radioulnar joint. The degree of swelling is variable. Ulnar sided wrist pain, exacerbated by ulnar

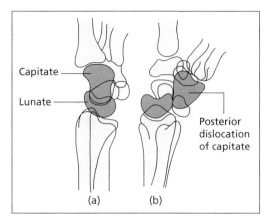

Capitate

Lunate

Posterior
dislocation
of capitate

(a)   (b)

Figure 8.16 Lateral views of the wrist: (a) normal left
and (b) abnormal right with perilunate dislocation.

deviation, may represent triangular fibrocartilage complex (TFCC) injury.

X Scaphoid views should be requested but will be normal in the presence of a sprain.

T× Suspicion of scaphoid injury should be treated
accordingly. Most patients with a sprained wrist settle
spontaneously if provided with a wrist brace for
10–14 days. Occasionally significant ligamentous damage will have been sustained leading to carpal instability
and long-term disability. Significant TFCC injury may
also cause prolonged symptoms. When symptoms are
not resolving after 2 weeks, the patient should be referred
for specialist advice. Arthroscopy or MR scan may identify lesions that are amenable to surgical repair.

Carpal tunnel syndrome

This is the most common form of entrapment neuropathy and most commonly occurs in women aged
40–60 years. The median nerve may be compressed
because its tunnel has become smaller (e.g. after a carpal
fracture) or the nerve has become larger (e.g. in leprosy).
However, the usual cause is that the contents of the carpal tunnel have expanded and the most common reasons for this are:

- interstitial fluid retention in pregnancy
- rheumatoid disease
- myxoedema
- acromegaly.

The patient complains of paraesthesia in the hand and
arm, typically the thumb, index, middle and part of the
ring finger. Symptoms classically awaken the patient in
the early hours of the morning and are relieved by hand

exercises or by hanging the arm out of bed. Examination
reveals anaesthesia and thenar muscle wasting in
advanced disease; otherwise, there is merely subjective
impairment of touch. Tinel's test and Phalen's test can be
used to elicit symptoms during examination. The upper
limb should be examined to exclude pathology of the
elbow, shoulder, thoracic outlet and cervical spine
because nerve entrapment at these points can produce
similar symptoms. Similar symptoms, with sensory
symptoms also including the palm, can occur with more
proximal median nerve entrapment due to pronator
syndrome.

X Radiographs are not generally indicated.
Electromyogram is diagnostic.

T× Temporary relief of symptoms may be achieved by
splinting the wrist with a removable brace at night. This is
particularly useful in pregnancy. Other patients should
be referred to the orthopaedic clinic for surgical release.

De Quervain's tenosynovitis

Inflammation of the tendon sheaths of extensor pollicis
brevis and abductor pollicis longus (at the volar side of
the anatomical snuff box) produces acute local tenderness. Pain extends over the dorsolateral aspect of the
forearm and is made worse by thumb movements. Ulnar
deviation, with the fist closed around the thumb
(Finkelstein's test) causes pain to the radial aspect of the
forearm.

T× Immobilisation (thus stopping repetitive hand and
wrist movements) will allow most cases to settle spontaneously. A replaceable splint is suitable. Referral back to
the patient's GP is appropriate, but some resistant cases
may require steroid injection or surgical division of the
stenosing tendon sheaths.

Peritendonitis crepitans

This condition is more common than de Quervain's tenosynovitis and involves the more proximal part of the
extensor tendons where there is no synovial sheath. The
patient, usually male, presents with pain on moving the
wrist. There may be a recent history of unaccustomed or
repetitive wrist movements. On examination, there is a
fusiform swelling over the radial side of the forearm, over
which crepitus may be felt when the wrist is moved.

T× The wrist should be rested in a removable splint during the day and NSAIDs should be supplied. With this
treatment, the condition usually settles within a few days.
In prolonged cases, physiotherapy with ultrasound treatment is helpful.

Trigger finger

This is another form of tenosynovitis, affecting the tendon sheath around flexor digitorum superficialis. It is most commonly caused by overuse or repetitive micro-injury to the sheath. Patients present with difficulty straightening or bending the affected finger, the finger locks in a flexed position then goes into extension with a painful snap.

Tx Immobilisation with splinting and NSAIDs initially. Referral back to the patient's GP is appropriate, but some resistant cases may require steroid injection or surgical management.

Avascular necrosis of the lunate

This is also known as Kienbock's disease. This condition is thought to be a long-term complication of repetitive minor wrist trauma causing loading on the lunate, without fracture. The patient presents with diffuse pain, which is worse on exercise; there is no recent history of injury.

XR The radiograph is diagnostic in advanced cases, but an MR scan may be required for definitive diagnosis of early disease. X-ray may show sclerosis, flattening and in severe cases fragmentation of the lunate.

Tx A wrist splint should be supplied and orthopaedic follow-up arranged; many of these patients will ultimately require operative intervention.

Osteoarthrosis of the wrist

This commonly involves the carpometacarpal joint of the thumb in older patients. It is often asymptomatic until minor trauma to the wrist causes pain in the joint. Symptoms suggest a scaphoid fracture, but this is unusual in elderly people.

XR Degenerative changes in the joint are obvious on radiographs.

Tx Symptoms are treated with a support bandage and NSAIDs, and the patient is referred to the GP.

Complex regional pain syndrome

Also known as Sudeck's atrophy, this syndrome is characterised by vasomotor disturbance of more than 6 months duration. It is a rare consequence of an often quite trivial wrist injury with symptoms out of proportion to the initial trauma. Of unknown aetiology, it may be related to inadequate mobilisation after injury. Pain is the dominant symptom throughout. The skin is hot and dry at first and the hand, and forearm are swollen.

XR The affected areas may appear osteoporotic on plain radiographs.

Tx The condition usually resolves spontaneously after many months. Physiotherapy gives symptomatic relief. Orthopaedic referral is essential.

VASCULAR PROBLEMS IN THE UPPER LIMB

Compartment syndrome in the forearm or hand → p. 112.

Deep vein thrombosis of the upper limb

Although uncommon, thrombosis of the axillary or subclavian veins may occur in the same way as deep vein thrombosis (DVT) of the leg. There may be a history of repetitive movements such as weight lifting or ten-pin bowling, and other risk factors are the same as for lower limb DVT. The patient complains of non-traumatic swelling of the arm, usually with some discolouration of the skin. DVT of the upper limb should not be confused with lymphoedema of the arm, which may follow infiltration or surgical clearance of the axillary lymph nodes in carcinoma of the breast.

Treatment of DVT → p. 110.

Ischaemia of the hand

Acute or subacute loss of blood supply to the hand may occur after accidental arterial injection of impure or insoluble substances (such as temazepam gel or plaster dust) into the arm almost always in the context of people who inject drugs. Ischaemia of a digit may occur after accidental injection with an adrenaline auto-injector.

Pain, pallor or discolouration of the hand that cannot be attributed to Raynaud's phenomenon requires an immediate opinion from a vascular surgeon (*also → p. 110*).

Problems with AV fistulas

Dialysis-associated steal syndrome: usually seen within the first month of AV fistula formation, it is characterised by cool, pale limb with absent or weak radial pulse which improves with compression of the dialysis access site. Vascular surgical input is required.

Haemorrhage: can rapid and difficult to manage due to the high arterial pressure within the graft. Measures to stop the bleeding can lead to thrombosis of the graft. An effective first step is to apply a bottle top over the bleeding point and hold tightly for 30 min with the limb elevated. A tourniquet may be needed if bleeding continues around the bottle top but should be a last resort. Renal and vascular teams should be involved. *Principles of applying a Pressure dressing →pp. 89 and 90.*

Achenbach's syndrome is a benign, although dramatic appearing condition in which sudden spontaneous bruising and burning or itching discomfort appears to the volar aspect of the finger. The fingertip is usually spared, and perfusion, temperature and function of the digit remain otherwise normal. The patient can be reassured.

Vibration White Finger is a secondary form of Raynaud's phenomenon precipitated by exposure to prolonged vibration (usually from hand-held power tools). Patients should be advised to limit the use of vibrating tools and use protective equipment such as anti-vibration gloves. Advise smoking cessation and keep hands as warm as possible to limit vasospasm. In severe cases, referral for consideration of calcium channel antagonists may be necessary.

9

The hand

Shah Rahman[1] and Sophie Jefferys[2]

[1] Oxford Deanery, Oxford, UK
[2] St Mary's Hospital, Imperial College Healthcare NHS Trust, London, UK

The hand is a vital and complex organ of function with important cosmetic impact. Its role in operating machines and using tools places it at a high risk of injury; 15% of all patients attending an emergency department (ED) have injured their hands.

IMMEDIATE ASSESSMENT AND MANAGEMENT

- Check the patient's general condition – perform an ABCDE assessment
- Make a quick local assessment
- Stop major bleeding by applying direct pressure; note a smaller area of contact allows maximum pressure
- Remove rings and bracelets
- Detect and document sensory loss
- Inject local anaesthetic, if necessary
- Take a history of the injury
- Take a brief past and social history
- Document the dominant hand
- Begin a detailed examination
- Obtain radiographs
- Keep elevated, where practicable.

Swelling

Swelling, which accompanies soft-tissue injury, will produce venous occlusion under constricting bands. This can lead to the interruption of arterial supply. Early removal of rings (and sometimes bracelets) is essential, using ring cutters if necessary.

Pain

Pain may be severe which heightens anxiety. Early injection of local anaesthetic (after examination of sensation) brings immediate relief. Digital nerve (ring) block and wrist block provide an effective means of anaesthetising larger areas. Subsequent cleaning and clinical and radiological examination can be carried out more carefully and therefore more accurately.

Cleaning

Cleaning can often be started by the patient over the sink. Industrial hand injuries are often extremely dirty. There is little point in applying a clean dressing to an oasis of sterile sutured skin that is surrounded by grease and grime. Make sure that the rest of the hand and forearm is cleaned. Cleaning by the patient after discharge will wet and contaminate the wound, potentially delaying healing.

History

The history may give important information on the extent of occult injury, e.g. contusion and devitalisation caused by crushing, direction of wounding, retained foreign bodies or injection of material through high-pressure hoses.

Social history should include occupation, smoking history and hand dominance. Past medical history should include peripheral vascular disease, diabetes, anticoagulant or steroid use, immunosuppression, use of walking aids and home support/functional baseline.

The RCEM Lecture Notes: Emergency Medicine, Fifth Edition. Edited by Catherine Williams and Amy Nickson.
© 2024 John Wiley & Sons Ltd. Published 2024 by John Wiley & Sons Ltd.
Companion website: www.wiley.com/go/LNEM5

Examination

Examination of the hand should follow the sequence: **look, feel, move, X-ray**. Findings should be recorded with the aid of drawings. Digits must be identified by name, i.e. **index, middle, ring** and **little** – rather than by number. Consider how best to describe anatomy in the context of volar/palmar or dorsal, ulnar or radial. POCUS (point of care ultrasound) can be used to rule in foreign bodies or cortical breaks, where needed.

WOUNDS TO THE HAND

General management of wounds → p. 410.
Small wounds and localised infections → Chapter 21 on p. 410.

In the hand, skin is at a premium and must be handled gently and conservatively; toothed forceps should be avoided. The main obstacles to wound healing are haematoma, infection and tension.

- Dead tissue must be excised, but the blood supply to the hand is good and may maintain flaps that would die elsewhere.
- Cleaning must be thorough. Gentle use of a toothbrush or a scrubbing brush is effective.
- Photographs, as per local policy, will help document the injury. Patients will often be able to photograph injuries on their own smart devices.
- Lacerations over the dorsum of the hand and knuckle area, sustained in a fight, are often inflicted by the opponent's teeth. They are human bites and must be treated accordingly (→ *p. 418*). Patients may be reluctant to admit they have been in a fight. Take particular care to examine the wound with the fist closed – there is a significant risk of MCP joint capsule penetration. They should be referred for formal washout by the orthopaedic team.
- Patients with open fractures should be given systemic antibiotics and referred for specialist care. Osteomyelitis or septic arthritis may not be apparent on a radiograph for the first 10 days after infection.
- All patients with hand wounds must be protected against tetanus, ensure patient's tetanus status is documented. (→ *p. 415*).
- The median nerve motor supply to the thenar muscles (→ *Box 8.6 on p. 123*) is very superficial and may be damaged by apparently minor wounds to the radial side of the palm.

- Adhesive, reinforced paper skin closures are not suitable for hand and proximal finger lacerations because they either restrict movement or impair blood supply, and they usually come off!
- Sutures to the palm that are too large (or badly placed adhesive strips) may cause skin overlap and a final, unacceptable, proud wound.

Injection injuries to the hand

Adrenaline Auto-injection injuries: As more patients are issued with self-injecting devices to treat anaphylaxis, accidental injections have become more common. Adrenaline auto-injectors (such as EpiPen, Emerade) contain either 0.15 or 0.3 mg adrenaline and so subcutaneous injection is rarely systemically dangerous. However, accidental injection into a digit may cause intense vasoconstriction and even irreversible tissue ischaemia. The affected finger may be pale and white with reduced sensation. Immediate aid can include immersing both hands in water as warm as tolerable to promote vasodilatation, and local anaesthetic infiltration. Local injection of phentolamine (1.5 mg with 1 mL 2% lidocaine) may be effective in reversing the adrenaline-induced vasoconstriction for up to 13 hours after the accidental injection. Note that UK production has been discontinued and stocks expired as of 2014. An opinion from a vascular surgeon may be required. Intravenous infusions of the prostacyclin analogue, iloprost, have also been used in this situation, as has stellate ganglion blockade. Calcium channel blockers and nitrates are ineffective. Further information is available from ToxBase/National Poisons Information Service.

High-pressure hose injection injuries: high-pressure hoses containing air, water, oil, grease and paint are used in many industries. Injection injuries from these tools can cause delayed but extensive soft-tissue damage. Skin penetration occurs easily (and often relatively painlessly) leaving minimal superficial injury and a normal-looking hand or finger. Initially, the injury may appear trivial but, within 24 hours swelling, paraesthesia and loss of function are apparent. Tissue necrosis follows and damage to deeper structures is often widespread. Radiographs may reveal particles or an air track. All of these injuries must be referred for inpatient treatment at the time that they are first seen. Laying open the track and removal of injected particulate matter are often required. Tetanus prophylaxis is essential.

Oil-based veterinary vaccine injection injuries: accidental self-inoculation of oil-based veterinary vaccine fluid leads to intense local pain. The wound may appear trivial but can lead to widespread necrosis. Referral is essential for observation, debridement and decompression if required.

Crush injuries of the hand

Inspection may not be a reliable guide to the extent of crushing. History can give valuable additional information.

XR This is almost always indicated.

TX If the whole hand has been crushed, e.g. between rollers, admission and elevation are necessary even if the initial examination does not reveal extensive injuries.

Check for signs of compartment syndrome in the hand compartments. Characterised by 'pain out of proportion', swelling and a 'claw-like' hand deformity, with severe pain on passive finger extension. Later signs include paraesthesia, paralysis and pulselessness.

Less extensive crushing injuries can be treated in the ED by:

- excluding injury to deep structures (radiological and clinical examination)
- providing local anaesthesia
- cleaning thoroughly
- delaying closure for 3–5 days until the oedema has settled.
- ensuring hand clinic follow-up.

Amputations of the fingers

These are common in many industries. Distinguish between crisp sharp injuries where the damage is usually immediately evident and crush or tearing injuries, where the damage is often hidden and has associated delayed complications.

XR This is necessary to exclude bony damage. If available, include substantial amputated tissue within radiographs taken.

TX Amputation of the digits proximal to the distal interphalangeal (DIP) joint may be suitable for reimplantation (→ p. 414). Amputated or partially amputated parts should be wrapped in saline soaked gauze, placed in plastic bag and then into a bag of ice.

Loss of more than the tip of the phalanx requires specialist opinion from a hand surgeon.

Amputations through the soft tissue of the fingertip can be left to close spontaneously. Cleaning must be vigorous and all dead tissue and dirt must be removed. The wound should then be covered with a non-adherent dressing and inspected not more than twice weekly. Antibiotics are not required unless there is bony involvement or infection is evident at the first dressing change. Exposed bone is best treated by referral for trimming.

Fingertip injuries that remain red, tender or swollen for more than 10 days may be developing osteomyelitis or septic arthritis. A radiograph may show early destruction of bone or loss of the joint space.

Partial avulsion of the fingertip

A combination of crushing and flexion of the fingertip (e.g. finger trapped by a door) may partially avulse the proximal end of the nail. There may be an associated crush fracture of the terminal phalanx (→ *Figure 9.1*). This injury is very common in children.

XR This should be obtained in all cases.

TX
Obtain adequate conditions for the repair. General anaesthesia may be necessary, but local anaesthesia with a ring block is usually adequate in adults (→ *Box 21.2 on p. 412*). *For sedation of children → p. 366.*

- Clean the area thoroughly.
- Restore the normal alignment of the finger. It may sometimes be possible to replace a nail with a firm distal attachment under the proximal skinfold; otherwise remove it. Do not leave the nail in an avulsed position because it will splint the bone and/or finger pulp in the same position.
- Maintain the alignment with sutures to the lateral lacerations if needed but do not suture the nail bed (→ *Figure 9.2*).
- Dress the finger with a non-adherent, antiseptic dressing.
- Provide adequate splintage. A Mallet splint may be slit dorsally for this purpose.
- Arrange follow-up according to local arrangement.

The tip of the finger will swell, but decompression will occur through the laceration.

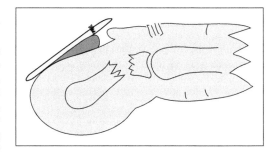

Figure 9.1 Crush–flexion injury to the fingertip.

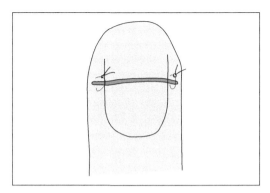

Figure 9.2 Position of sutures after removal of nail in crush–flexion injury.

Tendon injuries in the hand

Injuries to the tendons of the hand are common and often overlooked. Even the smallest wound to the skin may sometimes have allowed sufficient penetration to damage a tendon. Wounds involving glass or 'avocado-related' knife injuries are particularly sinister in this respect. Loss of function is the only reliable sign. Extensor tendon division is relatively easy to diagnose. *For the detection of flexor tendon damage → Box 9.1*. Also note the following:

- In the relaxed hand, the fingers tend to be held in increasing flexion from index to little finger. A pointing finger, which is out of line with this trend, suggests a flexor tendon or nerve injury.
- Partial division of a tendon may be overlooked initially, but subsequent rupture may occur. Suspicion of a tendon injury warrants referral for exploration.
- The relationship between a tendon and the overlying skin varies with joint position. This means that the damage to a tendon may not be immediately visible through a skin wound. The tendon must therefore be inspected during finger and wrist movements.

X̠ All wounds involving glass must have a radiograph taken.

T̠x Extensor tendons on the back of the hand may sometimes be repaired in the ED if a clean theatre and appropriate skills are available. Patients with other tendon injuries must always be referred. Minor degrees of tendon damage, involving less than a third of the diameter of the tendon, may be managed conservatively, but this needs experienced judgement.

Digital nerve injuries

Similar to tendon injuries, nerve injuries may not be immediately apparent. In both cases, deceptively small wounds can be sufficiently large to allow underlying

Box 9.1 The detection of flexor tendon injuries

Anatomy: flexor digitorum superficialis is used for fine movements. It has four fairly distinct muscle bellies. Each tendon inserts into the base of a middle phalanx. Flexor digitorum profundus is used for power grip. It arises as one muscle and is variably divided towards the musculotendinous junction. Each tendon inserts into the base of a distal phalanx.

Theory: hyperextension of one fingertip will stretch the entire profundus belly and preclude it from initiating flexion of any of the other fingers. Flexion of the unrestrained fingers can be achieved only at the proximal interphalangeal (PIP) joint by the action of more independent superficialis tendon.

Testing: for profundus assess active flexion at the DIP joint. For superficialis assess active flexion of the whole finger while the other fingers are hyperextended. Normally, flexion will occur at the PIP joint with the DIP joint remaining flaccid (profundus inactivated). If superficialis is divided, the whole finger will be flaccid.

damage. Distal sensation should always be tested prior to local anaesthetic and any complaint of changed sensation is taken seriously. Sometimes the patient complains of paraesthesia in the affected digit but retains crude awareness of touch as a result of apposition of the severed nerve ends – consider using two-point discrimination. The affected skin becomes dry 24 hours later and is evidently anaesthetised. Patients often describe the sensation of absent nerve conduction in terms of their last experience of it – as being injected by the dentist with local anaesthetic.

T̠x Neural injury distal to the PIP joint rarely warrants repair. Any resulting area of anaesthesia will become smaller with the passage of time as in-growth occurs from other nerves.

The digital nerve is more commonly damaged in its superficial position near the metacarpophalangeal (MCP) joint. Repair is indicated, especially if the anaesthesia is on the ulnar border of the little finger, the radial aspect of the index finger or the thumb. If in doubt, the patient should be referred for a specialist opinion. A repair within 72 hours aims to restore motor and sensory function and prevent a painful neuroma.

METACARPAL FRACTURES

Spiral fracture of the shaft of the metacarpus

This injury is produced by rotational forces on the finger. Rarely, it may be compound or multiple. The fracture is stable and usually undisplaced because of the integrity of the transverse metacarpal ligaments. Tendon and neurovascular damage are rare.

XR Anteroposterior and oblique views of the hand usually show the fracture clearly. Overlapping soft-tissue shadow or nutrient artery may be misinterpreted as an undisplaced spiral fracture.

TX Encourage movement but give a little support initially to alleviate pain. Follow-up should be in the fracture clinic or hand clinic.

Very rarely, rotational instability will result in persisting rotation of the finger, which is more easily detected on clinical than radiological examination – when the finger is fully flexed the tip is clearly malaligned. A specialist opinion is then necessary.

Transverse fracture of the shaft of the metacarpus

This injury is the result of direct trauma. It is often multiple and may be compounded with extensive soft-tissue damage. The inherent stability of the metacarpal arch is lost and so displacement is common.

XR Epiphyseal lines may be partially developed at the proximal end of the index finger metacarpus and are commonly misinterpreted as linear fractures.

TX This fracture requires immediate specialist attention. Internal fixation may be necessary to achieve stable reduction.

Fracture of the neck of the metacarpus

This is often termed the boxer's fracture, although most patients do not admit to fighting but to missing their opponent and hitting a brick wall. The fracture is usually of the little metacarpus, accounting for 25% of all metacarpal fractures, but injury to the ring or other metacarpal bones may also be seen.

> If the overlying skin is injured, it should be assumed that this is caused by contact with the opponent's teeth. This has the potential to develop the serious complications of a human bite, especially if there has been penetration of the MCP joint capsule (→ p. 418) and should be referred for formal washout and exploration in theatre by the orthopaedic team.

In the absence of a bite injury, associated damage to deep structures is unusual. The metacarpal head may be angulated. Pain and angulation cause an associated lag in extension of the corresponding finger.

XR The fracture is confirmed on oblique films of the hand, but may be missed on an anteroposterior (AP) film. Palmar angulation is best assessed with lines drawn through the medullary canal.

TX The second and third metacarpals usually require internal fixation. The fourth and fifth may be conservatively managed if the angulation in the neck is less than 40° and the shaft less than 20° with no rotation because remodelling will achieve good long-term function despite gross initial displacement. The patient should be warned that inability to extend the affected finger fully will persist for a few months, but that normal function can be guaranteed if the joints are mobilised as soon as possible. This explanation is an important part of the treatment. Most long-term complications are a direct result of immobilisation. Neighbour strapping (sometimes with a crepe bandage) and oral analgesia are supplied for use in the first few days and the patient should then be reviewed to ensure appropriate mobilisation by a therapist.

Any rotation, articular step-off greater than 2 mm or severe angulation >40° is not tolerated due to palmar pain and grip strength reduction. Severe angulation can be reduced with an ulnar block by stabilising the proximal part of the metacarpal dorsally and applying pressure to the head of the metacarpal from the palmar aspect. A short ulnar gutter or volar splint is required for 2–3 weeks followed by buddy strapping. A specialist opinion should be sought.

BONE AND JOINT INJURIES OF THE FINGERS

Dislocation of the MCP joint

Dislocation without fracture may occur in either direction. Importantly, the metacarpal head may 'button hole' through the articular capsule, which then shrinks around the metacarpal neck and prevents closed reduction.

Tx This dislocation should be referred for specialist advice. Open reduction may be necessary. The prognosis is usually good.

Ligament injuries of the MCP joint

Sudden sideways forces may cause ligamentous injuries at the index and little finger MCP joints.

XR Such injuries may be associated with minor flake fractures of the proximal phalanx – representing avulsion of the attachment of the collateral ligament – or with fractures of the base of the phalanx (→ *below*).

Tx These injuries resolve with conservative management unless the joint is grossly unstable, when open repair is indicated. Strapping the finger to its neighbour is sufficient. This allows flexion but prevents abduction. Follow-up by is advisable in the hand clinic.

Fracture of the proximal phalanx

Proximal phalanx fractures may occur through the base, shaft or neck. When open, they must be referred immediately for specialist treatment. Antibiotics should be started in the ED and anti-tetanus cover provided. Fractures into the joint require specialist referral.
Spiral fractures: these may produce rotational deformity, which is not always evident on a radiograph. Rotation is best detected clinically by noting the relative positions of the fingernails when the fingers are fully flexed into the palm. All the nails should lie in approximately the same plane with the fingertips pointing towards the palpable part of the radial artery. Rotational deformity, if found, requires a specialist opinion.
Fracture of the base of the proximal phalanx: this is most commonly seen, as a greenstick or buckle injury, in the little finger of children (→ *Figure 9.3*). The fracture is easily (and often) overlooked on a radiograph. Reduction may be achieved under local anaesthesia by inserting a cylindrical object, such as a pencil, into the cleft between the little and ring fingers and pushing the little finger towards the ring finger. A post-reduction radiograph is essential. Neighbour strapping is then applied and follow-up arranged.
Other metaphyseal fractures: fractures at the metaphyses through cancellous bone are usually stable and, if not significantly displaced, can be treated conservatively by neighbour strapping. Displaced metaphyseal fractures may be reduced under local anaesthetic by manipulation over a cylindrical object, such as a pencil as above.

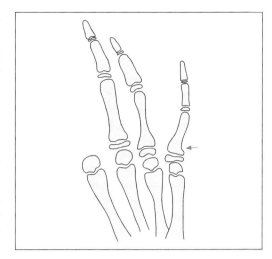

Figure 9.3 Greenstick fracture of the base of the proximal phalanx of the little finger.

Fractures in the cortical diaphysis: these are more often displaced and very unstable. Delayed displacement of apparently stable fractures may occur. They may require internal fixation and should be referred immediately for specialist input.

Proximal interphalangeal joint injuries

The PIP joint deserves careful consideration because:

1 It has the largest range of movement.
2 Long-term stiffness is a major disability.
3 Initial injury is often overlooked.
4 Delayed displacement of the extensor tendon can occur.

The extensor hood, volar plate and collateral ligaments may all be damaged without joint dislocation and assessment can be difficult.

> The ability to extend fully, or even slightly hyperextend, all of the joints (especially the PIP joint) of an injured finger is associated with good recovery. Failure to achieve a straight finger must be followed up because the flexion may become permanent.

XR Initial radiographs may look normal, even in the presence of a serious injury. Volar plate fractures are often missed.

Tx A patient with a PIP joint that is swollen or has a reduced range of movements should be followed up in a clinic. Swelling can take several months to settle.

The boutonnière deformity

Extensor hood and central slip rupture may go unrecognised (→ *Figure 9.4*). Extension may be possible initially because the lateral bands remain intact but, if the finger is not splinted, these gradually migrate laterally and, within a few days, lie anterior to the axis of the joint. The extensor mechanism now flexes the proximal joint, and by a compensatory device hyperextends the distal joint. This is a boutonnière deformity. To prevent this serious complication, all significant PIP joint injuries should be immobilised in extension and advice sought.

Dislocation of the PIP joint

Dislocation may occur in either direction, but is most commonly dorsal. Buttonhole entrapment of the head of the proximal phalanx in the disrupted volar plate (capsule) is particularly difficult to reduce and requires expert surgical skills to repair.

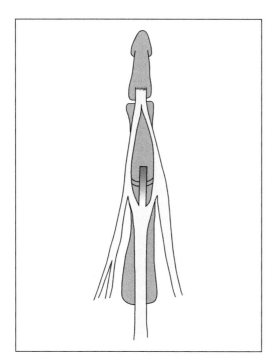

Figure 9.4 The extensor tendons of the finger. The central slip to the middle phalanx is shaded.

XR Radiographs should always be taken before reduction of any finger dislocation.

Tx Manipulation may be attempted under local anaesthesia but, if the dislocation does not reduce easily on the first attempt, the specialist advice must be sought. Repeated attempts at closed reduction will increase soft-tissue damage and make open repair more difficult. Closed reduction under digital nerve block or inhaled analgesia may be achieved by hyperextension, axial traction and flexion. If reduction is achieved, assess stability with gentle assessment of passive range of movement is achieved. Reduction must be confirmed with repeat X-rays. If closed reduction is immediately successful and examination does not reveal major ligamentous instability, the finger is held fully extended in a volar splint and strapped to its neighbour. The MCP joint must be left free to allow 90° of flexion. The patient is referred to the hand clinic.

Fractures of the intermediate phalanx

Fractures of the middle phalanx often extend into either joints and thereby produce an inherently unstable finger with a tendency to increasing deformity.

Tx These injuries must be referred for specialist advice, however small the fracture and however minimal the apparent displacement.

Dislocation of the DIP joint

The DIP joint has a smaller range of movement than the more proximal joints and injury to it is less often associated with major disability.

Dislocation of the DIP joint may be accompanied by a flake fracture from the adjacent bone. This may indicate collateral ligament injury if it is lateral, or long-tendon avulsion if more central.

XR Radiographs must precede attempts to reduce the dislocation and repeat clinical examination must follow successful reduction.

Tx Reduction is achieved by axial traction, without excessive force. Follow-up is required to ensure the return of full movement.

Mallet finger

Extensor tendon avulsion from the terminal phalanx produces a 'mallet' deformity. Passive movements are full and pain free, but there is no active extension at the DIP joint.

XR Radiographs should be taken to exclude other fractures. The presence of a small dorsal flake fracture improves the prognosis – the repair potential of bone is better than that of the extensor tendon.

TX The patient should be referred to the next hand clinic where a purpose-made hyperextension splint will be fitted. In the meantime, the DIP joint must be held continuously in full extension by a temporary plastic (Mallet) splint.

The splint may be changed occasionally to allow skin cleaning, but the finger must not be allowed to flex while unsplinted. Placing the hand on a flat surface, such as a table, during removal and cleaning will prevent this. After 6 weeks, the splint is worn only at night and during heavy manual work for a further month. Full return of active extension cannot be guaranteed. Functional disability is usually minimal even if no treatment is given, although there is also a cosmetic consideration. Some patients prefer to accept this outcome rather than suffer the restrictions imposed by a finger splint.

Fracture of the distal phalanx

These fractures are usually produced by crushing forces and are often comminuted. They may cause problems at the DIP joint when they extend across the articular surface but this is unusual. Bleeding is restricted by the fibrous loculi of the pulp space and by the nail to produce a subungual haematoma. Interstitial pressure quickly rises and the pain is severe.

TX Trephining the nail brings instant relief to the patient who has a haematoma under the nail. It is not contraindicated in the presence of a fracture. The nail itself is insensate and the blunt hot trephine produces a wide sterile hole compared with that produced by the tip of a drill.

A simple fracture of the terminal phalanx can be treated in a Mallet splint for 2–3 weeks until the pain has settled. More commonly, there is a soft-tissue injury, which demands more careful attention (→ *p. 134*).

THUMB INJURIES

Thumb injuries produce greater disability than similar injuries to the other digits because of impairment of pinch and grip. Principles of treatment are similar, but particular attention is given to the maintenance of length

after terminal injury and the ability to oppose and rotate the thumb against the other fingers.

> A thumb that can be flexed to touch the palm of the hand at the base of the little finger is unlikely to be severely injured.

Fracture of the thumb metacarpus

These fractures are often the result of an oblique abducting force and may be disabling. They usually occur through the proximal part or the base of the metacarpus. There is a painful swollen deformity at the base of the thumb but associated, deep, soft-tissue injuries are uncommon.

XR Epiphyseal lines may be partially developed at the distal end of the thumb metacarpus and are commonly misinterpreted as linear fractures.

TX If the fracture enters the carpometacarpal (trapezometacarpal) joint (Bennett's fracture dislocation), displacement is significant and reduction is then difficult. A Rolando's fracture is a comminuted Bennett's. The patient should be referred because internal fixation may be necessary. Closed manipulation may succeed but must be carried out by an experienced doctor. The fracture is usually held in a modified scaphoid plaster cast with the thumb abducted.

The more usual fracture through the metacarpal base, not involving the joint, is adequately treated in a scaphoid plaster cast. Reduction is not usually necessary.

Ligament injuries of the thumb MCP joint

Injury to the MCP joint of the thumb may be incapacitating because functional impairment is associated with thumb instability. The collateral ligaments or the MCP joint capsule may be extensively torn by forced extension or abduction. The ulnar collateral ligament is the most frequently damaged structure. Chronic injury to this ligament was common in gamekeepers. Skiers sustain an acute injury by pulling the thumb back in the ski-pole strap or artificial ski-slope matting during a fall – hence the term 'skier's thumb.'

Examination reveals specific tenderness over the palmar and web aspects of the MCP joint and pain on attempted abduction. There is usually a haematoma in the thenar area. The laxity of the joint may be compared with that of the opposite thumb. Instability is not always apparent because of the protective action of the thenar muscles.

XR Stress views may show subluxation of the joint or an avulsion fracture at the base of the proximal phalanx at the site of ligament insertion. Local anaesthetic around the metacarpus may be required to enable this procedure.

TX Surgical repair or plaster cast immobilisation may be indicated for significant ligamentous injury; specialist advice should be sought. Injuries to the MCP joint without either laxity or haematoma can be treated with a bandage thumb spica and review in hand clinic.

Other injuries to the thumb

Dislocation of the MCP joint: the dislocation may be reduced by axial traction under metacarpal ring block. The patient should then be referred to hand clinic because ligamentous instability or capsular damage may accompany the dislocation. A bandage thumb spica will give temporary support.
Fractures of the proximal phalanx: unstable or angulated fractures should be referred for reduction and fixation. This will include all fractures of the shaft. Undisplaced fractures of the base of the proximal phalanx can be treated with a bandage thumb spica and clinic review.
Dislocation of the interphalangeal joint: this can be reduced with axial traction under a ring block. A Mallet splint is then applied and fracture clinic review arranged.
Fractures of the distal phalanx: these fractures usually follow a crushing type of injury. Associated soft-tissue injury predominates. The treatment is the same as that for distal phalangeal injuries of the other fingers (→ p. 139).

Hand infections

Flexor tendon sheath infection

Infection of the flexor tendon sheath occurs most commonly following minor penetrating trauma. The affected digit will be erythematous, hot and painful. The presence of the four Kanavel's signs is strongly suggestive of a tendon sheath infection:

- Tenderness along the flexor sheath
- Fusiform swelling of the digit
- Pain on passive finger extension
- Flexed finger posture

Patients should be treated with intravenous antibiotics and referred to a hand surgeon or plastic surgeon for washout.

Deep hand space infections

The deep spaces of the hand include the mid-palmar space, hypothenar and thenar spaces. The mid-palmar space lies deep to the palmar aponeurosis and is a continuation of the carpal tunnel, the thenar space overlies adductor pollicis and the hypothenar space lies palmar to the 5th metacarpal. The thenar space is the most commonly infected.

The hand will be swollen, tender and erythematous. The concavity of the palm may be reduced due to swelling. Fingers are held in partial flexion with pain on passive extension (thumb – thenar space infection, little finger – hypothenar space infection, two to fourth fingers – mid-palmar space infection).

Patients should be treated with intravenous antibiotics and referred to a hand surgeon or plastic surgery for washout.

Felon → Chapter 21
Paronychia → Chapter 21

10

Burns, contamination and irradiation

Jodie Wilkinson
Northern Care Alliance, Royal Oldham Hospital, UK

LARGE BURNS

The skin is the largest organ of the body and constitutes a vital barrier against disease. It is also a major sense organ and has an important aesthetic role. Its damage is thus dangerous, painful and distressing. Thermal injuries may also involve the respiratory tract and lead to disturbances of metabolism and thermoregulation.

Immediate assessment and management

- Ensure an adequate airway. Give a high concentration of oxygen.
- Remove the source of the burn. Cut-off clothes but adherent clothing should not be peeled off.
- Flood the affected area with cold water if there is still evidence of heat transfer.
- Look for evidence of inhalation injury (→ *later*). If there is wheezing, give nebulised salbutamol.
- Measure the arterial blood gases and carboxyhaemoglobin level.
- Estimate the extent of the burn (→ *p. 142–144*). If more than 15% of skin area (or more than 10% in a patient <10 or >70 years), set up an intravenous (IV) infusion and take blood for haemoglobin, PCV (packed cell volume), urea and electrolytes (U&Es) and glucose.
- Monitor the pulse, BP (blood pressure) and SpO$_2$ (O$_2$ saturation). Alternative sites for pulse oximetry such as the nose, lips or tongue may be necessary.
- Assess the level of consciousness; if depressed consider carbon monoxide poisoning → *p. 300*.
- Obtain brief details of the incident and the patient.
- Obtain IV or IO access through unburned skin if possible. This is best secured using gauze in the first instance which can be subsequently replaced with sutures. Give adequate IV analgesia.
- Assess the depth of the burn (→ *p. 142*). If there are extensive, deep burns, cross-match blood.
- Cover burns with sterile towels, dry dressings or clear plastic food wrap.
- Insert a urinary catheter and measure the output of urine.
- Consider the possibility of other injuries. Associated injuries can comprise blast injuries sustained during an explosion or injuries sustained as the patient attempts to escape from a fire.

Inhalation injury

Inhalation of hot smoke and fumes is common in patients who have been confined in a burning environment such as a house fire. This may cause:

- direct thermal injury to the respiratory tract leading to upper airway oedema or obstruction
- inhalation of the products of combustion (carbon particles) and toxic fumes, leading to chemical tracheobronchitis, oedema and pneumonia
- carbon monoxide poisoning.

Direct thermal damage to the respiratory tract is uncommon in the otherwise minimally injured victim of a fire. In a more seriously burned patient, it may lead to

The RCEM Lecture Notes: Emergency Medicine, Fifth Edition. Edited by Catherine Williams and Amy Nickson.
© 2024 John Wiley & Sons Ltd. Published 2024 by John Wiley & Sons Ltd.
Companion website: www.wiley.com/go/LNEM5

severe oedema and a rapid onset of airway obstruction. This may also result from delayed sloughing of tracheal or bronchial mucosa. Such patients may need fibreoptic bronchoscopy.

The toxins present in fumes cause mucosal oedema, microvascular hyper-permeability, obstructive airway casts and surfactant dysfunction. Depressed epithelial integrity, loss of the mucociliary clearance mechanism, migration of upper airway secretions to the lower airway and immuno compromise predispose to bacterial colonisation and translocation. Thermal injuries can progress to acute respiratory distress syndrome.

Incapacity, which occurs quickly in domestic and industrial fires, is caused by a combination of hypoxia, carbon monoxide poisoning (caused by incomplete combustion) and hydrogen cyanide poisoning. Soft furnishings are a particular hazard, producing many toxic substances, including highly irritant and lethal hydrogen chloride.

Indicators of an inhalation injury include:

- History of exposure to fire in enclosed space
- Decreased ability to respond to fire, as may occur with small children, disabled or intoxicated patients
- History of impaired consciousness or confusion at any time
- Carbon deposits and acute inflammatory changes in the oropharynx
- Explosion with burns sustained to the head and torso
- Symptoms or signs of respiratory distress, including irritation of mucous membranes
- Stridor, hoarseness or aphonia
- Production of carbonaceous (black) sputum
- Burns around the lips, mouth, throat or nose, including singeing of nasal hairs and eyebrows
- Carboxyhaemoglobin level >10% in a patient who was involved in a fire.

Tx Consider the need for early intubation – before oedema of the upper airway makes this difficult or impossible. Request early senior anaesthetic advice. A large size endotracheal tube (size 8.0 mm or above) should be used as this will allow any subsequent bronchoscopy to be performed. The tube should be left long and uncut to allow for swelling of the face and airway.

Rapid sequence induction should be done with midline inline stablisation of the cervical spine if appropriate. Succinylcholine is safe to use in the first 24 hours after a burn, after this time, its use is contraindicated due to the risk of hyperkalaemia leading to cardiac arrest. This is thought to be due to the release of potassium from extra-junctional acetylcholine receptors and can persist for up to 1-year post-burn.

Management includes:

- Give high-concentration oxygen
- Give nebulised salbutamol for wheezing
- Check arterial blood gases and carboxyhaemoglobin

> Beware of conventional blood gas analyser readings in patients who may have high carboxy- or methaemoglobin levels. The oxygen electrode measures oxygen dissolved in plasma only and O_2 saturation is then calculated assuming all haemoglobin to be normal. Arterial O_2 pressure (PaO_2) and O_2 saturation may thus appear to be satisfactory despite very low total blood O_2 content.

- Request a chest radiograph
- Admit for 24 hours observation even if burns appear minimal.

Cyanide poisoning should be suspected in burn patients with an unexplained and persistent lactic acidosis, despite adequate fluid resuscitation.

Carbon monoxide poisoning → p. 300.
Cyanide poisoning → p. 303.

Assessment of a burn

Extent

The extent of a burn is estimated by using the rule of nines in adults (→ *Figure 10.1*). In children, the Lund–Browder chart is used to take account of the relatively larger head and smaller legs (→ *Figure 10.2*). As a useful guide, the surface area of the patient's own outstretched hand including the fingers is around 1% of the patient's body surface area.

> Do not take areas of superficial erythema into account when calculating the area of a burn. Make a note of these areas separately.

There is only a slight difference between the volume of fluid lost through partial-thickness and that lost through full-thickness burns, although the extent of erythrocyte destruction is greater in the latter.

Depth

The depth of a burn is a function of:

1 the temperature of the agent causing the burn
2 the length of time that it is in contact with the skin (i.e. the amount of energy transferred). Scalds are associated with a water temperature >50°C.

The depth of a burn is important in assessing the severity of the burn, planning for wound care and predicting

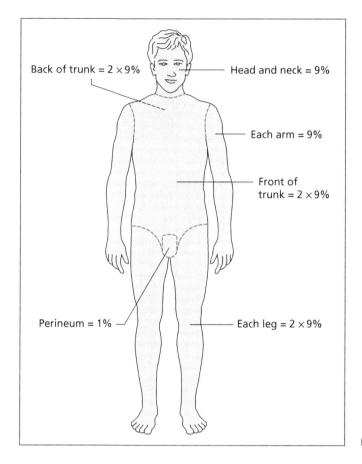

Figure 10.1 The 'rule of nines'.

functional and cosmetic results; however, it is often very difficult to estimate confidently the depth of a burn in the first few days.

The circumstances leading to the cause of the burn may help. A motorbike exhaust pipe burning through a leather boot may only inflict a superficial burn. Someone with epilepsy or alcohol problems who falls into a fire, or lies for an extended time against a domestic heater will sustain deeper burns. Elderly patients and those with peripheral neuropathy (e.g. people with diabetes) are at special risk. Electrical burns are usually very deep. Clothes closely applied to the skin, such as underwear, socks, belts and collars, tend to trap fluids and potentiate the severity of the burn locally.

Burns are categorised as follows:

- **Superficial** or first-degree burns (e.g. sunburn) expose intact nerve endings and are painful. They are characterised by erythema and the absence of blisters. They usually heal within a week without scarring.
- **Partial-thickness** or second-degree burns can affect the superficial dermal layer and have a red or mottled appearance with associated swelling and blister formation. The surface is hypersensitive and can have a wet, weeping appearance. These typically heal within 2–3 weeks with minimal scarring and full functional recovery.
- **Deep dermal burns**: Partial thickness burns can also affect the deep dermal layer leading to blistering and a dry, blotchy cherry-red appearance. Typically, this doesn't blanch, there is absent capillary refill and reduced or absent sensation. These injuries can take 3–8 weeks to heal with scarring and surgical treatment may be required for best functional recovery.
- **Full-thickness** or third-degree burns destroy nerve endings and are painless – testing the response to a pinprick may be helpful but is not always reliable. The skin can be dark and leathery or translucent, mottled and waxy in appearance.

Infection can easily convert a partial-thickness burn into a full-thickness injury.

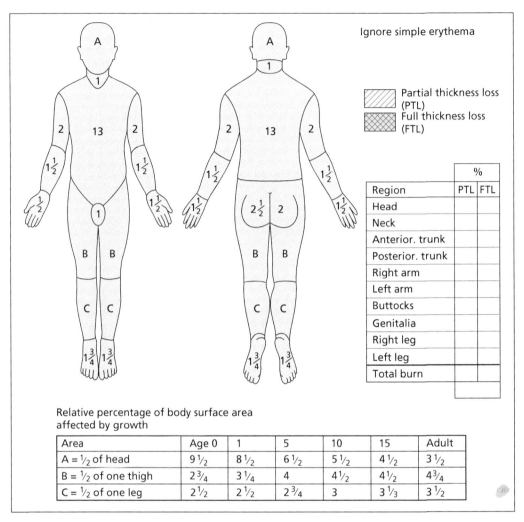

Figure 10.2 The Lund–Browder chart.

Region	PTL	FTL
Head		
Neck		
Anterior. trunk		
Posterior. trunk		
Right arm		
Left arm		
Buttocks		
Genitalia		
Right leg		
Left leg		
Total burn		

Relative percentage of body surface area affected by growth

Area	Age 0	1	5	10	15	Adult
A = ½ of head	9 ½	8 ½	6 ½	5 ½	4 ½	3 ½
B = ½ of one thigh	2 ¾	3 ¼	4	4 ½	4 ½	4 ¾
C = ½ of one leg	2 ½	2 ½	2 ¾	3	3 ⅓	3 ½

Treatment of burns

Flooding with cold water

The damage inflicted by hot fluids may be substantially mitigated by flooding the affected part with cold water. Pain is simultaneously reduced. Irrigation under running water for at least 20 min is effective in limiting the extent of the burn if carried out within the first 3 hours (but should commence as early as possible). Beware of hypothermia, especially in small children or elderly patients with large burns – attempt to 'cool the burn but warm the patient'. Any dry chemical powders should be brushed from the wound before the involved body surface area is rinsed with water. Cold water should not be applied to a patient with extensive burns (>10% total BSA).

> Never apply neutralising fluids to acid or alkali burns – the resulting chemical reaction is exothermic.

> 20 min cold water irrigation within 3 hours of a burn or scald reduces extent of burning by up to 80%.

Analgesia

Analgesia should be given early and always before transfer to another unit. It is usually underprescribed. The beneficial effects of morphine in small children greatly outweigh any haemodynamic side effects, but it is essential to calculate the initial dose using the patient's weight. Do not be afraid to give further doses as dictated by the state of the patient (→ *p. 10*).

Most significant burns need IV analgesia.

Tetanus

The tetanus status of all patients should be evaluated and tetanus immunisation given where appropriate.

Intravenous fluids

If the burn involves more than 15% of the skin (10% in children and elderly people) or involves the face (making oral feeding difficult), an IV line must be set up. It will be required for a few days and must be reliable and easy to maintain. Reduced immunological competence increases the risk of infection after burns. An aseptic technique must be used.

In patients with severe burns, evaluating the circulating blood volume is often difficult and there may be accompanying injuries that can cause hypovolaemic shock. Blood pressure measurements are also difficult to obtain and can be unreliable so monitoring of urine output is important and can reliably assess circulating volume. In children under 30 kg, a urine output of 1.0–1.5 mL/kg/hr is the aim and in adults 0.5–1.0 mL (use *ideal* body weight for these calculations). The initial intravenous fluid used should be Hartmann's solution or another balanced crystalloid.

Calculation of fluid requirements → Box 10.1.

Calculated fluids are required in addition to normal metabolic requirements. Fluid loss begins at the time of the burn.

Definitive care of large burns

Patients with large burns must not be kept in the ED for longer than it takes to:

- initiate resuscitation
- exclude, or treat, other major injuries

 Box 10.1 **Fluid replacement for burns**

- Intravenous fluids are required if more than a 15% surface burn (10% in those <10 or >70 years). Hartmann's solution or another balanced crystalloid should be used. An initial 10–20 mL/kg can be given whilst awaiting formal calculations.
- Isolated areas of erythema are not included in the calculation but cannot be ignored.
- No distinction is made between areas of full-and partial-thickness loss at this stage.
- Patients who have inhalational injuries in addition to skin burns initially require up to 40% more fluid.
- Fluid to be given must be calculated from the time of the burn rather than the time of arrival at hospital.
- The Parkland formula is used to calculate the amount of Hartmann's solution required in the first 24 hours following the burn:

$$\text{Weight}(\text{kg}) \times \text{Percentage burn} \times 4\,(\text{mL})$$

Half of this volume should be given during the first 8 hours and the remainder over the following 16 hours. Actual body weight should be used in this calculation.
- An additional amount will be required to satisfy the patient's normal fluid requirements (maintenance fluids for paediatric patients or about 1500 mL/day for a 70-kg man). This will be raised if there is pyrexia.
- Urinary output is the best way of monitoring fluid replacement. Plasma substitutes and blood will be required later on if there is a significant element of full-thickness burning.

- Establish monitoring and investigations
- Agree a treatment plan with the local burns unit
- Prepare for controlled transfer to the appropriate area.

The British Burns Association has referral criteria to specialised burns services (→ *Table 10.1*)

The specialised burns unit is often some distance from the ED and usually has a limited number of beds. It is inappropriate to transfer very severely burned elderly patients to specialised (and often distant) burns units when it is clear that they will die- discuss this decision with burns specialists and senior colleagues.

Table 10.1 Referral criteria for specialist burns services

Complex burn injuries include any of the following:

Extremes of age	Under 5yr or more than 60yr
Site involved (dermal or full-thickness loss)	Face, hands, perineum or feet
	Any flexure particularly the neck or axilla
	Any circumferential dermal or full-thickness burn of the limbs, torso or neck
Inhalation injury	Any significant such injury, excluding pure carbon monoxide poisoning
Mechanism of injury	Chemical injury (>5% TBSA)
	Exposure to ionising radiation injury
	High-pressure steam injury
	High-tension electrical injury
	Hydrofluoric acid injury (>1% TBSA)
	Suspicion of non-accidental burn injury; adult or paediatric
Size of skin injury with dermal or full-thickness loss	<16yr old with >5% TBSA
	16yr or over >10% TBSA
Pre-existing co-morbidities	Significant cardiorespiratory disease; diabetes; pregnancy; immunosuppression; hepatic impairment, cirrhosis
Associated injuries	Crush injuries; fractures; head injury; penetrating injuries

Before transfer check the following:

- The airway control is immaculate and unlikely to deteriorate.
- IV access is adequate and cannula fixed well in place.
- Fluid regimen is agreed and running.
- Monitoring equipment is suitable.
- Charts, notes and laboratory results are with the patient.
- Analgesia is satisfactory and can be topped up.
- Level of nursing/medical care required en route has been considered.

SMALL BURNS

Most burns under 10% of the body surface area can be managed on an outpatient basis. *Exceptions are discussed under Special burns → p. 147.*

Initial assessment and management

Initial action includes:

- the removal of the source of the burn
- flooding with cold water
- analgesia
- assessment of size, site and depth (a drawing is useful) → *p. 142–144.*

A temporary dressing, without medication, is applied once the burn area has been exposed and the patient is waiting for definitive care. Analgesia must be given as soon as possible, especially to children.

> Simple erythema is extremely painful. Even patients expected to go home after treatment may need parenteral analgesia.

The pattern of burning should be considered in the light of the history available. A scald from spilled water will produce a cascade effect, with streaks of burnt skin following the path of the falling fluid, possibly with increasing depth of injury where its flow has been held up by constricting clothes such as waistbands or socks. A scald with a glove or stocking distribution is unusual; either the patient has impaired peripheral or central pain perception or the limb was held underwater. In children, this type of appearance suggests non-accidental injury (→ *Box 10.2* and *p. 369*).

The depth of the burn influences long-term treatment and should be determined as soon as possible. Superficial erythema is initially painful, whereas full-thickness burns will be insensitive because the nerve endings have been destroyed. Most areas of most burns fall between these extremes and are termed partial-thickness burns.

If most of the dermal papillae and all of the skin appendages (hair follicles and sweat glands) are intact,

Box 10.2 Features of a burn that suggest non-accidental injury

- Glove or stocking distribution, especially if bilateral
- Involvement of buttocks or perineum
- Scalds with a clearly demarcated edge with no peripheral splash marks
- Small, even, rounded (cigarette tip) burns
- General features of history and presentation suspicious of non-accidental injury

there is a very good potential for spontaneous regeneration. The term 'deep dermal' is used to describe partial-thickness burns with only a few epidermal remnants remaining – usually around the necks of sweat glands and hair follicles. If the wound becomes infected, these cells may die, resulting in full-thickness skin loss. Prevention of infection is thus of paramount importance in deep dermal burns.

There is frequently a combination of partial- and full-thickness burning. The patient may consider the whole area sensitive and it is often difficult to determine the depth at the first examination. However, the distinction is usually unimportant in the very early stages of treatment. Most areas of full-thickness loss that require grafts are evident by 5–10 days. Electrical burns may be suitable for the specialised technique of immediate excision and grafting.

Dressing and follow-up of simple superficial burns

Skin debris and foreign material are removed with dilute antiseptic and cotton-wool balls. Small non tense blisters (<6 mm) should be left alone. Large and thin-walled blisters should usually deroofed, which also allows for full assessment of the wound base and depth of burn. Leaving parts of the devitalised skin can act as a nidus for infection.

A sterile, non-adherent or biosynthetic dressing is then applied. Antiseptic substances are not needed for most burns. Healing will occur more rapidly in a moist environment, but excess exudate should be kept away from the wound surface. A moist wound surface reduces damage to the new epithelium when the dressing is changed and is less painful.

The wound dressing can be covered with a more robust gauze for added protection. Limb burns should be elevated, but the patient is encouraged to move the burned part as much as possible. Stiffness will develop quickly and can be slow to resolve once established. Routine prophylaxis with antibiotics is not indicated.

The burn should be reassessed and redressed within 24–48 hours. Dressings should be changed no more than three times in the first week and less frequently thereafter. Most patients can be taught to dress small burns at home. Elderly patients can be treated at home by the district nurse or at the local health centre. All burns to special areas and full-thickness burns should be reviewed in the ED.

Once the wound has fully epithelialised and has thus become dry, it should be exposed to a clean environment but protected from dirt and friction by temporary dry dressings. A moisturising cream can be applied to replace the sweat gland secretions, which are often deficient for some months after burning. The patient should be warned that the skin will be especially sensitive to ultraviolet light throughout the following summer and high factor sunscreen should be applied regularly to exposed areas.

Skin grafting of burns

Some electrical burns are most effectively treated by initial excision and early grafting and are best referred immediately to a burns unit. However, most small, simple burns treated on an outpatient basis in an ED should be managed conservatively for at least the first 5 days.

Wounds under 2 cm in diameter usually contract and close spontaneously, even if there is full-thickness skin loss. Larger wounds will show evidence of marginal and focal epithelialisation. It should be possible to distinguish deep-dermal from full-thickness burns within 10 days of the injury. If the former remain sterile, thereby avoiding destruction of the epithelial remnants, they will heal spontaneously. The latter will require split-skin grafts.

SPECIAL BURNS

Burns to the face

Inhalation burns must be excluded ($\rightarrow$ *p. 141*). The patient may have deceptively good function when first assessed but can deteriorate over 24 hours. Swelling is a major problem:

- Patients with burns to the eyelids and cornea must be admitted to a specialised eye unit. Lid retraction may cause major problems. Apply an antibiotic (e.g. chloramphenicol) eye ointment before transfer.
- Burns around the mouth cause feeding problems. Inpatient care is usually required. The burns unit should be contacted for advice.
- Deep burns involving the nose and ear may destroy underlying cartilage and should always be referred for specialised care.
- Small partial-thickness burns of other areas of the face can usually be adequately treated on an outpatient basis, but should be discussed with burns specialists and may benefit from specialist follow-up. Chloramphenicol ointment should be prescribed if the burns have encroached on the periorbital area.

Burns to the hands

All but the smallest burns to hands should be discussed with a burns specialist. The fingers quickly stiffen up and the functional impact may be very significant.

Conventional bandages become very dirty, with an increased risk of infection. If the digits are affected, then individual dressings should be applied to each digit, a non-adherent anti-microbial dressing should be used with a secondary dressing of gauze swabs. The hands or feet should be bandaged into a position which will preserve function. Wounds need reassessing within 24–48 hours and all injuries that involve a joint should be referred for physiotherapy and specialist burns follow-up. Patients should also be encouraged to move the hand as much as possible.

Burns to the perineum

The perineum must be examined carefully. It is a common site for non-accidental burns. Any burns to the top of the thighs or on the buttocks, which cannot be adequately dressed, and all those nearer the perineum, which cannot easily be kept clean, must be managed in hospital and discussed with burns specialists. A short-stay ward may be appropriate, but extensive or full-thickness burns should be referred to the burns unit.

Circumferential burns

If a partial- or full-thickness burn extends completely around a limb, the distal circulation may become impaired. In this situation, any jewellery on the patient's extremities should be removed and the circulation and neurological status of the limb regularly assessed. Discuss such cases with a burns specialist. Minor degrees of venous obstruction can be treated by admission and elevation. Deep burns, which will quickly contract, may cause more serious obstruction. Similar complications may occur on the trunk causing respiratory distress, elevation of the head and chest by 20°–30° will help reduce neck and chest wall oedema. Escharotomy may be required if there is severe restriction of chest wall motion or in order to relieve circulatory compromise in a circumferentially burned limb. This procedure is associated with significant fluid loss and must not be undertaken without expert advice.

Fasciotomies are seldom required but may be needed to restore circulation in patients who have associated skeletal trauma, crush injury, high voltage electrical injuries and burns that involve tissue beneath the investing fascia.

Electrical burns

The body can act as a volume conductor of electrical energy and the heat generated results in thermal injury to tissues. Electrical burns are often more serious than they appear on the body surface. This is because there are different rates of heat loss from superficial and deep tissues, which allows for relatively normal overlying skin to coexist with deep muscle necrosis. Myoglobin released from damaged muscles may also lead to rhabdomyolysis.

Chemical burns

Acidic solutions produce painful coagulation burns, which are often self-limiting and superficial with the destruction of the surface epithelium and submucosa only. Concentrated and corrosive acids such as phenol and hydrofluoric acid (below) may cause deep burns with systemic absorption. Alkaline solutions produce deep, full-thickness liquefaction burns that can be surprisingly pain free at first. However, there is extensive damage that is due to solubilisation of proteins such as collagen, saponification of lipids and dehydration of tissue cells.

Tx No attempt should be made to neutralise chemicals on the skin (*except hydrofluoric acid*). Most neutralising reactions are exothermic and would cause an additional thermal injury. Dilution by continuous irrigation with water for at least 20–30 min (or until the pH of the burned area is normal) is the mainstay of treatment. Prolonged irrigation with cold water also reduces pain significantly. Caution must be exercised with young children who quickly become hypothermic. Systemic absorption of some chemicals (e.g. phenol) may be significant. Toxicological advice should be sought.

Hydrofluoric acid burns

Hydrofluoric acid (hydrogen fluoride or HF) is used extensively in industry and horticulture. Skin contact causes severe local tissue damage with a great deal of pain. The burn is deep and slow to heal. With solutions containing less than 50% hydrofluoric acid there may be a delay until the burn develops as follows:

- Anhydrous or >50% concentrations – immediate damage
- 20–50% concentrations – up to 8 hours delay
- <20% concentrations – up to 24 hours delay.

Even concentrations of acid as low as 2% may cause burns after prolonged skin contact. The severity of the hydrofluoric acid burn is proportional to the concentration of the acid, the duration of exposure and the rapidity of treatment with calcium gluconate.

Investigations: Significant absorption of fluoride ion through the skin causes hypocalcaemia, as well as hypomagnesaemia, hyperkalaemia and metabolic acidosis. Cardiac arrest may occur even with relatively small burn surface areas. The serum calcium and ECG should be checked in all patients with burns resulting from contact with hydrogen fluoride.

Tx Immediate irrigation of the contaminated area is essential and may be very effective. Pain, tissue destruction and hypocalcaemia can be reduced by converting the acid to its calcium salt. This is achieved by repeated application of calcium gluconate gel (marketed as hydrofluoric acid burn jelly). There is no exothermic reaction. The injection of 10% calcium gluconate around and under the burn is sometimes advocated for persistent pain in well-localised lesions. In severe cases of dermal pain, intra-arterial calcium gluconate has been used. This is given as 10 mL of 10% calcium gluconate diluted in 50 mL dextrose and infused into the brachial or radial artery over 3–4 hours.

It is important to use calcium gluconate not calcium chloride. Calcium chloride causes tissue necrosis and must not be administered subcutaneously and only calcium gluconate can be given intra-arterially.

White phosphorus burns

White (or yellow) phosphorus is commonly used in fertilisers, cleaning products, rodenticides, fireworks, military ammunitions and incendiary devices and may cause severe burns. Exposure to phosphorus can lead to hypokalaemia, hypocalcaemia and hypophosphataemia. In addition, toxic phosphorus pentoxide gas can be released, which is an irritant to the lungs.

Tx Injuries and burns that are contaminated with white phosphorus require special and unique management:

Remove contaminated clothing as the white phosphorus may re-ignite and set the clothing on fire. The burned area should be lavaged copiously to remove identifiable particles (which should be placed in water to prevent spontaneous combustion).

Phosphorus will fluoresce under ultraviolet light (wood lamp), and this will help identify phosphorus particles allowing the removal of any residual particles. The burned area must be kept covered with water or saline-soaked gauze to prevent further combustion.

A 1% copper sulphate ($CuSO_4$) solution rinse has previously been advocated to aid removal of the particles of phosphorus. Copper sulphate combines with phosphorous to create a blue–black cupric phosphide coating. This impedes further combustion and makes phosphorus particles easier to find. However, copper sulphate is toxic, and absorption can cause intravascular haemolysis and renal failure; silver nitrate may provide safer and more reliable antagonism of white phosphorus dermal absorption.

Chemical burns from giant hogweed

The plant *Heracleum mantegazzianum*, – better known as giant hogweed, is common in the British Isles and is found alongside roads, railway lines, rivers and footpaths, often in areas of wasteland. The plant is characterised by its size. Over a period of 4 years, it may grow up to 5 m in height, and it has a reddish-purple stem and spotted leaf stalks with fine spines that make it appear furry. The leaves may be up to 1.5 m in width with large white flowering heads. These characteristics make the giant hogweed plant irresistible to children who make swords and umbrellas from it.

Unfortunately, giant hogweed exudes a clear watery sap from its leaves and also from the stem in even greater quantities. This sap contains a glucoside called furanocoumarin, which renders the skin photosensitive to ultraviolet (UV) light. Exposure to sunlight after contact with the sap results in large painful blisters, burns and linear inflammation. This reaction usually appears within 15–20 hours of contact although it can occur up to 48 hours later. Damaged skin heals very slowly over at least 2 weeks, leaving residual pigmentation that can develop into chronic phytophotodermatitis. Inflammation may recur in sunlight for many months. Similar phytophotodermatitis can occur following an exposure to a range of other plants including lime juice.

Tx In the event of contact with giant hogweed sap, the skin should be washed immediately with soap and water and then covered to reduce the exposure to sunlight. Application of topical steroids, calamine lotion and anti-histamines can help alleviate itching. Otherwise, partial-thickness lesions are treated with dressings and analgesia until healing occurs. As the skin can remain photosensitive for several months or years, the patients should be advised to continue applying sunblock to the affected area.

Burns from hot tar

Hot bitumen solidifies on contact with the skin. Water should be applied at the site to hasten hardening and limit heat transfer. If the bitumen is still hot, then this should be continued for at least 20 min or until it has hardened and cooled.

The removal of bitumen from intact skin is controversial and does not appear to lead to quicker healing of the skin. Bitumen can be softened and removed by applying a lipid or polysorbate-based agent; this includes petroleum-based or polysorbate-based antibiotic ointments, liquid paraffin, sunflower oil and melted butter. However, this can take from 30 min up to several hours to work and reapplication and dressing changes may be required. Adherent material can be left in situ, and it will spontaneously detach after a few days; but if circumferential, then a longitudinal split in the bitumen should be made to prevent a tourniquet effect. Peeling or picking the bitumen should be avoided as this will increase the tissue damage.

ELECTROCUTION

High-voltage injury – >1000 V (including lightning)

A high-voltage electric shock usually occurs due to electrocution from a direct current (DC) which is common in industrial settings but can also occur from being struck by lightning. Injuries following a high-voltage exposure may result from the following:

- Falling or being thrown to the ground, causing secondary injuries
- Tetanic muscle contraction (more likely if exposed to AC current) which may prevent a patient from letting go, increasing the energy delivered to the body and causing fractures of long bones, crushed vertebrae and torn muscles
- Spontaneous ignition of clothing, causing burns
- Conduction of electricity through the body, causing entry and exit wounds and internal injuries
- Current passing along the surface of the body to earth, causing very deep burns over a large area of skin
- Current jumping from one part of the body to another, causing secondary exit and entry wounds.

A high-voltage injury may cause a respiratory or cardiac arrest. A respiratory arrest due to hypoxia can be a consequence of paralysis or tetanic contractions of the respiratory muscles. A cardiac arrest is usually the result of an adverse effect on the conducting system in addition to causing direct myocardial damage. High voltage or DC current usually causes asystole, whereas an AC current usually causes ventricular fibrillation. If this is successfully reversed or if the patient presents without having had a life-threatening cardiac dysrhythmia, it is unlikely that one will develop subsequently. Supraventricular tachycardia, atrial fibrillation, atrial tachycardias, junctional rhythms and first- and second-degree heart block have also been reported, but more commonly the ECG shows right bundle-branch block and/or ST changes. These changes may last for many weeks. Treatment is based on symptoms and clinical signs in the normal way. Myocardial ischaemia and infarction can occur as a result of coronary artery spasm and thrombosis. Troponin is the most specific cardiac injury marker.

If the current travels through the body, it naturally follows the path of least resistance. Nerves and blood vessels are good conductors. Increasing resistance is offered by muscle, skin, tendon, fat and bone in that order. Structures with high resistance will generate the greatest heat but, clearly, some tissues are more readily damaged by heat than others. Nerves, blood vessels, muscles and skin sustain most of the injury.

The entry point is typically charred and depressed. It becomes swollen very quickly, with the accumulation of extracellular fluid. The exit point has an explosive appearance – round or oval grey craters with no inflammatory changes. These increase in size over the first few days. Examining the entrance and exit burns can help predict the current pathway and therefore which internal structures may have been involved. It is important to remember that there is no correlation between the percentage of superficial burns and the degree of underlying tissue damage and the rule of nine should be used with caution. Muscle involvement is typically patchy, with swelling, necrosis and the later development of deep sepsis. Skeletal muscle damage can also lead to electrolyte disturbances and myoglobin release; rhabdomyolysis can result. Deep tissue injury in the extremities can lead to significant swelling and subsequent compartment syndrome.

In the peripheral nerves, axons are distorted and Schwann cells break down and coalesce. Spinal cord lesions are surprisingly common, often producing partial transections. Tetraplegia and paraplegia can occur, and these may be transient or permanent. Brain damage is unusual unless the head has been directly involved. When it does occur, it can manifest as loss of consciousness, amnesia, confusion, seizures and it can cause focal neurology. Keraunoparalysis (lightning paralysis) is a reversible, transient paralysis that is associated with sensory disturbances and peripheral vasoconstriction in lightning victims.

Blood vessels sustain endothelial damage and media degeneration. Thrombosis and late rupture can occur at sites distant from the entry point. Visceral lesions, which are often unrecognised, probably have a vascular aetiology. The most commonly affected visceral organs are the colon and small intestine.

Acute tubular necrosis is common. Inadequate volume replacement, myoglobinuria and direct damage to renal vessels probably all contribute to its development.

Cataracts are a well-recognised, late complication and late death is commonly caused by overwhelming sepsis.

Characteristic signs in patients struck by lightning → Box 10.3.

Tx

These patients should be assessed and treated as a trauma patient with cervical spine immobilisation.

> Box 10.3 **Characteristic signs of injury by lightning**
>
> - Damaged clothing
> - Linear surface burns or Lichtenberg figures (fern-like pattern on skin) that are pathognomonic
> - Tiny necrotic burns around the edges of the feet and toes
> - Ruptured tympanic membranes

Treatment in the ED is directed towards stabilisation of any life-threatening dysrhythmia and the early transfusion of crystalloid. Fluid loss cannot be calculated by burns formulae. The volume required is titrated against the patient's pulse, blood pressure, urine output and central venous pressure (CVP) if appropriate. Blood gases and plasma U&Es (including creatinine) should be measured. Acidosis is common in patients with extensive electrocution injuries.

The care of all patients who have been electrocuted must be discussed with a senior member of staff. Extensive soft-tissue injuries should be assessed in theatre. Tissue loss can be minimised by very early fasciotomy and removal of dead tissue. However, because of the patchy nature of the muscle involvement, this process is not as easy as with muscle damage resulting from direct injury. Occult visceral damage must also be considered.

Antitetanus prophylaxis is required for all patients.

Mortality is highest in lightning strikes (17.6%) compared with high voltage (5.3%) and low-voltage electrical injuries (2.8%).

Low-voltage injury – <1000 V

Domestic electricity supply is usually an alternating current (AC) and the typical household voltage is between 220 and 240 V at 50 Hz. As a result, low voltage burns of the type sustained from the domestic electricity supply are not usually associated with the above complications. However, the local burn is almost always full thickness and much deeper than it appears. The area of tissue necrosis may extend over the first few days. Senior advice should be sought. Early excision and grafting are often favoured by specialised burns units. Those patients who have sustained a low voltage injury and have a normal ECG, and no visible injuries can be safely discharged from the emergency department.

The use of electronic control devices such as Tasers has increased substantially in recent years. These devices deliver a temporary high voltage, low current electrical discharge that overrides natural muscle triggering mechanisms. A healthy individual who receives a single exposure is unlikely to suffer from significant consequences; however, those who receive multiple exposures are intoxicated and have multiple comorbidities are more likely to suffer deleterious effects. Injuries from being restrained and traumatic secondary injuries from falling after being tasered, particularly head injuries, need to be looked for and actively excluded. The Taser barbs themselves can also cause penetrating injuries and may need removing.

CONTAMINATION AND IRRADIATION

Contamination by toxic chemicals

Indicators of a chemical release include:

- Multiple casualties with similar non-traumatic symptoms and signs
- Unexplained symptoms including signs of skin, eye or airway irritation, breathing difficulties, nausea, vomiting, sweating, blurred painful vision, headache, disorientation, seizures or decreased level of consciousness
- The obvious presence of hazardous materials or unusual materials and equipment
- Unexplained vapour, mist clouds, oily droplets or films on surfaces of water
- Unexplained dead animals.

In the UK, expert advice can be obtained from the National Poisons Information Service and the Public Health England Centre for Radiation, Chemicals and Environmental Hazards. Ideally, any casualties should be decontaminated at the scene, but NHS secondary decontamination facilities will be needed to manage any casualties that have been transported directly to hospital or who have self-presented.

Tx in the ED The contaminated patient should be taken to a designated area. Disrobing is a critical step in the decontamination process and is very effective at reducing exposure to CBRN materials. Disrobing should be followed by dry decontamination for non-caustic chemical incidents. This can be performed using any dry paper tissue, towels or strips of blankets or sheets to blot the exposed skin; with care taken to avoid transferring contamination from one part of the body to another. If a caustic substance is involved, then wet decontamination should be carried out using water from any available source. Decontamination should follow the 'RINSE-WIPE-RINSE' method. Any contaminated areas should be rinsed with clean water or water-containing detergent, from the highest point downward; then the skin wiped with absorbent material and rinsed a second time with clean warm water. Ideally, self-decontamination by casualties is the best approach. If radioactive material is the source of the contamination, then a check for residual contamination should be performed and the decontamination repeated if required. Decontamination is not needed if the chemical agent released is a gas.

If volatile substances are involved, the hospital engineers must be alerted to prevent contamination of the air-conditioning systems. Staff should wear protective clothing; the risk for a health professional who uses standard precautions is likely to be tiny if not trivial. Some substances (e.g. phenol) may cause severe systemic poisoning by skin contact alone.

Contamination by radioactive substances

On average, there is one serious radiation incident – resulting in death or major radiation injury – in the world each year. In the last 50 years, there have been more than 200 incidents involving lost, stolen or misused sources of radiation. Recent anti-terrorist concerns include the possibility of exposure from a 'dirty bomb' (conventional explosive used to disperse radioactive material), a low-yield improvised nuclear device or a deliberately hidden source of radiation.

A person is contaminated when radioactive material is deposited on skin and/or clothing (external contamination) or into the body (internal contamination) by inhalation, ingestion or absorption via a wound.

Measurement of radioactivity and radiation → Box 10.5 on p. 153.
Types of ionising radiation → Box 10.4.

Symptoms and signs of external contamination

There may be no symptoms or signs although heavy contamination will provoke redness and burning of the skin. The patient must be informed about the importance of decontamination for both personal and public health reasons.

- A predetermined and separate entrance and treatment area for isolation and decontamination should be demarcated. This area must have a shower and

 Box 10.4 **Types of ionising radiation**

Ionising radiation is a form of energy that is emitted spontaneously by radioactive materials. It is invisible, odourless and tasteless. Natural radiation is present all around us: in air from cosmic rays, in the earth and building materials and in food and water. This comprises the background radiation to which we are all constantly exposed. Man-made sources of radiation and radioactive materials are used widely in medicine, scientific research, industry and radiographic detection systems.

- **Alpha particles** are heavy, highly charged and interact strongly with atoms. As a result, they lose momentum rapidly, can travel only very short distances and do not penetrate further than the outer layers of the human skin. Alpha emitters are hazardous only when inhaled, ingested, injected or absorbed through a wound
- **Beta particles** are also charged but interact less strongly with atoms than alpha particles. Consequently, they travel further and penetrate more: they can penetrate the dermis. Clothing (including standard personal protective equipment [PPE]) provides some protection against them. Beta particles can cause radiation skin injury on prolonged exposure but are hazardous to internal organs only when inhaled, ingested, injected or absorbed through a wound
- **Gamma rays** and their man-made equivalent, **X-rays**, are uncharged and so do not interact directly with atoms. They travel many metres in air and can easily penetrate the human body potentially causing organ damage. Their effects can be attenuated by dense materials such as concrete or lead shielding
- **Neutrons** are uncharged particles that travel far and penetrate everything except thick layers of concrete and water. They are highly damaging but only likely to be produced in the very early stages of a nuclear detonation or accident

water collection facility as detailed above. Floors of treatment and transit areas should be covered with disposable sheeting, as should non-disposable equipment. Air conditioning must be switched off and portable equipment removed.

Box 10.5 Measurement of radioactivity and radiation

Radiation is readily detectable with equipment, and contamination is easily measurable. Medical physics and nuclear medicine departments and frontline services all have equipment for detecting beta and gamma radiation and people trained to use it.

- **Radioactivity (and contamination by radioactive material) is measured in becquerels (1 Bq = 1 disintegration/s)**
- **The absorbed dose of radiation (the amount of energy absorbed per unit mass of tissue) is measured in grays (1 Gy = 1 J/kg tissue)**

Different types of radiation have different effects on human tissue. In equivalent dosages measured in grays, alpha particles and neutrons are more damaging than beta particles, gamma rays or X-rays in terms of the risks of cancer or of in heritable genetic defects. To account for this, the absorbed dosage is multiplied by a 'radiation weighting factor' to produce:

- **The equivalent dose (of an organ or tissue) is measured in sieverts (Sv). For X-rays, gamma rays and beta particles, the weighting factor = 1 and so 1 Gy = 1 Sv = 1000 mSv. Some organs are more radiosensitive than others (e.g. the bone marrow is more sensitive than the thyroid), and exposures are rarely uniform. Weighting the equivalent doses received by different organs and tissues during an exposure to allow for each organ's radiosensitivity, and then summing the results gives the effective dose. An estimate of the whole-body dose is helpful in estimating long-term cancer risk**

- Involved staff must wear theatre suits, long plastic aprons, caps, overshoes and two pairs of gloves.
- Patients and staff must not eat, drink or smoke within the designated area.
- There must be a place to decontaminate staff on arrival from the scene and before leaving the designated area. All personnel involved must be checked by the radiation protection adviser and should have a shower before leaving this area.
- Resuscitation is still the first priority but efforts must be made throughout to limit the spread of radioactive particles.

- Levels of radiation should be measured before and after decontamination.
- All clothing, swabs and fluids should be handled carefully and collected in labelled bags and containers. Removal of clothing can reduce external contamination by as much as 90%.
- Areas of the body unprotected by clothing take priority. Hands and nails should be cleaned with running water and surgical scrub for 5 min. Hair must be washed (with any shampoo) in a similar way; showers should not be taken while the hair is contaminated. The face should be cleaned and ears and eyes irrigated. The nose must be blown and the mouth washed out. Vacuum cleaning is sometimes recommended. If radiation monitoring confirms residual contamination of skin, then cleaning should be attempted with 5% potassium permanganate solution for 5 min. The brown staining is removed by the application of 5% sodium bisulphite. This system gives a visual confirmation of coverage and removal.
- Wounds must be covered before surface decontamination and later cleaned by direct irrigation.
- A member of staff should be tasked with recording all patient movements around the department.

Symptoms and signs of internal contamination

In 2006, a man died in a London hospital after unwittingly ingesting a drink containing polonium-210. This naturally occurring radionuclide has a half-life of 138 days. It undergoes decay by emitting alpha particles, accompanied by very low-intensity gamma radiation.

Ionising radiation kills cells and causes harm to tissues and organs (deterministic injury) or damages genetic material that increases the long-term risks of developing cancer and hereditary effects (stochastic risk). The increase in lifetime cancer risk for adult whole-body exposure is approximately 5% per Sv effective dose of radiation.

There may be no symptoms or signs but a deterministic injury should be suspected where there is

- any newly diagnosed acute bone marrow depression (leucopenia infection, thrombocytopenia, bleeding gums, nosebleed and bruising)
- burns, erythema or bullae with no history of heat or chemical exposure

- sudden, rapid hair loss especially if there is a relevant occupational history or unexplained nausea, vomiting or diarrhoea two to four weeks before onset
- when dealing with a bomb or other intentionally placed explosive device.

At high internal radiation doses, patients develop acute radiation syndrome (ARS) (→ *below*) and necrosis of internal tissues. However with substances that emit alpha particles (such as polonium-210) symptoms are more limited. The most common route for internal contamination is ingestion (often from contaminated hands), and then nausea, vomiting and diarrhoea are the initial symptoms. (These are also the early symptoms of classic radiation sickness.) Most ingested polonium-210 passes out of the body in the faeces but the urine and other body fluids will also be contaminated.

Measurement of radioactivity and radiation → Box 10.5.
Treatment of internal contamination by radioactive substances → p. 155.
Types of ionising radiation → Box 10.4.

It is important to distinguish between patients who have been contaminated by radioactive particles and those who have been irradiated. The former can spread radiation; the latter cannot. Some will be in both categories.

Exposure to radioactive substances (irradiation) and acute radiation syndrome

Radiation exposure occurs when all or part of the body is irradiated. Three key factors affect exposure: duration, distance and shielding. If the exposure time is halved, then the dose of radiation is halved. The inverse square law applies to distance: doubling the distance between the source and the body reduces the dose by a factor of four; trebling the distance between the source and the body reduces the dose by a factor of nine; and so on. In the same way that a patient who has had a radiograph presents no risk to others, radiation safety precautions are not needed for patients who have been exposed to radiation but are not contaminated.

At low doses of radiation that are equivalent to whole body doses of up to 1 Gy (equivalent to about 50 000 chest radiographs) there are no acute symptoms. The hazard is an increase in the lifetime risk of cancer that is quite modest compared with the 'background' cancer risk.

Many radiation accidents cause partial body injury: early erythema followed by bullae and, if severe, ulceration and necrosis (often of the hands). This may not necessarily progress to ARS. ARS follows a large, usually external exposure of all or most of the body to penetrating radiation (gamma rays, high-energy X-rays or neutrons) in a short time (seconds, minutes or hours). Symptoms of ARS occur in four phases: prodromal phase → latent period → illness → recovery or death. As the radiation dose increases, the prodromal and latent periods shorten and the severity of illness and the risk of mortality increase. Major trauma and radiation exposure interact synergistically on mortality.

If there are no symptoms (such as nausea or vomiting) in the first 6 hours after a suspected exposure, then serious acute radiation sickness is unlikely.

Features suggestive of significant penetrating irradiation that may progress to full radiation sickness include the following:

- A history of loss of consciousness (this suggests a high dose of radiation with a bad prognosis)
- Transient erythema after 24 hours
- Early nausea, diarrhoea and vomiting (especially within 1 hour of exposure)
- An early and dramatic fall in the white cell count.

Marked heterogenity of the distribution of the dose may result in non-classical pattern of injuries, for example a dose of 20+ Sv to a limb may cause only local injury without any haematopoietic or gastrointestinal effects.

Dose-related symptoms and signs of ARS → Box 10.6.

Tx

Assume that all patients are contaminated until you know that they are not!

Initial symptoms of ARS are non-specific and rarely immediately life threatening; treatment of other injuries therefore takes priority.

Box 10.6 Dose-related features of acute radiation syndrome

<1 Sv: usually asymptomatic
- Mild symptoms in up to 10% of people of episodic nausea and vomiting for 48 hours
- Slightly depressed white blood cell (WBC) count at 2–4 weeks post-exposure
- No fetal effects if the effective dose <100 mSv (100 000 mcSv) but counselling needed if pregnant and effective dose >100 mSv (100 000 mcSv).

1–8 Sv: haematopoietic syndrome
- Anorexia, nausea, vomiting and fatigue between 1 and 4 hours after exposure (the timing and severity are dose related)
- Latent period of between 2 days and 4 weeks and then
- Bone marrow depression (leukopenia and infection; low platelets and bleeding)
- Serial lymphocyte counts in the first 48 hours predict the severity
- Hair loss after 2 or 3 weeks after a dose of >3 or 4 Sv
- Lethal dose (LD) 50/60 is around 4.5 Sv without treatment.

>6 Sv: gastrointestinal syndrome
- Early nausea, vomiting, diarrhoea, anorexia and fatigue
- Latent period of up to 1 week and then
- Severe gastrointestinal (GI) symptoms (fever, abdominal pain, watery diarrhoea, GI haemorrhage, electrolyte imbalance and dehydration)
- Bone marrow depression (leukopenia and infection; low platelets and bleeding)
- LD 100 is about 10 Sv; death usually occurs within 2 weeks.

>20 Sv: central nervous system/cardiovascular system syndrome
- Burning sensation on the skin
- Almost immediate projectile vomiting and explosive bloody diarrhoea
- Headache, collapse, agitation, confusion and loss of consciousness
- May be a lucid interval (hours) and then
- Convulsions, coma, hypotension, shock and death within 2–3 days.

Early involvement of a multidisciplinary team with expertise in radiation medicine, health physics, haematology, gastroenterology, bone marrow transplantation, plastic surgery, public health medicine and toxicology is recommended.

- Commence standard resuscitation measures
- Do not handle unfamiliar objects or embedded fragments directly
- Relieve pain with morphine; give cyclizine or ondansetron for nausea and vomiting
- Obtain and record as much information as possible about the type and extent of the exposure to help assess the dose of radiation received.

Involve the local medical and/or health physics teams and local radiation safety officer urgently to arrange radiation screening of the patient.

- Take routine blood samples including a baseline full blood count
- Take WBCs every 3 or 4 hours for the first 12 hours after an acute exposure and then six hourly for the next 48 hours. A falling lymphocyte count is a sensitive indicator of incipient bone marrow failure, and early cytokine treatment is indicated if the count falls to $<1.5 \times 10^9$
- Arrange HLA typing and chromosome analysis (venous blood and nasal swabs)
- Test for internal contamination by faecal sampling or 24-hour urine collection.

Early expert advice (e.g. from departments of medical physics or nuclear medicine, the Health Protection Agency or the Ministry of Defence) is essential for formal radiation dose assessment and the management of internal contamination. The development of radiation sickness is a delayed phenomenon, and at-risk patients should be referred to the nearest oncology or haematology unit after discussion with the local radiation protection adviser. A history of irradiation should not delay surgery. As a result of the immunosuppressive effect of the radiation, if the dose is more than 1 Sv, all surgery should be carried out as soon as possible and certainly within 36–48 hours of the incident. If this is not possible, then recovery of the bone marrow must be awaited.

If a large number of patients have been affected by ionising radiation, then a system of triaging radiological injury severity according to signs, symptoms and initial lymphocyte count such as the European Society for Blood and Marrow Transplantation can be useful.

If the radiation dose received is calculable, then there is a stochastic risk of approximately 5% per Sv effective dose of radiation increase in lifetime cancer risk. However, no additional screening apart from that which is appropriate for the patient's age and sex is required.

Comparative doses of radiation → Figure 10.3.

- The average annual background radiation exposure in the UK = 2.2 millisievert

- The annual effective dose limit for a UK citizen = 1.0 millisievert

- The annual effective dose limit for a UK radiation worker = 20 millisievert

- Acute radiation sickness (whole body single dose) = 1,000 millisievert and above

- The LD 50/60 dose (50% mortality within 60 days if not treated) = approximately 4500 millisievert

- The LD 100 dose (100% mortality) = around 10 000 millisievert

- Chest X-ray (PA) = 0.02 millisievert
- Limb or joint X-rays (AP and lateral) = 0.12 millisievert
- Cervical spine X-rays (3 views) = 0.27 millisievert
- Abdominal or pelvic X-ray (AP) = 0.7 millisievert
- Lumbar spine X-rays (AP and lateral) = 1.0 millisievert
- CT scan of the brain = 2.0 millisievert
- CT scan of the abdomen or thorax = 8 to 10 millisievert

Figure 10.3 Comparative doses of radiation.

11

Cardiac arrest and cardiac dysrhythmias

Rob Summerhayes[1,2]

[1] Consultant in Pre-Hospital and Emergency Medicine, University Hospital Southampton
[2] Education Lead, Hampshire and Isle of Wight Air Ambulance

This chapter covers the essential theoretical and practical aspects of adult cardiac arrest and management of dysrhythmia. However, it does not claim to equip the reader with all the skills necessary to lead a resuscitation team. For this, it is essential to attend an Advanced Life Support (ALS) course or similar.

The protocols and algorithms in this chapter are taken from the guidelines published in 2021 by the Resuscitation Council (UK). As such they are consistent with the current recommendations of the International Liaison Committee on Resuscitation (ILCoR).

Cardiac arrest

Cardiac arrest is a sudden loss of blood flow to vital organs caused by the failure of the heart to pump effectively. It is a rapidly fatal requiring immediate cardiopulmonary resuscitation (CPR). CPR results in some (all be it limited) perfusion of those vital organs until definitive treatment can be provided.

For the purposes of managing cardiac arrest, it is divided into 'Shockable' and 'Non-Shockable' rhythms. The ALS algorithm (→ *Figure 11.2*) is based around this distinction which will be covered later in the chapter.

Interventions that contribute to a successful outcome after cardiac arrest are conceptualised by the Resuscitation Council as the 'Chain of Survival.'

- Early recognition of cardiac arrest and call for help
- Early CPR
- Early defibrillation
- Post resuscitation care.

This 'Chain of Survival' forms the structure of the start of this chapter:

Recognition of cardiac arrest → P. 157
CPR → P. 158
ALS and defibrillation → P. 158
Interventions during CPR → P. 161
Cardiac arrest in special circumstances → P. 165
Cardiac arrest in children → P. 169
Post resuscitation care → P. 170
Bereavement → P. 171

Recognition of cardiac arrest

A standardised approach should be taken to the assessment of a collapsed person.

1 **Safety**:
   Check it is safe to approach. Where there is a collapsed patient, a rescuer's attention is naturally drawn to the patient. It is important not to lose situational awareness and put oneself in danger – unlikely in hospital but a very real risk out of hospital.

2 **Stimulate**:
   Grasp the patient by the shoulder and give them a confident shake 'are you OK?' Follow this with a rapid 'Look, Listen and Feel' with a cheek over the airway looking down the body for chest rise and fall. This may indicate a patient is critically ill and there is a need for urgent help.

3 **Shout for help**:
   Ask someone to ensure appropriate help is coming (in the UK dial 999 in the community and 2222 in a

hospital). If the patient is unconscious, unresponsive and is not breathing normally (occasional gasps are not normal), start CPR.

> If there are any doubts about the presence of a pulse start CPR

Cardiopulmonary resuscitation (CPR)

The current guidelines emphasise that it is more important that people feel able to do something to help than they become focused on small details or concerned about causing harm. No greater harm can occur than failing to act when someone requires CPR and defibrillation. The community response to cardiac arrest remains critical to saving lives. Bystander CPR and use of an automated external defibrillator (AED) increase the chances of survival by two to fourfold. There is likely to be concern about doing 'mouth to mouth' or generating aerosol by ventilating a patient prior to healthcare professionals donning appropriate personal protective equipment. Therefore, chest compression-only CPR and the attachment of AED/defibrillator should be done until someone in the appropriate PPE arrives.

It is worth noting that the Resuscitation Council UK have de-emphasised feeling for the presence of a pulse in a collapsed patient, but if you are confident and trained to do so you may feel for a pulse to determine if the patient has a respiratory arrest rather than a cardiac arrest. If there are any doubts about the presence of a pulse start CPR.

Almost all resuscitation attempts start with Basic Life Support (BLS) → *Figure 11.1*.

BLS becomes (ALS) when a defibrillator is attached. → *Figure 11.2*.

The interventions that unquestionably contribute to improved survival after cardiac arrest are prompt and effective bystander CPR, uninterrupted high-quality chest compressions and early defibrillation for VF/VT (ventricular fibrillation/ventricular tachycardia). Although drugs and advanced airways are included as ALS interventions, they are secondary in importance to the high-quality, uninterrupted chest compressions and early defibrillation.

Advanced life support and defibrillation

BLS becomes ALS when a defibrillator is attached. → *Figure 11.2*.

The key decision point is differentiating shockable rhythms from non-shockable rhythms. However, cardiac arrest is a dynamic situation, and patients will often flip between shockable and non-shockable rhythms.

> *Drugs and advanced airways are included as ALS interventions, they are secondary in importance to the high quality, uninterrupted chest compressions and early defibrillation*

Shockable rhythms (VF/VT)

The first monitored rhythm is ventricular fibrillation or ventricular tachycardia (VF/VT) in approximately 20% of cardiac arrests. In arrests that start in a non-shockable rhythm about 25% convert to VF/VT at some stage during resuscitation.

High-quality chest compressions and early recognition and defibrillation of shockable is the key to improving survival rates.

The technique for safe defibrillation of the shockable rhythms should be learned and practiced on an Advanced Life Support Course.

Key points to management of the shockable rhythm are:

- Pauses in chest compressions to confirm VF or VT should be brief. Aiming for less than 5 seconds.
- Once VF/VT is identified chest compressions should be resumed immediately. All rescuers apart from the individual performing chest compressions should be told to 'stand clear'. Chest compressions should be continued while the defibrillator charges. Once the defibrillator is charged and the safety check is complete, the team member doing the chest compressions should also 'stand clear'. The shock is then safely delivered, and CPR immediately resumes.
- Chest compressions are immediately resumed after defibrillation (without first checking the rhythm or pulse) because:
  - o If defibrillation is successful, it is very unusual for this to be associated with the normal electrical rhythm to translate to a palpable pulse. The time taken for a palpable pulse to may be longer than 2 min in up to 25% of successful shocks.
  - o The delay introduced by trying to palpate a pulse will further compromise brain and myocardial perfusion if a perfusing rhythm has not been restored.
  - o If a perfusing rhythm has been restored, giving chest compressions for 2 min does not increase the chance of VF recurring.
  - o Post-shock asystole is relatively common. In this circumstance, compressions may usefully induce VF which can then be shocked at the next 2-min rhythm check.

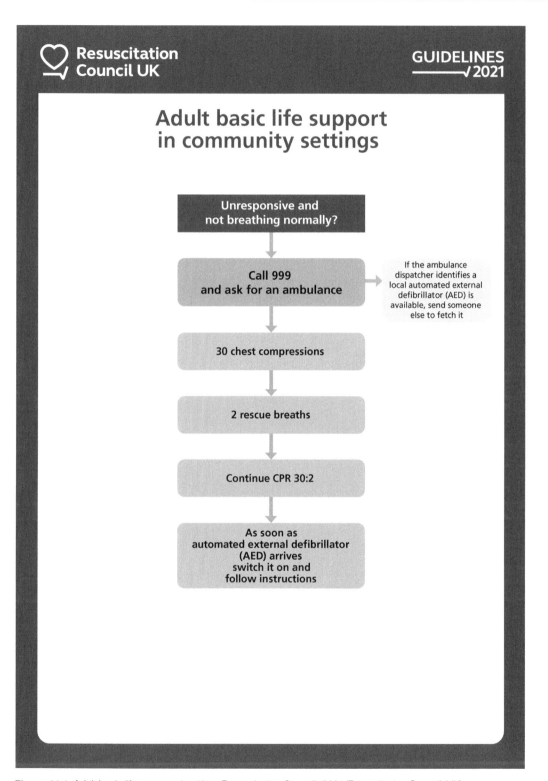

Figure 11.1 Adult basic life support algorithm. Resuscitation Council, 2021/Resuscitation Council (UK).

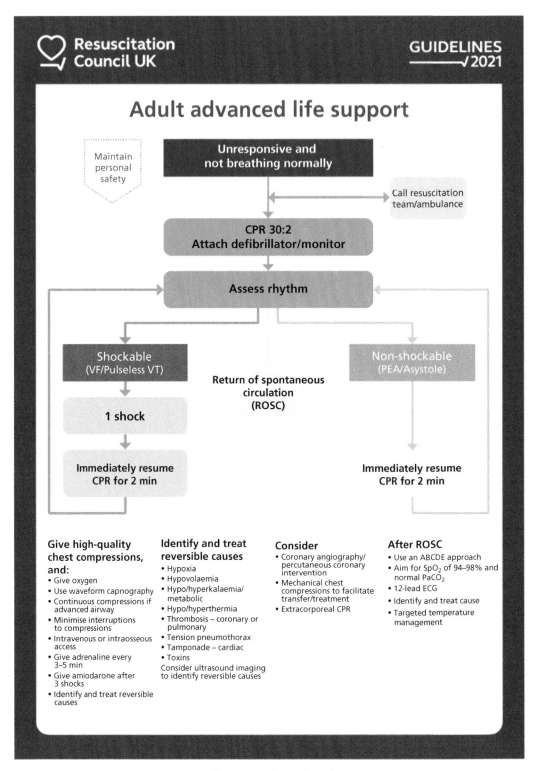

Figure 11.2 Adult advanced life support algorithm. Resuscitation Council, 2021/Resuscitation Council (UK).

Drugs in the shockable rhythm

The use of adrenaline, amiodarone and lidocaine are currently recommended by ILCoR. This is based largely on increased short-term survival, and there is a lack of evidence for increase in survival to hospital discharge.

Where there is a shockable rhythm, no drugs are given until after the third shock.

- **Adrenaline 1 mg**: Given after the third shock and then every 3–5 min (every other 2-min cycle).
- **Amiodarone**: 300 mg is given after the third shock with a further 150 mg that can be given if VF persists after the fifth shock.
- **Lidocaine**: 1 mg/kg is recommended as an alternative to amiodarone if amiodarone is not available. It is not recommended in addition to amiodarone.

Refractory VF/shock-resistant VF

Refractory VF refers to VF that persists despite shock delivery with the most commonly accepted definition being persistent VF despite ≥3 shocks.

- Continue effective CPR.
- Consider using a mechanical chest compression device such as LUCAS CPR and ResQPod impedance threshold device (the effectiveness of prolonged CPR dwindles as rescuers fatigue).
- Check the position and contact of the defibrillation pads and consider changing the pad position to anterior posterio.
- High-energy 'dual sequential' defibrillation using two defibrillators to deliver higher energy has been proposed and is in use in some systems. Evidence is limited and this is not currently recommended by ILCoR.
- Amiodarone should be administered after the third and fifth shock.
- Magnesium is often given in this circumstance. There is no robust evidence of an improved outcome.
- Consider attenuating the sympathetic drive that may be exacerbating the arrythmia. Esmolol (a beta blocker) and reducing adrenaline dosing are sometimes used in this circumstance although the evidence base is weak.
- Extracorporeal CPR (ECPR) should be considered in patients with a refractory arrythmia, few comorbidities and young age. ECPR is covered later in this chapter.

Non-shockable rhythms (PEA and asystole)

Pulseless electrical activity (PEA) is defined as cardiac arrest in the presence of electrical activity that would normally be associated with a palpable pulse. PEA can further be divided into 'true PEA vs pseudo PEA' by visualising the heart with ultrasound (→ *later*). True PEA is electrical activity but with no myocardial movement (cardiac standstill), whereas pseudo PEA is the presence of ventricular contractility visualised on ultrasound associated with electrical activity but without a palpable pulse. Pseudo PEA is associated with a better prognosis than true PEA and asystole, as it may represent a 'low flow', rather than 'no flow' state.

Asystole is the absence of electrical activity on the defibrillator. Ensure that this is not artefact (confirm that the defibrillator pads are attached to the patient, the defibrillator is set to read through the pads and that monitor gain is set appropriately). Check for the presence of regular p waves (p wave asystole) as this may respond to pacing.

The mainstay of management of both PEA and asystole is high-quality chest compressions, recognising and treating reversible cause (4Hs and 4Ts), obtaining an effective airway and vascular access.

Adrenaline 1 mg should be given as soon as vascular access has been obtained and then repeated every 3–5 min (every other 2-min cycle).

Interventions and considerations during CPR

Airway

During CPR, start with basic airway techniques and progress stepwise according to the skills of the rescuer until effective ventilation is achieved. If an advanced airway is required, only rescuers with a high tracheal intubation success rate should use tracheal intubation. The expert consensus is that a high success rate is over 95% within two attempts at intubation.

Aim for less than a 5 second interruption in chest compression for tracheal intubation.

Once a tracheal tube or a supraglottic airway (SGA) has been inserted, ventilate the lungs at a rate of $10\,min^{-1}$ and continue chest compressions without pausing during ventilations.

High-quality chest compressions

The importance of high-quality chest compressions cannot be overemphasised. In adults, they should be of 5–6 cm in depth ensuring full recoil between each compression at a rate of 100–120 per minute. Pauses in chest compressions must be kept to an absolute minimum (ideally <10 seconds).

Mechanical chest compression devices

Automated chest compression devises (e.g. LUCAS/Auto-Pulse) reliably give excellent quality chest compressions. However, they should not routinely replace manual chest compressions. The circumstances in which they are indicated are when good-quality manual compressions cannot be achieved, for example where a patient must be moved (e.g. from home to hospital) or for prolonged resuscitation attempts where rescuer fatigue will inevitably set in. Healthcare personnel who use these pieces of equipment must know their specific limitations, be able to apply them quickly and correctly in an emergency situation and be able to immediately restart manual CPR and troubleshoot if and when they malfunction.

End tidal CO_2 (etCO_2)

Waveform capnography is helpful in cardiac arrest and should be measured whenever there is an advanced airway *in situ*.

The role of capnography:

- Ensures correct placement of a tracheal tube in the trachea.
- Allows accurate monitoring of the respiratory rate during CPR which should be a rate of 10 min^{-1} once the airway is secured.
- May assist in identifying ROSC during CPR. An increase in end tidal CO_2 during CPR may indicate ROSC.
- Monitoring the quality of chest compressions. As depth and rate of chest compressions reduce so does etCO_2.

Reversible causes

Potential causes of cardiac arrest for which treatment exists must be considered during any cardiac arrest. For ease of memory, they have been divided into two groups of four known as the '4 Hs and 4 Ts'. → *see Figure 11.3*.

This list of eight conditions should be memorised and run through logically during the cardiac arrest and either excluded or treated.

When running through these causes in a cardiac arrest, try to start with the most likely causes first given the clinical scenario. This way therapy can be initiated in a timely fashion. (e.g. if someone has just collapsed after choking on a sausage don't start with toxins and end on hypoxia!)

- **Hypoxia**: Ensure the patient's lungs are ventilated with 100% oxygen. Confirm that the airway is being managed appropriately. Confirm that oxygen is connected and flowing.
- **Hypovolaemia**: Consider the possibility of an occult bleed (e.g. trauma, gastrointestinal bleeding or leaking

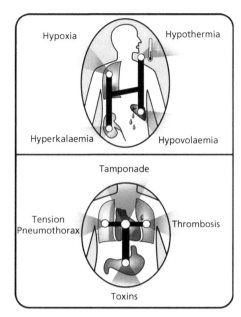

Figure 11.3 '4 Hs and 4 Ts'.

abdominal aneurysm). Obtain IV or IO access rapidly and treat with IV crystalloid or blood coupled with urgent interventions to stop bleeding.
- **Hyper/Hypokalaemia, Hypocalcaemia, Profound Hypoglycaemia**: These can be rapidly diagnosed by a point of care venous blood gas or suggested by the patient's medical history and ECG features.
- **Hypothermia**: This should be ruled out in any drowning, or a patient found in the cold. Do not rely on a tympanic thermometer if hypothermia is suspected – use a rectal or oesophageal probe.
- **Thrombus**: Consider acute coronary syndrome (ACS). If the history/ECG suggests ST elevation myocardial infarction, some systems have the capability for coronary angiography and stenting during CPR or after extracorporeal membrane oxygenation (ECMO) has been initiated, although this is uncommon.
Massive PE is another thrombotic reversible cause of cardiac arrest. If this is suspected, thrombolysis should be initiated and CPR should be continued for 60–90 min before termination of resuscitation efforts. This is another group of patients who could benefit potentially from extracorporeal CPR.
- **Tension pneumothorax:** The diagnosis may be suggested by the history (e.g. a patient with asthma or COPD with sudden onset shortness of breath and chest pain) and confirmed by examination or ultrasound. This should be decompressed immediately by needle or surgical thoracocentesis followed by chest drain.

- **Cardiac tamponade**: This is difficult to diagnose clinically during cardiac arrest but may be indicated by the history (penetrating chest injury, mediastinal malignancy and collapse after cardiac surgery). Point of care ultrasound (POCUS) can give a definitive answer. In the case of penetrating chest injury or collapse after surgery, resuscitative thoracotomy should be considered (*Chapter 6 → p. 83*). In the case of a medical cause of cardiac tamponade needle pericardiocentesis plus a fluid bolus may be sufficient to achieve return of spontaneous circulation (ROSC).
- **Toxins**: this is referring to poisoning. Collateral history is key in this circumstance. Consider the possibility of an intentional or accidental overdose, or exposure to environmental toxins. Where available appropriate antidotes or supportive therapy should be initiated. Prolonged resuscitation with a mechanical chest compression device or ECPR should be considered in this cohort as good outcomes are sometimes achieved after long periods of cardiac arrest. (*Chapter 15 Poisoning*)

Drugs used during CPR

Adrenaline

Adrenaline is a potent alpha- and beta-adrenergic agonist with a short half-life causing potent systemic vasoconstriction. The beta effects cause increased cardiac inotropy and chronotropy and therefore may increase cerebral and myocardial blood flow. However, there is evidence that suggest that it also increases increased oxygen consumption, may cause or exacerbate ventricular arrythmias, may cause transient hypoxaemia due to pulmonary arteriovenous shunting and may impair cerebral microcirculation.

There is good evidence that the use of adrenaline increases ROSC in the short term, but there is a lack of evidence of improved survival to hospital discharge.

Dosing
Shockable rhythm: 1 mg (10 mL of 1:10 000) IV Given after the third shock, repeated every 3–5 min.
Non-Shockable rhythm: 1 mg (10 mL of 1:10 000) IV Given as soon as IV access obtained, repeated every 3–5 min.

Amiodarone

Amiodarone is a membrane stabilising class III anti-arrhythmic drug.

It prolongs cardiac action potential and delaying refractory period. It delays K^+ efflux and depresses Na^+ and Ca^+ influx. It also has a negative inotropic and vasodilating effect due to partial antagonism of alpha and beta receptors.

Dosing
Shockable rhythm: 300 mg bolus IV given after the third shock. A second dose of 150 mg IV may be given if VF/VT persists after the fifth defibrillation.
Non-shockable rhythm: Not indicated

Calcium

Calcium plays a vital role in the cellular mechanisms underlying cardiac contraction. However, high concentrations may be harmful to ischaemic myocardium and brain parenchyma.

Dosing
Calcium is indicated if there is a PEA caused by hypocalcaemia, hyperkalaemia or if the patient has been poisoned with calcium channel-blocking drugs.
The dose is 10 mL of 10% Ca chloride or 30 mL of Ca gluconate which may be repeated if necessary.

Lidocaine

Lidocaine reduces ventricular automaticity and ectopic activity and increases the threshold for the development of VF. However, it also causes an increase in the energy required for defibrillation and the incidence of post-shock asystole. In addition, it is negatively inotropic. For these reasons, it is not routinely used for refractory VF/VT unless amiodarone is unavailable. The initial IV/IO dose for both adults and children is 1.0-1.5 mg/kg to a maximum total dose of 3 mg/kg in the first hour. Lidocaine and amiodarone should not be used together.

Magnesium

Magnesium is an important intracellular cation and co-factor. It facilitates neurochemical transmission. Indications for administration include polymorphic VT (torsade de pointes), digoxin toxicity, correction of hypomagnesemia especially is associated with arrythmias.

The usual dose of magnesium sulphate is 8 mmol (2 g or 4 mL of a 50% solution).

Further information about magnesium → *Box 11.7 on page 261*

Sodium bicarbonate

Cardiac arrest may lead to severe acidosis because of increased anaerobic metabolism and cessation of pulmonary gas exchange. Buffering acidosis with sodium bicarbonate is intuitive; therefore, it had been recommended as a first-line treatment for CPR. However, the best treatment for acidaemia in cardiac arrest is high-quality chest compressions and ventilation of the patient. Bicarbonate causes the generation of carbon dioxide, which diffuses into cells which may have the following effects:

- worsening intracellular acidosis
- negative inotropy
- left shift in the oxygen dissociation curve.

Dosing

Sodium Bicarbonate is indicated in cardiac arrest associated with:

- hyperkalaemia
- poisoning from sodium channel-blocking drugs (e.g. tricyclic antidepressants and propranolol).

1–2 mmol/kg. (50 mL of an 8.4% solution = 50 mmol)

Fluids

Infuse fluids rapidly if hypovolaemia is suspected. 0.9% sodium chloride or Hartmann's solution or blood products if major haemorrhage is suspected.

Fibrinolytics

These should be considered where the cardiac arrest is thought to be secondary to a massive pulmonary embolus. Alteplase or Tenecteplase may be used. The dosing of Alteplase in cardiac arrest is 50 mg IV bolus followed by 50 mg infusion.

CPR should be continued for 60–90 min.

Extracorporeal CPR (ECPR)

ECPR is a procedure in which ECMO is initiated emergently to restore tissue perfusion on patients who have had cardiac arrest. It has the potential to buy time allowing the treatment of a reversible cause of the initial cardiac arrest (e.g. coronary angiography and percutaneous coronary intervention [PCI], pulmonary thrombectomy for massive pulmonary embolism, rewarming after hypothermic cardiac arrest). To be effective, ECMO must be delivered soon after cardiac arrest (ideally <1 hour) in a selective group of patients. ECPR requires a highly skilled multidisciplinary team and costly equipment to both initiate and continue the therapy. Availability is therefore limited.

Ultrasound during CPR

POCUS is a well-established practice in emergency medicine and a core skill for emergency physicians. Focused echocardiography can be used during cardiac arrest and fits in the ALS algorithm during the pulse check. A designated sonographer can perform a rapid assessment and obtain information which can point to reversible pathology.

Echo in life support (ELS) is one of the competences to be obtained during specialty training in emergency medicine in the UK. This consists of a focused approach to echocardiography in the patient in arrest or peri arrest, not including the complex measurements and calculations of true echocardiography and instead seeking the answers to a few very specific questions.

There are doubts about the reliability of central pulse check during cardiac arrest, which makes the use of ELS vital. During resuscitation, access to parasternal area for image acquisition is problematic, there may be defibrillator pads and if using mechanical compression devices, it can be completely inaccessible. In this situation, a subxiphoid approach is preferred, and, if the view is unattainable (due to hyperinflation of stomach during bag mask ventilation, for example), an apical four chambers view can usually be obtained. It is important that ELS does not result in prolonged pauses in chest compressions. Probe positioning and acquisition of images during the pulse check should cause a pause of no more than 10 seconds. A video clip of the entire compression-free period can then be obtained for detailed review, while chest compressions are restarted.

There have been several proposed protocols for evaluation of the heart during cardiac arrest (FEEL, CAUSE, CASA and ShOC), some of them including peri-arrest period, some focussing on non-shockable rhythms only, but they all try to answer the same few questions:

1 Is the heart beating?
   - Cardiac standstill, also known as true asystole, is defined as the complete absence of any cardiac motion, including the ventricles, atria and valves.
   - Patients recognised to have standstill with concomitant electrical activity on the monitor are often described to have true PEA.
   - Pseudo-PEA is the presence of ventricular contractility visualised by ultrasound with electrical activity but no palpable pulse.

   This classification is important for prognostication, and the absence of coordinated cardiac activity proves to be an excellent predictor of failure to regain spontaneous circulation (negative predictive value 97%) with only a 0.6% survival to hospital discharge.

2 Is there a pericardial effusion causing tamponade (right ventricle collapse)?

3 Is there evidence of right ventricular strain?
   Right ventricle and atrium dilatation, 'D-sign' in parasternal short axis, paradoxical septum movement in diastole (indenting left ventricle) are all signs of right heart strain. Although these signs present an important prognostic role in the stable

patient with a pulmonary embolism, they have, in isolation, a weak positive predictive value for PE related cardiac arrest. All these signs can be found in hypovolaemia, hyperkalaemia, primary arrhythmias, pre-exiting chronic right ventricular strain and late into resuscitation of cardiac arrest of any other cause. Assessment of pre-arrest signs and symptoms (if known) and intra-arrest compression tests of femoral and popliteal veins (to confirm DVT) have been suggested in patients considered at high risk of pulmonary embolism.

4 Other non-cardiac structures to assess during cardiac arrest
- Pleural space for the presence of tension pneumothorax or a large amount of fluid to suggest haemorrhage/pleural effusion.
- Peritoneal space for the presence of free fluid to suggest haemorrhage/ascites.
- Abdominal aorta for the presence of ruptured aneurysm.
- Inferior vena cava (IVC) for intravascular fluid status (bearing in mind that IVC dilatation can happen due to increased intrathoracic pressure during mechanical ventilation and not due to volume overload).

If a return to spontaneous circulation ROSC is obtained, a more thorough ultrasound examination can be performed, including echo looking for regional wall motion abnormalities, evaluation of left ventricular function and lung ultrasound for cardiac failure and to guide resuscitation/post-arrest care.

There are several protocols for ultrasound assessment of the shocked (peri-arrest) patient, focussing on diagnosis of type of shock, possible causes and treatment options (→ see p. 250.)

Cardiac arrest in special circumstances

ALS requires tailoring in certain clinical contexts, these are known as 'special circumstances'. Here we will list these circumstances and the additional management required during cardiac arrest or in the peri-arrest patient.

1 Life-threatening electrolyte disorders
2 Poisoning
3 Asthma
4 Anaphylaxis
5 Pregnancy
6 Traumatic cardiac arrest
7 Drowning
8 Hypothermia.

Life-threatening electrolyte disorders

Potassium: Hyperkalaemia must always be excluded in patients with an arrythmia or cardiac arrest. Most patients will have ECG abnormalities if their potassium is >6.7 mmol/L. The effect of hyperkalaemia on cardiac conduction depends not only on the level of potassium but also the rate of increase. In the context of cardiac arrest secondary to hyperkalaemia, the potassium level is likely to be well over 6.5 and is usually associated with acute kidney injury. Cardiac arrest as a result of hyperkalaemia may occur with any presenting rhythm (PEA, VF, VT and asystole).

ALS needs to be modified with the following four steps in the context of hyperkalaemia:

1 Protect the heart: 10 mL 10% calcium chloride IV bolus – may be repeated.
2 Shift potassium into cells: 10 units short-acting insulin (e.g. actrapid) with 100 mL 20% glucose IV.
3 Give 50 mL 8.4% sodium bicarbonate IV if associated acidosis.
4 Remove potassium form the body. Consider dialysis if the above treatments are ineffective. The patient may need ECMO before dialysis can be attempted.

Hypokalaemia must always be excluded in patients with an arrythmia or cardiac arrest. Cardiac arrest as a result of hypokalaemia may occur with any presenting rhythm (PEA, VF, VT and asystole).

Many patients who are potassium deficient are also deficient in magnesium which is less easy to measure at the bedside. Magnesium is important for potassium uptake and for the maintenance of intracellular potassium levels. Therefore, replacement of magnesium is recommended alongside replacement of potassium in severe hypokalaemia.

In general terms, potassium should be replaced slowly (max 20 mmol/hr) but in an adult arrest/peri arrest situation it can be replaced at 20 mmol over 10 min followed by 10 mmol over 5–10 min with cardiac monitoring attached and via a central venous access if available.

Hypoglycaemia: may cause seizures and coma but is unlikely to cause cardiac arrest. However, it should always be checked in cardiac arrest and treated where it is found to be below 4 mmol/L.

Calcium: Hypercalcaemia causing ECG abnormality such as short QT/heart block/cardiac arrest should be treated with IV crystalloid.

Hypocalcaemia causing ECG abnormality such as short QT/heart block/cardiac arrest should be treated with 10–40 mL of 10% IV calcium chloride and 2 g magnesium sulphate IV.

Magnesium: Severe hypermagnesemia (>1.75 mmol/L) is usually iatrogenic (in the context of the large doses of magnesium given for, e.g. eclampsia). It causes muscle weakness, respiratory depression heart block and cardiac arrest. In addition to standard ALS 10 mL of 10% IV calcium chloride, saline diuresis and ECPR or haemodialysis should be considered.

Hypomagnesaemia (<0.6) may be associated with torsade de pointes and seizures. It should be treated with 2 g magnesium sulphate over 1–2 min in an emergency situation.

Poisoning

Poisoning remains a leading cause of cardiac arrest and coma in those under the age of 40. Intentional self-poisoning by recreational or therapeutic drugs is by far the commonest cause in the adult population but in the paediatric population the overdose is usually accidental. In the elderly patient consider drug toxicity caused by drug interaction, inappropriate dosing or deteriorating renal or liver function. Homicidal poisoning is uncommon.

The standard BLS and ALS principles and management apply to the poisoned patient with two caveats:

- Prolonged resuscitation and ECPR should be considered to 'buy time' to allow specific therapy to act or the effect of the toxin to 'wear off'.
- Amiodarone should be avoided in arrythmia secondary to poisoning by tricyclic anti-depressants and propranolol as the mechanism of toxicity in these circumstances is sodium channel blockade which will be exacerbated by the amiodarone.

Specific therapies for opiate, benzodiazepine, tricyclic antidepressant and stimulant overdose are covered in the toxicology chapter. *Chapter 15*

Asthma

Management of asthma → Chapter 13 pp. 213 and 351

Cardiac arrest secondary to asthma may be a terminal event as a result of hypoxaemia or may be a sudden event resulting from arrythmia. Underlying causes are:

- Severe bronchospasm and mucus plugging causing respiratory failure.
- Cardiac arrythmias caused by hypoxia and acidosis, stimulant drugs (such as aminophylline) or electrolyte abnormalities (particularly hypokalaemia).
- 'Breath Stacking' in the mechanically ventilated patient. A phenomenon caused by less air exiting the lungs than entering. This results in raised intrathoracic pressure which causes reduced venous return and eventually cardiovascular collapse. It is treated by disconnecting the patient from the ventilator and physically compressing the chest to allow exhalation.

- Tension pneumothorax (which may be bilateral). This needs to be actively excluded and, if in doubt, treated with needle and/or surgical thoracotomies.

Anaphylaxis

Anaphylaxis → p. 306

Adrenaline is the most important drug for the treatment of anaphylaxis. It suppresses histamine and leukotriene release. As an alpha receptor agonist, it reverses vasodilation and reduces oedema. It's beta agonist properties reverse bronchial constriction and increase myocardial contractility.

Occasionally, patients may succumb to the effects or anaphylaxis before adequate adrenaline is given and consequently sustain a cardiac arrest. If this occurs, CPR should be immediately commenced and 1 mg of IV (or IO) adrenaline should be administered.

Patients may have an extremely swollen airway making effective oxygenation and ventilation very challenging. Facemask ventilation and the use of supraglottic devises may be difficult or impossible. Involve a senior anaesthetist to manage the airway and if unsuccessful a surgical airway should be performed.

The collapsed anaphylactic patient is likely to be relatively intravascularly deplete and should be given a bolus of 500–1000 mL of IV or IO crystalloid.

Pregnancy

Cardiac arrest in pregnancy is rare occurring in 1 in 30 000 pregnancies. However, when it does occur, it is important for a clinician and the emergency department (ED) to be prepared.

Although the primary focus should be on the mother, it should not be forgotten that there is another potential life at stake. Resuscitation of the mother is performed in the same manner as in any other patient, except for a few adjustments.

- **Immediately get help:** ideally your team should include an anaesthetist, obstetrician and neonatologist.
- **Manually displace the uterus to the left**: After approximately 20 weeks gestation, the uterus is palpable at the level of the umbilicus and will press on the IVC impeding venous return and reducing the effectiveness of CPR and cardiac output. Displacement to the left improves venous return and therefore the effect of CPR.
- **Early tracheal intubation** is important as there is an increased risk of aspiration of gastric contents, increased oxygen demand of the pregnant patient, reduced functional residual capacity and functional residual volume are decreased resulting in hypoxia occurring rapidly after collapse.

- If the uterus is palpable above the umbilicus or the patient is known to have a gestational age above 20 weeks; prepare for resuscitative hysterotomy at the point of collapse as outcomes for both mother and child are time dependent. Ideally, the foetus should be delivered within 5 min of maternal arrest. The primary aim of resuscitative hysterotomy is to optimise resuscitation and survival of the mother; however, if delivery occurs rapidly and the infant is of a viable gestation, survival is a realistic possibility. *Resuscitative hysterotomy → Box 11.1*
- If the gestational age is 24 weeks or more, a team will need to be allocated to receive and attempt resuscitation of the foetus.
- The cause of cardiac arrest in pregnancy is the same as any female of childbearing age (e.g. trauma, poisoning and cardiovascular disease), in addition to this there are also obstetric related causes (haemorrhage, pulmonary embolism, eclampsia, sepsis, peripartum cardiomyopathy, anaesthetic complications and amniotic fluid embolism). These conditions are managed in the same way as the non-pregnant patient with the additional consideration of:
  - **Haemorrhage**: This may be antenatal or postnatal. Ectopic pregnancy, placental abruption, placenta praevia, placental increta, uterine rupture or postpartum haemorrhage caused by the '4Ts':
    Tone – uterine atony.
    Trauma – lacerations of the uterus, cervix or vagina.
    Tissue – retained placenta or clots.
    Thrombin – pre-existing or acquired coagulopathy.
    Tx Rapid fluid followed by balanced blood product resuscitation. Administer tranexamic acid. In postpartum, haemorrhage give oxytocin, ergometrine and prostaglandins. Perform uterine massage and bimanual compression of the uterus.
  - **Eclampsia**: Eclampsia is not a common cause of cardiac arrest but does cause cerebral agitation and seizures. It is treated with by managing the hypertension and an IV magnesium infusion. Magnesium overdose can occur, and in severe case, it can result in areflexia and cardiovascular collapse. (*hypermagnesemia → earlier*)
  - **Pulmonary embolism (PE)**: PE causes approximately 20% of maternal deaths. The use of fibrinolytic therapy needs considerable thought, particularly if a resuscitative hysterotomy will be performed. On balance, if the patient is in cardiac arrest, benefit of thrombolysis probably outweighs the risk.
  - **Amniotic fluid embolism**: Amniotic fluid embolus usually occurs immediately following delivery, though it can complicate pregnancy at any time. It is not a common complication but is associated with a high mortality. It is actually an anaphylactoid

---

 Box 11.1 **Resuscitative hysterotomy**

Prepare two resuscitation areas and three teams: two for the mother and one for the neonate.

- team to continue high-quality ALS
- team to perform procedure
- team to receive and manage resuscitation of neonate.

Call obstetrics and paediatrics/NICU for assistance early.

The indications for perimortem c-section are maternal cardiac arrest with gravid uterus above the umbilicus or known to be >20 weeks gestational age.

- Clean the skin
- Make a vertical incision from umbilicus to symphysis pubis (skin to peritoneum)
- Make a hole in the peritoneum just below the umbilicus with fingers and extend this with scissors
- Retract the urinary bladder inferiorly to avoid injury
- Make a small incision in the uterine fundus and extend this incision with scissors
- Deliver baby may need fundal pressure
- Clamp the cord with two clamps and cut between clamps
- Hand baby to designated team
- Deliver the placenta if possible with gentle cord traction – if it does not separate easily, leave in situ and await obstetric assistance
- Pack the uterus with sterile swabs pending the arrival of obstetric assistance.

---

reaction and not a true embolic event. When foreign debris from the amniotic fluid enters the maternal circulation, a systemic inflammatory response is initiated. Treatment is supportive based on ABCDE approach and correction of coagulopathy.

Traumatic cardiac arrest (TCA)

Traumatic cardiac arrest has a very high mortality, but when ROSC can be achieved, neurological outcome appears to be much better than in other causes of arrest. The history and scene may provide clues as to the cause of arrest. For example, a medical event (such as cardiac arrythmia/seizure) may cause a secondary traumatic event (e.g. road traffic accident). In these cases, traumatic injuries may not be the cause of arrest and so standard ALS with CPR and defibrillation are appropriate.

Commotio cordis is actual or near cardiac arrest caused by a blunt impact to the precordium resulting in ventricular fibrillation. It usually occurs during sport, most commonly baseball. Early defibrillation is essential.

Impact brain apnoea is frequently anecdotally witnessed in the pre-hospital arena following head injury. It is characterised by the cessation of spontaneous breathing following a blunt head injury. It is commonly accompanied by a catecholamine surge witnessed as hypertension followed by cardiovascular collapse. It is treated with simple airway manoeuvres and bag-mask ventilation and patients may go from being apnoeic and lifeless to alert and breathing in a few minutes.

The approach to a patient in traumatic cardiac arrest is similar to that of a medical arrest but the list of reversible causes in traumatic arrest is considerably shorter than the 4Hs and 4Ts of a medical arrest. → *Box 11.2 Reversible causes of cardiac arrest*

Chest compressions are still relevant in traumatic cardiac arrest but in circumstances where the cardiac arrest is due to hypovolaemia (in which case the patient may be in a 'low flow' state rather than true cardiac arrest) and where the patient has a cardiac tamponade or tension pneumothorax then chest compressions have a lower priority than the reversal of these pathologies (with thoracostomy, thoracotomy, haemorrhage control and transfusion)

Hypovolaemia

Uncontrolled haemorrhage is a common cause of TCA. At the same time as attempting to stop the haemorrhage, IV access should be obtained, tranexamic acid, warmed balanced blood transfusion (or if not possible warmed crystalloid) initiated and 10 mL of 10% calcium chloride should be administered.

Treat compressible external haemorrhage in a stepwise manner: direct pressure, topical haemostatic agents plus pressure dressings, large deep sutures where possible (e.g. scalp wounds), tourniquets. The tourniquet

Box 11.2 Reversible causes of traumatic cardiac arrest

- Hypovolaemia (major haemorrhage)
- Hypoxia
- Tension pneumothorax
- Cardiac tamponade.

should be applied as distally as possible and clearly marked with time of application.

Noncompressible haemorrhage is more difficult to treat: Broken limbs should be put in anatomical position and splinted. A pelvic binder should be applied (*Chapter 2 → P. 26*). Surgical control of bleeding (thoracotomy with compression of the descending aorta) or intravascular occlusion of the descending aorta (REBOA) should be considered.

Gaining IV access in TCA can be a challenge. If large bore peripheral IV access attempts fail after two attempts move to IO access, ideally in the humeral head as higher flow rates can be achieved and there is less chance of vascular disruption causing loss of precious volume into the extravascular space. If your team has the skills, a large bore central venous catheter can be placed to enable large volumes to be given rapidly.

Oxygen (Hypoxia)

Effective airway management is essential to maintain oxygenation and ventilation of the severely compromised trauma patient. Management with a supraglottic device such as i-gel is often an effective first step and can be upgraded to an endotracheal tube when clinicians with the correct skillset arrive.

In low cardiac output states, positive pressure ventilation causes further circulatory depression by impeding venous return to the heart. In cardiac arrest, it is important to aim for tidal volumes of 6 mL/kg and a respiratory rate of about 10 breaths/min.

Tension pneumothorax

13% of patients with traumatic arrest have a tension pneumothorax. Consequently, any patient in traumatic cardiac arrest should be presumed to have a tension pneumothorax until proven otherwise by decompression of the chest. *Tension pneumothorax Chapter 6 → p. 77*

Cardiac tamponade

In the context of trauma, cardiac tamponade occurs most commonly as a result of penetrating trauma (e.g. stabbing) but may also occur after blunt trauma when a broken rib penetrates the pericardium and myocardium.

The treatment of tamponade in a traumatic arrest is resuscitative thoracotomy *Chapter 6 → p. 83*.

Drowning

The approach to a drowning victim alters the start of BLS/ALS. Once arrest is confirmed, five initial ventilations are delivered. This is because most drowning victims will have sustained a cardiac arrest secondary to hypoxia. CPR at the standard adult or child ratios (30:2 or 15:2) should then be commenced.

Massive amounts of foam sometimes come from the airway of drowned patients. This is the result of surfactant mixing with aspirated water. Early intubation should be performed and the patient ventilated on 100% oxygen on a ventilator that can deliver PEEP as this will be required at up to 20 cm H_2O if the patient gets ROSC.

After prolonged immersion, most people will have become hypovolaemic. When the hydrostatic pressure of the water is removed as the victim is rescued, they may decompensate. Ensure that patients are rescued horizontally and give a rapid IV fluid bolus to correct the hypovolaemia.

Drowned victims are commonly hypothermic. Ensure they have a core temperature measured via an oesophageal, rectal or urethral catheter temperature probe.

Hypothermia

Hypothermia is defined as a core temperature of <35 °C and classified as:

Mild: 32–35 °C
Moderate: 28–32 °C
Severe: <28 °C

The following modifications to standard ALS should be made in the hypothermic patient:

- Check for signs of life, palpating a central pulse, for up to 1 min. The clinical assessment can be augmented by ECG monitoring, capnography and echocardiography. If there is any doubt, start chest compressions immediately.
- Consider using a mechanical chest compression device as the resuscitation may be prolonged.
- Do not delay careful tracheal intubation of the severely hypothermic patient, although this can cause ventricular fibrillation the benefit of effective oxygenation and ventilation outweighs the risk.

*Other adaptations in hypothermic cardiac arrest →
Box 11.3*

Cardiac arrest in children

This section is no substitute for doing an Advanced Paediatric Life Support Course where you will be equipped with skills and knowledge of how to prevent and manage paediatric cardiac arrest.

Hypoxia is the commonest cause of cardiac arrest in children, therefore oxygen delivery rather than defibrillation is the priority in paediatric arrest.

*Differences in ABCDE assessment of children Chapter 18
→ p. 342*

 Box 11.3 Adaptations in hypothermic cardiac arrest

Temperature	Drug modification	Defibrillation modification
<30 °C	Do not administer drugs	Defibrillate up to 3 times, if unsuccessful do not defibrillate again until temperature > 30
30–35 °C	Double interval between drug doses	Standard defibrillation regimen
>35 °C	Standard drug dosing	Standard defibrillation regimen

Airway: The children there is:

- Larger occiput. This results in the neck being flexed when a child is lying supine.
- Proportionally larger tongue
- High larynx
- Epiglottis which is long and stiff
- Narrowest portion is the cricoid cartilage (rather than the vocal cords)
- Small diameter of airways results in higher resistance to air flow and increased chance of airway obstruction
- Highly compliant trachea which can easily be obstructed by direct pressure or 'kinking'
- Short trachea which is in line with right bronchus making bronchial intubation much more likely than in an adult.

Consequently correct airway manoeuvring, placement of adjuncts that are sized correctly and involvement of a skilled operator to manage the airway is essential.

Breathing: Hypoxia is commonly the cause of cardiovascular collapse in children. Therefore, chest compression only CPR is discouraged and exhaled air resuscitation or use of high-concentration oxygen and bag-valve-mask should be used.

Paediatric CPR should always start with the delivery of five successful rescue breaths.

Circulation: Once the rescue breaths are given attention should turn to circulation. Failure of circulation is recognised by the absence of 'signs of life' after the initial rescue breaths. The absence of a central pulse or a heart rate of <60 is also an indication to start chest compressions.

> Even experienced healthcare practitioners can find it difficult to detect a pulse in a collapsed child, therefore unless you are certain that you can feel a pulse, start chest compressions.

In children, the chest compression to ventilation ratio is 15:2. Chest compressions should be at a rate of 100–120 per minute compressing one-third of the depth of the patient's chest and allowing full recoil between compressions.

PEA and asystole are the most common rhythms in paediatric cardiac arrest and 0.1 mg/kg adrenaline and a fluid bolus should be administered.

Disability: Babies and children are prone to hypoglycaemia when they are unwell so this should always be checked.

Exposure: Always fully expose critically ill children looking for clues as to the cause of their collapse, e.g. bruising suggesting non-accidental injury.

Post resuscitation care

The return of spontaneous circulation (ROSC) is an important step in the 'Chain of Survival'. The next challenge is to return the patient to a state of normal cerebral and haemodynamic function.

On recognition of ROSC, it is important to document the time, then do an A–E assessment of the patient with the aim of optimising physiology to provide optimal cerebral, myocardial and renal perfusion and assist the clearance of the toxic metabolites released from tissues which were poorly perfused during cardiac arrest.

After a short VF arrest, many patients will immediately return to normal cerebral function and physiology. These patients will not need tracheal intubation or sedation but will instead need a 12-lead ECG and consideration of immediate coronary angiography (see below).

Patients who have had a longer 'down time' are likely to be comatose or cerebrally agitated and will need intubation, ventilation and sedation prior to further investigation and intervention.

- **Airway**: The comatose or agitated patient should be intubated if this did not occur during the cardiac arrest. This facilitates controlled oxygenation and ventilation, protects against aspiration of gastric contents, aids in the control of seizures and temperature management.
- **Breathing**: Check the oxygen saturations, respiratory rate and end tidal CO_2.
  - Examine the chest looking for signs of injury (up to 70% of patients will have rib fractures as a result of CPR), which may cause a pneumothorax, or a flail segment. The endotracheal tube may be in a bronchus rather than trachea and consequently only one lung (usually the right) will be ventilated. Auscultate for crackles, the patient may have aspirated during the arrest or may now be developing pulmonary oedema.
  - An arterial blood gas should be checked. Hypoxaemia and hypercarbia are common after a cardiac arrest, both increase the likelihood of further cardiac arrest and secondary brain injury. Correcting by altering the ventilator settings aiming for a normal arterial pH, CO_2 and oxygen saturations of 94–98%. Also consider the electrolytes; potassium should be maintained between 4.0 and 5.0 mmol/L to reduce the chance of arrythmia and calcium which should be maintained above 1.0 mmol/L.
  - A chest X-ray should be performed to check the position of the ETT tube, lung fields, mediastinal and cardiac contour.
- **Circulation**:
  - Check blood pressure every 3–5 min, ensure ECG monitoring and the defibrillator remains attached as both the cardiac rhythm and cardiovascular status may remain unstable for some time as clearance of the toxic metabolites released from tissues which were poorly perfused during cardiac arrest occurs. Patients may need an adrenaline or noradrenaline infusion for this time period which can be run though a large peripheral vein.
  - If possible, site an arterial catheter to monitor beat to beat blood pressure and allow frequent measurement of arterial blood gasses. Consider placing a central venous catheter to allow safer administration of vasopressor drugs and a urethral catheter to measure urine output.
  - Record a 12-lead ECG as soon as possible. Refer patients with ST elevation or new left bundle branch block (BBB) for urgent PCI (or if this is unavailable within 120 min then consider thrombolysis).
- **Disability**: Check the blood sugar, pupillary responses, GCS and check to see if the patient can move all four limbs.
  - It is worth considering the comatose post cardiac arrest brain in the same way as one that has sustained a traumatic injury – it will swell after this insult. All the neuroprotective measures (*Chapter 3* → *p. 37*) that you would do after traumatic brain injury should be applied now.
  - Pupillary reaction is not a reliable indicator of neurological function following cardiac arrest (especially when adrenaline and/or atropine have been administered) and should not be used for prognostication in the first 24 hours.
- **Exposure**: Fully expose the patient looking for clues as to the cause of the arrest (e.g. evidence of injury or a

purpuric rash). Check the patient's temperature and start invasive temperature measurement using either an oesophageal or rectal catheter probe and initiate 'targeted temperature management' aiming for a temperature of 34–36 °C.

- Obtain collateral history from bystanders/friends/family and update them of the situation. If a patient's identity is unknown, the police can be called upon to help seek the next of kin.

Unless the cause of arrest is obvious, every patient should have an ED ultrasound, using the RUSH protocol or similar, which may demonstrate evidence of pulmonary embolus, hypovolaemia, cardiac tamponade and abdominal aortic aneurysm.

In addition to the RUSH ultrasound consider:

- Could this be cardiac? Get an ECG, echocardiogram and cardiology opinion.
- Could this be neurological? (e.g. subarachnoid haemorrhage) get a CT brain.
- Could this be vascular? (e.g. aortic dissection) Do a CT aortogram.
- Could this be a PE? Do a CT pulmonary angiogram.

Finally, ensure your documentation is up to date before transferring the patient to definitive or intensive care.

Unsuccessful resuscitation

Predicting the outcome from cardiac arrest is complex. There is no single prognostic factor or scoring system which is reliable.

The team leader must decide when it is appropriate to abandon attempts at resuscitation. This will require consideration of:

- The history of the current collapse and resuscitation
- Whether bystander CPR was performed
- The initial and subsequent rhythms
- The total time of cardiac arrest
- The clinical and ECG findings
- The patient's past medical history and functional status
- A point of care ultrasound
- A venous or arterial blood gas result
- The views of the other team members, including paramedics.

The team must also consider and attempt to reverse all reversible causes (4Hs and 4Ts) of arrest where relevant. These factors are combined to make a decision of potential survivability. Recovery is very unlikely in asystole that does not respond to 20 min of ALS. The British ambulance service uses 20 min of asystole as a criteria for 'Recognition of Life Extinct' (ROLE).

After a successful or unsuccessful resuscitation, a short debrief is valuable. Debriefing can include both clinical and emotional aspects and feedback from the relatives.

After some resuscitations, in particular those that are unsuccessful, staff may be distressed and in need of either formal or informal support. Everyone in the team should be aware of this and offered a referral to TRiM (trauma risk management) which should be made available in frontline healthcare organisations. It is a peer support system designed to help people who have experienced a traumatic, or potentially traumatic, event. After this initial assessment, the TRiM practitioner may be able to simply reassure and safety net the staff member or, with consent of the staff member, involve occupational health, the psychology team or chaplains.

Brain – stem death → p. 405.
Notification of death to the coroner → p. 404.

Care of suddenly bereaved individuals

The care of bereaved friends and family is as important as any other care delivered in the ED.

Death of a patient from a cardiac arrest in the emergency department is often sudden and commonly unexpected by the next of kin who may be ill prepared for it. Certain principles of care may make this terrible experience more bearable:

- Friends and family should be contacted promptly and dealt with as soon as they arrive at the ED. A designated (named) nurse should act as a liaison with the rest of the medical and nursing team. In an ongoing resuscitation, this nurse must make every effort to obtain up-to-date information for the relatives.
- Special facilities should be available for bereaved relatives, including a quiet, private room with a telephone, access to drinks and a toilet. The offer of making a cup of tea or coffee demonstrates compassion and is often very helpful for families in turmoil
- Arrangements must be made for relatives to get home safely and for care for those who are alone.
- When bad news is broken, it should be imparted gently and honestly, avoiding euphemism and over-involved medical explanations.

The family can be left to assimilate the news but should have another opportunity to ask further questions later on. Although the medical staff must be involved in the contact with the relatives, the breaking of bad news can be undertaken by any experienced member of the team.

- Both verbal and written information must be provided for the relatives concerning:
  - what to do next
  - coroner's procedures and the possibility of a post-mortem examination
  - helpful telephone numbers
  - a named contact in the ED or bereavement office with a phone number
  - details about any follow-up by a nurse or counsellor specialising in bereavement care.
- Other agencies must be informed of the death:
  In the hospital:
  - the IMEG (Independent Medical Examiners Group) must be informed of all NHS hospital deaths. They will scrutinise the medical record and discuss the case with the clinician involved. Their primary role is to ensure the organisation identifies and learns from avoidable deaths, but they also help clinicians decide what should be written on the death certificate and who should be referred to the coroner.
  - the medical records department
  In the community:
  - the deceased patient's GP
  - the police and social services need to be informed if there is an unexpected death of a child or violent death.

In most emergency departments, there is a bereavement checklist to ensure that all the above is performed.

Referring a Death to the Coroner→ Chapter 20 → p. 404

CARDIAC DYSRHYTHMIAS

This Section covers:

- General principles
- Bradyarrhythmias
- Tachyarrhythmias
- BBBs/Fascicular blocks/Pacemaker identification.

General principles

The treatment of all cardiac dysrhythmias should include:

- A structured ABCDE approach to the patient (→*Chapter 1*)
- Identification of adverse features:
  - **Shock:** (hypotension systolic BP < 90), pallor, sweating, cold extremities, thready or absence of peripheral pulse.
  - **Syncope**: Transient loss of consciousness (TLOC) because of transient loss of cerebral perfusion.

- **Heart failure** – Pulmonary oedema and/or raised JVP (distended liver in the infant).
- **Myocardial ischaemia:** Ischaemic pain or ECG changes consistent with ischaemia.

Extremes of heart rate – In addition to the above adverse features, it may be appropriate to consider extremes in heart rate as life-threatening features in themselves. However, this must be taken in context of the patient. Young fit patients can easily tolerate very high and very low heart rates whereas those with heart disease cannot:

Extreme tachycardia (above 150) results in reduced coronary blood flow as this occurs in diastole. Tachycardias are less well tolerated in the elderly and those with ischaemic or structural heart disease.

Extreme bradycardia (below 40) Patients with heart disease may not be able to compensate for the bradycardia by increasing stroke volume.

In an unstable patient, it is important to concentrate on early treatment to prevent deterioration rather than on prolonged attempts to identify a precise rhythm.

Treatment options depend on the clinical condition of the patient and the nature of the arrythmia. They are one of:

1. No treatment needed
2. Simple clinical intervention (e.g. vagal manoeuvres)
3. Pharmacological (drug treatment)
4. Electrical (cardioversion or pacing).

Bradyarrhythmias

Bradycardia is defined as a heart rate <60.

This may be physiologically normal for athletes/during sleep or may be an expected result of treatment with a beta or calcium channel blocker.

Pathological bradycardia may be caused by a conduction problem: malfunction of the SA node or from partial or complete failure of atrioventricular conduction. It is also worth noting that vagal stimulation causes bradycardia and occasionally syncope and that bradycardia may also be a peri-arrest finding secondary to hypoxia or hypovolaemia, particularly in children.

First-degree heart block

The PR interval is the time between the onset of the P wave at the sinoatrial node and the start of the QRS complex. It therefore represents a delay in conduction through the AV node and/or the bundle of His. First-degree heart block is defined as a PR interval > 200 ms (five small squares) and 'Marked first-degree heart block' is present if PR interval > 300 ms.

Causes of first-degree heart block include: Increased vagal tone, athletic training, inferior myocardial infarction, mitral valve surgery, myocarditis (e.g. Lyme disease), electrolyte disturbances (e.g. hyperkalaemia) and AV nodal blocking drugs (beta-blockers, calcium channel blockers, digoxin and amiodarone).

First-degree heart block may be a normal variant. It is usually an isolated finding that does not cause haemodynamic instability and rarely requires specific treatment.

Second-degree heart block

Second-degree heart block is present when some, but not all, P waves are conducted to the ventricles, resulting in the absence of a QRS complex after some of the P waves. There are three variations:

1 **Mobitz type 1 AV block**: (also called Wenckebach phenomenon)
   There is progressive lengthening of the P-R interval, then a failure of conduction. This is followed by a conducted beat with a normal P-R interval, then the lengthening process starts again. Its many causes include acute myocardial infarction (often inferior). If asymptomatic, this rhythm does not usually require immediate treatment. The need of treatment is dictated by the effect of the associate bradycardia on the patient and the risk of developing a more severe block or asystole (which is low unless the underlying cause is an acute myocardial infarct).
2 **Mobitz type 2 block**: the majority of beats are conducted with a constant P-R interval, but occasionally a P wave is not followed by a QRS complex 'a dropped beat'. People with a Mobitz type 2 block have a significant risk of developing a more severe block or asystole so should be closely monitored until a pacemaker is sited.
3 **Fixed second-degree**: (2:1 or 3:1) block: there are intermittent conducted and non-conducted atrial beats giving a ratio of P waves to QRS complexes of 2:1 or 3:1. This is usually a Mobitz type 2 block. Immediate

treatment decisions are determined by the effect of the associated bradycardia on the patient. The patient should be closely monitored whilst awaiting a pacemaker as there is a risk of third-degree heart block and asystole.

Third-degree heart block

Third-degree heart block is the impairment of conduction of electrical impulses from the atria to the ventricles (also known as 'complete heart block') → *see Figure 11.4*. There is no relationship between P waves and QRS complexes because atrial and ventricular depolarisation arises independently from separate 'pacemakers'.

A 'pacemaker' site in the distal His-Purkinge fibres or ventricular myocardium will produce broad QRS complexes with a rate of 30–40/min and is more likely to stop abruptly resulting in asystole. Less commonly there is narrow complex junctional escape rhythm. In this case, the 'pacemaker' is in the AV node or proximal bundle of His. This may result in a heart rate that is both adequate and regular and less likely to degenerate into asystole.

Complete heart block is usually a result of:

- Myocardial ischaemia
- Poisoning (including digitalis)
- Chronic heart diseases, especially aortic stenosis and congenital lesions
- Some acute infectious diseases, including rheumatic fever
- Complete heart block is commonly associated with an inferior infarction, it results from occlusion of the right coronary artery; the AV nodal artery is one of its branches.

Patients with complete heart block are often symptomatic as a result of their bradycardia and usually require immediate medical therapy as per the ALS bradycardia algorithm (→ *Figure 11.5*). They have a significant risk of asystole so should always be referred to a cardiologist for assessment and pacing.

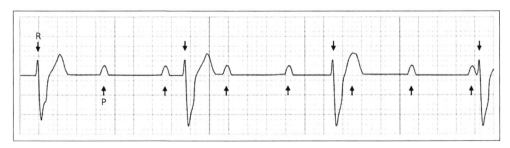

Figure 11.4 Complete heart block.

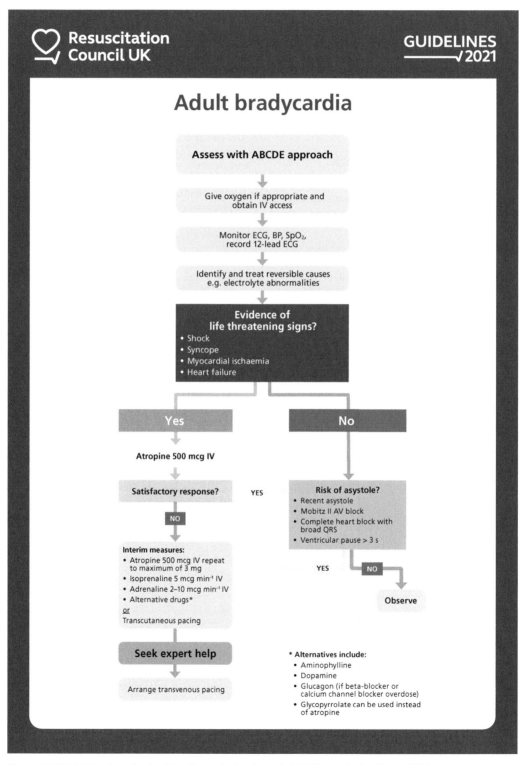

Figure 11.5 Adult bradycardia algorithm. Resuscitation Council, 2021/Resuscitation Council (UK).

Bradycardia in children

In paediatric practice, bradycardia is almost always a pre-terminal finding in patients with respiratory or circulatory insufficiency. ABC should always be assessed and treated before pharmacological or electrical management of the bradycardia is considered.

If there is hypoxia and signs of shock treat with:

- High concentration oxygen and effective ventilation. This may mean that bag valve mask ventilation or intubation and ventilation are required.
- If the above is ineffective slowly titrate adrenaline 10mcg/kg IV and then consider an adrenaline infusion.

If there has been vagal stimulation (e.g. suctioning the airway)

- Treat with adequate oxygenation and ventilation
- Give atropine 20mcg/kg (min dose 100mcg, max dose 600mcg)
- Atropine may be repeated at 5 min up to a max dose of 1 mg in a child and 2 mg in an adolescent.

If there has been poisoning seek expert help.

Agonal rhythm

Agonal rhythm occurs in dying patients it is slow and may be irregular both in morphology and rate. It is broad complex and does not usually generate a palpable pulse. An agonal rhythm is usually seen during the later stages of an unsuccessful resuscitation attempt and usually slows and degenerates into asystole. *Agonal rhythm → Figure 11.6*

Tachyarrhythmias

A pathological tachycardia may arise from atrial myocardium (atrial tachycardia/atrial fibrillation/atrial flutter), the AV junction (AVNRT/accelerated junctional tachycardia), the bundle of His or the ventricular myocardium (VT). When the tachycardia arises from above the bifurcation of the Bundle of His, it is 'supraventricular.'

QRS complexes will be narrow if ventricular depolarisation occurs normally, but will be broad if there is a BBB or if the electrical activity is transmitted through the ventricles themselves rather than the conducting system.

Sinus tachycardia is not an arrythmia. It is a response to a physiological, psychological or pathological stress (e.g. exercise, stress, blood loss, pain, etc.)

Tachyarrythmias can be divided into:

- Narrow complex tachycardias
- Broad complex tachycardias.

> Haemodynamic disturbance accompanying tachycardia often suggests a ventricular origin for the dysrhythmia but does not exclude a supraventricular cause.

Narrow complex tachycardia

This results from a supraventricular tachycardia with normal conduction to the ventricles. The rhythm may be irregular (atrial fibrillation or atrial flutter with variable block) or regular (atrial tachycardia, accelerated junctional rhythm (AJR) or SVT).

Narrow complex tachycardias are tolerated well by most patients, but if the rate is very fast or if there is underlying heart disease there may be decompensation.

> The human body responds to many different forms of illness with a tachycardia. If a patient has chronic AF, then he or she will develop fast AF rather than a sinus tachycardia in the context of fever, pain or intercurrent illness.

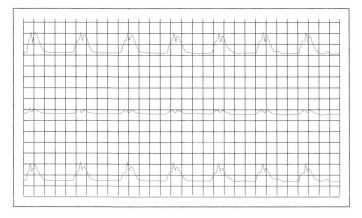

Figure 11.6 Agonal ECG rhythm.

Supraventricular tachycardia (SVT)

Although technically all non-sinus tachycardias that arise from above the bifurcation of the bundle of His are 'supraventricular tachycardias' most ED clinicians refer to: atrioventricular nodal re-entry tachycardia (AVNRT), atrioventricular re-entry tachycardia (AVRT) and AJRs as 'Supraventricular tachycardia' as they are all managed in a similar way on the ALS algorithm.

Atrioventricular nodal re-entry tachycardia (AVNRT): This is the most common type of regular narrow complex tachyarrhythmia and also the most common paroxysmal SVT → *see Figure 11.7*. It often occurs in patients with otherwise normal hearts and is thus relatively benign. The cause is a re-entrant circuit within the AV node.

Explanation of AV nodal re-entry circuits → Box 11.4

Atrioventricular re-entry tachycardia (AVRT): Re-entry involves an accessory pathway such as the Bundle of Kent in Wolff – Parkinson – White (WPW) syndrome. There is usually no visible atrial activity on the ECG. After resolution of the tachycardia, the ECG may show a short P-R interval and a delta wave (a slurred upstroke denoting pre-excitation) at the start of the QRS complex.

Accelerated junctional rhythm: AJR occurs when the rate of an AV junctional pacemaker exceeds that of the sinus node. This situation arises when there is increased automaticity in the AV node coupled with decreased automaticity in the sinus node → *see Figure 11.8*.

ECG features of an AJR:

- Narrow complex rhythm; QRS duration <120 ms (unless pre-existing BBB)
- Ventricular rate usually 60–100 bpm

> **Box 11.4 AV nodal re-entry circuits**
>
> In the normal AV node, there are two pathways along which the atrial impulse can travel – a slow pathway with a short refractory period and a fast pathway with a longer refractory period. The two unite to become the bundle of His. During normal sinus rhythm, the atrial impulse travels along both pathways but completes its journey via the fast pathway only because the slow pathway has already become refractory.
>
> In AVNRT, a premature atrial beat occurs at a crucial time and the impulse finds the fast pathway to be still refractory and so travels along the slow pathway. When it gets to the point where both fast and slow pathways join to form the bundle of His, the fast pathway has recovered from its refractory period and the impulse travels backwards up it. This establishes a re-entry circuit and is the mechanism in 90% of patients with AV nodal tachycardia. In the other 10% of patients, a premature ventricular beat is the source of the problem and a slow – fast circuit is set up – the reverse of the situation described above. As a result of the normal anatomy involved, affected individuals are often young and healthy with no detectable heart disease.

- Retrograde P waves may be present and can appear before, during or after the QRS complex. They are usually inverted in inferior leads (II, III and aVF), upright in aVR+V1
- AV dissociation may be present with the ventricular rate usually greater than the atrial rate.

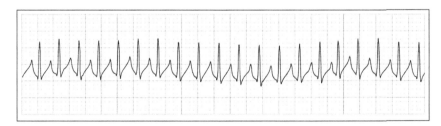

Figure 11.7 The AVNRT ECG is regular with no visible atrial activity. LITFL.

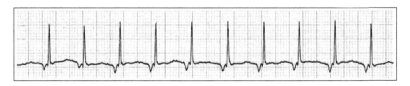

Figure 11.8 Accelerated junctional rhythm. Note the retrograde P waves. LITFL.

Causes of accelerated junctional rhythm include anything that disrupts electrical activity in the SA node. Common causes include:

- Digoxin toxicity (= the classic cause of AJR)
- Beta-agonists, e.g. isoprenaline, adrenaline
- Myocardial ischaemia
- Myocarditis
- Cardiac surgery.

Atrial tachycardias

Atrial tachycardia: is caused by a single ectopic focus.

Multiple causes including: digoxin toxicity, atrial scarring, stimulants including cocaine, caffeine and alcohol. The atrial rate is more than 100 beats/min, and the P wave morphology and axis is abnormal (e.g. inverted p waves in inferior leads) due to ectopic origin. However, the p waves have an isoelectric baseline (unlike atrial flutter).

Atrial flutter: The atria 'flutter' at around 300 beats/min and 2:1 or 3:1 atrioventricular block occurs to give rates of up to 150–160 complexes/min. The ECG should show regular atrial activity at a rate of 300 bpm, loss of the iso-electric baseline and 'saw-tooth' pattern of inverted flutter waves in leads II, III and aVF. If adenosine is administered or a vagal manoeuvre performed, flutter will not usually cardiovert (unlike AVNRT), although typically there will be a transient period of increased AV block during which flutter waves may be unmasked.

Within the ED atrial flutter should be managed in a similar way to atrial fibrillation. *See below.*

Atrial fibrillation (AF): AF is the most common sustained arrythmia. It's prevalence doubles with each decade of life beyond the age of 50, rising to 9% of the population at the age of 80. The heart rate is irregular in both rhythm and morphology. AF usually appears as a narrow – complex tachycardia on ECG but, if there is aberrant (i.e. abnormal) conduction such as a BBB, then broad complexes may be seen.

Atrial fibrillation may be caused by distention or hypertrophy of the atria, metabolic derangement (e.g. low potassium), toxins (e.g. alcohol) and physiological stress (e.g. infection in the elderly) → *see Box 11.5.*

Box 11.5 **'I match up' a mnemonic that lists the more common causes of AFs**

Infection (particularly in the elderly)
Mitral valve disease/myocardial ischaemia/ infarction
Alcohol
Thyrotoxicosis
Cardiomyopathy
Hypertension
Unknown ('Lone AF')
Pulmonary (pulmonary embolus, pneumonia and malignancy).

Treatment of regular narrow complex tachycardia

A regular narrow complex tachycardia is either a sinus rhythm (which is managed by addressing the underlying cause) or one of the regular supraventricular tachycardias (AVNRT/AVRT/AJR/atrial tachycardia or atrial flutter).

Resuscitation Council (UK) algorithm for the treatment of tachycardia in adults summarises the management strategy (with a pulse) → *Figure 11.9 Adult Tachycardia Algorithm.*

If there are life-threatening features, then a synchronised shock should be delivered.

The majority of patients presenting with a narrow complex tachycardia will not be haemodynamically unstable. So vagal procedures and medical management can be undertaken.

- Vagal manoeuvres include carotid sinus massage, or a modified Valsalva manoeuvre.
- **Modified valsalva**: The patient asked to blow into a manometer at a pressure of 40 mmHg, in the semi-recumbent position but immediately at the end of the strain, the patient is laid flat and has their legs raised by a member of staff to 45° for 15 seconds.
- Adenosine is effectively a 'chemical shock' – immediate effect, short acting and relatively safe in both stable and unstable patients. The initial dose is 6 mg for an adult which is given as a rapid IV bolus – use a large 'flush' to get the drug to the heart quickly. Some patients experience an unpleasant sensation with administration of adenosine and should be warned of this but reassured that it is only short lived.

If the first dose of adenosine proves to be ineffective, up to two further doses (of 12 and 18 mg, respectively) may be given at 2 min intervals.

Patients after heart transplantation or who are taking dipyridamole or carbamazepine may be very sensitive to the effects of adenosine and should be given an initial dose of 3 mg. Adenosine should be avoided in patients with WPW syndrome or brittle asthma.

If adenosine is contraindicated or the patient would prefer a different agent then verapamil can be used to perform the cardioversion. Verapamil should be avoided if the patient is on a β blocker, has a history of heart failure, impaired LV function, atrial flutter/fibrillation with an accessory pathway.

The above management will terminate almost all AVNRTs or AVRTs within seconds. Failure to terminate a regular narrow complex tachycardia with adenosine suggests the presence of atrial tachycardia or atrial flutter.

Infants with SVT

Infants with a tachydysrhythmia may present with a sudden onset of poor feeding, tachypnoea, pallor and lethargy. SVT is the most common non – arrest

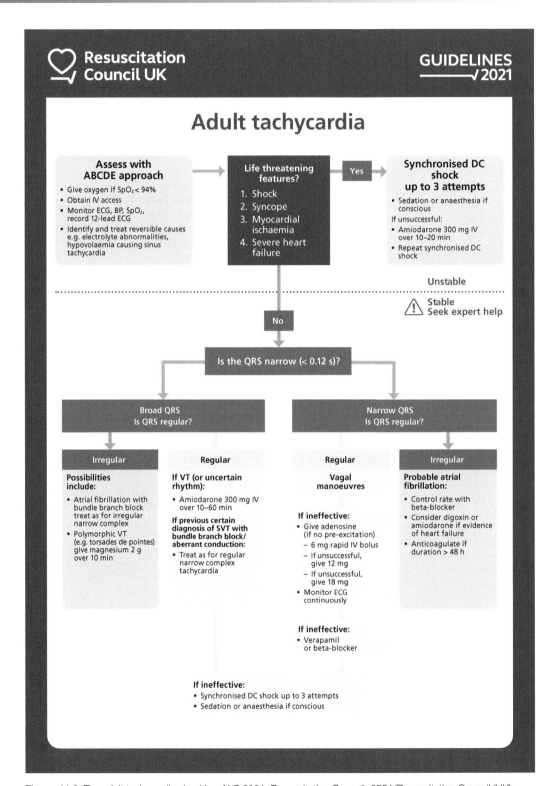

Figure 11.9 The adult tachycardia algorithm ALS 2021. Resuscitation Council, 2021/Resuscitation Council (UK).

arrhythmia of infancy and may give rise to cardiogenic shock. Heart rates range from 220 per min to as high as 300 complexes per min. As infants are unable to perform the vagal manouvres, an alternative first line is to try applying an ice-cold cloth on the face for 30–40 seconds. Adenosine can be used if this fails – 100–200 mcg/kg.

Management of atrial fibrillation (AF)

The management of acute atrial fibrillation is summarised in → *Figure 11.10. Management of Acute Atrial Fibrillation*.

When faced with a patient in new fast atrial fibrillation the key questions are

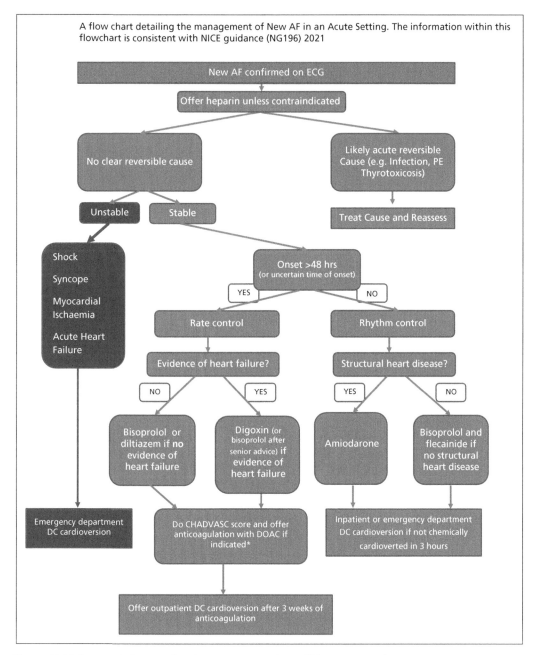

A flow chart detailing the management of New AF in an Acute Setting. The information within this flowchart is consistent with NICE guidance (NG196) 2021

Figure 11.10 A suggested approach to the management of new AF in an acute setting.

1 Is there a secondary and reversible cause for example pneumonia, hyperthyroidism, alcohol excess, pulmonary embolus? This underlying cause should always be looked for and treated before specific rate or rhythm control therapy is started.
2 Is the patient unstable with signs of shock/syncope/myocardial ischaemia/acute heart failure? In which case they should be immediately sedated and electrically cardioverted.
3 Has the patient been in AF for less than 48 hours? In which case acute rhythm control can be attempted either using drugs or electricity.
4 Has the patient been in AF for more than 48 hours? In which case they should be pharmacologically rate controlled.
5 Does the patient need anticoagulation? AF is a significant risk factor for stroke. In the acute phase patients should be offered a dose of heparin unless it is contraindicated. Patients should then have their stroke risk calculated using the CHA_2DS_2-VASc score → see Table 11.1, bleeding risk calculated using the ORBIT score and anticoagulated if the risk of stroke outweighs the risk of bleeding → see Box 11.6.

Broad complex tachycardias

Broad complex tachycardias (QRS duration >120 ms) may be ventricular in origin or may be a supraventricular rhythm with aberrant conduction (i.e. a BBB).

In an unstable patient with adverse features the distinction between will not affect the immediate treatment. A synchronised cardioversion should be delivered.

If a patient has a broad complex tachycardia with no adverse features the next step is to determine whether it is regular or irregular.

Table 11.1 CHA2DS2VASC Score for stroke risk in atrial fibrillation

Congestive heart failure		1
Hypertension		1
Age	<65	0
	65–74	1
	>75	2
Diabetes Mellitus		1
Stroke/TIA/Thromboembolism history		2
Vascular disease		1
Sex	Female	1
	Male	0
Total Score		/9

Box 11.6 Anticoagulation in patients with AF

Offer anticoagulation with a direct – acting oral anticoagulant to people with atrial fibrillation and a CHA_2DS_2VASc score of two or above, taking into account the risk of bleeding.

Consider anticoagulation for men with atrial fibrillation and a CHA_2DS_2VASc score of one, taking into account the risk of bleeding.

Apixaban, dabigatran, edoxaban and rivaroxaban are all recommended as options.

Do not offer anticoagulation to people aged under 65 years with AF and no risk factors other than their sex (that is a CHA_2DS_2VASc score of zero for men or one for women)

Regular broad complex tachycardia

This may be ventricular tachycardia (VT) or an SVT with aberrant conduction. If unsure of the underlying rhythm then the safest option is to treat the patient for VT.

Ventricular tachycardia

This is a sign of a heart that is 'irritable' or has disordered conduction caused by intrinsic damage, electrolyte disturbance or drugs. High rates may cause a variable loss of cardiac output although this feature alone does not distinguish VT from SVT. The ECG shows a regular broad complex tachycardia (QRS > 120 ms) at a rate of >120 beats/min. Independent P waves may be seen that are unrelated to the QRS complexes; fusion beats can also occur. VT may be monomorphic or polymorphic depending on the origin. VT always has the potential to degenerate into ventricular fibrillation (VF) and so treatment must not be delayed.

Patients with VT and no pulse

These patients should receive immediate CPR and defibrillation at the earliest opportunity.

Patients with VT and adverse features

For patients with adverse features such as:

- Shock
- Syncope
- Myocardial ischaemia
- Acute heart failure.

Treatment is synchronised cardioversion (starting with 120–200 J) under sedation.

- Treat hypokalaemia with KCl and MgSO4 if the serum potassium is known to below 4.0
- IV amiodarone 300 mg over 20–60 min followed by an infusion of 900 mg over 24 hour
- Get specialist input and consider repeated synchronised DC cardioversion if VT persists. Treatment with other drugs (e.g. lidocaine, procainamide, flecainide or sotalol) or overdrive pacing may be suggested by the cardiology team.

Stable patients with VT

- Treat hypokalaemia if the serum potassium is below 4 (with IV potassium and magnesium)
- IV amiodarone 300 mg over 20–60 min followed by an infusion of 900 mg over 24 hour.
- Sedation and synchronised DC shock if VT persists.

Regular broad complex tachycardia of uncertain origin

In a clinically stable patient with no adverse features, adenosine can be given to a patient with a broad – complex tachycardia of uncertain origin. This constitutes a useful diagnostic test – in SVT the ventricular rate will usually slow after adenosine whereas in VT the heart rate will continue unchanged.

However, only use this strategy in patients with a regular rhythm. In fast AF occurring in patients with an accessory AV pathway, as in Wolff-Parkinson-White Syndrome, when a AV node is blocked there may be a worsening of the tachycardia and degeneration into VF as the anomalous accessory pathway is left unchallenged by normal conduction through the AV node.

Irregular broad complex tachycardia

This is most likely to be atrial fibrillation with a co-existing BBB. Other possible causes are AF with an accessory pathway such as Wolff-Parkinson-White Syndrome or polymorphic VT. AF with aberrant conduction does not usually cause haemodynamic instability, however patients with polymorphic VT (Torsades De Pointes) are usually unstable.

Torsade de pointes

This is a variety of polymorphic VT where the fast ventricular complexes vary from beat to beat, as if the electrical axis is twisting around a fixed point (→ *Figure 11.11*). There is usually an underlying prolongation of the Q–T interval, caused by drugs (especially the selective serotonin reuptake inhibitors) or electrolyte disturbance (e.g. hypokalaemia). The condition may occur in patients who have taken the antihistamine terfenadine in overdose or in combination with any of the following interacting substances:

- Erythromycin, clarithromycin or related macrolide antibiotics
- Ketoconazole, itraconazole or related imidazole antifungal drugs
- Concentrated grapefruit juice.

Patients with cardiac or hepatic disease are especially at risk.

Episodes of torsade de pointes are usually self-limiting but may progress to VF. Treatment is with IV magnesium (→ *Box 11.7*) or β blockers. Antiarrhythmic drugs such as lidocaine, quinidine, sotalol and amiodarone may further increase the Q–T interval and thus worsen the condition. Overdrive pacing may be required to prevent rapid relapse.

Long Q–T syndromes

A long Q–T interval may be acquired or, in very rare cases, congenital. For the commonest acquired causes of a long Q–T syndrome → *Box 11.8*. Consequent ventricular dysrhythmias may cause palpitations, syncope or even sudden death. The Q–T interval must be corrected for heart rate and is then called the QTc.

This calculation is usually performed automatically by modern ECG machines. The normal QTc is 0.38–0.46 seconds. To make a confident 'eyeball' diagnosis, the Q–T

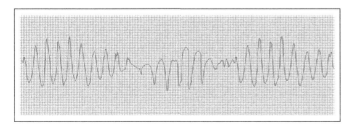

Figure 11.11 ECG trace of Torsades de pointes.

Box 11.7 **Magnesium therapy**

Intravenous magnesium may sometimes be helpful in the control of certain resistant ventricular dysrhythmias such as

- VT secondary to hypokalaemia
- VT that is resistant to DC shock
- Torsade de pointes
- Some tachycardias that are secondary to the effects of drugs including digitalis, antiarrhythmics and occasionally tricyclic antidepressants.

The dose is 4–8 mmol magnesium (diluted to 20 mL with saline) administered intravenously over 5–10 min; 1 g magnesium sulphate contains 4 mmol magnesium ion and a 50% solution contains approximately 2 mmol/mL. Transient flushing – sometimes accompanied by hypotension – is to be expected in almost all patients. The total dose of magnesium may be up to 16 mmol, followed by an infusion of 2.5 mmol/h.

Children: IV magnesium sulphate 25–50 mg/kg over several minutes; maximum dose 2 g.

Box 11.8 **Acquired causes of a long Q–T interval**

- **Drugs:** antiarrhythmics, antidepressants, antihistamines, antimalarials, phenothiazines, organophosphates and high-dose methadone (the commonly used SSRI antidepressants citalopram and escitalopram are both associated with dose-dependent Q–T interval prolongation)
- **Electrolyte disturbances:** hypokalaemia, hypocalcaemia or hypomagnesaemia
- **High-protein liquid diets and other dietary factors**
- **Coronary ischaemia, myocarditis and severe heart failure.**

interval should be around half a second (0.48 second or 12 small squares on the ECG).

Identification of pacemakers

The increasing complexity and diversity of pacemakers have necessitated the use of an identification system. An original three-letter code, which was agreed by the International Association of Pacemaker Manufacturers,

Table 11.2 **Pacemaker codes**

Position of letter	Meaning of letter
First	Identifies chamber(s) paced (V = ventricle; A = atrium; D = dual)
Second	Identifies chamber(s) sensed (V = ventricle; A = atrium; D = dual; 0 = none)
Third	Describes the pacemaker's response to sensed impulses (T = triggered; I = inhibited; D = dual; R = reverse)
Fourth	Describes programmable functions
Fifth	Describes tachydysrhythmia control functions

has been expanded into a five-letter code to enable description of newer programmable units (→ *Table 11.2*). A simple pacemaker is described by the code VVI (ventricular pacing which is inhibited by sensed ventricular impulses).

Bundle branch block

BBB of recent onset after MI is associated with a less favourable prognosis and, in the case of left BBB (LBBB), is an ECG indication for reperfusion therapy (→ *p 182*). As a rough guide, a broad RSR (M – shaped) pattern in V1 is caused by right BBB (RBBB) and a similar pattern in V6 indicates LBBB. (*For further information about the ECG diagnosis of BBB → Table 11.3 and Figure 11.12*) The further interpretation of BBB requires an expert opinion.

Bifascicular block

This results when only half of one bundle branch is conducting normally. There is most usually a combination of RBBB with left anterior hemiblock, which appears as left-axis deviation on the ECG. A quick way to check for this common type of bifascicular block is to look for a broadened M pattern in V1 and a deep S wave that is bigger than the R in II. This conduction disturbance

Table 11.3 **ECG diagnosis of bundle-branch blocks** (*also → Figure 11.12*)

RBBB	LBBB
QRS >120 ms	QRS >120 ms
Secondary R wave in V1, V2 and V3	Broad monophasic R wave and absence of Q wave in I, V5 and V6
Wide S wave in I, V5 and V6	ST and T in opposite direction to QRS

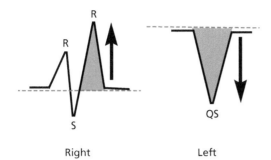

V1

R

R

S

QS

Right   Left

Figure 11.12 Differentiation of RBBB and LBBB using the morphology of V1.

may cause drop attacks in the same way as complete heart block.

Patients with evidence of either trifascicular (bifascicular block with a degree of AV block) or bifascicular disease after MI may require prophylactic cardiac pacing, particularly if there is history of syncope.

Intraventricular abnormalities of conduction

These may cause notching of the QRS complex but do not require treatment.

12

Chest pain

Vivek Chhabra and Amy Nickson[1,2]

[1] Emergency Medicine Consultant, York and Scarborough Teaching Hospitals NHS Foundation Trust, Calderdale and Huddersfield NHS Foundation Trust, UK
[2] Sexual Offences Examiner, Lancashire SAFE Centre, Preston, UK

Chest pain is one of the most common presentations to the emergency department (ED). The patient is worried because they know that chest pain occurs in a heart attack. The doctor is conscious that 'time is muscle' in the case of a heart attack and that there are a wide range of serious pathologies to be considered, e.g. pulmonary embolism (PE), pneumothorax, aortic dissection and life-threatening upper gastrointestinal emergencies. To complicate matters further, symptoms of myocardial infarction (MI) and PE can be very different from the classic descriptions in the textbooks.

Patients reporting chest pain are usually advised to attend ED promptly by telephone advice lines and primary care services as well as friends and relatives. Chest pain accounts for more than 20% of all medical admissions in the UK. Despite that, acute myocardial infarction (AMI) is still missed, estimated in various studies to occur in between 2% and 10% of chest pain patients.

If there are any immediately obvious symptoms or signs of serious illness or if the patient looks unwell:

- Connect the patient to monitoring devices – ECG, BP and SaO_2.
- Administer a high concentration of oxygen by mask if the SaO_2 (arterial oxygen saturation) is <94% on air.
- Obtain venous access and take blood for routine tests including initial troponin assay.
- Request an urgent chest radiograph (CXR) and consider the need for other imaging.
- Consider the need for oral aspirin, sublingual nitrates and intravenous morphine and titrate according to response along with intravenous emetics, if needed.

> Beware of the middle-aged man who wants you to make a diagnosis of indigestion.

IMMEDIATE ASSESSMENT AND MANAGEMENT

- Perform an ABCDE assessment → *Chapter 1*.
- Reassure the patient.
- Allow the patient to sit up or lie in the position they feel most comfortable.
- Obtain a 12-lead ECG immediately (within 5–10 min of arrival) and interpret it at once. If there are changes that, when combined with the clinical picture, indicate the need for reperfusion therapy (ST-segment elevation myocardial infarction [STEMI] or STEMI equivalents → *later*) manage and treat without delay (→ *p. 187*).

Further assessment

Ask about

- Duration of pain
- Nature of pain including radiation and whether constant or intermittent (→ *Later*)
- Relationship of pain to breathing, coughing or moving
- Precipitating factors, including exercise, stress or exposure to cold.
- Relieving factors, such as rest, change in position and use of glyceryl trinitrate (GTN)

The RCEM Lecture Notes: Emergency Medicine, Fifth Edition. Edited by Catherine Williams and Amy Nickson.
© 2024 John Wiley & Sons Ltd. Published 2024 by John Wiley & Sons Ltd.
Companion website: www.wiley.com/go/LNEM5

Be aware that GTN will relieve the pain of oesophageal spasm and response or otherwise to GTN is not a useful diagnostic test.

- Similarity of pain to previous events (e.g. MI or angina)
- Accompanying symptoms such as sweating, nausea, vomiting, flatus or general malaise
- Shortness of breath
- Collapse or blackout, however, transitory
- Palpitations
- Medical history including risk factors for coronary artery disease, connective tissue disease and arteriopathy like stroke, peripheral vascular disease
- Family history, alcohol, smoking and erectile dysfunction in males < 50 yrs of age. Sedentary life style or excessive and strenuous physical activity

Look for

- Pallor, sweating or cyanosis
- Abnormal pulse or BP
- Raised jugular venous pressure (JVP) or dependent oedema
- Added heart sounds
- Changed respiratory rate and pattern
- Low SaO_2 on air
- Reduced air entry and abnormal breath sounds
- Abdominal tenderness – especially epigastric and renal (which may mimic chest pain) and hepatic discomfort (congestive heart failure).

Pallor and sweating usually indicate serious illness.

MI AND THE ACUTE CORONARY SYNDROMES

Coronary heart disease (CHD) has been the leading cause of death worldwide for at least 30 years and is now killing more people than ever before. One in six deaths globally are caused by CHD which is also now the biggest cause of premature mortality worldwide.

Despite advances in medical care, CHD still remains one of the UK's leading causes of death and the most common cause of premature death, causing one death around every 8 min and admission of one patient to hospital with a heart attack every 5 min. Thirty per cent of people experiencing their first MI will die!

The three major risk factors for CHD are smoking, hypertension and hyperlipidaemia. The disease progresses faster in the presence of diabetes and obesity and doubles in incidence in those who are physically inactive. However, the presence or absence of these risk factors has very limited utility in ruling in or out acute coronary syndromes in the acute setting, as people with no obvious risk factors are still more likely to die of an MI than from any other cause.

People with South Asian ethnicity in the UK are at a particularly higher risk of coronary disease due to central obesity and diabetes but may have a lower mortality once coronary disease has manifested.

CHD begins several decades before the acute event with the formation of atherosclerotic plaques. Seventy-five per cent of fatal coronary thromboses occur when there is a sudden rupture of the thin fibrous cap covering an inflamed, lipid-rich plaque leading to platelet aggregation followed by vasospasm. Activation of the coagulation cascade then leads to the conversion of fibrinogen to fibrin, which is responsible for the subsequent stabilisation of the fragile thrombus. Within 30 min of complete coronary occlusion, MI develops, progressing from the subendocardium to the subepicardium.

The term 'acute coronary syndrome' (ACS) describes a continuum of conditions that are associated with acute myocardial ischaemia as a result of interruption of the coronary blood supply. The syndromes range from unstable angina to full-thickness MI (also described as occlusive MI).

Diagnosis of acute coronary syndromes and evolving MI

Definitions

A myocardial infarct is defined by a rise in cardiac troponin with at least one value above the 99th percentile and at least one of the following:

- Symptoms of ischaemia
- New significant ST-segment-T wave changes or new left bundle branch block (LBBB)
- Pathological Q wave changes in the ECG
- Imaging evidence of new loss of viable myocardium or new regional wall motion abnormality
- Identification of an intracoronary thrombus by angiography.

Symptoms

Be aware that 'typical' descriptors of cardiac pain such as 'heaviness' or 'pressure' are not highly predictive of MI. It is often reported that women and elderly patients present with 'atypical' pain, however in reality, the classical description of cardiac pain is inadequate. Cultural and linguistic differences in patient's description of pain contributes to the difficulty in differentiating cardiac from non-cardiac chest pain based on its nature.

Descriptors of pain such as 'sharp' and 'stabbing' perform relatively better and significantly *decrease* the likelihood of chest pain representing an MI, however, are insufficient in isolation to rule out ischaemia. Chest pain which is worse than previous angina or similar to previous MI is highly suspicious for cardiac ischaemia. As are symptoms such as sweating, pallor, nausea or general malaise.

> There is no such thing as 'non-cardiac sounding' chest pain.

Coronary thrombosis may also present without pain ('silent MI'), or with complications of MI (e.g. left ventricular failure [LVF]), with an acute confusional state or history of collapse in elderly people.

Be wary of the middle-aged man with 'indigestion', especially when there is no significant history of dyspepsia. A few days history of vague retrosternal pain in these patients is much more likely to be the warning pains that often predate an MI. Recurrent belching in these patients is a sign of autonomic disturbance and as such may accompany an infarction. Symptomatic relief from antacids should not reassure the clinician that this is not ischaemic pain.

Some patients present with very atypical pain, in both site and character, e.g. pain localised to the abdomen or to the one shoulder or arm or just one of the fingers alone. Many experienced doctors have sent such patients home who have later proved to have an MI or died.

Signs

There are no reliable signs to distinguish MI from other causes of pain. Cardiogenic shock, acute pulmonary oedema or dysrhythmia makes the diagnosis much easier, but physical examination of the patient is often normal. Pallor and sweating should never be ignored; they point to autonomic disturbance. The heart rate may be fast, slow or average. Likewise, the BP may be raised or low but is often normal. A slow heart rate often occurs in an inferior MI because the right coronary artery that supplies this area also supplies the conducting system. (In addition, it delivers blood to the posterior myocardium and the right ventricle, although in some patients the circumflex branch of the left coronary artery is responsible for much of this territory. The anterior and lateral myocardium is invariably supplied by the left anterior descending artery.)

Risk stratification in chest pain

The chest pain history, examination, serum biomarkers and the ECG are often used together to predict the likelihood of ACS or non-ACS, using validated tools. The ED clinician's job is to carefully apply these tools to the patient in front of them, whilst also strongly considering other potential causes of their pain.

Investigations in MI/ACS

ECG within 5–10 min of arrival is essential along with review of pre-hospital ECG's if available. Figure 12.1 illustrates the range within which a normal axis lies. A repeat ECG after 20 min may also help for establishing dynamic changes in high-risk chest pain.

Cardiac dysrhythmias → p. 172.
ECG changes in other acute coronary syndromes → p. 193.
ECG diagnosis of STEMI and indications for thrombolysis → below.

> A normal ECG does not exclude an MI.

CXR is usually normal.

Routine blood tests should be taken, for FBC, U&Es, LFTs, calcium, serum glucose and high sensitivity Troponin I or T

Cardiac markers in ACS → p. 191.

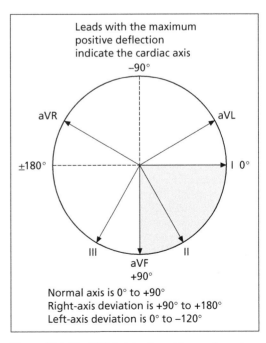

Figure 12.1 The ECG limb leads and the cardiac axis.

ECG diagnosis of occlusive MI requiring immediate reperfusion therapy

Complete coronary occlusion causes an evolving MI that can be averted by timely reperfusion therapy. In the UK, primary percutaneous coronary intervention (PPCI) is preferred over thrombolysis, although thrombolysis should be considered if PPCI is not available within 2 hours of first medical contact.

When chest pain is accompanied by the following ECG patterns, immediate reperfusion been shown to be of benefit. These patterns are

1 ST elevation MI (STEMI)
2 STEMI equivalents
3 New left bundle branch block (LBBB).

ECG changes in STEMI

ST-segment elevation signifies complete occlusion of a major coronary artery and accounts for 30–40% of classic MIs. The occlusion/infarction sequence classically begins with subtle alterations in the T wave. These hyper-acute T waves are tall, peaked and broadened with a loss of clear demarcation from the ST segment (→ Figure 12.2).

Elevation of the ST segment ('convex-upwards') soon follows in leads that face the area of injury; reciprocal ST depression may also occur. Abnormal Q waves, which signify myocardial necrosis, may be present in the first ECG but in most cases do not appear for hours or even days after presentation. These pathological Q waves are wide (0.04 second – one small square – or more) and deep (4 mm or a quarter of the size of the subsequent R wave). They result from potentials that are transmitted through an electrical window of inexcitable myocardium and so suggest the presence of complete (transmural) rather than partial-thickness (subendocardial) damage (→ later). Severe intracellular disturbance may cause a similar picture. Finally, as the ST segment returns to the baseline, symmetrically inverted T waves appear. The timing and magnitude of all of these ECG changes vary greatly from patient to patient.

The site of a typical transmural infarction may be localised from the position of the ECG changes:

- **Anterior**: V1, V2, V3, V4
- **Lateral**: V5, V6
- **High lateral**: I, aVL
- **Inferior**: II, III, aVF (additional ST elevation in V4R [a right-sided V4] suggests infarction of the right ventricle → Box 12.1 and p. 195).

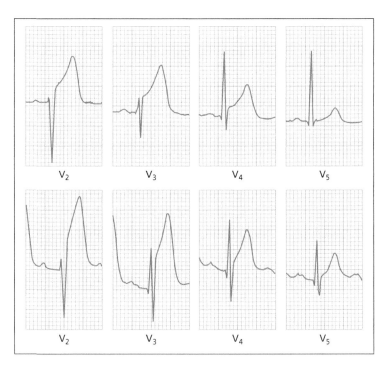

Figure 12.2 Two examples of hyperacute T waves in acute MI.

> **Box 12.1 ECG signs of true posterior and right ventricular MI**
>
> *Posterior infarction*
> - Tall R wave in the anterior leads (V1–V3)
> - ST depression in the anterior leads (V1–V3), i.e. there is a mirror image of the usual Q wave and ST elevation pattern (→ *Figure 12.3*). Flip test: Turn the ECG over 180 degrees to look at the back of the upside-down paper against a bright light source to see the "flipped" ST elevation in V1 – V3 with Q waves
> - ST elevation in posterior chest leads
>
> *Right ventricular infarction*
> - ST elevation in V4R
> - ST elevation in V1–V3 (and eventually Q waves in these leads)
> - ECG changes of inferior MI

ECG changes that meet defined criteria for the diagnosis of STEMI need initiation of reperfusion therapy:

1 ST elevation of at least 2 mm in two adjacent precordial (chest) leads (V2–V6) or
2 ST elevation of at least 1 mm in two limb leads (I, II, III, aVL or aVF).

ECG changes in STEMI equivalents

These represent patterns of ECG changes that represent major coronary artery occlusion without fulfilling the above STEMI criteria.

1 Wellen's syndrome
  This pattern often occurs in a patient with an episode of resolved chest pain and can be associated with a normal baseline troponin. It is characterised by biphasic T waves or deeply inverted T waves in V2 and V3. It represents critical stenosis in the left main stem or left anterior descending (LAD) artery (→ *Figure 12.3*).
2 De Winter's T waves
  Tall prominent 'hyperacute' T waves are seen in the precordial leads with preceding ST depression. This represents acute LAD obstruction and will morph into an anterior STEMI pattern if untreated (→ *Figure 12.4*).
3 Posterior MI
  Isolated posterior infarction is rare and usually occurs as part of a posterolateral or inferoposterior picture (→ *Figure 12.5*).

ECG signs of true posterior and right ventricular MI → Box 12.1.

An isolated posterior infarct may be hard to diagnose on a conventional 12-lead ECG, it can be more reliably seen on a 15-lead or a 17-lead ECG. A 15-lead ECG has been described that utilises V4R and two posterior leads (→ *Figure 12.6*). This technique increases the detection of ST elevation in MI by about 10%. The extra three leads should be obtained when the standard 12-lead ECG shows either ST depression in the anterior chest leads or equivocal right-sided or inferior changes. Low-voltage ST elevation of just 0.5 mm in the posterior chest leads is sufficient to diagnose a posterior STEMI and initiate reperfusion therapy.

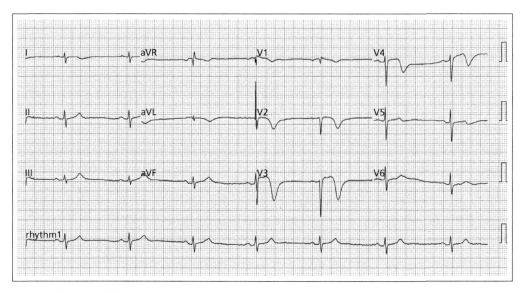

Figure 12.3 12-lead ECG of Wellen's syndrome – demonstrating biphasic and deeply inverted T waves in V2–V4.

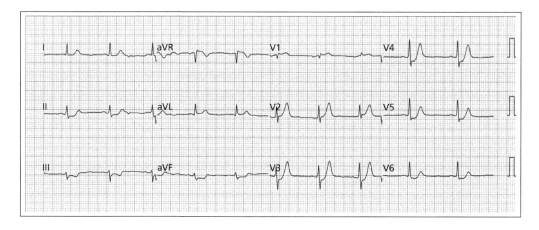

Figure 12.4 12-lead ECG of De Winter's T waves, best seen in V3 and V4.

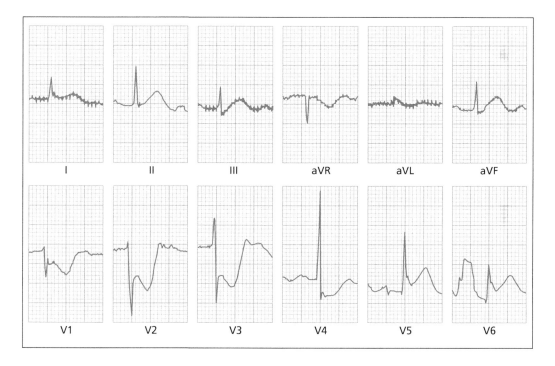

Figure 12.5 12-lead ECG of a true posterior infarction.

ECG changes in LBBB with MI

Patients with LBBB have a much worse prognosis with acute MI than patients with normal ventricular conduction, whether the LBBB is pre-existing or new. However, these patients (who account for around 0.5% of all patients with infarcts) have been shown to benefit greatly from reperfusion therapy. Consequently, in the presence of new LBBB, it is essential to refer promptly. In pre-existing LBBB, three ECG criteria (the Sgarbossa criteria) have been shown to have value in the diagnosis of MI (→ Box 12.2).

Diagnosis of LBBB → Table 11.3 on p. 182.

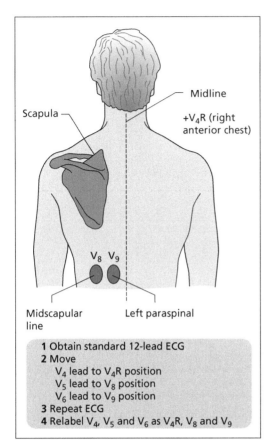

Midline

Scapula

+V₄R (right anterior chest)

V₈ V₉

Midscapular line

Left paraspinal

1 Obtain standard 12-lead ECG
2 Move
  V_4 lead to V_4R position
  V_5 lead to V_8 position
  V_6 lead to V_9 position
3 Repeat ECG
4 Relabel V_4, V_5 and V_6 as V_4R, V_8 and V_9

Figure 12.6 How to record a 15-lead ECG.

Box 12.2 ECG diagnosis of MI in the presence of LBBB – Sgarbossa criteria

Three ECG criteria have been shown to be useful in the diagnosis of MI in patients with LBBB:

1 ST-segment elevation of ≥1 mm in ≥1 lead that is concordant with (in the same direction as) a positive QRS complex
2 ST-segment depression of ≥1 mm in lead V1 or V2 or V3 (concordant change)
3 ST elevation of ≥5 mm in ≥ 1 lead that is discordant with (in the opposite direction from) a negative QRS complex

Criteria 3 has been modified in the Smith–Sgarbossa criteria to:

Proportionally excessive discordant ST elevation – defined as >25% of the depth of the preceding S wave.

Treatment of ST elevation MI (STEMI)

The following section applies to new LBBB as well as STEMI equivalents.

- All alert and conscious patients with suspected ACS including STEMI shall be given Aspirin 300 mg after excluding allergy/hypersensitivity (if allergic clopidogrel 300 mg can be substituted) along with 800 mcg (2 puffs) of sublingual GTN.
- Having made the diagnosis of an evolving MI requiring immediate reperfusion therapy, the emergency treatment detailed below must not delay preparations for PPCI.
- Oxygen by mask and IV access.
- Continuous monitoring of vital signs and ECG.
- Analgesia – IV morphine 5–10 mg or diamorphine 2.5–5 mg.
- Antiemetic if vomiting (e.g. IV metoclopramide 10 mg).
- Patients undergoing PCI are given prasugrel 60 mg or ticagrelor 180 mg. Clopidogrel 300 mg only if already on any oral anticoagulant.
- Prasugrel is not recommended for patients who are aged >75 years, weigh <60 kg or who have a history of transient ischaemic attack (TIA) or stroke.
- Nitrates are used for persistent pain. Buccal GTN is a convenient and effective alternative to IV nitrates. The initial dose is 2 mg, but this may be increased to 3–5 mg if necessary, in the carefully monitored patient. A sublingual aerosol spray of GTN can be useful for a quick effect (two puffs = 800 mcg). *For GTN infusions → p. 220.*

Treatment of NSTEMI and ACS → p. 193.
Thrombolysis → p. 191.

Reperfusion therapy for STEMI

There are two possible reperfusion treatments:

1 **Primary percutaneous coronary intervention (PPCI)**: coronary angioplasty should take place within 90 min of arrival in hospital ('door-to-balloon' time) or within 120 min of first medical contact ('call-to-balloon' time). As a treatment standard, PCI should not be delayed for more than 60 min after the time that thrombolysis could have been given. PCI is a very effective therapy but system constraints may limit its delivery. If a patient of STEMI walks in or brought by ambulance to a hospital without PCI facility, then the aim is to dispatch the patient within 30 min of arrival, to the centre with PCI facility whilst managing cannulation, analgesia and antiplatelet therapy. The system of referral varies by centre, but there should be a 'hot

line' for discussing cases, including those where the diagnosis is uncertain.

2 **Immediate thrombolysis** (→ *p. 183*): thrombolysis should start within 20–30 min of arrival in hospital ('door-to-needle' time) or within 60 min of first contact with the emergency services ('call-to-needle' time). Local factors and protocols will control which of the above two treatments is most suitable for a particular patient. If the patient's chest pain started more than 3 hour before arrival (a delayed 'pain-to-needle' time), then primary PCI is much more effective than thrombolysis. In the remote settings in certain parts of world, fibrinolytic drugs may be the only possible means of reperfusion.

Contraindications of fibrinolytic therapy → Box 12.3.
Standard regimens of fibrinolytic drugs → Box 12.4.

'Golden Hour' for reperfusion therapy starts at the onset of pain. The resolution of chest pain and reduction in ST elevation suggest reperfusion.

> Outcomes with PCI for opening closed arteries are far better than thrombolysis along with lower risk of complications.

Biochemical markers of myocardial damage

The cardiac specific troponins T and I (cTnT and cTnI) are proteins that are released into the bloodstream by damaged heart muscle. The cardiac isoforms of both troponins are specific and are not found in skeletal muscle or other tissues. They are used for three main purposes:

1 To confirm or exclude the diagnosis of an ACS
2 To quantify the extent of myocardial damage and thus allow for risk stratification
3 To assess reperfusion and reinfarction.

Troponins have diagnostic sensitivities for acute MI, which approach 100%. With highly sensitive (HS) troponin assays, the maximum sensitivity occurs 3 hours after the onset of symptoms – which means a blood sample taken at that time is very useful.

Use of troponin levels to guide safe discharge of patients from hospital, however, in patients with dynamic ECG changes and chest pain, cardiology input must be taken irrespective of the initial troponin result.

False-positive HS troponin levels: increased troponin can occur in patients who do not exhibit the clinical features of an ACS. These false-positive results can lead

Box 12.3 Contraindications to thrombolytic therapy

This is not an exhaustive list.

Absolute contraindications
- Known coagulation defects or bleeding diatheses
- Recent haemorrhage, significant trauma or surgery (including dental extraction)
- Haemorrhagic stroke or stroke of unknown causation at any time
- Ischaemic stroke in last 6 months
- History of central nervous system (CNS) damage, aneurysm or neoplasm
- Intracranial surgery or significant head injury within the last 3 weeks
- Severe uncontrolled hypertension
- Acute pericarditis or bacterial endocarditis
- Active pulmonary disease with cavitation
- Aortic dissection
- Active peptic ulceration
- Gastrointestinal bleeding within last 4 weeks
- Acute pancreatitis
- Severe liver disease
- Oesophageal varices
- Visceral neoplasm with increased risk of bleeding
- Heavy vaginal bleeding
- Coma
- Previous allergic reaction to drug (streptokinase)

Cautions/relative contraindications (balance risk–benefit for each patient)
- Current oral anticoagulant therapy
- Recent non-compressible arterial or central venous puncture sites
- Traumatic resuscitation
- TIA in last 6 months
- Diabetic retinopathy (small risk of bleeding only, so not a major contraindication)
- Hypertension (systolic BP >180 mmHg)
- Abdominal aortic aneurysm
- Genitourinary (GU) bleeding in the last 10 days
- Pregnant or <1 week postpartum

to situations where a raised troponin is difficult to interpret along with other clinical conditions in which raised troponins have been identified (→ *Box 12.5*).

Timing of the release of the three main cardiac markers into the bloodstream after ischaemic chest pain → Figure 12.7.

Box 12.4 Thrombolytic regimens for STEMI

Tenecteplase (TNK-tPA)
Weight adjusted regime of single IV bolus over 10 seconds + IV 2.5 mg Fondaparinux:

- 30 mg if weight <60 kg (6 ml)
- 35 mg if weight 60 kg to <70 kg (7 ml)
- 40 mg if weight 70 kg to <80 kg (8 ml)
- 45 mg if weight 80 kg to <90 kg (9 ml)
- 50 mg if weight ≥90 kg (10 ml)

Alteplase (tPA)
IV bolus followed by infusion to maximum dose of 100 mg over 90 min + heparin for 24–48 hours. If not using a special programmable syringe driver:

- Draw up 50 mg of alteplase into each of two 50-mL syringes
- Give an IV 15-mg bolus from the first syringe
- Infuse 50 mg (the entire contents of the second syringe) over 30 min, using an infusion pump
- Infuse the remainder of the first syringe (35 mg) over the next 60 min.

For patients <65 kg give a 15-mg IV bolus, then 0.75 mg/kg over 30 min and then 0.5 mg/kg over 60 min.

 Box 12.5 Other conditions associated with a raised troponin level

Cardiac conditions
- Myocardial contusion (raised troponin is not a sensitive indicator of trauma but has a high positive predictive value)
- Heart failure
- Cardiac arrhythmias
- Myocarditis and cardiomyopathy
- Structural heart disease (e.g. aortic stenosis)
- Coronary artery spasm
- Cardiac surgery and post-transplantation
- Cardiac electrophysiological procedures and pacing (not DC cardioversion)
- Myocardial drug toxicity

Non-cardiac conditions
- Renal failure (most common reason for a false positive)
- Critical illness (sepsis/shock)
- Hypertensive emergencies
- Aortic dissection
- Pulmonary embolism (associated with large emboli and right ventricular damage)
- Pulmonary hypertension
- Acute neurological event (e.g. SAH)
- Non-cardiac surgery
- Rhabdomyolysis
- Infiltrative disease (e.g. sarcoidosis)

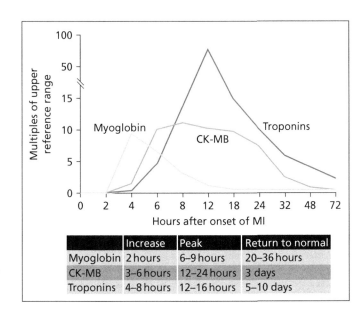

Figure 12.7 The release of the three main cardiac markers into the bloodstream after MI.

	Increase	Peak	Return to normal
Myoglobin	2 hours	6–9 hours	20–36 hours
CK-MB	3–6 hours	12–24 hours	3 days
Troponins	4–8 hours	12–16 hours	5–10 days

Acute coronary syndromes without ST elevation

ACS without ST elevation comprise a continuum from unstable angina (UA) through to non-ST elevation MI (NSTEMI). Sensitive markers of myocardial damage (such as troponins) have revealed that there is no real qualitative difference between the various diagnostic labels. There is an underlying critical but incomplete occlusion of one or more coronary arteries. The ECG may show ST depression and/or T-wave inversion but is often completely normal. ST depression carries a worse prognosis (*significance of T-wave inversion on a 12-lead ECG → Table 12.1.*) The diagnosis of myocardial necrosis may be made from the ECG alone (especially in the case of certain patterns such as subendocardial infarction) but more commonly depends on the presence of raised levels of serum cardiac markers. With the aid of troponin levels, unstable angina may be somewhat arbitrarily differentiated from NSTEMI.

Irrespective of time of onset of chest pain blood samples for HS troponin should be taken at presentation and a repeat might be needed to calculate Δ – which is the proportional change in troponin between the 1st and 2nd samples and can be a rise or fall. A Δ of >5 is significant value.

A 2nd blood sample may not be required when 1st HS troponin is negative (<5 ng/L) and the patient is deemed to be very low risk using either TIMI, T-MACS, EDACS or HEART risk scores (→ *Box 12.6*). The choice of decision aid will depend on local guidelines and pathways. Patient and their relatives are the most important members of our team and must be involved in the decision-making process, especially since many chest pain patients are discharged without a definitive diagnosis. It can be helpful to calculate the score with the patient and explain what the findings mean. Some patients may wish to stay for a second troponin 'just to be safe', whereas others may be happy to accept a level of risk.

Subendocardial infarction

Although pathological and electrical findings do not correlate exactly, established MIs may be classified by ECG into two broad groups: Q-wave and non-Q-wave infarctions. Patients with ECGs in the latter group have smaller infarcts and a lower initial mortality, although they have a high risk of further (usually Q-wave) infarctions. Transmural (full thickness) damage to the myocardium (e.g. untreated STEMI) is usually associated with the development of Q waves and/or the loss of R-wave voltages, whereas incomplete infarction of the ventricular wall leads to prolonged ST and T-wave changes (→ *Box 12.7*). This subendocardial infarction accounts for about 25% of all classic infarcts and represents the most severe end of the ACS spectrum, just before STEMI. It results from either diffuse three-vessel disease or a single severe stenosis.

Tx of ACS without ST elevation

- Oxygen and IV access
- *Continuous monitoring* of vital signs and ECG
- *Analgesia* – IV diamorphine 2.5–5.0 mg with an antiemetic if vomiting (e.g. IV metoclopramide 10 mg)
- *Antiplatelet therapy* – aspirin 300 mg and clopidogrel 300 mg by mouth. *For glycoprotein(GP) IIb/IIIa inhibitors → p. 195.*

  Aspirin induces a long-lasting functional defect in platelets by blocking the arachidonate metabolism (thromboxane A_2-dependent platelet aggregation). After ACS, it is continued for life in a dose of 75 mg daily. There are only a few contraindications to aspirin – known hypersensitivity, bleeding peptic ulcer and severe liver disease. Clopidogrel is a thienopyridine that inhibits ADP-induced platelet aggregation. In patients with ACS, it provides an additional 20% relative risk reduction over and above aspirin for MI, CVA and death. The loading dose is 300 mg, followed by 75 mg a day for 12 months. The onset of action of clopidogrel is delayed for 2–4 hours.
- *Antithrombin therapy*

  Low-molecular-weight heparins (LMWHs) are more effective in ACSs than standard unfractionated heparin. They have a higher plasma availability and better factor Xa inhibition. The prolonged half-life and more predictable kinetics allow them to be given subcutaneously without monitoring of clotting parameters. The best evidence is for fondaparinux 2.5 mg SC or enoxaparin 1 mg/kg if the patient has renal failure. If the patient is on a DOAC or Warfarin and comes

---

Table 12.1 Significance of T-wave inversion on a 12-lead ECG

Leads with T-wave inversion	Significance
AVR only	Normal
V1 only	Occurs in 20% of normal adults and most children
V1 and V2	Occurs in 5% of normal adults and many children
V3–V6	Always abnormal in adults
I and II	Always abnormal in adults
AVL, AVF and III	May be normal if the T-wave axis is similar to the QRS axis

Abnormal T-wave inversion may be due to ischaemia, strain or pericarditis.

Box 12.6 **ACS and chest pain decision tools**

TIMI – (thrombolysis in myocardial infarction) risk score for UA/NSTEMI

- Age ≥65 years
- Aspirin (or clopidogrel) use in last 7 days
- Prolonged or recurrent angina in past 24 hours
- Known CAD (e.g. >50% stenosis of a vessel, prior angioplasty or stent, prior bypass [CABG], documented prior MI, stable angina with +ve ETT)
- ST changes of at least 0.5 mm in at least 2 leads of the ECG
- Positive biochemical cardiac marker
- At least 3 risk factors
  - Hypertension/BP >140/90
  - Smoker
  - High cholesterol
  - Diabetes
  - Family history of CAD male <55, female <65

Fulfilling none or just one of these criteria gives a 14-day risk of MI or death of 5% and further risk stratification must be done by using another risk score or as per institutional guidelines.

T-MACS (Troponin-only manchester acute coronary syndrome) decision aid

- ECG ischaemia
- Worsening or crescendo angina
- Pain radiating to right arm or shoulder
- Sweating observed
- Hypotension (systolic BP <100 on arrival)
- HS troponin T level

A computer-based programme like MDCalc is needed to calculate the risk of ACS of major adverse cardiac event (MACE) within the next 30 days. If all of the criteria are negative with a HS troponin T<6.6 ng/L, the risk will come out as 'very low' or 1%.

EDACS (Emergency department assessment of chest pain score)

- Age in years
- Sex female 0 point, male +6 point
- Sweating no 0 point, yes +3 points
- Pain radiates to arm, shoulder, neck, or jaw no 0 points, yes +5 points

- Pain occurred or worsened with inspiration no 0, yes -4 points
- Pain is reproduced by palpation no 0, yes -6 points

Low risk group patients score <16 with no ischaemic changes on ECG and both 0-hr and 2-hr troponin negative.

HEART (history, ECG, age, risk factors, troponin) pathway for early discharge in acute chest pain

- History
  - Slightly suspicious   0 point
  - Moderately suspicious   1 point
  - Highly suspicious   2 points
- ECG (1 point: No ST depression but LBBB, LVH, repolarisation changes (ex: digoxin); 2 points: ST depression/elevation not due to LBBB, LVH, or digoxin)
  - Normal   0 point
  - Non-specific repolarisation abnormality   1 point
  - Significant ST deviation   2 points
- Age
  - <45 years   0 point
  - 45–64 years   1 point
  - ≥65 years   2 points
- Risk factors (HTN, hypercholesterolemia, DM, obesity (BMI >30 kg/m²), smoking (current, or smoking cessation ≤3 months), positive family history (parent or sibling with CVD before age 65); atherosclerotic disease: prior MI, PCI/CABG, CVA/TIA or peripheral arterial disease)
  - No risk factors   0 point
  - 1–2 risk factors   1 point
  - ≥3 risk factors or artherosclerotic disease   2 points
- Troponin
  - ≤normal limit   0 point
  - 1–3 × normal limit   1 point
  - >3 × normal limit   2 points

A low score (0–3 points) estimates a 0.9–1.7% risk of MACE and can be calculated using MDCalc.

 Box 12.7 **ECG signs of subendocardial infarction**

- ST-segment depression (earliest change)
- Reduction in size of R wave
- Deep symmetrical negative T wave

Unlike the more common transmural infarction, subendocardial infarction does not result in

Q waves. The ECG changes are usually reflected in multiple leads but are especially frequent in the precordial leads. Exact location of the infarct site is difficult or impossible.

with ACS, continue DOAC or Warfarin, start aspirin (clopidogrel if allergic) but do not give LMWH.

- *Nitrates*

For GTN infusions → p. 220.

- *Glucose and insulin infusion*
  Patients with diabetes and MI have double the mortality of those who do not have diabetes. In addition, there is experimental and limited clinical evidence that routine administration of glucose and insulin may improve metabolism in ischaemic myocardium. This treatment is inexpensive and should be given to all patients with either known diabetes or a blood sugar >11 mmol/L on admission.

- *β Blockers*
  If not contraindicated, early administration of a β blocker is recommended for all patients with MI or other ACS. A slower heart rate results in better coronary artery filling. Calcium antagonists are an alternative if β blockers are contraindicated.

Inpatient treatment: all patients with MI or a suspected ACS require admission to hospital for monitoring, 6 or 12-hour troponin measurement and specialist assessment. Risk factor modification, optimisation of BP control and lipid-lowering therapy will then be considered. Ideally, an echocardiogram and coronary angiography will be performed.

ACE inhibitors: these drugs are of benefit to all patients with MI who have no contraindications, especially those with hypertension or poor LV function. Treatment with an angiotensin-converting enzyme (ACE) inhibitor should be started within 24 hours of the acute episode and continued for at least 6 weeks. A raised troponin is strongly associated with a reduced ejection fraction and so is used in some centres as an indication for ACE inhibitor therapy.

Glycoprotein IIb/IIIa inhibitors: platelets are a key element of the thrombus formation in ACS. Their initial aggregation is caused by the formation of fibrinogen bridges between surface receptors. The glycoprotein (GP) IIb/IIIa inhibitors (abciximab, eptifibatide and tirofiban) are the most potent inhibitors of platelet aggregation available and work by blocking the binding of fibrinogen to these receptors. Abciximab is a monoclonal antibody, which binds to GP IIb/IIIa receptors, and should be used only once in an individual patient. This group of drugs is used, under specialist advice:

1. In ACSs without persistent ST elevation (usually eptifibatide or tirofiban)
2. As an adjunct to primary PCI (especially in patients with diabetes or undergoing complex procedures) (usually abciximab).

Unfortunately, GP IIb/IIIa inhibitors have been shown to cause increased bleeding when combined with fibrinolytic drugs.

CRUSADE score
Useful to stratify risk for major bleeding in a subgroup of patients e.g. frail elderly patients with diabetes, renal or heart failure presenting with NSTEMI or STEMI, prior to initiation of treatment.

Treatment of complications of MI

The outcome after acute MI is in part determined by the characteristics of the patient. Advanced age, diabetes, renal insufficiency and previous MI or CVA all contribute to a less favourable outcome.

Right ventricular infarction

This accompanies around a third of inferior MIs and causes the non-specific triad of hypotension, raised JVP and clear lung fields. ST elevation in V4R is very suggestive of the diagnosis; ST elevation in V1–V3 is also often present (→ *Box 12.1*). Echocardiography may confirm the diagnosis. Right ventricular preload must be maintained carefully with IV fluids along with urgent cardiologist involvement and vasodilators should be avoided.

Sinus bradycardia

This is common with inferior infarction because the inferior myocardium shares its blood supply with the right ventricle, posterior left heart and conducting system. (The sinoatrial [SA] node is supplied by the right coronary artery in 55% of patients and by the circumflex artery in the remaining 45%. The AV node is served by the right coronary artery in 90% of cases with just 10% of patients having a circumflex supply). At heart rates >45 beats/min, sinus bradycardia is best just observed, but below this it starts to cause hypotension and faintness. IV atropine is effective (adult dose: 200–2000 mcg depending on the response). Tachycardia may reduce coronary perfusion while increasing oxygen demand and is thus to be avoided.

Left ventricular aneurysm

This occurs in 5% of MIs (usually large transmural anterior infarcts). Unsurprisingly, it decreases cardiac output and increases mortality by a factor of 6. Thrombus may form inside the aneurysmal sac. A CXR may show cardiomegaly, and there may be persistent ST elevation on the ECG. Echocardiogram is required for a definitive diagnosis. Treatment is symptomatic together with anticoagulation.

Free wall rupture of the ventricle

This is seen after 5% of MIs, 90% of cases occurring within 14 days of infarction. Acute tearing chest pain is followed by collapse, profound shock, pulseless electrical activity (PEA) and death. Ruptured ventricle is thought to be responsible for 10–20% of post-MI deaths. Subacute free wall rupture causes a rapid-onset tamponade.

Ventricular septal rupture (acute ventricular septal defect or VSD)

This occurs in 1% of MIs, usually in the first week. The patient experiences a sudden onset of chest pain and shortness of breath. On examination, there is biventricular failure and shock. A harsh pansystolic murmur is present in 90% of cases with a systolic thrill in 50%. Echocardiogram confirms the diagnosis. Treatment of the heart failure is aimed at keeping the patient alive while waiting for immediate surgical repair of the defect.

Acute mitral regurgitation

This occurs in 1% of MIs, usually in the first week. It is caused by LV dilatation, papillary muscle dysfunction or papillary muscle rupture. The clinical presentation ranges from tachycardia and LVF to shock and PEA. There is usually a soft pansystolic murmur. A CXR shows pulmonary oedema; echocardiogram confirms the diagnosis. Temporary medical management of the heart failure should precede immediate valve replacement surgery.

Cardiac arrest → p. 157.
Cardiogenic shock → p. 251.
Dysrhythmias → p. 172.
LVF and acute pulmonary oedema → p. 219.
Pericarditis → p. 199.

Type 1 and type 2 MI

Type 1 – primary event, with coronary artery involvement and atherothrombotic plaque rupture or erosion.

Type 2 – secondary event, acute imbalance in myocardial O_2 supply and demand due to illnesses causing hypoxia, tachyarrhythmia and hypotension, e.g. by anaemia, sepsis or arrythmia. The myocardial injury is similar even though the coronary arteries are without atherothrombosis and the one-year mortality is higher than Type 1 MI. **Tx** – aspirin 300 mg PO (Clopidogrel 300 mg if allergic to aspirin) and treatment of the underlying disease.

Cocaine and chest pain

Cocaine can cause chest pain due to myocardial ischaemia or MI due to release of catecholamines, increased O_2 demand, coronary vasospasm and thrombosis. Also, by its effect on connective tissue of aorta and by instigating abrupt and severe hypertension, cocaine can increase the propensity of aortic dissection. The other causes of chest pain like pneumothorax and pneumomediastinum may manifest due to respiratory toxic effects of cocaine inhalation.

All patients of chest pain with cocaine as primary cause may need repeated doses of intravenous benzodiazepine besides treating the identified associated complications

with O_2, GTN and aspirin along with angioplasty or thrombolysis if ECG suggests acute MI. Beta blockers are to be avoided in these patients due to risk of paradoxical hypertension and increase coronary vasoconstriction (→ *p. 292*).

Chest pain post coronary interventions

Patients may present to emergency department after undergoing coronary stenting or after major thoracic surgery including coronary artery bypass grafting (CABG). The pain in such situations could be due to blockage of stent or grafted vessels and could be due to infection of the wound.

Angina pectoris (stable angina)

> Cardiac pain occurring at rest is always worrying. A couple of attacks of resting pain (i.e. unstable angina) commonly occur a few days before a fatal infarction.

The pain of angina pectoris is cardiac pain and thus is identical to that described above for MI. Even the intensity of the pain apparently overlaps that experienced in some infarctions. Angina arises from heart muscle, which is working too hard for its available blood, and hence oxygen supply. As such, it must be differentiated from the pain felt in myocardium that is losing its blood supply, i.e. infarcting.

> A patient with cardiac pain that has lasted for more than 20 min should be admitted to hospital.

To diagnose stable angina confidently the following should be confirmed.

- The patient is known to suffer from angina.
- The pain lasts only a few minutes.
- There are no atypical accompanying features, e.g. sweating.
- There is no increase in the frequency of the attacks, i.e. the patient is not developing crescendo angina.
- The pain is precipitated by the usual factors (e.g. exercise) and it is not becoming unstable angina.
- Relief from the pain is spontaneous or by GTN.
- The ECG is unchanged.

> If this episode is so typical, why did the patient come to hospital? Resolve this question before discharge.

Tx

Treatment of unstable angina → Acute coronary syndromes on p. 193.

Patients with stable angina of short duration can be allowed to go home if the above criteria are met. GP follow-up should be arranged who may consider coronary calcium scan in borderline risk patients.

OTHER SERIOUS CAUSES

OF CHEST PAIN

1 Pulmonary embolism (→ *Chapter 13 p. 227*)
2 Dissecting aneurysm of thoracic aorta
3 Pericarditis (→ *p. 199*)
4 Pneumothorax (→ *p. 201*)
5 Pneumomediastinum by oesophageal or tracheal tear (→ *p. 203*)
6 Pancreatitis (→ *p. 316*).
7 EVALI - E-cigarette, or vaping, product use–associated lung injury

Dissecting aneurysm of the thoracic aorta

Acute aortic syndrome includes acute aortic dissection, intramural thrombus, penetrating atherosclerotic ulcer and aortic injury due to blunt trauma. Although aortic dissection (AD) is relatively rare (around 1 in 10 000 ED attendances or 1 AD:200 ACS), the consequences of missing the diagnosis are catastrophic, with the clinician pickup rate being 15-43%. Mortality for Type A dissection (which involves ascending and the arch of aorta) increases by 1% for every 1 hour that the diagnosis is delayed.

Aortic dissection involves splitting of the tunica media to form a true lumen and a false lumen after a tear in the tunica intima. It can be classified into Type A and Type B using the Stanford and DeBakey systems (→ *Figure 12.8*) depending on whether the ascending or descending aorta is involved (or both).

The classical presentation is of sudden severe, central chest pain radiating to the back between the scapulae but this is relatively rare. Patient can belong to any age group and may be asymptomatic or complain of non-specific

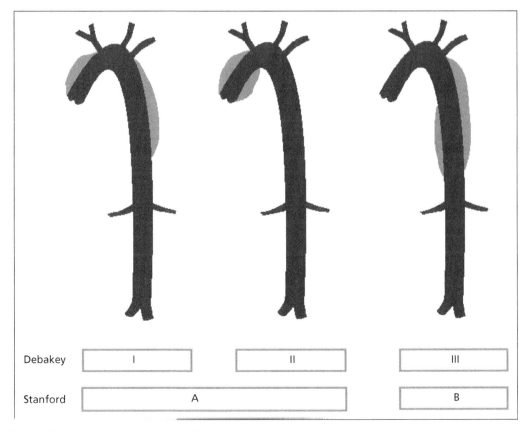

Figure 12.8 Stanford and DeBakey classification of aortic dissection.

chest pain, epigastric pain, acute abdomen (85%), back pain or come with features of stroke, syncope, heart failure and limb ischaemia or a mix of these symptoms.

In view of the above, a thorough history is very important and the following points shall alarm the clinician:

- Very sudden, often severe 'thunderclap' chest, back or abdominal pain which often resolves or is improved by the time the patient attends the ED. Many of these patients are previously fit and well and have never been to hospital. They may have called an ambulance because of the severe nature of the pain.
- Pain is often maximal at onset.
- The pain could be transient in nature, and it could recur in a different place (e.g. back, abdomen). Beware of symptoms 'above and below' the diaphragm.
- Some symptoms may not quite fit or the patient may have experienced transient neurological symptoms associated with the chest pain.
- Patients may present with 'chest pain and something else', e.g. chest pain and headache, chest pain and neurological symptoms, chest pain and syncope.
- The patient may have a feeling of 'impending doom'.

Clinical examination may be fully normal but occasional presence of the high-risk signs below may help clinically suspect the diagnosis; however, absence of these signs does not exclude aortic dissection:

- pulse deficit in either arm - difference in count between heart beat and peripheral pulse
- a systolic blood pressure difference between the arms (often quoted as a difference in systolic of >20 mmHg – however, approximately 10% of people with hypertension have a significant difference between arms)
- chest pain plus a focal neurological deficit
- the presence of a new aortic murmur
- hypotension
- shock.

Risk factors for aortic dissection include:

- Previous history of aortic dissection, know aneurysm or aortic surgery.
- Hypertension (often undiagnosed)
- Connective tissue disorders (e.g. Marfans, Loeys Dietz, Ehlers Danlos, Turners syndrome)
- Family history of dissection or sudden unexplained death
- Bicuspid aortic valve, aortitis and coarctation of the aorta
- Pregnancy
- Polycystic kidneys.

However, the diagnosis is still possible despite absence of all of these risk factors.

Fatality in young and middle-aged women with Turners syndrome presenting with chest pain is very high, as this diagnosis is simply not considered despite

the risk for acute aortic dissection being increased by >100 fold.

Investigations: A 12-lead ECG will help exclude other diagnoses, e.g. STEMI, unstable angina. However, patients with ST changes on the ECG may have concomitant aortic dissection and should be discussed with senior ED and cardiology colleagues.

The initial lab results may be normal; however, there is small role of D-Dimer in the same way it is used in excluding PE, when the pre-test probability of aortic dissection is low and hence a negative D-Dimer test may help exclude this diagnosis. One can assess pre-test probability by using the Aortic Dissection Detection Risk Score (ADD-RS) ($\rightarrow$ Table 12.2).

Patients with an ADD-RS score of 1 or less should be considered for D-Dimer testing while others should go on to definitive imaging of the aorta.

Chest X-ray films have no role in the diagnosis of acute aortic dissection, unless there are no CT scan facilities in which case the thoracic artery dissection in some patients may show wide superior mediastinum, left pleural effusion, left pleural 'cap', trachea moved to right, blurred aortic outline and left main bronchus moved down.

Table 12.2 Aortic dissection detection risk score ADD-RS

High-risk features

High-risk conditions	Marfan's syndrome
	Connective tissue disorder, e.g. Ehlers Danlos
	Family history of aortic disease
	Known thoracic aortic aneurysm
	Known aortic manipulation, e.g. surgery, PCI
High-risk pain features	Chest, back or abdominal pain described as • Abrupt in onset • Severe in intensity and • Sharp, ripping or tearing in nature
High-risk examination features	Evidence of perfusion deficit, e.g. pulse deficit, BP difference between the arms or focal neurological deficit
	Murmur of aortic regurgitation (not know to be old)
	Hypotension or shock states

Low risk (score 0): no high-risk features present

Intermediate risk (score 1): any single high-risk feature present

High risk (score ≥2): two or more high-risk features present

Treatment: In a patient with clinical suspicion of aortic dissection based on the history and examination (+/– carefully selected investigations), an urgent CT aortic angiogram (CTA) should be arranged.

Meanwhile, oxygen, monitoring and IV access shall be gained immediately and blood samples sent to the laboratory for routine tests and cross-matching, while the patient is given IV analgesia (e.g. morphine). Until the diagnosis is confirmed, all such patients should be managed in a high dependency area (e.g. resuscitation room, CCU, HDU)

Patients need aggressive management of hypertension (systolic blood pressure above 120 mmHg) aiming for a systolic blood pressure of between 100 and 120 mmHg. This is typically achieved with an infusion of labetalol. This should be started in the ED without delay. Treating pain with opiates and maintaining a calm reassuring environment will also help control the BP. Glyceryl trinitrate infusion can be added if BP control is proving challenging.

Patients who are hypotensive (systolic blood pressure <100 mmHg) should NOT have aggressive fluid therapy, but all should have large bore intravenous access. Onset of profound shock may be due to cardiac tamponade (→ *p. 111*) in type A aortic dissection, for which 'controlled' pericardial drainage of blood may help attain SBP of 90 mmHg, while preparing for surgery, in these very unstable patients.

Patients with Type A dissection should be referred to the cardiothoracic surgeons and managed as per their advice which is likely to involve transfer to a cardiothoracic centre.

Patients with Type B dissection should be referred to vascular surgeons and often admitted to a high dependence area capable of arterial line monitoring for blood pressure control. The vascular surgery team shall lead discussions with appropriate specialties (e.g. interventional radiology, cardiology and intensive care) and coordinate patient management.

Pericarditis

Pericarditis presents as sharp, persistent midsternal chest pain, which varies in intensity with body position. The pain may be worsened by inspiration, swallowing, exercise and lying down. It is usually said that the pain is relieved by sitting and leaning forward. However, even the reverse can occur – exacerbation of the pain with flexion of the trunk. Radiation of the pain to the superior part of trapezius muscle is very suggestive of pericarditis. A rub is sometimes heard during part of the cardiac cycle and is often loudest at the left sternal border.

Causes

Most cases are caused by infection of which viruses are by far the most common, followed by bacterial infections, TB and fungi. Other causes include:

- MI
- PCI (percutaneous coronary intervention)
- paraneoplastic syndromes like carcinoma of breast or bronchus
- uremia
- collagen vascular disease like SLE, PAN and rheumatoid arthritis
- rheumatic fever
- post cardiac surgery or radiotherapy
- trauma
- drugs such as methyldopa, minoxidil, hydralazine, procainamide, isoniazid and cyclosporin.

Stages of pericarditis

The four stages of pericarditis are classically associated with particular ECG changes but these are seen in their totality in <50% of patients:

Stage 1: widespread ST elevation and PR depression with reciprocal changes in aVR (1–2 weeks) (→ *Figure 12.9*)
Stage 2: normalisation of ST changes; generalised T wave flattening (1–3 weeks)
Stage 3: flattened T waves become inverted (3 to several weeks)
Stage 4: ECG returns to normal (several weeks onwards)

Investigations

The ECG classically shows widespread, modest (0.5–1 mm) and concave ST elevation and PR depression (in all ECG leads except aVR and V1 which may show reciprocal ST depression and PR elevation). The ST and PR changes are relative to the baseline formed by T-P segment. Sinus tachycardia is also commonly present. There are no pathological Q waves.

> PR depression can also be seen in 12% of patients with STEMI.

Spodick sign: 80% of patients' ECGs in stage 1 pericarditis reveal at least two leads with down sloping of TP segment of at least 1 mm – best seen in lead II and lateral precordial leads.

Echocardiography may detect an effusion.

Other relevant investigations are CXR, FBC, U&Es, CRP, troponin and blood cultures if sepsis is suspected.

The two common differentials of these ECG changes are:

- Benign early repolarisation (BER)
- STEMI

The ECG features discussed in → *Table 12.3* may further help with better diagnoses.

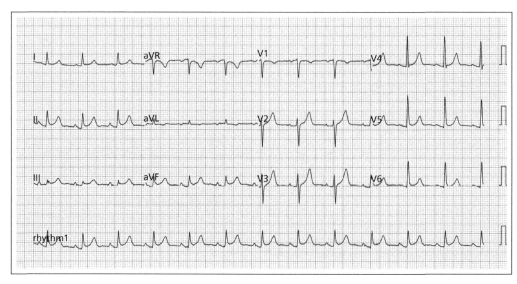

Figure 12.9 ECG showing classic ST and PR changes of pericarditis.

Table 12.3 Comparison of ECG changes seen in benign early repolarisation (BER), pericarditis and STEMI

ECG in BER	ECG in pericarditis	ECG in STEMI
• ST elevation in precordial leads only • Absent PR depression • Prominent T waves • V4 lead may have characteristic 'fish-hook' sign – notched J-point elevation • Non-progression in ECG changes over time	• ST elevation is generalised • PR depression in many leads • Normal T wave amplitude • No 'fish hook' in V4 • Slowly evolving dynamic ECG over time	• ST elevation with reciprocal depression (in leads other than aVR and V1) • ST elevation greater in lead III than lead II. • Convex up or horizontal ST elevation

So, when considering an ECG diagnosis of pericarditis note the following:

– PR depression in multiple leads is suggestive of pericarditis; however, 12% of patients with STEMI may have associated PR depression due to atrial infarction.
– Spodick's sign on ECG can be seen in 29% of patients with pericarditis compared to 5% of patients with STEMI and hence may help when seen in conjunction with other ECG features, if present.

However, if feeling uncertain (not uncommon), ask for senior advice and document for repeat/serial ECG after 20 min interval from the first one and obtain serial troponin levels.

Tx Treatment of viral pericarditis (the most common form seen mostly in previously well young or middle-aged adults) is with non-steroidal anti-inflammatory drugs (NSAIDs) and colchicine, to avoid the development of myocarditis and constrictive pericarditis. Diclofenac 75 mg IM may be given in the ED. Patients should be advised to rest and withdraw from sporting activity.

Patients may need hospitalisation depending on the clinical severity and/or outcome of investigation results or referred for review and follow-up in SDEC/EAU (Same Day Emergency Care/Emergency Assessment Unit) facility by acute medical physicians or cardiologists. Patients with fevers, immunosuppression and elevated troponin should be admitted, as should those with non-viral causes such as uraemia.

Post-infarction pericarditis is seen in 5–20% of patients with transmural MI. The incidence is halved by the use of fibrinolytic drugs. There may be a low-grade fever and an echocardiogram may show an effusion. Post-infarction pericarditis is treated with high-dose aspirin. (NSAIDs and steroids can interfere with myocardial healing.)

Dressler's syndrome occurs in 1–5% of patients 1–3 months post MI. It is thought to have an autoimmune origin. Pericardial effusion is rare in Dressler's syndrome. This type of pericarditis is also treated with aspirin and referred to cardiologists.

Myocarditis and endocarditis → p. 252.

Pneumothorax

Pneumothorax is the leaking of air into the pleural space between the lung and chest wall due to rupture of a small area of either normal lung (as in trauma) or abnormal lung tissue such as a subpleural bleb or a bulla. The pressure caused by leaked air leads to partial or total collapse of the lung and depending on severity patients may present with mild to severe pleuritic chest pain along with sudden breathlessness.

Early treatment options include observation, aspiration or intercostal drain insertion depending on the severity of presentation, size of the pneumothoraces and presence of underlying lung disease.

There are varieties of pneumothorax along with special situations as described below:

1 **Spontaneous pneumothorax**: primary or secondary
2 **Tension pneumothorax**
3 **Traumatic pneumothorax**: open or closed
4 **Iatrogenic**: post bronchoscopy, CT-guided lung biopsy
5 **Pneumothorax mimic (pseudo-pneumothorax)**: bulla in COPD patients, resected lung and skin-fold pneumothorax
6 **Pneumothorax in special situations**, e.g. background of lung resection, bullous COPD, small asymptomatic pneumothorax prior to intubation or transfer by road or air.

Spontaneous pneumothorax is usually caused by rupture of a small area of abnormal lung tissue such as a bulla or subpleural bleb. This may be precipitated by increases in intra-alveolar pressure such as may occur with exertion or coughing. The patient complains of a sudden onset of pleuritic pain, but this may not be severe. The degree of shortness of breath depends on the size of the pneumothorax. There may be a history of a previous episode. Clinical signs like hyper-resonance to percussion and diminished air entry over the affected lung depend on the amount of pulmonary collapse.

Primary spontaneous pneumothorax generally occurs in young healthy adults, and they can tolerate a large air leak without showing any signs of distress.

Secondary spontaneous pneumothorax is generally seen in elderly population with background of emphysema, pulmonary fibrosis or other underlying lung disease in whom even a small pneumothorax can precipitate respiratory failure. However, it may also happen in any age in patients of TB, asthma, Marfan's syndrome, cystic fibrosis, sarcoidosis, bronchial carcinoma and oesophageal rupture.

Tension pneumothorax causes life-threatening dyspnoea and shock. It is more common after trauma but can happen in other circumstances as well as in the presence of intermittent positive pressure ventilation (IPPV) or iatrogenically after central venous line insertion. Traditional teaching tells us that chest X-ray should never be used to diagnose tension pneumothorax; however, since most EDs have the ability to obtain a film in resus within minutes, many get diagnosed this way (→ *Figure 12.10*). For the management of tension pneumothorax → *p. 77*.

Traumatic pneumothorax can be caused by external trauma like penetrating or blunt injuries to chest causing open or closed pneumothorax, respectively, or can be caused by barotrauma by IPPV or during diving, flights or high altitude. Though most traumatic pneumothoraces will need chest drain insertion, the management may require immediate decompression in tension pneumothorax but could be conservative in a subset who are at the other end of spectrum. A CT scan is a better modality than chest X-ray for investigation of chest trauma as it will easily demonstrate even small pneumothoraces along with other injuries which may influence further interventions like chest drain. Also, it may help decide conservative management in patients who have isolated chest injury with small closed traumatic pneumothorax (→ *see also Chapter 6*).

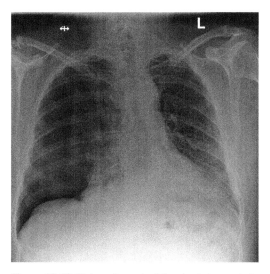

Figure 12.10 Plain radiograph of the chest demonstrating a large right pneumothorax which is beginning to cause tracheal and mediastinal shift to the left.

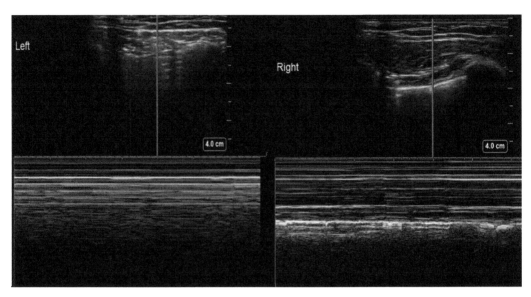

Figure 12.11 POCUS image in M-mode showing pneumothorax ('barcode sign') on the left versus normal lung ('seashore sign') on the right.

Investigations

Chest X-ray

A standard erect posteroanterior (PA) projection has the sensitivity of 92% for detection of pneumothorax, whilst in a supine film the pickup of pneumothorax may be limited to 50%.

Rotate the digital image/X-ray film by 90° and then look at the border of the lung fields in between the rib spaces, especially in the apices. Occasionally, the pneumothorax is visible only medially, in the cardiophrenic angle when it is loculated. If the chest X-ray is normal despite a high degree of clinical suspicion, then a lateral chest or lateral decubitus radiograph can be requested. Using the chest X-ray, the size of a pneumothorax is described as either 'small' or 'large', depending on the distance between the lung edge and the chest wall 'at the level of the hilum', which is an estimate based on the assumption that lung collapse is symmetrical. If this gap is <2 cm across, then the pneumothorax is classified as small; a rim of 2 cm or more defines a large pneumothorax because a 2 cm pneumothorax has been calculated as being equivalent to a 50% loss of lung volume.

POCUS (point of care ultra sound)

Owing to its convenient bedside location and increased sensitivity in the supine patient, POCUS may be of utility in patients who are unable to sit up or as part of the rapid assessment of shock where tension pneumothorax is a potential cause. If there is pneumothorax 'in the area directly under the probe', then the ultrasound will show:

1 Loss of lung sliding
2 Loss of characteristic B-lines
3 Increased clarity of A-lines
4 'Barcode' sign on M-mode (→ *Figure 12.11*).

CT chest

Is the gold standard. Ideal in cases of acute trauma or other situations when erect chest X-ray is not possible. CT is also used to differentiate a pneumothorax from complex bullous lung disease or previous lobectomy, or when the lung fields are obscured by surgical emphysema.

Tx

- Apply monitoring and secure IV access
- Apply O2 to maintain SpO_2 94–98%, (88–92% in COPD patients)
- Aspiration of a pneumothorax → *Box 12.8*
- Insertion of a chest drain tube → *Figure 6.2 on p. 76.*

Most patients with a primary pneumothorax do not have a persistent air leak. Moreover, it has been shown that the risk of recurrence is less if a chest drain tube is not inserted.

Box 12.8 Pneumothorax aspiration technique

- Locate the second intercostal space in the midclavicular line with patient sitting in upright position (an axillary approach is an alternative in 5th intercostal space with patient lying with the pneumothorax side upwards)
- Infiltrate local anaesthetic down to the pleura
- Enter the pleural cavity with a cannula and withdraw the needle (the cannula should be 16 FG or larger and at least 3 cm long)
- Connect the cannula to a 50-mL syringe via a three-way tap
- Begin aspirating air from the pleural cavity. Aspiration should be discontinued if the patient becomes distressed or coughs excessively or if >2.5 L (50 mL × 50) is aspirated
- Obtain a repeat chest X-ray

Patients with 'high-risk' features should proceed straight to a drain (if the pneumothorax is large enough for one to be safely inserted) and hospital admission:

- Hemodynamic compromise (tension pneumothorax)
- Significant hypoxia
- Bilateral pneumothorax
- Underlying lung disease
- >50 years of age with significant smoking history.

Stable patients with well controlled pain and minimal dyspnoea can be managed in one of three main ways depending on their preference:

1 **Patient wishes to avoid procedures:** manage conservatively with short inpatient stay, or regular outpatient review (every 2–4 days) if an ambulatory pathway is available.
2 **Patient wishes for rapid relief of symptoms**: discharge with ambulatory pneumothorax device such as Rocket Pleural Vent™ – review as an outpatient every 2–3 days.
3 **Patient wishes for rapid symptoms relief (but no provision of ambulatory device or outpatient pathway)**: needle aspiration followed by repeat chest X-ray. Proceed to drain if no improvement. If there is improvement following aspiration, patient can be discharged with review as an outpatient in 2–4 weeks.

On discharge, advise the patient to return if symptoms worsen and not to fly or go diving for at least 6 weeks.

For chest drains, catheter-over-guidewire (Seldinger technique) sets (10–14 Fr) are used in the management of pneumothoraces. Check for any anticoagulants or known coagulopathy disorder before the intervention. The instillation of intrapleural local anaesthetic has been shown to reduce the pain caused by a chest tube *in situ*. 20–25 mL of 1% lidocaine (200–250 mg) is injected after insertion of the tube and then 8-hourly as required.

Patients with pneumothoraces that fail to expand should be referred to a respiratory physician who may indicate for suction to be applied to the drainage bottle (high volume, low pressure of up to 20 cm H_2O).

Spontaneous absorption of pneumothoraces does occur but can take several weeks as the pleura is, for obvious functional reasons, resistant to gas exchange in either direction. Around 1.5% of the volume of each pleural cavity can be absorbed per 24 hours. High-flow oxygen increases this rate by a factor of 4 (but only during the period of administration).

Tx of complex or loculated pneumothorax

Radiologically (CT) guided aspiration may be required. Never aspirate or drain a pneumothorax if you feel this is unsafe based on patient factors or radiological image – seek expert help!

Pneumomediastinum

This is an under-recognised condition caused by the same factors that give rise to pneumothorax. The two may coexist. The most common symptom is discomfort in the neck, although chest pain is also frequently experienced. Hamman's sign, a pathognomonic crunching sound synchronising with the heart beat due to heart beating against air-filled tisuues, is heard in less than 50% of cases.

Investigations: Diagnosis is by chest X-ray. Pneumomediastinum is usually unilateral, whereas air in the pericardium is seen all around the heart border.

Tx This consists of analgesia and observation while awaiting spontaneous resolution.

Pleurisy

Inflammation of the pleura causes a characteristic, unilateral, sharp pain, which is worse with movements of the lungs (i.e. deep breathing and coughing). Patients often describe it as being like a knife. Pyrexia is common; a pleural rub is not.

Investigations: A CXR is usually normal but may show an area of underlying pneumonia or an accompanying (small) pleural effusion.

Tx Most minor cases of pleurisy are viral in origin. Antibiotic therapy is given as for other chest infections (→ *p. 220*). Analgesics will be required; the addition of NSAIDs may sometimes help.

Tracheitis

In adults, tracheitis causes central chest pain of a burning nature, which is worse with deep breathing. The patient may be dyspnoeic, pyrexial and with stridor coughing purulent phlegm.

Tx This is directed at the underlying infection.

Bacterial tracheitis in children (a much more severe illness) → *p. 349.*

Oesophagitis

Reflux oesophagitis and oesophageal spasm cause central chest pain, which is sometimes relieved by GTN. Relief also occurs with simple antacids, suppression of acid production being the main treatment. Unfortunately, there is often no easy way to differentiate this condition from MI and thus caution is always needed (→ *p. 185*).

Rupture of oesophagus

These patients may present with chest, back/neck pain due to traumatic or spontaneous rupture of oesophagus (Boerhaave's syndrome) usually after a violent vomiting episode. Signs of shock and subcutaneous emphysema may be noted clinically and on chest X-ray and CT which may also show pneumomediastinum, pleural effusion and pneumothorax. ECG is normal. Treat in resus with O_2, IV analgesics, fluids and antibiotics while treating other injuries and refer to cardiothoracic surgeons.

Shingles

Shingles is the infection of a peripheral sensory nerve by the chickenpox virus. It spreads from the dorsal root ganglion where the virus has remained dormant since primary infection.

> A patient with shingles can infect others – causing chickenpox. Shingles is the result of autoinfection and thus cannot be 'caught'.

The burning pain of herpes zoster infection always predates the characteristic vesicular rash by a day or two. A thoracic nerve is often affected by shingles causing chest pain and initially the diagnosis can be very elusive. A vague red patch may sometimes be seen in the early stages of the disease, hence always ensure to examine the skin.

Tx Treatment with aciclovir should be started as soon as possible. The adult dose is 800 mg 5 times daily for 7 days. This treatment is thought to reduce the severity of postherpetic neuralgia, a difficult and time-consuming condition to treat. Concurrent administration of amitriptyline may reduce the severity of neuralgia further.

Musculoskeletal chest pain

Pain in the chest wall is usually worsened by movements of the trunk such as sitting up and by deep breathing and coughing. It may also be related to movement of the arm at the shoulder joint. Sometimes the pain radiates down the arms, but systemic features are usually absent. Areas of tenderness are common but by no means inevitable. However, one needs to be cautious, especially in middle and elderly age group patients especially females, where patients with ACS may have chest pain worse on movements with the element of reproducible tenderness.

The problem otherwise may emanate from the muscles (viral myalgia or Bornholm's disease) or from the costal cartilages (Tietze's syndrome). Rib and muscle injuries can also present as unexplained chest pain. Such injuries often go unnoticed during sporting activities or periods of intoxication. Rib fractures caused by prolonged coughing is another cause of chest pain.

Tx Treatment of musculoskeletal pain consists of analgesia and reassurance.

Rib fractures → *p. 76.*

Intra-abdominal causes of chest pain

Upper abdominal conditions such as pancreatitis, peptic ulceration, cholecystitis and renal colic can sometimes present as pain in the chest (→ *Chapter 16*).

EVALI - E-cigarette, or vaping, product use–associated lung injury.

An easily misdiagnosed serious inflammatory lung condition in vaping young adults which can masquerade initially as innocuous musculoskeletal chest pain with some dyspnoea and cough due to pneumonitis and then rapidly evolve into life threatening chest sepsis type presentation due to pneumonia and other systemic features. Imaging reveals ground glass opacities in lungs and the mainstay of therapy is prolonged glucocorticoids and hospitalisation.

13

Respiratory distress

Amy Nickson

Emergency Medicine Consultant, Royal Bolton Hospital, Bolton, UK
Sexual Offences Examiner, Lancashire SAFE Centre, Preston, UK

There are more emergency admissions in the UK for respiratory disease than for any other type of illness. It is responsible for 12% of urgent admissions to hospital.

THE UPPER AIRWAYS

The upper airways are very vulnerable to both infection and obstruction. Their clearance and maintenance are the primary concern in any patient with respiratory distress.

Choking

Choking is the result of complete or near-complete obstruction of the upper airways by foreign or ectopic material. It is most common in children and elderly people.

> Some elderly patients who present with inhalation of foreign material have had a stroke whilst eating.

The patient may grip the throat with one hand and the wrist with the other ('the universal choking sign'). Collapse with cyanosis while eating may mimic myocardial infarction (the 'café coronary').

Tx Get help. Encourage coughing in the responsive patient.

Resuscitation Council (UK) algorithms for the treatment of choking in adults and children → Figures 13.1 and 13.2.

Advanced life support when there is ineffective coughing, or apnoea:

1 Back blows ×5
2 Abdominal thrusts (children and adults) or chest thrusts (infants) ×5
3 Direct laryngoscopic removal of foreign material
4 Surgical bypass of the obstruction.

Blind probing with a finger is contraindicated because it may force a foreign body further down the narrow respiratory tract.

Notes on 1–4 above:

1 In children, back blows can be administered with the child prone and the head lower than the trunk. In adults, the most suitable position is with the patient standing upright. Sequences of five blows or thrusts are recommended.
2 An obstructing foreign body may be expelled by means of abdominal thrusts, also known as the Heimlich manoeuvre (→ *Box 13.1*). The liver and spleen are less well protected by the ribs in infants, making the abdominal thrusts relatively dangerous and less likely to be effective.
3 If the above fails and the patient becomes unresponsive, direct laryngoscopy may allow visualisation of the obstruction and then its removal by suction or with Magill's forceps.
4 The cricothyroid membrane is the recommended site for an emergency surgical airway because a tracheotomy is difficult and time-consuming to perform. Needle cricothyroid puncture is an alternative to direct surgical cricothyroidotomy. However, ventilation can then be achieved only with high-pressure oxygen and not with a bag and mask.

The RCEM Lecture Notes: Emergency Medicine, Fifth Edition. Edited by Catherine Williams and Amy Nickson.
© 2024 John Wiley & Sons Ltd. Published 2024 by John Wiley & Sons Ltd.
Companion website: www.wiley.com/go/LNEM5

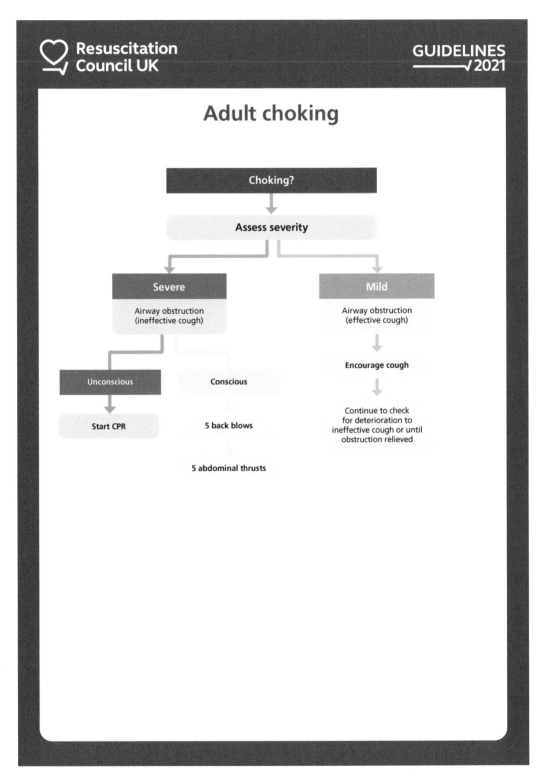

Figure 13.1 Treatment of a choking adult. Resuscitation Guidelines. Reproduced with the kind permission of the Resuscitation Council (UK).

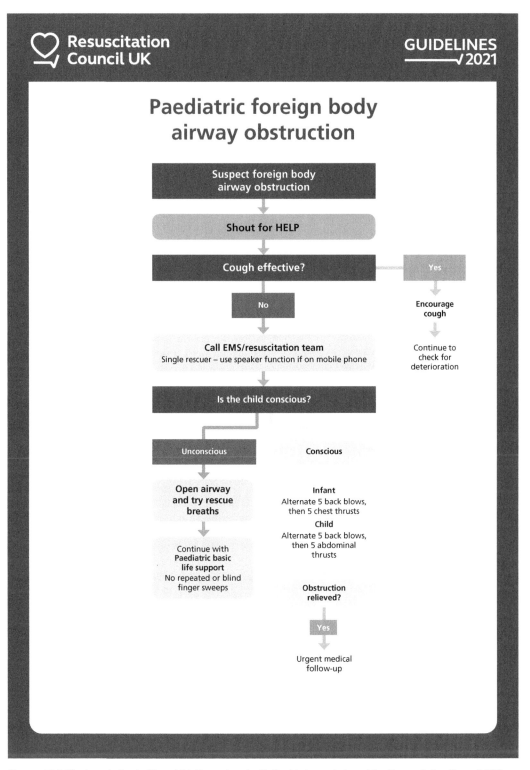

Figure 13.2 Treatment of a choking child. Reproduced with the kind permission of the Resuscitation Council (UK).

> **Box 13.1 Performing abdominal thrusts**
>
> *Patient standing*
> Place your arms around the patient's waist from behind. Grip your wrists together directly beneath the xiphisternum and then give five short, sharp 'bear hugs' up into the epigastrium.
>
> *Patient lying*
> Stand or kneel astride the patient's pelvis. Place the heel of one hand in the epigastrium and reinforce it with the other hand. Then give five short sharp thrusts upwards and backwards.

Cricothyroidotomy → p. 23.
Needle cricothyroid puncture → p. 23.

Post-asphyxia care

Most choking occurs in the community, hence patients who are brought to ED following choking will either now be in cardiac arrest due to failed attempts to dislodge the foreign body or failure to recognise choking, or will still have dyspnoea or decreased conscious level following dislodgement. Those who achieve return of circulation should be admitted, often to the ICU. Those who remain dyspnoeic or have a depressed level of consciousness should, in most cases, be ventilated. Cerebral oedema is common after severe asphyxia; neuroprotective measures should be instigated. Pulmonary oedema may complicate prolonged obstruction.

Stridor and partial upper airway obstruction

Partial obstruction of the extrathoracic airways – at or above the cricoid ring – causes stridor, which is a harsh, high-pitched noise during inspiration. Intrathoracic obstruction typically causes expiratory wheezing. Characteristically, the patient with partial upper airway obstruction sits forward on outstretched arms or elbows (the 'tripod position'). Other signs of partial obstruction of the upper airway are:

- drooling of saliva
- hoarseness
- rattling noises in the upper airway
- snoring and seesaw respiration (in the unresponsive patient).

Maintenance and protection of the airway → Chapter 1, pp. 1–3.

> Cessation of stridor may indicate sudden complete obstruction.

The causes of partial obstruction of the upper airway are:

- the tongue and soft tissue of the airway, in a patient with low GCS
- inhaled foreign body, including blood and vomit
- allergic swelling of the airway (including insect stings)
- burns to the airway
- other direct trauma to the airway, which may occur after attempted hanging or a blow to the throat (note that dislocation of the cricoid cartilage may occur in children)
- infection of the larynx (including the epiglottis) or of the trachea
- infection of the mouth, tonsils or pharynx
- tumour and strictures
- infection superimposed on congenital abnormality in a small infant. Congenital abnormalities of the airway usually present in the first few weeks of life but should be considered up to the age of 6 months.

XR Radiographs should be obtained only in a stable, calm, well-oxygenated patient with an uncertain underlying diagnosis. The only appropriate films are anteroposterior (AP) chest and lateral soft-tissue view of the neck, performed in the ED, and these have limited utility.

A widened soft-tissue shadow on the lateral view of the neck may represent a retropharyngeal abscess or a swollen epiglottis. A coin in the trachea will have passed through the vocal folds in the sagittal plane and will thus appear end-on as a vertical line on an AP chest X-ray. In contrast, a coin in the oesophagus usually lies in the coronal plane (circular shaped on AP chest X-ray).

Special problems in children

1 The flow in any tube is proportional to the fourth power of the radius. Hence, any reduction in the size of the child's small upper airway will have a much greater effect on airflow than a similar reduction in an adult.
2 Any stimulus is likely to cause increased distress, crying and consequent clinical deterioration. Therefore, interventions such as venepuncture should not be undertaken until specialist help has arrived. Pulse oximetry is useful in the interim.

Tx If there is marked stridor and cyanosis:

- Call for expert help immediately (senior anaesthetic and ENT specialists)

- Prepare difficult airway equipment and set up for emergency cricothyroidotomy. If the patient is not too distressed by it, clean and mark the location of the cricothyroid membrane on the neck.
- Reassure the patient and allow any position of comfort
- Give 100% oxygen or, better still, Heliox (70% helium with 30% oxygen) (helium has better flow characteristics than nitrogen or oxygen and may reduce airflow resistance)
- Try nebulised adrenaline (5 mg) as a temporary measure
- Consider parenteral adrenaline for allergic swelling.

> Do not examine the mouth or throat – any stimulus will increase the risk of complete obstruction.

If no help is available and the patient is about to die:

- Attempt laryngoscopy and endotracheal intubation preferably with a video laryngoscope and bougie. Foreign material can be removed with suction and Magill's forceps. If the anatomy of the pharynx is distorted by oedema, ask a colleague to squeeze the chest; escaping air bubbles will help to identify the position of the upper larynx.
- Have a second clinician preparing to perform cricothyroidotomy (→ pp. 22-23).

In less urgent cases:

- Reassure the patient and allow a position of comfort
- Give oxygen
- Give IV antibiotics if bacterial neck space infection is suspected (patient appears toxic and may have meningism, torticollis, trismus, external neck swelling and redness and lymphadenopathy)
- Refer to ENT, with a view to performing nasoendoscopy of the upper airways in the resuscitation area.
- CT scan of the neck with contrast is the gold standard test, if the patient is stable enough and able to lie supine.

Allergic swelling of the upper airways → p. 306.
Angioedema → p. 274.
Diphtheria → p. 439.
Epiglottitis in adults → p. 439.
Inhalational burns → p. 141.
Ludwig's angina → p. 440.
Peritonsillar infections → p. 439.
Retropharyngeal abscess → p. 440.
Stridor in children → p. 348.

THE LOWER AIRWAYS AND LUNGS

The restoration of adequate breathing is a priority, which is second only to the maintenance of a clear airway.

Respiratory arrest

Isolated respiratory arrest or failure of ventilation in the presence of a clear airway and a central pulse occurs in four main circumstances:

1 Poisoning with opiates (→ p. 291)
2 General brainstem depression (e.g. drugs, stroke, head injury)
3 Respiratory failure with CO_2 narcosis (→ p. 211)
4 Neuromuscular paralysis.

The treatment is artificial ventilation with 100% oxygen until the underlying cause can be remedied.

Initial assessment and management of acute breathlessness

- Assess for signs of airway obstruction.
- Check adequacy of breathing:
  1 Are there regular breaths?
  2 What is the rate of breathing? It should be between 12 and 20 per minute
  3 Is there symmetrical chest rise and fall?
  4 Is the patient working hard and using accessory muscles?
  5 Can they talk?
- If breathing is slow, irregular or inadequate, support ventilation with bag-valve-mask or Mapleson C ('Waters') circuit. Call for help.
- Otherwise, give oxygen by mask and apply a pulse oximetry probe. Aim for SaO_2 of 94% initially, unless there is information available that tells you they have a history of type 2 respiratory failure – then aim for 88–92% → Box 13.2 oxygen delivery systems.
- Expose and examine the chest.
  1 Are there signs of chest injury?
  2 Is the trachea in the midline
  3 Is there audible bilateral air entry?
  4 Are there added sounds?
  5 Is the percussion note normal?
- Evaluate the effectiveness of breathing:
  1 What are the oxygen saturations?
  2 Is the patient cyanosed?
  3 Is the patient alert and oriented?
  4 Are there signs of shock?

Box 13.2 Oxygen delivery systems

Nasal cannulae provide oxygen at adjustable flow rates in litres of oxygen per minute (L/min). The actual FiO_2 (fraction of inspired oxygen) delivered by nasal cannula is somewhat variable, dependent on the depth (tidal volume) and rate that the patient breaths and whether they have their mouth open. They have the benefit of being more comfortable and less 'claustrophobic' for patients.

Venturi masks have the advantage of delivering oxygen at a specific fixed concentration (FiO_2): 24% (blue), 28% (white), 31% (orange), 35% (yellow), 40% (red), 50% (pink) and 60% (green). This makes it easier to calculate P/F ratios (see Box 13.3) and to wean down in a stepwise manner.

Non-rebreather masks have an added reservoir bag which fills with oxygen whilst the patient exhales and then empties when the patient inhales the contents. Therefore, providing a much higher FiO_2; up to ~95% in a well fitted mask pulled tightly to the face.

High flow nasal cannulae (HFNC) can deliver flow rates of up to 60 L/min of oxygen and an FiO_2 of up to 100%. They also warm and humidify the gases, provide some positive end expiratory pressure (PEEP) and help with alveolar opening.

Below is the approximate FiO_2 delivered by devices at different flow rates.

Device	O₂ Flow L/min	Approximate FiO₂ (%)
Nasal cannulae	1	24
	2	28
	3	32
	4	36
	5	40
	6	44
Face mask	4–5	40
	6–7	50
	8–9	60
Non-rebreather mask	10–15	60–95%

5 Check the blood gases. Is the patient adequately exhaling CO_2?
- Consider immediate therapy for wheezing or pulmonary oedema.
- Obtain a chest X-ray, bloods and ECG – do not forget glucose – DKA can mimic respiratory distress.
- Obtain a history and complete a full examination of the patient.

Like pain, shortness of breath must be relieved as soon as possible after initial assessment.

Investigations in respiratory distress

Chest X-ray (PA if possible)

An anteroposterior supine chest X-ray taken on the trolley in the resuscitation room may be necessary in a critically ill patient but is a poor substitute for a posteroanterior erect film because:

- the mediastinum and heart size are magnified
- fluid levels are not identified
- the penetration is often inappropriate
- the film is often rotated or incomplete
- there is a potential radiation hazard to staff.

Twelve-lead ECG

A rhythm strip from a three-lead ECG is insufficient for diagnostic purposes in a patient who may have subtle changes of myocardial ischaemia or pulmonary embolism.

Pulse oximetry

Measurement of SaO_2 is extremely useful as it provides constant, non-invasive evaluation of oxygenation and pulse rate. However, there are some drawbacks:

- It does not assess pH and $PaCO_2$ which may both be abnormal in the presence of normal oxygen saturation.
- SaO_2 is inaccurate in the presence of carboxyhaemoglobin (COHb), (house fires, faulty gas heaters, heavy smokers).
- Pulse oximetry underestimates hypoxaemia in patients with dark skin.

On a supine chest X-ray, an effusion or haemothorax may mimic diffuse lung changes (→ p. 74).

Arterial blood gases

Arterial blood sampling in the conscious patient should be performed with local anaesthetic, using intradermal and subcutaneous lignocaine through a small needle (25G orange). In many cases, venous blood gas (VBG) is adequate and less uncomfortable for the patient. Venous pH has sufficient agreement with arterial pH for it to be an adequate alternative in most situations, and if the $PaCO_2$ is normal or low, this has excellent sensitivity for ruling out arterial hypercapnia. However, if $PaCO_2$ is elevated on VBG, correlation with arterial PCO_2 is poor.

Estimation of the expected partial pressure of oxygen in an arterial blood gas sample → Box 13.3.

Respiratory failure

This is defined as the inability of the respiratory system to adequately oxygenate the body or failure to eliminate CO_2 from deoxygenated blood. The primary pathology occurs either within the lungs or in the respiratory muscles.

Type I respiratory failure

This is the failure of *oxygenation*, with a low PaO_2 (<60 mmHg or 8 kPa at sea level) and a normal or low $PaCO_2$. When a healthy person is given lower and lower

Box 13.3 **Estimation of the expected partial pressure of oxygen in an arterial blood gas sample**

With healthy lungs, the PaO_2 in (mmHg) should be approximately equal to 5 times the percentage of oxygen in the inspired gases (FiO_2), i.e. expected PaO_2 (mmHg) = $5 \times FiO_2$ (%).

For example, breathing room air with healthy lungs, the expected PaO_2 = $5 \times 21\%$ = 105 mmHg.

To convert to kPa, divide by 7.6:
105/7.6 = 13.8 kPa

Another way of expressing this is with the P/F ratio, which is a widely used clinical indicator of the severity of hypoxaemia.

P/F ratio = PaO_2/fraction of inspired O_2

For example – a patient with PaO_2 of 10 kPa on 80% FiO_2: 10/0.8 = 12.5.

Acute respiratory failure is defined by P/F ratio of <40 in kPa (or <300 in mmHg).

concentrations of oxygen, they begin to lose rational thinking, then become agitated, confused and then comatose. Where there is disease in the lungs, there is an accompanying sensation of dyspnoea and air hunger, caused by a complex feedback loop between chemoreceptors in the carotid body and mechanical receptors in the lungs and chest wall.

The underlying physiology is often a ventilation/perfusion mismatch, where there are areas of lung being perfused by blood that are not being ventilated due to lung disease processes. This leads to shunting of deoxygenated blood back into the arterial system. Typical examples are pulmonary oedema and pneumonia. As there are areas where gas exchange does not occur, 100% inspired oxygen is unable to completely correct shunting and so there will be a low P/F ratio (a big drop between the FiO_2 and PaO_2). Management involves administration of high concentrations of oxygen and attempted improvement of the underlying lung disease which may involve positive pressure ventilation to recruit and splint open airways.

Continuous positive airway pressure (CPAP) is a way of delivering positive end expiratory pressure (PEEP), which helps open bronchioles and alveoli and can reduce intrapulmonary shunting. It is delivered via a tight-fitting face mask or a hood. Indications for CPAP include acute pulmonary oedema, Covid-19 pneumonitis, lung contusion and obstructive sleep apnoea.

In the case of pulmonary embolism, the opposite type of ventilation/perfusion mismatch occurs. Ventilated lungs are unable to oxygenate blood due to failure of perfusion. (*PE →p. 227*).

Type II respiratory failure

This is failure of *ventilation*, whereby low PaO_2 (<60 mmHg or 8 kPa) accompanies a raised $PaCO_2$ (>45 mmHg or 6 kPa). Meaning that the patient is unable to adequately increase their minute ventilation (i.e. depth and rate of breathing) to exhale CO_2. The most common cause is COPD (→ *p. 216*). Other causes include:

- paralysis, weakness or fatigue of the respiratory muscles
- restrictive lung disease
- chest deformity, especially with superadded infection
- morbid obesity
- depression of the respiratory centre by sedative/opiate drugs or CNS pathology.

As $PaCO_2$ levels rise, the patient's conscious level will begin to drop, as will their respiratory drive and a downward spiral to coma and respiratory arrest begins. Hypercapnia is associated with increased cerebral blood flow and raised intracranial blood pressure so can contribute to worse outcomes in patients with brain injury or illness.

Patients with chronic hypercapnia have compensation at the kidneys, where extra H^+ is excreted, causing a rise in plasma bicarbonate concentration. Hence, in a patient with COPD you may be alerted that the $PaCO_2$ level is above their usual tolerance if they are drowsy, and the pH of the blood is below 7.35.

Treatment aims in type II respiratory failure are to increase minute ventilation by reversing causes of CNS depression or by supporting respiration until the underlying cause can be treated. Respiratory support can be provided in two main ways:

- Non-invasive ventilation (NIV) is also known as non-invasive positive pressure ventilation (NIPPV) or bilevel positive airway pressure (BPAP). This offers the benefits of avoiding a general anaesthetic and the associated risks, and allows the patient to take short breaks for food and comfort. The main drawback is the uncomfortable feeling of the tight mask and the pressure of air being forced in. Starting pressures low and working up, can help, as can some support and reassurance and a small dose of anxiolytic medication. It is not suitable for patients who cannot protect their airway. *For the use of NIV → Box 13.4.*
- Invasive ventilation requires an endotracheal tube or tracheostomy tube. Patients will require sedation and paralysis for intubation and admission to ICU. Once intubated, patients can breathe spontaneously with some pressure support, can have the whole respiratory process taken over for them (controlled mandatory ventilation CMV) or a combination of the two (synchronised intermittent mandatory ventilation SIMV). There are significant risks to being sedated and intubated, such as ventilator-associated pneumonia (VAP), muscle wasting and weakness, haemodynamic instability, pain, agitation and ICU delirium to name just a few. It is a 'life-prolonging' treatment which temporarily improves ventilation whilst the underlying cause gets better. Hence, it is not a suitable treatment for patients whose cause of respiratory failure is not going to get better.

Acute respiratory distress syndrome (ARDS)

ARDS is defined by the Berlin criteria:

- bilateral diffuse opacities on chest X-ray or CT
- not due to cardiogenic pulmonary oedema
- occurring within 1 week of a clinical insult
- with PaO_2/FiO_2 ratio <300 (<40 when calculated in kPa) (→ *see Box 13.3*)

 Box 13.4 Use of non-invasive ventilation

Indications for NIV

- COPD with pH <7.35, pCO_2 >6.5 and RR >23 after bronchodilator therapy and controlled O_2
- Neuromuscular disease or chest wall deformity with pH<7.35 and pCO_2 >6.5
- Obesity hypoventilation with pH <7.35, pCO_2 >6.5 and RR >23
- Cardiogenic pulmonary oedema unresponsive to CPAP

Absolute exclusion criteria

- Severe facial deformity
- Facial burns
- Fixed upper airway obstruction

Relative exclusion criteria (NIV may still be suitable if considered to be the patient's ceiling of care)

- pH <7.15
- GCS <8, confusion or agitation
- Pneumothorax without a chest drain
- Recent facial, oesophageal or gastric surgery
- Uncontrolled vomiting
- Bowel obstruction
- Respiratory arrest

Commence NIV starting with 4 cmH$_2$O expiratory PAP (EPAP) and 10 cmH$_2$O inspiratory PAP (IPAP)

Increase IPAP slowly in 2 cmH$_2$O increments (up to a maximum of 25 cmH$_2$O) to obtain inspiratory time <33% of total respiratory time (Ti TOT)

There is hypoxia, diffuse lung inflammation and decreased lung compliance. Examples of typical triggering events include:

- Sepsis
- Trauma
- Pancreatitis
- Transfusion
- Drowning or aspiration
- Burns

Management involves treated the underlying cause and usually admission to ICU for intubation and ventilation. Patients are typically ventilated with low tidal volumes, to prevent overdistension of lungs and further injury, so a degree of hypercapnia is permitted.

Foreign bodies in the lower airways

Sudden onset of coughing and wheezing may accompany aspiration of a foreign body into the lower airways. The right main, intermediate or lower bronchi are the most likely sites for obstruction to occur. Peanuts and toy fragments are the most commonly inhaled objects in children; bony food particles, broken teeth and small dental instruments predominate in adults. The presence of a unilateral wheeze, recurrent infection or other atypical symptoms and signs may suggest the possibility of an intrathoracic foreign body.

XR Chest X-rays detect <20% of foreign bodies, but may reveal indirect findings in about 40% of the cases, such as hyperinflation. CT remains the ideal test when suspected.

TX All patients with confirmed foreign body should be referred for bronchoscopy.

Foreign bodies in the oesophagus and gastrointestinal tract → p. 437.
Foreign bodies in the upper airways → p. 206.

Asthma in adults

Asthma continues to be a major health problem in the UK, 8 million people, or 12% of the population. It is responsible for the deaths of around 1200 people each year. Patients with severe asthma and one or more adverse risk factors have a higher risk of death. *For risk factors for developing near fatal or fatal asthma → Box 13.5.* However, around 90% of asthma attacks that are severe enough to require admission to hospital develop relatively slowly over a period of 6 hours or more. Therefore, there is usually enough time for effective action.

The clinical features of asthma result from a reversible inflammatory obstruction of the lower airways, which has three main components:

1 Hyperreactivity and spasm of the bronchial smooth muscle
2 Oedema of the walls of the bronchi
3 Increased production and retention of secretions.

Asthma is caused by a type 1 hypersensitivity, or IgE-mediated response to a wide variety of substances, commonly house-dust mite faeces and pollen. A viral infection is a common trigger for an acute exacerbation; exercise is responsible for around 40% of attacks. Thunderstorm asthma is a phenomenon where the air flow and pressure changes during a thunderstorm cause pollen and fungal particles to be broken up leading to multiple attendances shortness of breath in patients with asthma and hay-fever.

> A pneumothorax may occasionally be the cause of an acute deterioration.

 Box 13.5 **Patients at risk of developing fatal or near fatal asthma**

Patients with a combination of one or more indicators of severe asthma:

- Previous near fatal asthma (e.g. required ventilation or had respiratory acidosis)
- Previous admission for asthma (especially if in the last year)
- Repeated attendances at ED for asthma (especially if in the last year)
- Asthma treatment requiring three or more classes of medication
- Heavy use of β_2 agonists

And one or more adverse risk factors:

- Non-adherence with treatment and monitoring
- Self-discharge from hospital
- Psychiatric illness including depression and self-harm
- Current or recent major tranquilliser usage
- Alcohol or drug abuse
- Learning difficulties
- History of abuse in childhood
- Employment and income problems
- Severe domestic, marital or legal stress
- Social isolation
- Denial of illness
- Obesity

Dyspnoea and wheezing are the predominant features. Bronchodilators may control these symptoms, but it is steroids that modify the underlying inflammatory processes.

Ask about

- When this attack started
- Improvement or deterioration in symptoms
- The patient's assessment of severity
- What triggers an attack and how often
- Recent hospital admissions
- Any ICU admission
- Why this time was chosen to come to hospital; this is an important discriminator when considering discharge
- Previous and current drug use, especially steroids and theophyllines
- Other conditions, including upper respiratory tract infections and pregnancy.

If nebulised drugs were given before hospital arrival by the paramedics, precise details and initial peak flow rate should be noted.

Examination begins while taking the history and setting up the nebuliser.

Look for

- Difficulty with speech – spontaneous sentences or single words?
- Reduced peak expiratory flow rate (PEFR). *For predicted values of PEFR for adults → Figure 13.3 and Box 13.6*
- Tachycardia and tachypnoea
- Indrawing of ribs, flaring of nostrils and use of accessory muscles
- Signs of pneumothorax
- Poor audible air entry
- Agitation, confusion or drowsiness
- Exhaustion
- Pyrexia
- Cyanosis.

> Less wheezing than expected on auscultation may indicate less air movement, not less asthma.

Box 13.6 Predicted peak expiratory flow rates for adults of average height (in L/min)

Age (years)	15	20	30	40	50	60	70
Male		550	590	630	630	610	580	540
Female		460	480	500	480	460	430	410

The standard deviation (SD) of these values is 48 L/min for men and 42 L/min for women. Values of PEFR up to 2 SD less than predicted are within normal limits.

Investigations in asthma

Chest X-ray is not indicated routinely in acute asthma. It should be requested only in cases of suspected pneumothorax, pneumomediastinum, pneumonic consolidation or inhaled foreign body. Patients with life-threatening asthma or failure to respond to treatment will also require a chest X-ray.

Arterial blood gas analysis is required only in patients with features of life-threatening asthma and in those with an SaO_2 (on pulse oximetry) <92%. There is usually a low $PaCO_2$ due to hyperventilation and a low PaO_2 caused by ventilation–perfusion mismatch. A normal $PaCO_2$ is worrying and a high $PaCO_2$ (>40–45 mmHg or 5.3–6.0 kPa) indicates respiratory muscle fatigue and impending respiratory arrest. Electrolyte estimation is important as hypokalaemia can occur. A raised white cell count is to be expected with catecholamine release and steroid therapy. Theophylline levels can be measured in patients who are taking regular methylxanthines at home.

The PEFR should be measured in all patients and used as a guide to treatment. PEFR expressed as a percentage of the patient's previous best value is the most useful clinical parameter. In its absence, PEFR expressed as a percentage of the patient's predicted value is a reasonable guide. *For predicted values of PEFR for adults → Figure 13.3 and Box 13.6.*

Life-threatening asthma (PEFR 33% of best or predicted)

Features include:

- altered conscious level
- silent chest
- cyanosis

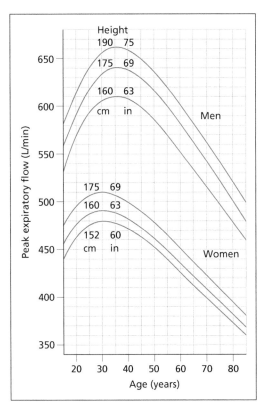

Figure 13.3 Predicted peak expiratory flow rates in adults.

- poor respiratory effort
- arrythmia
- hypotension
- exhaustion.

Pulse oximetry and arterial blood gas analysis show:

- $SaO_2 < 92\%$
- $PaCO_2$ within the normal range of 4.6–6.0 kPa (35–45 mmHg) – higher than this is considered 'near fatal' asthma
- $PaO_2 < 8$ kPa (60 mmHg) irrespective of oxygen therapy

Tx

- Obtain anaesthetic/intensive care help immediately in life-threatening asthma.
- Give a high concentration of oxygen (at least 60%) via a well-fitting facemask. The aim is to keep the SaO_2 between 94% and 98%.
- Monitor SaO_2, ECG and BP.
- Give salbutamol 5 mg (or terbutaline 10 mg) nebulised by oxygen with a flow rate of at least 6 L/min. Add ipratropium 500 mcg to the same nebuliser. (This anticholinergic drug has been shown to produce additional bronchodilatation to that produced by β_2 agonists alone, leading to faster recovery times and shorter durations of admission.)
- Give prednisolone 40–50 mg by mouth. If the patient cannot swallow oral medication or is vomiting, give IV hydrocortisone 100–200 mg 6-hourly. (Prednisolone 10 mg is roughly equivalent to hydrocortisone 40 mg.) Steroids should be continued for at least 5 days or until full recovery.
- Repeat the salbutamol/terbutaline after 15 min. (The β_2 agonists can be administered almost continuously; the ipratropium may be repeated at 4–6 hour intervals.)
- Give a single dose of magnesium sulphate 2 g by IV infusion over 20 min. *For further information on magnesium → p. 261.*
- Consider the use of IV salbutamol 200 mcg or IV terbutaline 250 mcg (given slowly over 10 min) for those patients in whom inhaled therapy cannot be used reliably.
- Consider (after consultation with a senior) the use of IV aminophylline. This may benefit occasional patients with life-threatening asthma who are resistant to standard therapies. A loading dose of 5 mg/kg is given over 20 min with ECG monitoring. This is followed by an infusion of aminophylline of 0.5–0.7 mg/kg per hour. The loading dose is omitted in patients who are already taking oral methylxanthines.

Failure to recognise and act on the need for ventilation is the main preventable cause of death in asthma.

Intubation and ventilation may be required. All patients who are failing to respond to treatment should be referred to ICU. This includes patients with worsening PEFR, deteriorating blood gases or acidosis, exhaustion, confusion or drowsiness. Some evidence suggests that IV ketamine is a useful adjunct/induction agent as it has some bronchodilating properties.

Ventilating a patient with severe asthma can be difficult. Patients can develop hyperinflation or 'air trapping' and barotrauma such as pneumothorax. Intubation should not be delayed, however, in the unconscious patient or those with poor respiratory effort. Hypoxic brain injury occurs in as little as 4 minutes!

IM and IV adrenaline is often used in a critical situations, as there is some evidence that a proportion of critically unwell patients with 'acute asthma' actually have anaphylaxis →*see Box 13.7 differential diagnosis of wheeze.*

Despite theoretical reasons for its efficacy, Heliox (helium and oxygen mixture in a 70:30 ratio) has not been shown to be of conclusive benefit in asthma. Similarly, non-invasive ventilation (NIV) is not recommended for the unstable patient with acute asthma.

Severe asthma (PEFR between 33% and 50% of best or predicted)

Features include:

- inability to complete a sentence in one breath
- respiratory rate ≥25 breaths/min
- pulse rate ≥110/min.

 Box 13.7 Differential diagnosis of wheeze

- Asthma
- COPD
- Anaphylaxis
- Foreign body
- Vocal cord problems (or may cause stridor)
- External compression of bronchi (e.g. lymph node, goitre or tumour)
- Heart failure
- Eosinophilic granulomatosis with polyangiitis (EGPA)
- Gastro-oesophgeal reflux
- Bronchitis and bronchiolitis
- Inhalation injury (chemical or gastric contents)
- Loeffler syndrome (typically presents with transient radiographic infiltrates and an elevated eosinophil count due to hypersensitivity to helminth infection)
- Carcinoid syndrome (facial flushing, diarrhoea, tachycardia)
- Scombroid poisoning

Tx The patient should be treated as described for life-threatening asthma above, although IV magnesium should be given only if there is a poor response to inhaled bronchodilators. Aminophylline is unlikely to be considered. Admission is required to an area with monitored beds.

Moderate asthma (PEF between 50% and 75% of best or predicted)

The patient can finish a sentence and has no features of severe asthma.

Tx
- Give salbutamol 6–10 puffs using an inhaler and large volume spacer and give prednisolone 40–50 mg orally
- Wait 15–30 min after the initial treatment and then repeat the PEFR.
- If the patient is worse and PEFR <50% treat as severe asthma. If better and PEFR >75% consider discharge (→ below). If PEFR is still between 50% and 75% repeat the salbutamol.
- If repeated doses of β_2 agonist have been needed, the patient should be observed until doses can be spaced at least 4 hours apart.

Mild asthma (PEFR >75% best or predicted)

- The patient can talk normally.

Tx The patient should be given his or her usual bronchodilator and then kept under observation for at least 30–60 min. If the PEFR remains >75% consider discharge (→later). If the PEFR falls, treat as described in the appropriate section above.

Asthma in pregnancy

The physiological changes in pregnancy can be associated with a worsening or improvement of asthma symptoms. Uncontrolled asthma is associated with maternal and foetal complications so acute severe asthma is pregnancy should be treated vigorously. Give drug therapy as per non-pregnant patients, including steroids and magnesium. Obstetric review and continual foetal monitoring are recommended for pregnant women with acute severe asthma.

Discharge of a patient with asthma

Most patients who are sufficiently ill to request emergency help with their chronic condition will require oral steroids (as well as inhaled steroids and bronchodilators as part of a long-term management plan). Prednisolone 40–50 mg given orally for 5 days is usually adequate.

> Around 15% of patients with asthma who are discharged from hospital reattend within 2 weeks.

Advise patients on how frequently to use their β_2 agonist and when to seek help. Printed leaflets are perfect for this purpose. Patients who return to the ED after discharge should be automatically admitted. The patient's GP should be informed of the attendance and arrangements made for primary care follow-up within 48 hours.

Asthma in children aged <5 years → p. 351.
Predischarge checklist for moderate and mild asthma →
  Box 13.8.

Acute exacerbations of chronic obstructive pulmonary disease

Chronic obstructive pulmonary disease (COPD) is the fifth biggest cause of mortality in the UK and is responsible for millions of lost working days and a huge amount

 Box 13.8 Predischarge checklist for moderate and mild asthma

Mild–moderate asthma
- The patient is stable over at least 1 hour of observation
- The PEFR is at least 75% of normal for the patient
- The patient has both oral steroids and inhaled bronchodilators to take home
- The patient understands his or her condition and treatment and can use the inhalers satisfactorily
- Follow-up is arranged (e.g. by the GP within 48 hour)
- There is good home support

Relative contraindications to discharge of a patient with asthma
- Remaining significant symptoms
- Concerns about compliance
- Psychological problems or learning difficulties
- Poor social circumstances or lives alone
- Presentation at night
- Previous ICU admission for asthma
- Previous severe attacks needing hospitalisation
- Already on steroids
- Pregnancy
- Drug-induced attack

of suffering. It is characterised by reduced respiratory function due to a combination of destruction of alveoli (emphysema) and obstruction of bronchioles by a chronic inflammatory process (bronchitis). The airflow obstruction is usually progressive, not fully reversible and relatively unchanged over a period of several months. Most patients have a chronic productive cough, which is worse in winter. There is no single diagnostic test for COPD, but airflow obstruction is suggested by a forced expiratory volume in 1 second (FEV_1) of <80% of the predicted value for that patient or a FEV_1/FVC (forced vital capacity) ratio below 0.7.

Patients with COPD have varying combinations of chronic bronchitis and emphysema. However, the two classic descriptions of 'blue bloaters' and 'pink puffers' does not accurately describe the spectrum of lung pathologies. Instead, it is thought that COPD represents a variety of different phenotypical responses to inhaled toxins such as cigarette smoke. Defining and recognising these phenotypes can help direct ongoing management of patients, for instance, those with 'asthma-COPD overlap' phenotype respond well to corticosteroids, whereas management for the 'frequent exacerbator' will focus on long term anti-inflammatory treatments.

Acute deterioration that precipitates ED attendance is usually associated with:

- increased dyspnoea
- purulent sputum
- increased sputum volume.

This is frequently the result of superadded infection. Other causes include chest injury, inappropriate sedation and uncontrolled oxygen therapy. A cough fracture may also precipitate deterioration.

Exhaustion is a common feature, with the patient sitting up using accessory muscles of respiration. Confusion and shortness of breath may make a detailed history difficult to obtain.

> The risk of dying from an exacerbation of COPD is closely related to the development of a respiratory acidosis, the presence of other serious illnesses and the need for ventilatory support.

Cor pulmonale is suggested by the combination of peripheral oedema, raised venous pressure, a systolic parasternal heave and a loud pulmonary second heart sound.

Investigations:
- Pulse oximetry will demonstrate a low oxygen saturation in most patients with COPD. Some patients may have a resting SaO_2 <90% even when stable.

- Analysis of blood gases will usually confirm hypoxia with rising hypercapnia and respiratory acidosis. The blood gas analysis should be repeated after 30–60 min of treatment.
- Full blood count, electrolytes, chest X-ray and ECG must be obtained together with the past medical notes.
- Plasma theophylline levels should be measured in all patients who are taking regular methylxanthines.
- Sputum should be sent for microscopy and culture in patients with purulent sputum
- Take blood cultures in patients with pyrexia or sepsis.

Tx

Immediate treatment: the patient should be sat up and given controlled oxygen by facemask to keep the SaO_2 around 90% ($\rightarrow$ Box 13.2 – oxygen delivery systems).

Bronchodilators: Nebulised β_2-adrenoceptor agonists (salbutamol 5 mg or terbutaline 10 mg), will treat any reversible element of the COPD and can be repeated similarly to asthma. Nebulised ipratropium bromide 500 mcg is also helpful. This antimuscarinic bronchodilator has a delayed onset of action of up to 30 min but lasts for 3–6 hours. If the patient is hypercapnic or acidotic, the nebuliser should be given with air.

After consultation with senior staff, IV aminophylline may be considered for patients who have a poor response to nebulised bronchodilators. A loading dose of 5 mg/kg is given over 20 min, followed by an infusion of aminophylline of 500 mcg/kg per hour. Take great care if using aminophylline in patients who are already taking oral methylxanthines at home and check interactions with their other medications.

Oxygen: the administration of a high concentration of oxygen in patients with COPD may cause respiratory depression, CO_2 narcosis and coma. It used to be said that the normal hypercapnic drive to breathe could be abolished by chronic hypercapnia and the theory ran that the patient was then reliant on the less sensitive hypoxic drive to stimulate respiratory effort.

In actual fact, the clinical deterioration that may follow oxygen therapy is almost certainly due to ventilation/perfusion mismatch and the Haldane effect:

- Usually, the capillaries vasoconstrict around poorly ventilated alveoli to divert blood to well ventilated alveoli where carbon dioxide can be removed. Applying high flow oxygen will cause these capillaries to dilate, but the deoxygenated blood that passes through will not be ridded of its CO_2.
- Chronically desaturated haemoglobin can carry more CO_2, so if provided with excessive oxygen, the Hb becomes saturated and cannot transport as much CO_2 which is then carried freely in the plasma, decreasing the pH.

The bottom line is this; hypoxia kills patients, so give oxygen then review and monitor regularly. For most patients with COPD, the target should be SaO_2 of between 88% and 92%.

Steroids: it is now recognised that almost all patients with an acute exacerbation of COPD benefit from high-dose steroids (prednisolone 30 mg daily) for 5–7 days. For patients who are unable to take tablets in the ED, IV hydrocortisone 100 mg should be given.

Antibiotics: In the presence of purulent sputum, anti-bacterial therapy is required. *Haemophilus influenzae, Streptococcus pneumoniae* and *Moraxella catarrhalis* are typical pathogens in COPD and so amoxicillin or doxycycline are suitable first-line antibiotics. Patients with consolidation on chest X-ray should be treated as pneumonia (→ p. 220).

Admission to hospital: the decision to admit a patient with COPD to hospital depends on a variety of both clinical and social factors as well as the availability of a specialist home-based care team. *For factors that suggest that a patient with an exacerbation of COPD should be admitted to hospital → Box 13.9.*

Respiratory support: subsequent therapy depends on the clinical findings, further history and the results of blood gas analysis. The presence of an acidosis (pH <7.35) is usually a bad sign and is now regarded as an indication for non-invasive ventilation (NIV) (→ Box 13.16). The respiratory stimulant, doxapram, is occasionally used if NIV is unavailable. If the pH falls to <7.25 or the $PaCO_2$ rises to >80 mmHg (10.6 kPa), or if the patient becomes drowsy or exhausted, ICU specialists should be involved with a view to instituting intubation and intermittent positive-pressure ventilation (IPPV).

Box 13.9 Factors that suggest that a patient with COPD should be admitted to hospital

- Difficulty coping at home, living alone or in poor social circumstances
- Poor or deteriorating general health
- Poor activity or confined to bed
- On long-term oxygen therapy
- Significant co-morbidity (especially cardiac disease and type 1 diabetes)
- Rapid rate of onset of exacerbation
- Severe breathlessness or cyanosis
- Worsening peripheral oedema
- Acute confusion or otherwise impaired level of consciousness
- SaO_2 <90%, pH <7.35 or PaO_2 <7 kPa
- Chest X-ray changes suggestive of infection or other new pathology

---

Decision making:

In patients with severe and end-stage COPD, intubation and admission to ICU is unlikely to be in their best interests, as they would be subjected to prolonged suffering without promise of a meaningful quality of life or survival at the end. An important part of the ED clinician's job here is to gather information about the patient's wishes as well as their baseline function and frailty score. One should discuss with the patient and their family about the possibility, if NIV does not provide any improvement, that end of life care and symptomatic relief will be offered. Many patients are absolutely clear that their wish is to avoid further episodes of NIV or ventilation, and they should be supported in this decision.

Bronchiolitis in children → p. 350.
Respiratory failure → p. 211.

Acute exacerbations of bronchiectasis

Around 1 in 1000 adults in the UK has bronchiectasis, often as a result of childhood infections, cystic fibrosis, immunodeficiency or rheumatoid disease. However, in 50% of patients, no cause or associated condition is found. It is believed that the bronchi are dilated and destroyed by a cycle of recurrent infection, inflammation, excessive production of mucus and reduced mucus clearance. Patients have chronic symptoms of dyspnoea and a productive cough; their sputum is mucopurulent. Some patients may present to an ED with an acute exacerbation, usually brought about by infection. Symptoms include worsening breathlessness, increased coughing and sputum production, haemoptysis (usually not severe), chest pain, fever, malaise and lethargy. Chest signs may be minimal; low-pitched crackles may be heard. In severe disease, finger clubbing and respiratory failure are seen.

Ix: Chest X-ray shows the characteristic changes of bronchiectasis in only 50% of patients:

- Thickened bronchial walls seen as parallel 'tramlines' or ring-shaped opacities
- Cystic lesions with fluid levels
- Areas of collapse and scarring.

Send sputum samples for culture.

Tx Treatment includes oxygen, nebulised saline, physiotherapy (postural drainage and percussion) and antibiotics. If likely pathogens are not known from previous sputum cultures, amoxicillin 500 mg three times daily is given for 14 days. For more severe exacerbations, blind prescription of broad-spectrum anti-pseudomonal antibiotics should be considered. Intubation and ventilation may be required. Excessive secretions tend to limit the effectiveness of non-invasive ventilation (NIV) in bronchiectasis, but it can be warranted in patients who are fatigued with respiratory failure.

Interstitial lung disease

ILD refers to more than 200 chronic lung disorders which have thickening of the lung interstitium as the common factor. The most common types are idiopathic pulmonary fibrosis (IPF) and sarcoidosis. IPF has a very poor prognosis, with a mean survival of 3 years from diagnosis. Acute dyspnoea in a patient with ILD is commonly due to:

- Infection
- Pulmonary embolism (PE): (patients with ILD have a higher risk than those with cancer)
- Pulmonary hypertension (→ p. 231)
- Congestive heart failure
- Diffuse alveolar haemorrhage
- Pneumothorax

Chest X-ray often shows diffuse ground glass abnormalities, which makes the diagnosis of new changes quite difficult, hence CT scan is often used to evaluate for consolidation, PE and new malignancy.

At the point of needing intubation and ventilation, these patients usually have a very poor prognosis and are unlikely to survive an ICU admission. The treatment will involve supplemental O_2, antibiotics, steroids (depending on the cause of ILD) and sometimes a trial of NIV.

Pulmonary oedema

Fluid may collect in the lung tissue for a variety of reasons, the most common being left ventricular failure (LVF). Pulmonary oedema may also be associated with the following:

1 Over-transfusion and excessive fluid therapy
2 Smoke and other noxious gas inhalation (→ p. 141 and 303)
3 Acute traumatic brain injury (neurogenic pulmonary oedema → p. 38)
4 Intracranial haemorrhage (neurogenic pulmonary oedema → p. 238)
5 Shock from any cause (acute respiratory distress syndrome ARDS → p. 212)
6 Ascents to high altitudes (→ p. 247).

Acute pulmonary oedema causes symptoms and signs of hypoxia:

- Rapidly increasing shortness of breath, which is worse on lying down
- Tachypnoea and laboured breathing (stiff waterlogged lungs)
- Pallor and sweating: ECG stickers and cannula dressings may not stick
- Tachycardia

- Anxiety and distress
- Depression of consciousness (mostly caused by CO_2 narcosis).

The hypoxia leads to a vicious cycle of worsening myocardial performance and increasing oedema. On auscultation there are widespread crackles. These make the diagnostic gallop rhythm difficult to hear. Classic pink, frothy sputum is uncommon. Peripheral oedema and a raised jugular venous pressure (JVP) indicate associated right heart failure. There may be a history of ischaemic heart disease, orthopnoea or paroxysmal nocturnal dyspnoea. Chest pain results from either angina secondary to the hypoxia or from a myocardial infarction (MI) that precipitated the LVF.

'Cardiac asthma' describes the wheeze that these patients may develop if oedema causes significant airway obstruction.

Ix: Arterial blood gases will show a variable degree of hypoxia, hypercapnia and acidosis.

B-type natriuretic peptide (BNP) is a cardiac hormone produced by the heart in response to ventricular stretching. BNP can be used to help differentiate cardiac failure from COPD and other causes of dyspnoea. A BNP level <100 ng/L (NT proBNP <300 ng/L) rules out acute heart failure as a cause.

Point of care ultrasound (POCUS) of the lung fields will reveal 'B-lines' suggestive of the presence of interstitial pulmonary fluid. *Radiological changes in pulmonary oedema → Box 13.10 and Figure 13.4.*

Tx

- Sit the patient up, if possible.
- Give a high concentration of oxygen by mask or via a continuous positive airway pressure (CPAP) circuit at 5 cmH₂O pressure initially (→ *below*).
- Establish IV access and take blood gases.

> **Box 13.10 Radiological changes in pulmonary oedema**
>
> - Widened vascular markings in the upper lung fields due to diversion of blood (upper lobe diversion)
> - Air bronchogram
> - A widened mediastinum with spreading (bat's wing) shadows
> - Horizontal lines in the lower lobes (Kerley B lines)
> - Small pleural effusions
> - Cotton-wool shadows throughout the lung fields
> - Cardiomegaly

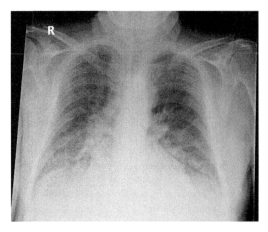

Figure 13.4 Chest radiography in pulmonary oedema – portable, erect AP film.

- Start monitoring SaO_2, ECG and BP.
- Request a chest X-ray and ECG.
- Treat acute arrhythmias ($\rightarrow$ *p. 172*).
- If the patient has a history of fluid retention or weight gain, give IV furosemide in 20–40 mg boluses and consider the need for a urinary catheter.
- Start nitrate therapy to further reduce venous return. Several alternative routes are effective ($\rightarrow$ *Boxes 13.11 and 13.12*). GTN must be used with care because it may worsen hypotension and tachycardia.
- Avoid opiates – which can worsen outcomes, in the acute phase.
- If the patient has low blood pressure, treat for cardiogenic shock ($\rightarrow$ *p. 251*)

Intubation and positive-pressure ventilation (IPPV) may be required in a rapidly deteriorating patient.
CPAP and NIV: in acute pulmonary oedema, CPAP and NIV (BPAP) help to alleviate respiratory distress and improve outcomes. They work in several ways:

- Positive airway pressure restores functional residual capacity by improving alveolar recruitment and splinting.
- Increased intrathoracic pressure reduces preload by decreasing venous return.

 Box 13.11 Alternative routes for GTN administration in LVF

1 GTN spray one to two puffs (= 400–800 mcg) or equivalent tablet sublingually, followed by a GTN 10 mg transdermal patch
2 GTN 5 mg buccal tablet, followed by a second tablet in the opposite buccal sulcus, if necessary, after 3–5 min
3 GTN infusion 10–200 mcg/min $\rightarrow$ *Box 13.12*

 Box 13.12 Intravenous infusion of GTN

- Make 50 mg of GTN solution up to 50 mL with 0.9% saline in a large syringe in an infusion pump (i.e. mix a 1 mg/mL solution).
- The IV dose of GTN is from 0.6 mg/h to 12 mg/h (equivalent to 10–200 mcg/min)
- Start the infusion at 1.5–3.0 mL/h and adjust this dose by a factor of two every 15–30 min according to the patient's clinical condition

---

- Afterload is lowered by increasing the pressure gradient between the left ventricle and the systemic circulation, which may contribute to an increase in stroke volume.
- NIV can improve hypercapnia in patients with type 2 respiratory failure

NIV $\rightarrow$ Box 13.4 on p. 212.

Pneumonia

This is the most common serious infection seen in adults in the ED and may be fatal even in people who have been previously healthy. Complications include sepsis, lung abscess, empyema and respiratory failure. The outcome is greatly improved by early treatment with appropriate antibiotics. The patient with pneumonia presents with a short history of fever and productive cough ('rusty' sputum with *Streptococcus pneumoniae* infection). There may be tachycardia, shortness of breath and pleuritic chest pain. Findings on examination vary from obvious lobar consolidation to minimal crepitations. Symptoms may be less specific in elderly people, such as lethargy and confusion. Children may present with abdominal pain ($\rightarrow$ *p. 353*). Pneumonia is defined as severe (with a mortality rate in excess of 10%) if two or more of the following 'CURB 65' criteria are present:

- **C**: new confusion
- **U**: urea >7 mmol/L.
- **R**: respiratory rate >30 breaths/min
- **B**: systolic BP <90 mmHg or diastolic BP <60 mmHg
- **65**: age >65 years.

This is used to predict mortality and thus suggest the need for admission. It can also be used to guide the prescription of antibiotics. The risk of death rises to 40–60% in patients with scores of four or five.

Patients with diffuse or bilateral changes on chest X-ray should be admitted and treated aggressively even if their CURB-65 score is 0.

Community-acquired pneumonia

The most common pathogens isolated in community acquired pneumonia are *S. pneumoniae* and *Haemophilus influenzae*, however, in most patients no pathogen is found. TB and AIDS may both present as an acute community-acquired pneumonia.

Acute infection complicating COPD → p. 216.
HIV infection → p. 337.
Legionnaires' disease → p. 223.
Pneumonia in children → p. 353.
Atypical pathogens → p. 223.
TB → p. 225.

Patients at an increased risk of pneumococcal infection

Patients who have had a splenectomy, no matter how long ago, are at a high risk of developing overwhelming pneumococcal infection. Similarly, some other conditions may cause a functional hyposplenism:

- Sickle cell disease and thalassaemia
- Coeliac disease
- Systemic lupus erythematosus
- Lymphoma and leukaemia
- Other immunodeficiencies.

Such patients should have received pneumococcal vaccine and must be regarded with a high level of suspicion whenever they develop a pyrexia or acute respiratory symptoms.

Investigations: A chest X-ray may show a variable picture; a classic lobar atelectasis is unusual. *For the appearances of lobar collapse-consolidation on chest X-ray → Figures 13.5, 13.6 and 13.7.* Identification of the causative organism will be aided by the cultures of blood (taken before the administration of antibiotics) and sputum and pneumococcal and legionella urinary antigen tests. Blood specimens should also be taken for a full blood count, blood chemistry, C-reactive protein and arterial blood gases. Consider testing for HIV (→ p. 337).

Tx

- Sit the patient up and give a high concentration of humidified oxygen.
- Start IV rehydration.
- Monitor SaO_2, ECG and BP.
- Consider immediate transfer to the ICU if the PaO_2 cannot be maintained above 60 mmHg (8 kPa). (This level of desaturation is regarded as respiratory failure → p. 211.)
- Give antibiotics based on CURB-65 score and local guidelines. In patients who do not have signs of severe sepsis (→p. 250) await radiological confirmation of the diagnosis prior to starting antibiotics.

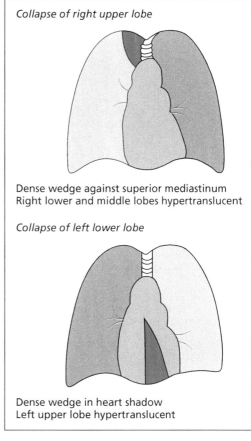

Collapse of right upper lobe

Dense wedge against superior mediastinum
Right lower and middle lobes hypertranslucent

Collapse of left lower lobe

Dense wedge in heart shadow
Left upper lobe hypertranslucent

Figure 13.5 Appearance of lobar collapse on a chest X-ray.

- If the infection is not severe and the patient has not been previously treated in the community, amoxicillin 500 mg–1 g three times daily by mouth (for 7 days) is an appropriate antibiotic. For patients who are allergic to penicillins, clarithromycin or doxycycline can be used.
- All patients with a severe community-acquired pneumonia (*CURB-65 of ≥2*) should be given IV co-amoxiclav 1.2 g three times daily with IV clarithromycin 1 g twice daily from the first presentation for 7–10 days.
- Prescribe analgesia for pleuritic chest pain.

Almost all patients who present to hospital with pneumonia will require admission, but in those who appear well, with no hypoxia or tachycardia, a CURB-65 score of 0 and no unstable co-morbidities, discharge home may be appropriate. Remember to give smoking cessation advice to those who smoke.

Patients with consolidation on chest X-ray should have a follow up X-ray in 6–8 weeks to check for resolution and ensure that the opacities are not due to underlying malignancy.

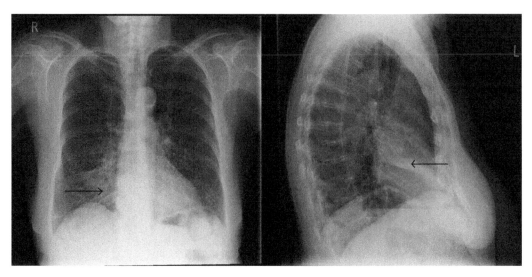

Figure 13.6 Radiological appearances of right middle lobe collapse on AP and lateral films.

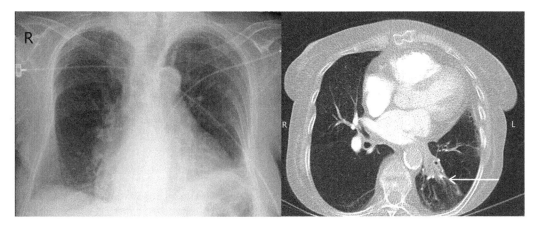

Figure 13.7 Subtle chest X-ray appearance of consolidation behind cardiac shadow, demonstrated more clearly on CT thorax.

Explain to patients that after starting treatment they should steadily improve but should return to ED should they feel more unwell or dyspnoeic. Most people can expect that by:

- 1 week: fever has resolved
- 4 weeks: chest pain and sputum production have reduced
- 6 weeks: cough and shortness of breath have improved
- 3 months: respiratory symptoms have resolved but fatigue may persist
- 6 months: should feel back to normal

Hospital-acquired pneumonia This is defined as a pneumonia that occurs after at least 48 hours in hospital and so should not usually present to ED. However, patients may present from institutions such as nursing homes where hospital-type opportunistic organisms are found. A wide variety of pathogens are causal including Gram-negative bacilli and *S. pneumoniae*. Early-onset hospital-acquired pneumonia (i.e. occurring within 5 days of admission) can be treated with co-amoxiclav. Late-onset infection requires an anti-pseudomonal penicillin combination (e.g. piperacillin with tazobactam) or a quinolone (e.g. ciprofloxacin).

Atypical pathogens are characterised as those which are difficult to diagnose and do not respond to usual first-line antibiotics for community-acquired pneumonia. Treatment is with clarithromycin or doxycycline.

- **Mycoplasma pneumoniae**: epidemics spanning three winters occur every 4 years in the UK. Extra-pulmonary manifestations of mycoplasma infection include skin rashes, musculoskeletal pain, gastrointestinal upset, haemolytic anaemia and neurological disease.
- **Chlamydia pneumoniae**: tends to occur in outbreaks within closed communities
- **Chlamydia psittaci:** infection is acquired from birds and animals, but human-to-human spread may occur
- **Coxiella burnetii ('Q fever')**: cases frequently occur in April to June related to lambing and calving season. Outbreaks occur in relation to animal exposure but <10% of patients had occupational exposure. Q fever in pregnancy, whether symptomatic or asymptomatic, may result in miscarriage or adverse pregnancy outcomes.

Pneumocystis jirovecii pneumonia (formerly known as *Pneumocystis carinii* pneumonia or PCP – this acronym is still in use) is a fungal infection frequently associated with HIV (→ *p. 337*). The chest X-ray shows diffuse, bilateral interstitial changes. The diagnosis may be confirmed by culture of sputum or broncho-alveolar lavage specimens. PCP is treated with co-trimoxazole 120 mg/kg per day in two to four divided doses either by mouth or intravenously.

Aspiration pneumonia is associated with impaired airway reflexes from a wide variety of causes including depressed consciousness, neurological disease and general debilitation. Radiographic changes are often inconclusive or delayed for several hours after aspiration. Consolidation appears most usually in the right upper or middle zones. Pathogens in this situation include *S. pneumoniae*, *Klebsiella pneumoniae* and anaerobic bacteria. IV co-amoxiclav 1.2 g 3 times daily is recommended.

Clearance and protection of the airway → pp. 2 and 205.
Prophylaxis of gastric acid aspiration in pregnant patients with major trauma → p. 32.
Respiratory failure → p. 211.

Legionnaires' disease is caused by infection with the Gram-negative organism *Legionella pneumophila*, which is harboured in institutional water systems. The disease is spread by airborne droplets, most commonly to middle-aged men in warm conditions. There may be a history of a recent stay in a hotel, hospital or travel abroad. Legionnaires' disease starts with a flu-like illness and then develops into a severe chest infection, often with accompanying gastrointestinal features. Symptoms and signs include:

- fever and rigours
- pleurisy and haemoptysis
- abdominal pain, diarrhoea and vomiting
- a relative bradycardia.

Ix: These may reveal:

- raised WCC with neutrophilia and lymphopenia
- low plasma sodium (<130 mmol/L)
- proteinuria and haematuria
- unilateral patchy shadowing (often confined to a lower lobe) and pleural effusions on chest X-ray.

The specific urinary antigen test is diagnostic (although the result is not available immediately).

Tx Oral or IV fluoroquinolone is the first-line antibiotic, e.g. ciprofloxacin 500 mg twice daily. Ten or more days' treatment may be required. Legionnaires' disease is notifiable in the UK (except in Scotland).

Covid-19

Covid-19 is the illness associated with the novel coronavirus known as severe acute respiratory syndrome coronavirus 2 (SARS-CoV-2). The virus was first seen during an outbreak of respiratory illness in the Wuhan area of China in November–December 2019. Cases continued to spread outside of the area and then throughout the world. As worldwide case numbers increased, the World Health Organisation (WHO) declared a pandemic on 11 March 2020. By the end of 2022, there had been over 649 million cases and 6.6 million deaths globally.

Scientific consensus is that SARS-CoV-2 is zoonotic in origin; however, the source of the original outbreak is yet to be conclusively determined. The first dose of vaccine outside of a clinical trial was given on 8 December 2020, to a 90-year-old woman in the UK. Since then, over 13 billion doses have been given worldwide.

Symptoms of Covid-19 infection are:

- Fever
- Cough
- Fatigue
- Loss of taste and smell
- Conjunctivitis
- Sore throat
- Headache
- Muscle and joint pains
- Rashes
- Nausea, vomiting and diarrhoea.

Transmission is through infectious respiratory particles. The main complications of Covid-19 are 'Covid pneumonitis' or acute respiratory distress syndrome (ARDS), thromboembolism and post-covid-19 syndrome ('long covid'). People aged 60 years and over, and those with underlying medical problems like high blood pressure, heart and lung problems, diabetes, obesity or cancer, are at higher risk of developing serious illness. Approximately 15% of patients require oxygen and 5% need intensive care, although this has changed with different variants of the virus.

Severe respiratory disease usually presents with breathlessness and low SaO_2, around 7–10 days after the onset of the above symptoms. Tissue samples of affected lungs show diffuse alveolar damage, consistent with ARDS but with a higher thrombus burden in pulmonary capillaries.

In children, a rare complication is a severe inflammatory syndrome a few weeks after infection (PIMS-TS). This is thought to be a form of vasculitis, and symptoms overlap with Kawasaki disease. Patients present with a persistent fever and a range of other symptoms including abdominal pain.

Ix: Infection can be detected in nasal and throat swabs by bedside antigen tests (lateral flow test) and laboratory PCR testing. Chest X-ray can be normal or show bilateral patchy infiltrates. FBC may show lymphopenia.

Tx: Assess the patient with appropriate personal protective equipment on

- Apply oxygen via a non-rebreather mask and titrate to keep SaO_2 >92%
- Escalate to CPAP if still hypoxic
- Prone positioning can benefit oxygenation (in both awake and intubated patients)
- Refer to intensive care those needing CPAP or high FiO_2 – very frail and multi co-morbid patients are unlikely to survive an ICU admission with Covid-19 and consideration should be made to the appropriate ceiling of care for that individual.

Specific treatments for Covid-19 are constantly changing and updating (see local guidance) but may include:

- Dexamethasone for patients needing admission to hospital and supplemental oxygen
- Baricitinib for patients requiring supplemental oxygen who are already receiving dexamethasone
- Tocilizumab or sarilumab for patients needing CPAP or ventilation
- Remdesivir for patients requiring oxygen who have creatinine clearance >30 mL/min and Alanine aminotransferase <5 times upper limit of normal.

Consider a 5-day course of nirmatrelvir and ritonavir (Paxlovid) or Molnoparivir for adults with COVID-19 who:

- do not need supplemental oxygen for Covid-19, and
- are within 5 days of symptom onset, and
- are thought to be at high risk of progression to severe Covid-19.

Covid-19 is associated with increased risk of venous thromboembolism (VTE) meaning all patients admitted to hospital should receive prophylactic low-molecular-weight heparin (LMWH), unless contraindicated. A negative D-dimer appears to be effective in ruling out VTE; however, most patients with active Covid-19 infection have high D-dimer levels. Depending on bleeding risk, some patients may be commenced on treatment dose LMWH, whereas others will need radiological confirmation of the VTE (*Pulmonary embolism → p. 227*). This is an area of ongoing research.

A rare complication of covid vaccination is vaccine-induced thrombocytopaenia and thrombosis (VITT), causing cerebral and other deep vein thromboses. VITT is probable in patients with thrombosis, thrombocytopaenia and a very high D-dimer.

Post-Covid-19 syndrome is characterised by symptoms such as fatigue, breathlessness, palpitations, 'brain fog', joint and muscle pains and dizziness for over 12 weeks after Covid-19 infection.

Influenza

Every winter in the UK, during a 6- to 8-week period, influenza is associated with a sharp increase in both mortality and hospital admissions. At this time, consultations for respiratory illness may increase up to 10-fold. In an average year, an estimated 2000–3000 people die in the UK from influenza-related causes; in years with major epidemics, there have been over 20 000 excess deaths. People at an increased risk from influenza (and who should be vaccinated against it) include those who are aged ≥65 years, residents in long-term care and people with certain chronic illnesses including:

- respiratory disease (especially COPD and asthma)
- heart disease
- renal disease
- immunosuppression (from any cause and including asplenia)
- diabetes.

The symptoms of influenza are relatively non-specific – pyrexia, malaise, anorexia, myalgia, nausea and coughing.

Tx The treatment of influenza is mostly symptomatic – fluids and antipyretic analgesics. However, during an epidemic, high-risk patients in the groups listed above who present within 36 hours of the onset of symptoms should be considered for antiviral therapy. For adults and children >40 kg, oseltamivir 75 mg is given by mouth twice daily for 5 days. An alternative for patients >12 years is zanamivir 10 mg by inhalation twice daily for 5 days.

Avian influenza (bird flu) is a disease of birds caused by influenza viruses that are closely related to human influenza viruses. It is an important disease economically for farmers because of losses in poultry flocks. Transmission to humans in close contact with poultry or other birds occurs rarely and only with some strains of avian influenza, (e.g. subtype H5N1). The potential for transformation of avian influenza into a form that both causes severe disease in humans and spreads easily from person to person is a great concern for world health.

Tuberculosis

Every year 10 million people develop tuberculosis (TB), mostly in low- and middle-income countries. The causative organism of TB, *Mycobacterium tuberculosis*, is an obligate parasite with no free-living saprophytic forms. It is capable of both intracellular and extracellular existence. Other mycobacteria (e.g. *Mycobacterium avium-intracellulare*) are increasingly recognised as human pathogens, which cause both pulmonary and systemic disease. High-risk groups for TB (and other mycobacterial infections) include the following:

- Children and young adults
- Immigrants from high-risk countries (the countries with most cases are Bangladesh, China, India, Indonesia, Nigeria, Pakistan, Philippines and South Africa.)
- People with poor socio-economic status
- Residents of prisons, nursing homes and other institutions
- Individuals who are dependent on alcohol or use IV drugs
- People with HIV and other causes of immunodeficiency
- People with some chronic illnesses (e.g. diabetes)
- People on long-term steroid therapy
- Health-care providers.

Patients with pulmonary TB may present to an ED with chronic respiratory symptoms, general illness, night sweats and weight loss. Sometimes TB may be an incidental finding on a chest X-ray. Suspect TB in a patient who has had multiple courses of antibiotics with only transient improvement, and those with a cough for more than three weeks with haemoptysis.

> A person with undiagnosed smear-positive pulmonary TB infects around 10 other people each year.

Investigations: The chest X-ray in primary TB is likely to show changes in the lower lobes with mediastinal or hilar lymphadenopathy and, sometimes, a pleural effusion ($\rightarrow$ *see Figure 13.8*). Post-primary TB is caused by either reinfection or reactivation of a primary lesion (tubercle bacilli can remain dormant but viable in the body for many years). The altered immune response of the host results in a different radiographic picture:

- Disease in the upper lobe or superior segments of the lower lobes
- Pleural effusions and cavitating lesions
- Pneumonic consolidation, nodules or miliary spread.

In immunodeficient patients (e.g. those with HIV), mycobacterial infection causes lymphadenopathy and minimal changes on a chest X-ray and is more likely to cause disseminated TB.

Definitive diagnosis is made by detecting acid fast bacilli in a bodily fluid (e.g. sputum, lymph node aspirate), by microscopy, nucleic-acid amplification (NAAT) or culture (which can take several weeks to yield a result). Multiple samples of sputum taken at different times are more likely to achieve a positive result.

Tuberculin skin testing (TST, or Mantoux test) and interferon-γ-release assay (IGRA) assess for the bodies response to tuberculous antigens but cannot differentiate

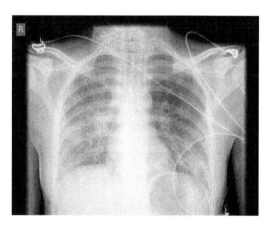

Figure 13.8 Appearance of Tuberculosis on a chest X-ray with bilateral changes.

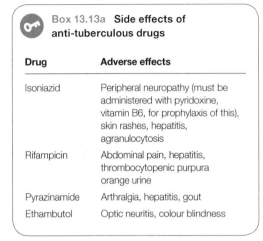

Box 13.13a **Side effects of anti-tuberculous drugs**

Drug	Adverse effects
Isoniazid	Peripheral neuropathy (must be administered with pyridoxine, vitamin B6, for prophylaxis of this), skin rashes, hepatitis, agranulocytosis
Rifampicin	Abdominal pain, hepatitis, thrombocytopenic purpura orange urine
Pyrazinamide	Arthralgia, hepatitis, gout
Ethambutol	Optic neuritis, colour blindness

between latent and active infection. A negative test does not rule out TB either. TST can be affected by previous vaccination with BCG.

Tx Patients with suspected TB should be referred to a respiratory physician for specialist treatment. In the UK, antimicrobial therapy is with four drugs (rifampicin, isoniazid, pyrazinamide and ethambutol) for 2 months and then two drugs (rifampicin and isoniazid) are given alone for another 4 months (→ *see Box 13.3a*). TB is a notifiable disease throughout the UK.

Collapse of the lung (atelectasis)

Segmental collapse is generally a result of sputum retention or infection. Lobar collapse occurs with pneumonia, TB, malignancy and foreign body aspiration. The treatment of collapse is that of the primary condition. → *Figures 13.5 and 13.6*

Pleural effusion

Usually presents as breathlessness with or without pleuritic chest pain but can be asymptomatic if small. Typical findings include reduced breath sounds and dullness to percussion to the base of one lung field, with typical chest X-ray findings of 'whited out' lung field and meniscus sign (slants upwards towards lateral wall). There needs to be around 250 mL of fluid before a blunted costophrenic angle is evident on plain erect chest X-ray. Point of care ultrasound (POCUS) is more sensitive, capable of detecting as little as 5 mL of fluid in experienced hands (→ *see Figure 13.9*).

Pleural effusions are categorised as transudates (associated with increased capillary hydrostatic pressure or decreased osmotic pressure) or exudates (associated

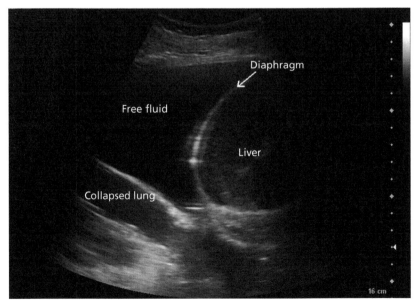

Figure 13.9 POCUS image of right sided pleural effusion using curvilinear probe.

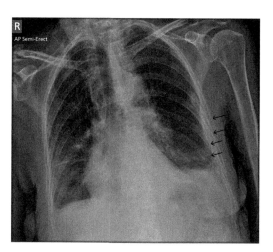

Figure 13.10 Chest radiograph of a patient treated initially for infection but was found to have haemothorax due to multiple left rib fractures (denoted by arrows).

Box 13.13b **The causes of pleural effusion**

Transudative (<25 g/L protein, pleural: serum protein ratio <0.5)
- Heart failure (most common)
- Liver failure
- Renal failure/nephrotic syndrome
- Hypothyroidism
- Meig's syndrome – pleural effusion and ascites due to benign ovarian tumour
- Ovarian hyperstimulation syndrome
- Post coronary artery bypass surgery – small left pleural effusion is common

Exudative (>35 g/L protein, pleural: serum protein ratio >0.5)
- Pneumonia (empyema)
- Malignancy
- Mesothelioma
- Tuberculosis
- Pulmonary embolism
- Rheumatological conditions, e.g. rheumatoid arthritis and SLE
- Drugs – such as tyrosine kinase inhibitors (Pneumotox app. has information on drug causes)

with altered permeability of pleural membrane and capillary walls to proteins) →*Box 13.13b causes of pleural effusion*.

It is important for the ED clinician to also consider traumatic haemothorax as a cause, especially in frail or older patients, those on anticoagulation and those who are unable to relay the history of events (→ *see Figure 13.10*). Aortic dissection can cause left-sided effusion (a haemothorax) as can Boerhaave's syndrome/spontaneous oesophageal rupture (gastric contents).

Tx Pleural aspiration should not be undertaken for bilateral effusions where transudative causes are suspected. Instead, the focus should be on treating the underlying cause. Diagnostic tap (preferably ultrasound guided) can be performed where the cause is uncertain. Samples should be sent for protein, glucose, LDH, pH, white cell count, microscopy and culture and cytology. Milky aspirate suggests chylothorax due to disruption of lymphatic drainage; request cholesterol and triglycerides to be performed on samples. Where effusions are too small to safely tap, the patient will need admission or outpatient follow-up for a CT scan.

Large effusions, causing respiratory compromise, may need a chest drain inserting. This should be performed under ultrasound guidance, and Seldinger-type drains are recommended (10–14F). (*Chapter 6 → p. 76*)

Pulmonary embolism

The overall incidence of PE in the UK is 60–70/100000 people per year with an in-hospital mortality rate of around 10%. *For recognised risk factors for VTE → Box 13.14.* About 50% of PEs occur in patients already in hospital or long-term care, 25% in patients with other recognised risk factors and the final 25% are idiopathic (unprovoked). Without prophylaxis, up to 50% of patients undergoing major orthopaedic surgery, around 25% of general surgical patients and almost 20% of general medical patients will have a VTE. Thromboprophylaxis with heparin reduces these figures by around 50%.

DVT → p. 110.

Over 90% of patients with PE are breathless or have a raised respiratory rate (>20 breaths/min). Only 3% will not have dyspnoea, tachypnoea or pleuritic chest pain. Haemoptysis occurs in around 10% of cases of PE, but isolated haemoptysis is usually due to another cause. A fifth of patients with a PE have a cough. Areas of crepitus or a pleural rub is sometimes heard, as is a pulmonary flow murmur. Thrombosis of the deep veins may be present but is usually occult.

For patients with suspected PE, a two-level Well's score should be calculated (→ *Box 13.15*). For patients

Box 13.14 **The risk factors for venous thromboembolism**

Major risk factors **(relative risk = 5 to 20 fold)**
- Pregnancy or puerperium
- Major abdominal or pelvic surgery (usually procedures lasting >30 min)
- Major orthopaedic surgery (e.g. hip or knee replacement)
- Malignancy (especially advanced or metastatic or in the abdomen/pelvis)
- Lower limb fracture (especially with cast)
- Previous proven VTE
- Thrombotic disorders including known thrombophilias
  - Protein A, C and S deficiencies
  - Factor V Leiden
- Varicose veins
- Reduced mobility (hospitalisation or other institutional care and especially critical care admission)

Minor risk factors **(relative risk = 2 to 4 fold)**
- Age >60 years
- Oral contraceptives and hormone replacement therapy (*also → Table 7.2 on p. 109*)
- Chronic diseases (e.g. COPD, infection, metabolic diseases, renal dialysis and neurological disability)
- Anti-phospholipid syndrome
- Central venous catheter in situ
- Previous superficial venous thrombosis or phlebitis
- History of VTE in a first-degree relative
- Dehydration
- Injecting drug use
- Obesity (body mass index [BMI] >30 kg/m²)
- Long-distance sedentary travel (both by air and by road)

Box 13.15 **Well's score for PE and PERC criteria**

Well's score
- Clinical features of DVT (minimum of leg swelling and pain with palpation of the deep veins) – 3 points
- Heart rate >100 bpm – 1.5 points
- Immobilisation for more than 3 days or surgery in previous 4 weeks – 1.5 points
- Previous DVT or PE – 1.5 points
- Haemoptysis – 1 point
- Cancer (receiving treatment within the last 6 months or palliative) – 1 point
- Alternative diagnosis is less likely than PE – 3 points

A score of >4 means PE is 'likely'.
A score of ≤4 mean PE is 'unlikely'.

PERC criteria
- Age <50 years
- Pulse <100 bpm
- $SaO_2 \geq 95\%$
- No haemoptysis
- No oestrogen use
- No surgery or trauma requiring hospitalisation within 4 weeks
- No prior VTE
- No unilateral leg swelling

All criteria fulfilled means PE can be 'ruled out'. Do not use the tool in patients with thrombophilia, cancer, beta blocker use, pregnancy and post-partum. Be cautious when using in patients with an amputated leg or obesity/chronic oedema where new swelling may be more difficult to detect.

scoring 'likely', a CT pulmonary angiogram should be performed. If scoring 'unlikely' a D-dimer test should be performed. D-dimer is a breakdown product of cross-linked fibrin which is sensitive, but not specific for VTE – hence a good 'rule out' test. Unfortunately, it becomes even less specific with increasing age, hence age-adjusted cut offs can be used to increase specificity. A positive D-dimer will require further investigation with CTPA, a negative result rules out PE.

Another tool called PERC (PE rule-out criteria) can be used for patients with a symptom of PE, e.g. pleuritic chest pain, where the clinician feels PE is unlikely to be the cause. A patient fulfilling all PERC criteria is thought to have <2% chance of PE. This is where the point of equipoise is thought to lie between the harm of investigating (radiation, anaphylaxis to contrast) and the harm of not investigating (missing a PE).

Other investigations that are performed to look for alternative diagnoses and to help risk stratify the severity of a PE:

- FBC/WCC (to look for infection and severe anaemia) and blood chemistry should be requested. Baseline renal and liver function tests as well as prothrombin time (PT) and activated partial thromboplastin time (aPTT) should be performed prior to starting anticoagulants.

- Blood gases and SaO_2 may show hypoxia on air but not usually with small pulmonary emboli. Measurement of the blood gases is not indicated if there is a normal SaO_2 on air.
- Around a third of patients with a moderate or large pulmonary embolus have a raised troponin level. This is associated with right ventricular strain (*see massive and submassive PE below*)
- Investigations for occult cancer in idiopathic VTE (present in 7–12% of such patients) are indicated only if the presence of malignancy is clinically suspected or suggested by a chest X-ray or blood tests. Tests for thrombophilia are indicated in patients aged <50 years with recurrent PEs or a strong family history of thromboembolic disease.
- ECG may be normal; any changes are the result of right heart strain (→ *Box 13.16 and Figure 13.11*).
- Chest X-ray is often unremarkable, occasionally there may be segmental collapse, localised absence of vascular markings, pleural effusion, an area of peripheral infarction ('sail' shadow) or a prominent pulmonary artery.
- Identification of a deep vein thrombosis (DVT) will help in the diagnosis of PE (→ *p. 110*). Duplex ultrasound is the investigation of choice.
- POCUS can be used in experienced hands to look for signs of right heart strain in PE such as right

ventricular dilation and 'D' shape flattening of the intraventricular septum.

- For patients with an allergy to contrast or severe renal impairment, a ventilation/perfusion single photon emission CT (V/Q SPECT) is the scan of choice instead of CTPA.

Massive and sub-massive pulmonary embolism: sometimes, the presenting symptoms of PE are collapse, syncope, hypotension, shock or even cardiac arrest. *Massive PE* (sometimes referred to as 'high risk') is defined as PE with shock or systolic BP <90 mmHg and mortality is estimated at 18–30%. Intravenous thrombolysis with alteplase or tenecteplase is recommended for patients with massive PE and those in cardiac arrest

Box 13.16 **ECG signs of PE**

- Sinus tachycardia (most common positive finding)
- T wave inversion in leads V1–V4, III and aVF
- Right axis deviation >90°
- New atrial fibrillation
- Incomplete or complete right bundle branch block (RBBB)
- P pulmonale in II and III
- S1, Q3, T3 (an S wave in lead I and a Q wave with T-wave inversion in lead III)

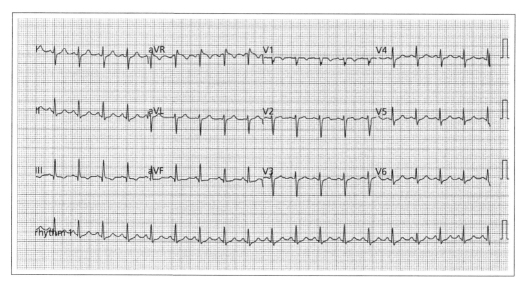

Figure 13.11 ECG of a patient with sub-massive PE, demonstrating sinus tachycardia, right axis deviation and S1, Q3, T3 pattern.

suspected to be due to PE. When the cause of cardiac arrest is unknown; however, thrombolysis does not appear to improve outcomes. In out-of-hospital cardiac arrest, if thrombolysis is to be given, it should be as soon as possible to increase the likelihood of a positive outcome. Ten per cent of patients will have a major bleed following thrombolysis and 1.5% will have a haemorrhagic stroke. EDs with access to interventional radiology and techniques such as catheter-directed thrombolysis and clot retrieval may consider these treatments as an alternative.

Sub-massive PE (or 'intermediate risk') has no shock but has signs of right heart strain on ECG or demonstrated by a raised troponin, raised BNP or dilated right ventricle on CT or echocardiogram. Further research is needed to determine the use of thrombolysis at either normal or half doses, to prevent the feared complication of pulmonary hypertension in these patients.

Suspected PE in pregnancy: PE is the leading direct cause of maternal mortality in the UK. Pregnancy is associated with a 4–6-fold increased risk of VTE and the puerperium with a 20-fold increased risk. D-dimer and risk stratification tools are not validated and should not be used during pregnancy. If a pregnant woman presents with symptoms of PE, she should have an ECG and chest X-ray. If there are also symptoms of DVT, a compression duplex ultrasound should be performed next, and if positive; treatment can be commenced. If there are no features of DVT, then a V/Q scan or CTPA should be performed (CTPA is preferred when the chest X-ray is abnormal.)

V/Q scan gives a slightly higher dose of radiation to the foetus compared to CTPA (~0.5 mGy versus ~0.1 mGy), chest X-ray is even less (<0.01 mGy). A foetal dose of 100 mGy confers a 1% overall risk of childhood cancer (the baseline risk for any child is 0.2%), and CNS malformations start to occur at doses of 100000 mGy. CTPA is thought to increase the mother's breast cancer risk by around 13.6% above her background risk, so a 25-year-old with a 10-year risk of 0.1% will now have a 0.1136% chance. Hence, the risk of either of these scans is bound to be less than missing a potentially life-threatening PE.

Treatment is with LMWH (*for dosing* → *see Box 13.17*) as other oral anticoagulants are contraindicated. All pregnant women being admitted or investigated for suspected PE should have obstetric input prior to discharge. Unfractionated heparin will be the first-line choice of treatment in pregnant and postpartum women with *massive* PE, but in the deteriorating or peri-arrest patient, thrombolysis should still be considered. Management should involve senior clinicians from medical, obstetric and intensive care teams. A resuscitative hysterotomy should be performed within 5 min if cardiac arrest occurs and the pregnancy is more than 20 weeks (*see Chapter 11 page 167*).

 Box 13.17 Anticoagulant dosing in PE

Enoxaparin
- 1.5 mg/kg is given subcutaneously every 24 hours.
- 1 mg/kg every 12 hours for PE in patients with risk factors such as obesity, cancer or symptomatic or recurrent PE.
- In pregnancy, 1 mg/kg twice daily is used (based on pre-pregnancy weight).
- In patients with severe renal impairment (i.e. creatinine clearance CrCl <30 mL/min), 1 mg/kg every 24 hours

Tinzaparin
- 175 units/kg once daily (same in pregnancy)

Dalteparin
- 200 units/kg daily or 100 units/kg twice daily if patient at risk of bleeding or pregnant

Apixaban (direct inhibitor of activated factor X)
- 10 mg twice daily for 7 days and then 5 mg twice daily for 3 months

Rivaroxaban (direct inhibitor of activated factor X)
- 15 mg twice daily for 21 days and then 20 mg daily for 3 months (to be taken with food)

Dabigatran (direct thrombin inhibitor)
- 150 mg twice daily (110 mg twice daily in over 75-year-olds, renal impairment and patients taking verapamil)
- Should only be given after 5 days of a parenteral anticoagulant

Edoxaban (direct inhibitor of activated factor X)
- 60 mg daily (30 mg daily if CrCl 15–50 mL/min, weight <60 kg or concomitant use of P glycoprotein inhibitors (such as erythromycin, ciclosporin, dronedarone, quinidine or ketoconazole)
- Should only be given after 5 days of a parenteral anticoagulant

Seek specialist advice before starting these treatments in patients with gastrointestinal cancer or recent GI bleeding, recent brain surgery of intracranial haemorrhage. *For reversal of DOACs →Chapter 14 p. 272*

Tx

Initial treatment: includes oxygen and analgesia.

Anticoagulation: should be started before imaging in patients with high clinical probability of PE. A DOAC (direct oral anti-coagulant) is preferred except in severe renal failure (creatinine clearance <15 mL/min), and antiphospholipid syndrome where LMWH then warfarin is preferred (→ *see Box 13.17*). Standard unfractionated heparin is a less convenient and requires frequent monitoring but is useful in patients where immediate reversal may be needed, e.g. patients with bleeding risks or those who have had thrombolysis. An initial IV loading dose of 75 units/kg is followed by a continuous IV infusion of 18 units/kg/hour.

Thrombolysis: may be considered for massive life-threatening emboli. IV alteplase 10 mg is given over 1–2 min followed by an IV infusion of 90 mg over 2 hours (maximum dose 1.5 mg/kg in patients <65 kg). Tenecteplase 30–50 mg is given over 10 seconds. Thrombolysis is followed by unfractionated heparin but without the loading dose. An IV bolus of alteplase 50 mg can be administered during cardiac arrest, due to PE or if cardiac arrest is thought to be imminent.

Admission to hospital: this is required for most patients with PE. A proportion of patients can be managed in the community, but this depends on local protocols and services. The simplified PE severity index (sPESI) is a tool that can be used to select patients at lower risk of complications that might be suitable for outpatient investigation and treatment. One of more of the following means 'high risk':

- Age >80 years
- History of cancer
- History of chronic cardiopulmonary disease
- Heart rate ≥110 bpm
- Systolic BP <100 mmHg
- SaO_2 <90%

The decision to investigate and manage patients as an outpatient should be made by a senior clinician and only where provisions exist for follow-up within 24 hours.

Pulmonary hypertension

Pulmonary hypertension (PH) is defined as an elevated pulmonary artery pressure >25 mmHg and encompasses four types of disease process:

- Pulmonary arterial hypertension (PAH)
- Left-sided heart disease
- Chronic respiratory disease and/or hypoxia
- Chronic thromboembolic pulmonary hypertension

The common emergencies related to PH are described as 'CRASH'; chest pain, right ventricular failure, arrythmias, sepsis and haemoptysis. Many of the usual resuscitative measures, such as IV fluids and positive pressure ventilation are not tolerated well by patients with PH and can trigger a downward spiral of haemodynamic collapse. Give oxygen, consider early administration of antibiotics and cardioversion of any tachyarrythmias. Use fluid boluses very cautiously and consider noradrenaline followed by dobutamine or milrinone for cardiogenic shock.

Patients known to a specialist PAH centre should be discussed with them. Ensure that patients continue to receive their important medications for PH (e.g. sildenafil, epoprostenol, iloprost and bosentan), noting that some of these are delivered by continuous infusion.

Hyperventilation syndrome

Although some people are prone to attacks of hyperventilation, it is rare for significant psychiatric disease to be the cause. There is usually underlying anxiety and social stress.

The patient becomes increasingly frightened by an apparent inability to breathe adequately. Attempts to breathe rapidly result in dizziness and further anxiety. Tachypnoea blows off CO_2 and the resultant respiratory alkalosis causes a fall in ionised calcium. Paraesthesia in the fingers and around the mouth, chest tightness and palpitations are common consequences.

Tx Investigation should accompany treatment; calm reassurance is essential. Organic respiratory problems, such as spontaneous pneumothorax, PE or salicylate poisoning, must be ruled out. This will certainly entail physical examination and pulse oximetry. ECG, chest X-ray and blood gas analysis may also be needed in some cases. Any condition causing tachypnoea can cause respiratory alkalosis, e.g. pulmonary embolism, severe pain and salicylate toxicity.

Encourage the patient to take slow deep breaths using counting and coaching methods. Benzodiazepines can be used if the acute situation is severe. Once the patient is feeling better, explore their current concerns and anxieties and give advice and reassurance about the condition.

Other causes of respiratory distress

If struggling to find the cause of respiratory distress in a patient with normal chest exam, X-ray and ECG, think – *could it be one of these rarer causes*?

- Diabetic ketoacidosis → *pp. 255*
- Other metabolic acidosis – e.g. salicylate poisoning → *pp. 263 and 280*
- Carbon monoxide poisoning → *pp. 300*
- Severe anaemia

- Inhalation of fumes, smoke and other gases → *pp. 141 and 303.*
- Cardiac tamponade → *pp. 253*
- Valvular disease → *pp. 251*
- Myocarditis → *pp. 252*
- Anaphylaxis → *pp. 306*
- Upper airway mass
- Neuromuscular disease (e.g. Guillain Barre syndrome, Myaesthenic crisis)
- Increased intra-abdominal pressure (e.g. ascites, abdominal compartment syndrome)
- Rib fractures

Spontaneous pneumothorax → p. 201.

Vaping refers to the use of an electronic device that turns liquid into a vapour by heating it so the user can inhale. The liquid typically contains propylene glycol, vegetable glycerine, flavourings and nicotine. There have been cases of e-cigarette and vaping associated lung injury (EVALI) in the USA and one case in the UK with a fatal outcome. Many of the cases in USA were using tetrahydrocannabinol (THC) liquids, which are illegal in UK. Any suspected cases should be reported via MHRA yellow card scheme:

1 Using e-cigarette or vaping in 30 days prior
2 Pulmonary infiltrates on chest X-ray or CT scan
3 Absence of respiratory infection
4 No evidence of alternative diagnosis (e.g. cardiac, autoimmune).

Haemoptysis

Patients may present with haemoptysis as an isolated symptom. The blood is usually coughed up in a small quantity mixed with sputum. History and examination must aim to exclude serious illnesses such as chest infection, pulmonary oedema, PE, TB or malignancy. FBC, ECG and chest X-ray should be performed on all such patients with the same aim. Ensure there are no bleeding sources in the upper airways, e.g. post-tonsillectomy bleed. Patients who are then found to have no other apparent abnormalities can be referred back to their GP for further management or under 2 week wait for lung cancer if over 40 years. Most haemoptysis in young people is idiopathic.

Troublesome cough

Other causes of cough to consider include:

- Allergies and postnasal drip
- Gastroesophageal reflux
- Lung cancer
- Smoking
- ACE inhibitors
- Pertussis (whooping cough) – suggested by a cough lasting more than 14 days with paroxysms of coughing, vomiting with coughing or a whooping sound.

14

Collapse and sudden illness

Amy Nickson

Emergency Medicine Consultant, Royal Bolton Hospital, Bolton, UK
Sexual Offences Examiner, Lancashire SAFE Centre, Preston, UK

COLLAPSE

The term 'collapse' can be used to describe a variety of different conditions or healthcare events. It can be a sudden deterioration in health, an inability to maintain an upright posture, an episode of transient loss of consciousness or even a state of emotional or physiological shock.

The priorities in patients who present with a sudden onset of illness or who have collapsed are to:

- start resuscitation
- seek out reversible conditions and treat them
- begin a structured assessment.

Assessment and management of the collapsed patient

Details of immediate assessment and management applicable to all emergency patients are given in *Chapter 1*. The same structured system can be used for the collapsed patient.

A – Airway

- Clear the airway with suction or other physical means.
- Maintain the airway by positioning or using airway adjuncts.
- Protect the airway by positioning the patient in the recovery position and having suction available.

- Consider the need for endotracheal intubation.
- Protect the cervical spine if the history is unknown, vague or suggests the possibility of trauma.
- Consider specific treatment for foreign body obstruction ($\rightarrow$ *p. 205*) or anaphylaxis ($\rightarrow$ *p. 306*).

B – Breathing

- Assess at the adequacy of respiration and consider the need for immediate ventilation.
- Establish monitoring (SaO_2, BP and ECG.)
- Give oxygen if the O_2 saturation (SaO_2) is <94% on air.
- If the SaO_2 is low or if there is a suggestion of CO_2 narcosis, check the blood gases.
- Commence therapy to relieve hypoxia and dyspnoea; consider specific treatment for:
  - cardiorespiratory problems (severe left ventricular failure, chronic obstructive pulmonary disease [COPD], asthma, pneumonia, pulmonary embolism and spontaneous pneumothorax $\rightarrow$ *Chapter 13*)
  - CO_2 narcosis $\rightarrow$ *p. 211*
  - anaphylaxis $\rightarrow$ *p. 306*.

C – Circulation

- Establish venous access and give intravenous (IV) fluids as necessary.
- Examine the cardiovascular system and assess heart rate and BP.
- Consider the possibility of acute haemorrhage

- Consider specific treatment for:
  - cardiothoracic problems (myocardial infarction [MI], pulmonary embolism → *page*; dysrhythmia → *Chapter 11*)
  - abdominal problems (gastrointestinal bleed, intra-abdominal bleeding or sepsis → *Chapter 16*)
  - anaphylaxis → *p. 306.*

D – Disability

- Record the level of consciousness.
- Look at the pupils, muscle tone and reflexes and record any localising signs.
- Run your hands over the scalp to discover any swelling or bleeding.
- Look for photophobia, neck stiffness and purpura.

A decreased level of consciousness indicates that something is wrong with the brain or its fuel supply. It may be:

1 Poisoning or gross metabolic disturbance (including CO_2 narcosis and hypothermia)

2 Cerebral injury or pathology (head injury, intracranial bleeding, thrombosis, embolism, infection, swelling, tumour, fitting, etc.)

3 Failure of the brain's fuel supply (hypoxia, hypovolaemia, cerebral ischaemia or hypoglycaemia)

Common causes of sudden collapse with coma → Box 14.1.

E – Environment and exposure

- Take the temperature (tympanic or rectal).
- Remove clothing (but keep warm), examine the whole patient – front and back. Search the clothing for treatment cards, drugs, suicide notes and identification.
- Consider specific treatment for:
  - hypothermia → *p. 247*
  - infection
  - hyperpyrexia → *p. 249.*

Box 14.1 Common causes of sudden collapse with coma

- Subarachnoid haemorrhage
- Brainstem cerebral vascular accident (CVA)
- Hypoglycaemia
- Poisoning (e.g. tricyclic antidepressants)
- Head injury

F – Fits

- Control any tonic–clonic activity with benzodiazepines (→ *p. 243*).
- Protect the tongue from the teeth with a Guedel airway.

G – Glucose

Check the blood sugar in any patient who is unresponsive or behaving strangely and administer IV glucose if necessary.

H – History

- Get as much detail as possible from bystanders, ambulance crew and relatives. The essentials are AMPLE (→ *p. 10*).
- Obtain hospital records.

I – Immediate analgesia and investigations

- Give analgesia, if required, and look for the cause of any pain.
- Request a chest X-ray.
- Obtain an ECG.
- Take blood for full blood count (FBC), urea and electrolytes (U&Es), glucose, C-reactive protein (CRP) and lactate (causes of raised lactate see *Box 14.2*). Consider also requesting a serum osmolality. The osmolar gap is a useful and easily available indicator of toxic and metabolic disorders → *Boxes 14.3 and 14.4.*
- Consider the need for a nasogastric tube and/or a urinary catheter in all unresponsive patients.
- Consider the need for radiographs of the hips and pelvis in any older person who has collapsed or been found on the floor.

Box 14.2 Causes of an elevated lactate (LLACTATESS)

- **Liver:** hepatic impairment will reduce lactate clearance
- **Lung:** lactate is released from the lung in acute lung injury
- **Accelerated glycolysis:** adrenergic drugs, e.g. salbutamol
- **Congenital disease:** mitochondrial disease and inborn errors of metabolism
- **Toxins:** both therapeutic and otherwise, e.g. toxic alcohols and cyanide
- **Anaerobic metabolism:** from global or local tissue underperfusion, e.g. ischaemic bowel
- **Thiamine deficiency:** common in nutritional deficiency and alcohol excess, thiamine is a

cofactor for pyruvate dehydrogenase, deficiency increases lactate production
- **Efflux of lactate** to the extracellular space due to alkalosis. High lactate is commonly seen in psychogenic hyperventilation
- Sepsis: predominantly as a result of tissue hypoperfusion
- Seizures

 Box 14.3 **The osmolar gap**

This is useful as a screening test for osmotically active poisons in the bloodstream and in the search for a cause for a metabolic acidosis.

Osmolar gap is the difference between lab-measured serum osmolality and calculated serum osmolarity.

Measured serum osmolality is normally 280–300 mosmol/L (measured by freezing point osmometry).

Calculated serum osmolarity is twice the serum sodium concentration plus the glucose and the urea levels (in mmol/L).

$$\text{Calculated osmolarity} = (2 \times Na^+)$$
$$+ \text{glucose} + \text{urea}$$

This is a simplification of a more accurate formula:

$$\text{Calculated osmolarity} = (1.86 \times Na^+)$$
$$+ \text{glucose} + \text{urea} / 0.93$$

If the osmolar gap is >10, then there are probably abnormal osmotically active substances in the bloodstream such as:

- ethanol
- methanol
- ethylene glycol
- mannitol.

These are all substances with a small molecular weight. Even in poisoned patients, most other drugs do not achieve a high enough molar concentration to contribute to osmolality, which depends purely on the number of molecules present.

The osmolar (or more correctly osmolal) gap should be interpreted cautiously in the critically ill patient because circulatory failure may cause it to increase. Hyperosmolar IV infusions, ketoacidosis and chronic (but not acute) renal failure may do the same.

 Box 14.4 **The anion gap**

The anion gap refers to the concentration difference between the measured serum cation (sodium) and the measured serum anions (chloride and bicarbonate). It is normally 12 mmol/L (±2). An anion gap of >20 is definitely abnormal.

$$\text{Anion gap} = Na^+ - (Cl^- + HCO_3^-)$$
$$= 10 - 14 \text{ mmol} / L$$

An increased anion gap suggests an underlying metabolic acidosis – usually as a result of poisoning, renal failure or excess production of lactate or ketones. This is because, in metabolic acidosis, excess acids are titrated by bicarbonate, the level of which then falls – resulting in an increase in the calculated anion gap. *Metabolic acidosis → p. 263.*

Poisoning

Treatment of poisoned patients → Chapter 15.

Unexplained collapse with generalised or bizarre signs must always raise the possibility of poisoning, even if this is denied.

Collapse in children

Collapse in children usually accompanies overwhelming pathology such as shock, respiratory failure or intracranial infection.

Meningococcal septicaemia → p. 354.
Miscellaneous paediatric conditions → Chapter 18.
Paediatric resuscitation → p. 168.

Collapse in elderly people

Collapse in elderly people is common and complex because of the following:

1 Homeostatic mechanisms and physiological reserves are impaired – a relatively small change in health can cause sudden decompensation of an already failing system.
2 Lack of social support and delayed access to carers may prevent timely interventions.
3 Elderly patients are often taking a multiplicity of drugs.
4 The patient often presents with global vague problems (e.g. 'off legs') rather than specific and localised abnormalities.

The cause of a sudden deterioration in an elderly patient may not be immediately apparent from the history or clinical examination. For this reason, most collapsed older patients will need investigation before discharge to exclude diagnoses such as the following:

- MI or pulmonary embolism
- Heart block or other dysrhythmia
- Pneumonia, pyelonephritis or other infection
- Gastrointestinal bleeding or other blood loss
- Anaemia or renal failure
- Chronic subdural haemorrhage or CVA
- Fractured neck of femur.

FBC, standard blood chemistry, glucose, ECG and CXR are essential. CRP, plasma calcium and osmolality are useful in non-specific illness.

Patients who have been found lying on the floor are often cold, dehydrated and frightened; they often need admission for further assessment and stabilisation. Looking for precipitating illness and resulting injuries means a thorough, top-to-toe examination is required. The plasma creatinine kinase should be measured and the urine tested for myoglobin.

NEUROLOGICAL PROBLEMS

Acute confusional states → *p. 375.*

Transient loss of consciousness

Transient loss of consciousness (TLOC) is a common presentation to ED, it affects almost half the population at some point in their lives. The main categories of TLOC are syncope (global cerebral hypoperfusion), neurological (seizure) and psychological (encompassing non-epileptic attack disorder and narcolepsy).

A careful history is essential to ascertain the following:

- What the patient was doing at the time of the syncope
- What posture they were in
- What warning signs were experienced
- Whether the person feels that they were fully recovered
- The past medical history and medications.

'Red flag' symptoms include:

- TLOC during exertion
- Dyspnoea, chest pain or headache
- TLOC in patients over 65 with no prodrome
- Tongue-biting, incontinence or post-ictal drowsiness/confusion
- Family history of sudden cardiac death before age 40

Information from observers and paramedics can be extremely useful in this respect.

Subsequent examination and investigations can be tailored to the likely causes of the syncope as suggested by the history. Every TLOC patient should have at least an ECG and some will need blood tests and measurement of lying and standing BPs. Be aware that some patients will falsely attribute the 'fall' to tripping or slipping, perhaps to prevent 'all the fuss'. Remember, when a person trips, they usually put out their hands to stop the fall. Look for the presence (or absence) of abrasions to the palms.

Syncope can be broken down further into three main types:

Vasovagal syncope: There should be a history of some warning symptoms before the faint, such as feeling hot, sweaty and seeing spots in the vision. There is usually a vagal trigger, such as the sight of blood, cervical or bowel wall stretch, coughing or emotional distress. A mild degree of bradycardia is a common finding even when the patient appears to have fully recovered. Often, a vasovagal faint will be accompanied by brief convulsive movements – an 'anoxic' fit. The patient can be reassured and discharged if there is a good history of a simple faint and a full and rapid recovery (although many patients report feeling 'worn out' afterwards).

Orthostatic syncope is caused by postural hypotension with light headedness and TLOC within a few minutes of standing. It can be diagnosed if there is a drop in systolic blood pressure upon standing of >20 mmHg (or a drop in diastolic BP >10 mmHg). Be aware, this might not always be present by the time the patient reaches hospital, especially if they have had something to eat and drink and been outside in the cool air. The first BP reading should be taken after the patient has been lying supine for 5 min and then the second reading is taken after 3 min of standing. Postural hypotension is often associated with medications such as vasodilators, antihypertensives and antidepressants or conditions with autonomic dysfunction such as diabetes or Parkinson's disease. Dehydration, sepsis, pulmonary embolism and acute haemorrhage can also present with TLOC resembling orthostatic syncope, but these patients are likely to have ongoing abnormal observations.

Cardiac syncope is the most important and not to be missed cause of TLOC. It is caused by a non-sustained episode of serious arrythmia, such as ventricular tachycardia (VT), ventricular fibrillation (VF), complete heart block or sinus pauses. In people over 45 years, this is most commonly due to ischaemic heart disease, and in people under 35 years it is due to inherited arrhythmogenic conditions such as Brugada syndrome. Patients with cardiac syncope often have no preceding symptoms and usually recover quickly. They may have had multiple episodes before seeking medical attention. Beware of syncope during exertion or where there is a family history of sudden death.

Table 14.1 **ECG Changes to consider in Syncope 'WOBBLER'**

W	Wolff–Parkinson–White syndrome	Short PR interval, delta wave
O	Obstructed AV pathway	Heart blocks
B	Brugada syndrome	Coved ST segment elevation >2 mm in >1 of V1–V3 followed by a negative T wave
B	Bifasicular block	Right bundle branch block with left or right axis deviation.
L	Left ventricular hypertrophy – consider aortic stenosis and hypertrophic cardiomyopathy (HOCM)	S wave depth in V1 + tallest R wave height in V5 and V6 >35 mm, often with ST depression and T wave inversion in lateral leads
E	Epsilon wave – characteristic finding in patients with arrhythmogenic right ventricular dysplasia (ARVD)	Small deflection ('blip' or 'wiggle') buried in the end of the QRS complex – best seen in ST segment of V1 and V2
R	Repolarisation abnormality	Long QT or Short QT intervals

A worrying history for cardiac syncope or an abnormal ECG (→ *Table 14.1*) should prompt referral for telemetry monitored observation, echocardiogram and review by a cardiac electrophysiologist.

Headache

Headache is a relatively common presentation to ED and has many causes, including several serious, life-threatening conditions. Fortunately, the vast majority are primary headaches, such as migraine or cluster headache, but missing a more serious cause such as sub-arachnoid haemorrhage (SAH) can be catastrophic.

Common pathological causes of a headache → Box 14.5.

'Red flag' features in the history of a patient with a headache include:

- sudden onset of symptoms
- neck stiffness and photophobia
- confusion or decreased conscious level
- fit or loss of consciousness
- visual loss or other visual change
- other neurological symptoms
- pain worse on waking, straining or leaning forwards
- worst-ever headache
- first severe headache in a patient aged >35 years
- pregnancy and postpartum
- new headache in a patient with a ventriculoperitoneal (VP) shunt.

 Box 14.5 **Causes of a headache**

- Tension headache
- Migraine/cluster headache
- Subarachnoid haemorrhage (SAH)
- Other intracranial bleed
- Pre-eclampsia
- Cerebral venous sinus thrombosis
- Post head injury headache
- Intracranial infection
- Systemic febrile illnesses
- Space-occupying lesion
- Temporal arteritis

- Malignant hypertension
- Hypercapnia/hypoxia
- Poisoning (CO_2, nitrates)
- Glaucoma
- ENT infection, e.g. sinusitis
- Dental problems
- Neck problems
- Cerebrospinal (CSF) fluid leakage
- Dehydration
- Psychogenic factors, including anxiety and depression

The examination of a patient with a headache should record the following:

- Cortical functioning/Glasgow Coma Scale (GCS)
- Gross neurological state
- Pupillary signs
- Fundoscopy
- The presence or absence of meningism or neck tenderness
- Temperature
- The presence or absence of rashes
- Otoscopy
- Blood pressure
- Palpation of the scalp and sinuses for tenderness

XR CT is a useful first-line investigation of a headache with red flags. A negative scan within 6 hours of pain onset has good sensitivity for ruling out SAH.

TX Most patients will just want the pain to be better, so analgesia should be prioritised.

Head injury

Chronic subdural haematoma → p. 46.
Management of patients with head injuries →Chapter 3 on p. 34.

Head injury must be considered as the cause of loss of consciousness or amnesia when a patient has collapsed without witnesses.

Subarachnoid haemorrhage

Primary SAH occurs in 1 in 1000 adults. Most (80–85%) of these bleeds are caused by the rupture of saccular ('berry') aneurysms, usually situated around the circle of Willis or one of its major branches. In the remaining 15–20% of cases, no aneurysm is detected and are often due to other disorders affecting the blood vessels (such as arteriovenous malformations).

If untreated, SAH has a one-year mortality of 65% (compared with 18% if the aneurysm is treated).

SAH usually presents as one of the following:

1 Sudden collapse with a depressed level of consciousness with or without convulsions and/or vomiting
2 Sudden onset of severe occipital headache ('thunderclap' headache) with or without other neurological features. There may be a history of recent 'warning' episodes of headache. The patient may be feeling much better at the time of ED examination.

Meningism is often present even in the comatose patient although neck pain and photophobia are not essential for the diagnosis. Lateralising signs are usually 'soft' or absent.

Fundoscopy of comatose patients with SAH may reveal preretinal (subhyaloid) haemorrhages; this sign is pathognomonic.

Investigations: Non-contrast CT scan of the brain is more than 98% sensitive at detecting subarachnoid blood. It also shows the amount and distribution of the blood and complications such as surrounding oedema, hydrocephalus or ischaemic damage. Larger bleeds or those with extension into the brain parenchyma almost always yield a positive result. However, the sensitivity of CT falls to less than 50% after a week and the blood may have been completely reabsorbed by 10 days.

When the history is suggestive of SAH and the CT scan is delayed >6 hours after the onset of headache and is negative, lumbar puncture may be required. This should not be performed until at least 12 hours have elapsed since the onset of symptoms. A bloody tap can be distinguished from true SAH by levels of red cells that remain constant in successive collection tubes and by the presence of breakdown products of haemoglobin such as xanthochromia. MRI, conventional catheter angiography and MR/CT angiography are all used as further investigations for aneurysm, once SAH is confirmed.

TX
- ABCs
- Terminate convulsions
- Check the blood sugar
- Refer the patient to the general physicians/ neurosurgeons as appropriate.

The calcium antagonist nimodipine (60 mg every 4 hours) is used to prevent the development of secondary cerebral ischaemia due to vasospasm. This occurs in 50% of patients, usually in the first 5–10 days after the bleed.

Intracranial infection

Impaired consciousness and pyrexia suggest intracranial infection. Meningitis is the most common cause and may be associated with infection elsewhere. Encephalitis (usually herpetic) may present as confusion, disorientation, drowsiness or bizarre behaviour.

Encephalitis → p. 356.
Features and treatment of both bacterial and viral meningitis → pp. 355 and 356.
Prophylaxis of meningitis contacts → p. 355.

> Neck stiffness is absent in up to 30% of cases of bacterial meningitis.

Meningococcal disease is especially important for ED personnel to recognise because very early treatment (with IV antibiotics, fluids and ventilation) improves the prognosis. In the UK, cases of meningococcal infection usually rise in the autumn and reach a peak early in the New Year. This annual rise in cases starts in university students, although the highest incidence rates are in children aged <2 years. Muslim visitors to Saudi Arabia for the Hajj or Umrah pilgrimages are also at risk of meningococcal infection.

Other types of intracranial infection include abscesses and collections, often due to spread from ENT infections, seeding from intravenous drug use or immunosuppression such as HIV. CNS tuberculosis, cerebral malaria and neurocysticercosis are associated with travel to endemic areas. Ensure that you gather information on patients' social and travel history.

Meningococcal disease → p. 354.

Temporal arteritis

Cranial or giant cell arteritis is a panarteritis of unknown aetiology, which affects medium-sized vessels, particularly cranial branches. Affected arteries are thickened and tender and thrombosis may occur. The condition is related to polymyalgia rheumatica and is predominantly seen in patients aged >60 years (and almost never in people aged <50).

Temporal arteritis – the most common manifestation – starts with an acute onset of headache. There is a sharp, burning pain over the temporal artery, which may be locally tender or even pulseless. Neurological signs are caused by ischaemia in the territory of other inflamed arteries:

- **Visual impairment**: which may progress to blindness caused by ischaemia of the optic nerve and retina
- **Ophthalmoplegia**: due to ischaemia of the ocular motor nerves
- **Pain on eating**: due to masseter claudication
- **TIA/stroke**: caused by involvement of branches of the vertebral or carotid arteries.

Systemic malaise and weight loss sometimes occur. In many cases, the features are atypical.

Investigations: A raised erythrocyte sedimentation rate (ESR) suggests the diagnosis, but a normal ESR does not exclude it. Plasma CRP is also elevated in most cases. Serial ESRs and biopsy of the superficial temporal artery may be required.

Tx As soon as the diagnosis is suspected, oral prednisolone, 40–60 mg daily or parenteral methylprednisolone, 1 g IV (if visual symptoms) should be given.

> The primary aim of treatment in temporal arteritis is to prevent the occurrence of permanent neurological damage, especially blindness.

Migraine

The first severe attack of migraine usually occurs in the teenage years or early 20s. There may be an isolated unilateral throbbing headache (common migraine), or a more complicated syndrome preceded by some form of aura (classic migraine). In the latter case, the headache may be accompanied by:

- gross malaise
- pallor and tremor
- nausea and vomiting with gastric stasis
- visual disturbance such as scintillating scotoma (a blind spot in the visual field with surrounding flashing or wavy lines)

- abdominal pain
- focal neurological signs such as paraesthesia and numbness or even hemiparesis.

Over half of all patients with migraine have a family history of the condition and many suffered from travel sickness as children. Episodes of migraine may last for hours or even days. Those attacks that are atypical in severity or duration should be given special consideration.

Tx First-line treatments are with paracetamol, NSAID and aspirin (900 mg). If a patient is vomiting use an antiemetic such as metoclopramide or prochlorperazine and an alternative route of NSAID (e.g. ketorolac 60 mg IM or diclofenac 100 mg PR). Triptans such as sumitriptan are specific treatments for migraine (→ *Boxes 14.6 and 14.7*) but are not effective in every patient. Opioids are not recommended for treating migraine.

 Box 14.6 **Use of sumatriptan**

Oral dose = 100 mg, repeated after 2 hours if needed, max 300 mg/24 hours
Subcutaneous dose = 6 mg, repeated after an hour if needed, max 12 mg/24 hours
Intranasal dose = 20 mg repeated after 2 hours if needed, max 40 mg/24 hours
Sumatriptan may cause:

- lethargy
- dizziness or vertigo
- sensations of warmth
- feelings of pressure or heaviness in any part of the body

 Box 14.7 **Contraindications to sumatriptan**

- Known hypersensitivity to the drug
- Ischaemic heart disease
- Conditions predisposing to ischaemic heart disease
- Prinzmetal's angina/coronary artery vasospasm
- Poorly controlled hypertension
- Patients taking monoamine oxidase inhibitors, selective serotonin reuptake inhibitors (SSRIs) or lithium
- Pregnancy or lactation
- Children
- Age >65 years

Cluster headache

This is a related condition that is more common in men and is often misdiagnosed. There is severe unilateral facial pain (orbital, supraorbital or temporal) with lacrimation and rhinorrhoea. Each attack starts abruptly and lasts from 15 min up to 3 hours. In over 80% of patients, the headaches 'cluster' into episodes over a period of a few weeks before there is a time of remission. Abortive treatment is usually with high-flow oxygen or triptans but to prevent more episodes in this cluster a preventative medication such as verapamil should be started.

Cluster headache is a member of a group of comparatively rare conditions called trigeminal autonomic cephalalgias. They are characterised by severe unilateral pain in a trigeminal distribution and are associated with ipsilateral cranial autonomic features. Paroxysmal hemicrania is another member of the group with similar features to cluster headache although attacks are shorter, more frequent and more common in women.

Tension headache

This is the most common cause of a headache, occurring more often in females than in males. Symptoms may persist for several days and occur up to 14 days/month. The pain is usually described as a tight cap or band pressing around the head. Nausea and difficulty getting to sleep may also be experienced. There should be an absence of any headache red flags → p. 237

Tx The patient has often found that simple analgesics have not relieved the pain. Non-steroidal anti-inflammatory drugs (NSAIDs) may help, as may paracetamol and caffeine combinations, but opioids should be avoided to prevent medication overuse headache (MOH).

Brainstem stroke

Sudden catastrophic collapse may be caused by haemorrhage into or infarction of the brain stem. There will be:

- coma
- small fixed pupils (exclude narcotic/opiate poisoning)
- few, if any, lateralising signs.

Respiration continues but other brainstem functions and reflexes are attenuated. The prognosis is grave.

XR It is important to make an accurate diagnosis as soon as possible with a CT scan.

Tx As soon as the prognosis is assured, the relatives must be gently informed. The patient should be admitted to a bed and kept comfortable while nature takes its course.

End of Life care and DNACPR → pp. 16 and 171
Care of bereaved relatives → p. 171
Diagnosis of brainstem death → p. 405

Ventriculoperitoneal shunts

VP shunts are tubes which drain CSF from the ventricles into the peritoneum, for patients with congenital or acquired hydrocephalus. There is usually a valve or reservoir which is palpable just behind the patient's ear. Complications include infection (in a newly placed shunt) and obstruction/blockage. The common presenting features of shunt complications are vomiting, lethargy and headache. A CT head scan is the usual first-line investigation to check for increasing ventricle size. A shunt series involves plain radiographs of the neck, chest and abdomen to track the route of the shunt and look for kinks. Early consultation with a neurosurgeon is required when shunt malfunction is suspected.

Cerebrovascular events

Cerebrovascular disease is the fourth most common cause of death in the UK and the single most common cause of severe disability.

> Collapse associated with unilateral abnormal neurological signs is most commonly caused by a stroke or a TIA (→ *later*). The distinction between the two overlapping conditions is impossible in patients who are not already recovering when seen.

Most CVAs (80%) are a result of thrombotic or embolic cerebral infarction rather than haemorrhage. The most common causes of emboli are atrial fibrillation (AF), mural thrombosis and valvular heart disease, and these emboli lodge in the large cerebral arteries, particularly the middle cerebral arteries. Atherosclerosis causes both intracerebral thrombosis and thromboembolism from the internal carotid arteries.

The Oxford or Bamford system of stroke classification defines a total anterior circulation stroke as having three components: contralateral motor or sensory deficit, homonymous hemianopia and higher cortical dysfunction such as dysphasia and visuospatial disturbance. The combination of any two of these features is called a partial anterior circulation stroke. A posterior circulation stroke may manifest itself as cerebellar ataxia or brainstem signs or isolated homonymous hemianopia. Occlusion of deep perforating arteries (which arise from both the anterior and posterior circulation and supply the white matter of the cerebral hemispheres and brain stem) causes a lacunar stroke. This leads to pure motor, pure sensory or mixed sensorimotor deficit.

Stroke mimics are events causing similar symptoms but with a global cause such as hypoglycaemia or profound hypotension, where treatment of this will resolve the neurological features.

> A patient who complains of vague unilateral symptoms must be taken seriously.

A stroke causes loss or disturbance of motor and sensory function. In the very early stages, spinal reflexes are usually depressed although the plantar response may be extensor. Severe hypertension may be present but intervention to lower it in the ED is contraindicated because this may precipitate further cerebrovascular damage.

Investigations: Routine blood tests including glucose and ECG should be performed. Brain imaging should be undertaken as soon as possible in all patients, certainly within 24 hours of the onset of symptoms unless there are good clinical reasons for not doing so. The brain scan must be performed urgently if the patient has:

- a known bleeding tendency or is taking anticoagulants
- a depressed level of consciousness
- a severe headache at the onset
- an uncertain diagnosis or atypical features (most doctors would consider age <60 years as atypical)
- unexplained, progressive or fluctuating signs
- papilloedema, neck stiffness or fever
- indications for thrombolysis or thrombectomy (→ *later*).

> Non-contrast CT is most useful for excluding intracerebral haemorrhage and conditions such as brain metastases. It should be performed as soon as possible. However, it has a low sensitivity (around 26%) for detecting early ischaemia when compared with MRI (83%).

Tx
- Give oxygen, if required, to maintain the SaO_2 >94%.
- Monitor vital signs.
- Do not routinely lower BP in the acute phase of an ischaemic stroke unless there are specific circumstances such as hypertensive encephalopathy or aortic dissection. Patients who are to receive intravenous thrombolysis will need blood pressure reduction to 185/110 mmHg.
- Patients with haemorrhagic stroke should have blood pressure control with a goal of 140 mmHg systolic. *Hypertensive emergencies→ p. 253.*

- Check the blood sugar and urgently treat hypoglycaemia.
- Establish IV access and give maintenance IV fluids. The patient should be kept nil by mouth until there has been a proper assessment of the airway and swallowing reflexes.
- Treat pyrexia which is associated with a worse outcome, possibly because of its effects on free radical production or cerebral metabolism.
- Admit the patient to hospital for assessment and rehabilitation – usually in a specialist stroke unit.

Anticoagulants are usually prescribed for all patients with persistent or paroxysmal AF. Other patients with an ischaemic stroke require antiplatelet therapy with aspirin 300 mg daily for 2 weeks.

For the mechanism of action of other antiplatelet drugs → p. 193.

Thrombolysis for stroke

Thrombolysis with alteplase is felt to be beneficial if given within 4.5 hours of an ischaemic stroke in selected patients, under the instruction of a stroke specialist. The aim is to limit the size of the cerebral infarct and thus improve the functional outcome. Alteplase (tPA) is given intravenously over 60 min in a dose of 900 mcg/kg (to a maximum of 90 mg). The initial 10% of the dose should be given by bolus injection and the remaining 90% by infusion. A CT brain scan must be performed before thrombolysis to exclude intracerebral haemorrhage.

General contraindications to thrombolysis › Box 12.3 on p. 191.
Specific contraindications to the use of thrombolysis in ischaemic stroke → Box 14.8.

> **Box 14.8 Specific contraindications to the use of thrombolysis in ischaemic stroke**
>
> *Also → p. 191 for the general contraindications to thrombolysis.*
>
> - Onset of symptoms more than 4.5 hours previously or unclear time of onset
> - Previous stroke within the past 3 months
> - History of stroke in patient with diabetes
> - Evidence of intracranial haemorrhage
> - Seizure at onset of stroke
> - Systolic BP >185 mmHg or diastolic BP >110 mmHg
> - Platelet count below 100×10^9/L
> - Treatment with anticoagulant

Thrombectomy for stroke

Thrombectomy together with IV thrombolysis can be performed within 6 hours of stroke in patients with a confirmed proximal anterior circulation occlusion, or within 24 hours where there is potential to salvage brain tissue on CT perfusion or diffusion-weighted MRI scans.

Hyperacute Stroke Units are set up to deliver these treatments throughout the UK and you should familiarise yourself with your local referral pathway.

Transient ischaemic attack

A TIA is defined as an abrupt loss of focal cerebral or monocular function with symptoms lasting <24 hours which, after adequate investigation, is presumed to be caused by embolic or thrombotic vascular disease.

> There is no qualitative difference between a TIA and an ischaemic stroke. Truly transient cerebrovascular events last for only a matter of minutes!

The risk of having a stroke after a hemispheric TIA is over 5% in the first 7 days, with the greatest risk occurring in the first 72 hours. In addition, a TIA is a marker for general vascular disease. Half of all TIAs are caused by the thromboembolic complications of arteriosclerosis in the arteries that supply the brain; emboli from the heart account for a further 20%.

The diagnosis of TIA is based on the history. Symptoms – usually loss of function – are of sudden onset and are maximal from the start (→ *Box 14.9*). As TIAs are focal events, global symptoms such as lightheadedness, dizziness and syncope are rarely consistent

---

> **Box 14.9 Symptoms of a TIA**
>
> TIA in the carotid territory (80% of TIAs):
>
> - Unilateral paresis
> - Unilateral sensory loss
> - Aphasia
> - Monocular visual loss
>
> Vertebrobasilar TIA:
>
> - Bilateral or alternating weakness or sensory loss
> - Bilateral visual loss/hemianopia
> - Two or more of the following: vertigo, diplopia, dysphagia, dysarthria and ataxia

---

with the diagnosis. The following predisposing factors should be sought:

- AF or other source of cardiac embolism
- Hypertension
- Carotid disease (bruits)
- History of smoking
- Hypercholesterolaemia.

Investigations: All patients should have a routine blood tests (FBC, ESR, U&Es, LFTs [liver function tests], glucose, random cholesterol and ECG). An urgent CT scan of the brain should be considered for patients who have a bleeding disorder or are taking an anticoagulant. Carotid duplex scan is usually requested from the TIA clinic.

Tx Once the symptoms are clearly resolving, oral aspirin (300 mg) should be given to all patients in whom it is not contraindicated. Admit to hospital patients who have had more than one TIA in a week. Other patients may go home, provided there are arrangements for assessment by a specialist service within 7 days of the TIA at the latest.

Driving after a stroke or TIA

The UK Driver and Vehicle Licencing Agency (DVLA) rules on fitness to drive state that a patient with a diagnosis of stroke or TIA must not drive for at least 1 month. He or she may resume driving after this time if his or her clinical recovery is judged to be satisfactory and he or she has not had any fits. There is no need to notify the licencing authority (DVLA) unless there is a residual neurological deficit 1 month after the episode. A patient with multiple TIAs will require an attack-free period of 3 months before resuming driving and must notify the DVLA.

Transient global amnesia

Transient global amnesia (TGA) describes a sudden and temporary loss of memory in an otherwise well patient who is fully conscious throughout the episode. Distant memories are preserved, as is immediate recall of current events. The patient often repeatedly asks questions about how they got here and what happened today. There is complete recovery within 24 hours (and usually much sooner). TGA is of unknown aetiology and carries no increased risk of CVA or other illness although there is a small risk of recurrence. The main known risk factor is a history of migraine. Management focusses on excluding other conditions and reassuring the patient.

Acute vestibular syndrome (vertigo)

Acute vestibular syndrome is described as an acute onset of rotational dizziness and nausea which is worse on moving the head, associated with a clinical finding of nystagmus. The causes are usually split into central (i.e. cerebellar causes) and peripheral (i.e. vestibular or inner ear).

Acute, constant symptoms are most commonly due to vestibular neuronitis, a viral or post-viral inflammatory disorder affecting the vestibular portion of the eighth cranial nerve. The nystagmus is horizontal with a fast phase beating away from the affected side. Only a small proportion of cases are due to inflammation of the labyrinth, i.e. labyrinthitis, and are associated with concurrent hearing loss and sometimes pain. Hearing loss is actually more indicative of a central cause as these are more common than labyrinthitis, which is typically over-diagnosed.

The central causes of acute vertigo (which includes cerebellar infarct and haemorrhage) are the cause of vertigo in up to 25% of adults over the age of 50 presenting to the ED. The patient may have other cerebellar signs such as dysarthria and ataxia or headache if there is acute haemorrhage. The nystagmus may be vertical or horizontal and can change direction with gaze. The patient may have risk factors such as hypertension or AF. Frequently, it is difficult to differentiate between those with peripheral and central causes.

A full neurological examination including HiNTS exam (see → *Box 14.10*) can help differentiate patients with central and peripheral causes, but it is important to consider posterior circulation stroke in all patients with risk factors and those who are unable to stand or walk.

- After a few seconds, quickly uncover the eye and look for a small vertical corrective movement
- Realigning of the eye vertically is concerning for a central pathology.

Investigations: Patients with acute vertigo should have an ECG and blood glucose. CT scan is often used as first-line imaging modality for suspected central vertigo, but has a poor sensitivity, so MRI is usually warranted where suspicion is high.

Tx Symptomatic treatment is usually with antihistamines such as cinnarizine and dimenhydrinate, benzodiazepines such as diazepam and antiemetics such as prochlorperazine. There is some evidence for the use of steroids and vestibular exercises for vestibular neuronitis.

Episodic vestibular syndrome may be due to vestibular migraine, benign paroxysmal positional vertigo (BPPV), TIA and Meniere's disease. BPPV is characterised by the ability to reproduce nystagmus and vertigo on Dix-Hallpike test and is treated using maneuvers such as Epley. Remember that patients with all causes of vertigo will have worsening of symptoms with head movements, and BPPV should only be diagnosed if they feel completely normal between short lived episodes.

Also → CVA and TIA on pp. 240 and 242.

 Box 14.10 **HiNTS exam**

Head-impulse test

- Gently move the patient's head side to side asking them to focus on your nose
- When their neck muscles are relaxed, turn the head 20° to each side rapidly then to the midline
- A corrective saccade (a beat of nystagmus whilst the eyes 'catch up') is a positive head-impulse test and reassuring for a peripheral problem.

Assessment of nystagmus

- Assess the eye movements in all directions looking at the direction of nystagmus (it can help to focus on a conjunctival blood vessel)
- Nystagmus that changes direction with gaze is highly suspicious for a central cause.

Test of skew

- Cover one of the patient's eyes with your hand and ask them to look at your nose

---

Convulsions (seizures)

Treatment of fits in children → p. 356.

Fits occur when there is one of the following:

- **Deprivation of cerebral fuel supply (anoxic convulsion):**
  - hypoglycaemia or hypoxia
  - transient dysrhythmia or cardiac arrest
  - syncope
- **Cerebral irritation:**
  - head injury
  - cerebral tumour or infection
  - poisoning
  - fever in children
- **Primary epilepsy**
- **Withdrawal of sedatives**: alcohol or drug withdrawal.

A fit causes a dramatic increase in the cerebral metabolic demand for oxygen and also partial airway obstruction and decreased ventilation. Hypoxia must be prevented by urgent airway control and rapid treatment of the fit before elucidation of the underlying cause can be undertaken.

Tx

- Protect or remove the patient from harm.
- Check for a pulse and breathing and attach monitoring.
- Give high-concentration oxygen by facemask. Never attempt to force open the airway by inserting a wedge in the mouth – use a Guedel airway once the jaw has relaxed.
- Obtain venous access.
- Give IV lorazepam (initially 0.1 mg/kg for adults, max 4 mg). If IV access cannot be obtained, then diazepam can be given rectally. Repeat once after 5–10 min.
- If the patient is pregnant or recently post partum and give IV magnesium sulphate 4 g IV.

When the fit has stopped:

- place the patient in the recovery position
- monitor vital signs
- check the blood sugar
- start investigating the circumstances that led to the fit and perform a full physical examination.

If the fit is not terminated, move to second-line agents and call for urgent help – an anaesthetist may be needed.

- **Levetiracetam**: 60 mg/kg (max 4500 mg) IV
- **Phenytoin or Fosphenytoin**: immediate loading dose of 20 mg/kg (max 1500 mg) by IV infusion at a rate of no more than 50 mg/min (or 1 mg/kg per min)
- **Valproate**: 40 mg/kg (max 300 mg) IV

As soon as it becomes apparent that more than one drug is required, consideration should be given to the need for rapid sequence induction and intubation. This usually entails intensive care unit (ICU) admission for sedation, paralysis and ventilation.

Serial seizures without full recovery should be treated as aggressively as status epilepticus as ongoing cerebral ischaemia is a strong possibility.

A fully recovered patient with known epilepsy may go home under the following circumstances:

- There are no unusual features in this episode.
- They remain well after 2 hours observation.
- There is social support at home.
- The GP is informed of the discharge.
- The usual drug supply is available.

Non-epileptic attack disorder

Also known as psychogenic seizures or functional seizures, they consist of transient episodes of reduced consciousness and involuntary movements. Patients often have a history of severe psychological trauma. There is no single feature that can reliably differentiate this condition from epileptic seizures in the ED, although there may be recall of events, forced eye closure, pelvic thrusting and an absence of intraoral injury. The lactate will be typically normal compared to the raised levels seen with other types of seizure.

Patients are not faking these episodes or looking for attention, nor should they be subjected to painful stimuli in an attempt to 'fool them'. Maintain a calm environment and gently provide reassurance that they are safe and being looked after. If there is uncertainty about the diagnosis, treat as for convulsions and refer on to a neurologist or 'first fit clinic'.

Peripheral neuropathies and similar conditions

There are many causes of conduction failure of the peripheral nerves including drugs, diabetes, infections, vitamin deficiencies and alcoholism. Many cases are idiopathic. Guillain–Barré syndrome is the most common type of acute polyneuropathy in the UK → *later*.

Isolated peripheral neuropathies may follow stretching or compression of nerves due to injury or local tissue swelling. Radial nerve palsy (wrist drop) and foot drop sometimes present to an ED. Both conditions should be treated by splintage and referral for investigation.

Acute (transverse) myelitis may look similar to a polyneuritis. It causes a specific sensory level with bilateral leg weakness and bladder and bowel dysfunction.

Functional neurological disorder (FND) typically presents with one or more symptoms of altered motor or sensory function with no medical explanation. Emphasis should go towards diagnosing this condition through positive findings rather than attempting to rule out other conditions with multiple investigations. Often there are inconsistent examination findings, for example a patient may have difficulty dorsiflexing the foot while supine but be able to stand on their heels without difficulty. There are some validated tests to help identify FND such as Hoover's sign, where weakness in hip extension becomes normal when the patient concurrently flexes the contralateral hip against resistance. Patients will usually require evaluation by a neurologist experienced in diagnosing this condition, but the ED doctor can explain that this is the condition the patient probably has and the exam finding that lead to this conclusion. Explain that FND occurs when the nervous system is not damaged but is having difficulty 'getting signals through'.

Multiple sclerosis (MS) is not a peripheral neuropathy but may be mistaken for one because the multiple central nervous system (CNS) lesions responsible are scattered in both time and place. MS may present with a vast array of different neurological features including loss of vision, diplopia, spastic weakness of the legs, numbness and paraesthesia, sphincter disturbance, painful flexor spasms and cerebellar signs (vertigo, tremor and nystagmus).

Botulism → p. 246.
Myasthenia gravis → below.
Poliomyelitis → p. 266.
Tetanus → pp. below and 415.

Guillain–Barré syndrome (acute polyneuritis)

Guillain–Barré syndrome is an ascending polyneuritis of unknown aetiology, which has an annual incidence of 1–2 cases per 100 000. It is the most common form of acute peripheral neuropathy in the UK; however, only around 25% of patients are correctly diagnosed on their first visit to ED.

There are at least four clinicopathological subtypes. Most cases (85%) are described as 'acute inflammatory demyelinating polyradiculoneuropathy'. Between 25% and 30% of patients require artificial ventilation. Mortality rates range from 3% to 6% overall but rise to around 20% in ventilated patients.

The features of Guillain–Barré syndrome develop over the course of a few days or sometimes several weeks. There may be a history of a preceding infection (most commonly cytomegalovirus or *Campylobacter jejuni*) and then severe backache before the development of neurological symptoms and signs as below:

- Paraesthesia with minimal or no sensory loss starting symmetrically in fingers and toes
- Progressive, symmetrical, ascending weakness, which may include ocular, bulbar and respiratory muscles. The initial complaint is often difficulty climbing stairs.
- Greatly diminished or absent tendon reflexes
- Autonomic disturbances such as tachycardia, cardiac dysrhythmias and labile blood pressure.

Motor involvement (which may be either proximal or distal) usually predominates over sensory loss (often distal). Of the cranial nerves, the facial nerve is the most commonly affected.

Investigations: The cerebrospinal fluid (CSF) usually contains an increased amount of protein with normal cell counts. Differential diagnoses should be excluded (botulism, cauda equina, myasthenia gravis, transverse myelitis, poliomyelitis and tick paralysis.) Patients should be tested for HIV. Spirometry is useful to assess the degree of respiratory impairment.

Tx If the condition is clinically suspected, then the patient must be admitted to hospital. Intensive care is appropriate if there is bulbar or respiratory weakness

or autonomic signs. Most cases of Guillain–Barré syndrome recover spontaneously over several weeks. Immunotherapy with intravenous immunoglobulin or plasma exchange has been shown to hasten recovery but corticosteroids do not help. Residual disability is found in 20% of those patients who survive the illness.

Tetanus

Gas gangrene (Clostridium perfringens infection) → p. 274.
Prophylaxis against tetanus infection in wounds → p. 415.

Infection is caused by contamination of a wound with the spores of the bacillus *Clostridium tetani*. Days or even weeks after infection, local multiplication of the organism occurs with release of its neurotoxin, tetanospasmin. Even the most trivial of wounds can introduce tetanus into the body, but some wounds carry a particularly high risk of infection. (*Factors that help to identify tetanus-prone wounds → p. 416*). The incubation period of tetanus is between 4 and 21 days (usually about 10 days), and the case fatality rate is almost 30%. Tetanus is a notifiable disease.

Active immunisation against tetanus was adopted nationally in the UK from 1961. Most cases in the UK are in older adults and people who inject drugs.

It is important to understand the mechanism of action of tetanus toxin. In the ventral horn of the spinal cord, negative feedback loop neurons (Renshaw cells) limit the activity of the α-motoneurons. Tetanus toxin preferentially prevents discharge from GABA inhibitory interneurons in spinal cord and brainstem leading to unrestricted motor nerve activity and autonomic instability. Strychnine (and brucine) compete with glycine for its receptors on the α-motoneurons and thus cause a very similar clinical picture.

Acute dystonic reactions ('oculogyric crises') → p. 307.
Meningism → p. 355.
Hypocalcaemia → p. 260.
Trismus from facial infection→ p. 440 may also mimic tetanus.

The clinical features of tetanus can progress slowly over as much as 2 weeks. In the usual order of appearance, they are as follows:

- Stiff muscles near the wound (or injection site)
- Jaw stiffness and trismus ('lock-jaw')
- Abdominal rigidity
- Progressive painful muscle spasms (the fixed mocking grin caused by facial muscle tightening is known as the 'risus sardonicus' and extensor spasms of the back, neck and limbs are called opisthotonus)
- Dysphagia and respiratory difficulty
- Autonomic dysfunction.

Consider the diagnosis of tetanus in injecting drug users presenting with muscle stiffness or muscle spasms.

Tx Supportive therapy is essential, with special attention given to the airway, respiration and autonomic activities. High doses of IV benzodiazepines or general anaesthesia with neuromuscular blockade is usually required to control spasms. The tetanus bacillus is sensitive to both benzylpenicillin and metronidazole. Immunoglobulin against tetanus toxin (HTIg) 100–300 IU/kg is given intramuscularly in multiple sites. Suspicion of tetanus infection should provoke a discussion with a specialist in infectious diseases. Strychnine poisoning is treated with similar supportive and relaxant therapy.

Botulism

Botulinum toxin is one of the potent poisonous substances known to humans.

Food-borne botulism: the features of botulism typically begin between 12 and 36 hours after ingestion of contaminated food, frequently home-canned goods. The earliest symptoms are usually gastrointestinal (nausea, vomiting and abdominal pain) and neurological (dysfunction of the cranial nerves).

Wound botulism: this variant of botulism has been seen in people who inject drugs, probably as a result of contaminated drugs. Unlike the classic food-borne disease (which is caused by the ingestion of preformed toxin), wound botulism occurs when the spores of the anaerobic bacterium *Clostridium botulinum* contaminate a wound, germinate and produce toxin *in vivo*.

Infant botulism: Infants typically present with constipation and poor feeding followed by progressive hypotonia and weakness. Ask about ingestion of honey.

Botulinum toxin blocks the release of acetylcholine from the neuromuscular junction and characteristically causes a descending flaccid paralysis:

- Dysphonia, dysarthria and dysphagia (in >95% of cases)
- Blurred or double vision and ptosis (in >90% of cases)
- Dizziness and general muscle weakness (in >70% of cases)
- Immobility and respiratory distress.

Patients are afebrile with no sensory loss and no confusion. Autonomic signs include dry mouth, dilated pupils/blurred vision, constipation and urinary dysfunction; postural hypotension may also occur. Surprisingly, deep tendon reflexes are preserved. Diagnosis can be confirmed in a reference laboratory using serum, stool or contaminated food samples but may take 4–6 days to yield results. Hence treatment should be started based on clinical symptoms and signs.

Tx Ventilatory support may be required, as may surgical debridement of wounds. *C. botulinum* is sensitive to benzylpenicillin and metronidazole. Botulinum antitoxin should always be given because it is effective in reducing both the severity and the duration of symptoms.

CONDITIONS RELATED TO ENVIRONMENT AND EXPOSURE

Conditions caused by diving

Decompression sickness

Decompression sickness or 'the Bends' may occur up to 48 hours after diving, 90% develop symptoms within 6 hours. It is caused by nitrogen (which has been dissolved in the blood under pressure) coming out of solution and forming bubbles in the bloodstream and tissues if the diver emerges too quickly. The patient may present as a collapse without offering a history of recreational diving because many people do not appreciate the potential for delayed onset of symptoms. There is an increased risk with longer and more frequent dives. There is:

- malaise
- joint pains
- itching and rashes (cutis marmorata)

In severe cases, there are signs and symptoms of cardiopulmonary, vestibular and CNS involvement such as:

- chest pain
- dyspnoea, coughing and haemoptysis
- hypertension or hypotension
- tinnitus or deafness
- nausea, vertigo and nystagmus
- headache
- behavioural changes and altered consciousness
- convulsions.

In the presence of rapid ascent there may also be pulmonary barotrauma leading to pneumothorax or even arterial gas embolism and stroke symptoms.

Tx
- Start high flow oxygen regardless of the patient's sats
- Rule out pneumothorax with a chest X-ray
- Commence IV fluid resuscitation
- Control fits and agitation.

Discuss the patient with a specialist in diving and hyperbaric medicine. Recompression in a hyperbaric chamber may be required. The National Diving Accident

Helpline can be contacted 24 hours a day, 365 days a year, on 07831 151523.

Altitude-related illness

Barometric pressure falls logarithmically with increasing altitude. The partial pressure of oxygen (21% of barometric pressure) falls at the same rate. At 19 000 ft (5800 m), these pressures are 50% of their values at sea level, falling to 28% at the summit of Mount Everest. The ambient temperature also drops by 6.5°C with every additional 3300 ft (1000 m) in altitude. The complex physiological changes of acclimatisation include increased minute ventilation, increased sympathetic tone, increased pulmonary vascular resistance and, after several weeks, an increased haematocrit.

Acute mountain sickness: This affects around 75% of people who ascend rapidly to heights of more than 10 000 ft (3000 m) above sea level and even troubles 20% of people at just 7500 ft (2300 m). It is usually defined as a headache accompanied by any of the following symptoms: nausea, vomiting, malaise, fatigue, lethargy, anorexia and insomnia. Sleep may be disturbed by periodic breathing or even apnoea. Acute mountain sickness (AMS) usually resolves within 3 days of arriving at altitude but sometimes leads to life-threatening cerebral or pulmonary oedema. The causes of these altitude-related illnesses are poorly understood. There is some genetic predisposition associated with capillary leakage, fluid retention and stimulation of chemoreceptors in the presence of hypoxaemia. The risk is increased with rapid ascents and failure to acclimatise. All patients will have a low SaO_2. It is said that AMS can be minimised by 'climbing high and sleeping low'.

High-altitude cerebral oedema: the most severe manifestation of altitude sickness is acute cerebral oedema, which can be overwhelming if untreated. It is thought to have the same pathophysiology as AMS and may represent the extreme form of the condition. In addition to the usual symptoms of mountain sickness, there is a progressive deterioration in mental status with ataxia and, in some cases, focal neurological deficits. Eventually, coma supervenes.

High-altitude pulmonary oedema: this is seen in 2–4% of climbers once 14 000 ft (4300 m) is reached and is the most common medical cause of death at altitude. Atmospheric hypoxia is thought to cause pulmonary hypertension, uneven perfusion and capillary leakage. The first symptoms are cough and tachypnoea, followed by increasing dyspnoea and cyanosis.

High-altitude retinal haemorrhages: are usually asymptomatic and resolve spontaneously.

Tx Sufferers must be advised to stop and rest immediately before the condition worsens. Oxygen, analgesics and antiemetics should be given and descent arranged. A reduction in altitude of as little as 1500–3000 ft (450–900 m) may be all that is required. Acetazolamide 125–250 mg twice daily may be given to increase the rate of acclimatisation. High-altitude cerebral oedema is treated with dexamethasone 4 mg (by any route) every 6 hours and hyperbaric therapy (in a portable unit such as a Gamow bag) if available. Patients with high-altitude pulmonary oedema should be given oral nifedipine 10 mg 4-hourly (or 30 mg extended release twice daily) and hyperbaric therapy, in addition to standard treatments for the oedema.

Other risks in climbers

These include hypothermia, frostbite, UV keratitis, exacerbation of pre-existing diseases and, of course, trauma.

> British expeditions to peaks higher than 23 000 ft (7000 m) have experienced death rates of 4.3 per 100 climbers.

Hypothermia

Hypothermia is defined as a core temperature <35°C:

- Mild hypothermia – <35°C
- Moderate hypothermia – <32°C
- Severe hypothermia – <28°C.

Core temperature must be measured with a device accurate for low readings.

There are three main types of accidental hypothermia:

1 **Acute (immersion) hypothermia**: heat production is overwhelmed by sudden cold stress (immersion, lying injured in snow)
2 **Acute (exhaustion) hypothermia**: cooling occurs only as energy reserves are exhausted (endurance sports, outdoor pursuits and immersion in relatively warm water)
3 **Subacute (urban) hypothermia**: the victim has been exposed to moderate cold for days, often with several predisposing factors (elderly, alcohol dependent, illicit drug use, homelessness). Rising energy costs are likely to increase the incidence of this condition.

> Up to 3% of medical patients admitted to UK hospitals during winter months have core temperatures <35°C.

There are several important haemodynamic changes in hypothermia:

- Profound vasoconstriction occurs. This is accompanied by a diuresis.
- Fluid moves into the extracellular compartment and cells.
- Immersion in water causes hydrostatic compression of the body – an effect similar to vasoconstriction and hence removal from water may cause 'rescue collapse'.
- As the core temperature decreases, bradycardia occurs followed by ventricular fibrillation and asystole.

The reversal of these effects during re-warming creates a danger of fluid overload. *For causes of death in hypothermia → Box 14.11.*

> **Box 14.11 Causes of death in hypothermia**
>
> - Hypovolaemia and circulatory collapse
> - Fluid overload leading to cardiac failure and pulmonary or cerebral oedema
> - Ventricular fibrillation
> - Hypoxia
> - Continued cooling and cardiac standstill
> - Underlying pathology that predisposed patient to hypothermia (e.g. poisoning or CVA)

Hypothermia also induces metabolic and neurological upset:

- There is both respiratory and metabolic acidosis. Serum potassium levels rise.
- As the body temperature falls, carbohydrate is progressively replaced by fat as the metabolic fuel. Insulin resistance develops but the blood sugar level may be high or low.
- Coagulopathy can occur due to the disruption of coagulation enzymes.
- Pancreatitis may occur.
- Haemolysis may rarely occur in patients with cold agglutinin disease.

- CNS symptoms include memory impairment, slurred speech, ataxia and coma. Patients may exhibit paradoxical undressing.

Tx Hypothermia is a reversible condition. Recovery has been reported from core temperatures as low as 13.7°C. Cardiovascular complications may make re-warming hazardous, but if normothermia can be regained patients rarely show any residual stigmata in the CNS or elsewhere.

- Remove clothing, especially if wet.
- Institute careful monitoring with rectal or oesophageal temperature probes and 3 lead ECG.
- Treat the patient gently – the most common precipitant of VF in hypothermia is mechanical movement of the body.
- Start passive re-warming:
- Gently dry the skin.
- Wrap the patient in blankets.
- Cover the scalp with a hat or blanket.
- Establish an IV line, although fluid therapy must be carefully monitored.
- Take blood for baseline full blood count, glucose, U&Es, coagulation and amylase.
- Consider parenteral thiamine for malnourished patients and those with high alcohol intake.
- Obtain an ECG. It may show bradycardia and a characteristic notching of the S wave (usually seen best in V4) referred to as a J wave (present in 80% of patients with severe hypothermia) → *Figure 14.1*
- Consider coincidental injury. Bruising and swelling are slow to appear in hypothermia and examination may be deceptively normal. The skin will be susceptible to burns and pressure effects because of its poor blood supply.
- Consider active methods of re-warming (→ *Box 14.12*) in elderly patients with a core temperature <32°C and in younger patients with a temperature <30°C. ICU-level monitoring and facilities for ventilation must be available for these groups. Patients with the slow-onset (subacute) type of hypothermia (invariably elderly people) should probably be re-warmed at a rate no faster than 0.5°C/h to avoid the risk of pulmonary and cerebral oedema.

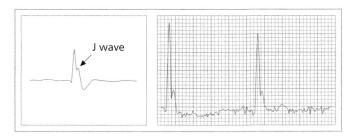

Figure 14.1 J waves on the ECG in hypothermia.

Box 14.12 **Re-warming in hypothermia**

Re-warming may be of two main types:

- **Passive re-warming**: insulation and other measures to prevent further heat loss
- **Active re-warming**: heat supplied to the surface or the core of the body

Active external re-warming

- Heat packs applied to axillae and groins
- Heat lamps
- Forced air systems – such as Bair Hugger™

Active core re-warming
This is more effective and logical than surface warming and should be employed in severe hypothermia. Techniques include the following:

- Airway warming: warm, moist air is supplied from a humidifier.
- Warmed IV fluids – warmed to 44° through peripheral or central line.
- Gastric, bladder or peritoneal lavage with warm saline
- Extracorporeal blood warming: this requires specialised facilities

Hypothermic patients with no detectable cardiac output

Diagnosis of arrest (feeling for a central pulse) should take place over about 60 seconds. The depressed circulation is difficult to assess; inappropriate cardiopulmonary resuscitation may precipitate VF.

Ventilation and chest compressions should be started. The compliance of the lungs, heart and chest wall is decreased in hypothermia.

> The administration of warm (40°C) IV fluids is attractive but technically difficult to achieve because the high flows and volumes required may lead to fluid overload.

Defibrillation for VF is less effective as the core temperature falls – especially to <28°C. Thus, it is usually recommended that, if there is no response to the initial three shocks, subsequent attempts at defibrillation are delayed until the core temperature rises to >30°C.

Metabolism of drugs is impaired in hypothermia and toxic accumulation of drugs may thus occur. For this reason, it is usually recommended that adrenaline and other drugs are withheld until the patient's core temperature

reaches 30°C. At this point, the interval between drug doses is doubled (adrenaline is given every 6–10 min) until at least 32°C has been reached.

Resuscitation efforts can often be long, with episodes of return of circulation alternating with pulselessness. Insertion of an arterial line may help detect loss of output and monitor beat to beat blood pressure. Use of a mechanical CPR machine will help avoid fatigue within the resus team. Consider extracorporeal membrane oxygenation (ECMO) if available.

Apparently dead patients may be hypothermic but recoverable, especially children. The heart can still be working even if this is clinically undetectable. Patients who may have suffered from hypothermia must therefore be re-warmed to at least 32° before assessing viability. There are reports of patients surviving after more than 6 hours of CPR!

Cardiac arrest → Chapter 11.

Hyperpyrexia and hyperthermia

Hyperpyrexia is defined as a core temperature in excess of 41°C. This can result from three main causes:

1 Febrile illnesses
2 Exposure or environmental (see heat stroke below)
3 Hyperthermic conditions.

In a fever, the thermoregulatory set point of the hypothalamus is raised. This usually causes temperatures of between 38 and 41°C, and rarely up to 42°C – a response that may be protective against some infectious diseases. Hence, the effect of antipyretics, such as paracetamol, which reset the temperature control mechanism. Cooling measures alone are relatively ineffective and short-lived.

Hyperthermia is a condition in which there is an imbalance between heat production and heat loss. Urgent treatment is required to lower the temperature; however, antipyretics will have no effect. Brain damage continues throughout the period of hyperpyrexia.

Causes of hyperthermia include the following:

- The extreme effects of drugs (e.g. anticholinergics, sympathomimetics, serotonin syndrome)
- Idiosyncratic reactions to drugs (e.g. neuroleptic malignant syndrome and malignant hyperthermia → *p. 281*; ecstasy and other stimulant drugs → *pp. 292*)
- Tetanus and other severe tonic–clonic conditions (→ *p. 245*)
- Thyroid storm → *p. 257*, phaeochromocytoma or adrenal crisis
- Excessive exercise, exhaustion and dehydration (heat exhaustion → *below*)

- Combinations of the above (e.g. febrile illnesses accompanied by convulsions or profound dehydration; stimulant drugs and prolonged dancing with an inadequate fluid intake).

> If the patient's temperature is >42°C, then hyperthermia is the likely diagnosis rather than fever.

Treatment of hyperthermia → p. 281.

Heat exhaustion and heat stroke

Heat exhaustion results from a combination of excessive exercise, exhaustion of energy stores and dehydration. Symptoms include headache, malaise, nausea, vomiting, faintness and muscle cramps. Core temperature is usually <41°C and mental status is unaffected. Treatment is rest, cooling, fluids and glucose. In most cases, the condition runs a benign course and does not lead to a hyperpyrexic emergency.

Heat stroke leads to temperatures >41°C, with tachycardia, tachypnoea and hypotension. Patients may have altered mental status, seizures or coma. Patients should be rapidly cooled with ice bath immersion if available. Otherwise, use cold IV fluids, ice packs and spray the skin with water whilst directing fans at the patient.

CARDIOVASCULAR PROBLEMS

Anaphylaxis → p. 306.
Cardiac dysrhythmias → p. 172.
Dyspnoea → Chapter 13 on p. 209.
Myocardial infarction → p. 185.
Pulmonary embolism → p. 227.

Shock

Shock is a state of inadequate perfusion of vital tissues. This may be caused by inadequacies in the pump (heart), the delivery system (blood vessels) or the perfusing fluid (blood). Compensatory mechanisms are activated in response to reduced tissue perfusion. The sympathetic nervous system vasoconstricts and increases myocardial contractility. This is followed by renin–angiotensin–aldosterone-mediated retention of fluid and salt by the kidneys. Hypotension occurs when these mechanisms have been overwhelmed or unable to respond (e.g. older age, medications such as beta-blockers or adrenal insufficiency).

There are four basic types of shock:

1 **Cardiogenic shock:** pump failure
2 **Hypovolaemic shock**: decreased blood volume
3 **Distributive shock**: leaky or dilated blood vessels
4 **Obstructive shock**: physical obstruction to the flow of blood, e.g. tension pneumothorax or tamponade.

In reality, there often exists a mixture of these types. For instance, in septic shock, there is vasodilation and maldistribution of fluid, but there may also be elements of cardiac depression due to myocyte dysfunction, and hypovolaemia due to sweating and reduced oral intake.

Point of care ultrasound (POCUS) can be a useful tool, in experienced hands, to differentiate some of the important causes of shock in the collapsed patient. A typical approach would be as follows:

- Assess left ventricular contractility and look for signs of right heart dilation and tamponade
- Assess inferior vena cava (IVC) size and collapsibility
- Assess lung fields for signs of pneumothorax
- Assess abdominal aorta for aneurysm
- Assess right and left upper quadrants and suprapubic region of abdomen for free fluid.

Anaphylactic shock → p. 306.
Hypovolaemic, septic and cardiogenic shock → below.
Neurogenic shock → p. 54.

Hypovolaemic shock

Loss of blood or other body fluid may result in hypovolaemic shock. The patient will often appear pale and have cool, mottled skin. They may complain of thirst. As the degree of shock progresses the blood pressure will drop and the patient will become agitated, then confused and then unresponsive.

Tx
- Insert two large IV lines. Short thick lines are the best.
- Cross-match blood.
- Institute full monitoring, consider invasive blood pressure measurement with an arterial line.
- Give IV fluids or blood in boluses of 10–20 mL/kg.
- Look for the cause of the shock, in particular;
  - Pregnancy test in women of childbearing age, considering ruptured ectopic
  - Blood in the mouth or melaena in GI haemorrhage
  - Blood loss in trauma
  - Fluid loss from stomas or sweating
- Insert a urinary catheter and monitor output.

Sepsis and septic shock

Sepsis is the body's overwhelming and life-threatening response to infection that can lead to tissue damage, organ failure and death. People at particular risk of sepsis are those who:

- are very young (<1 year) and very old (>75 years)
- are immunosuppressed
- are pregnant or post-partum
- have recently had surgery, burns or large wounds
- have indwelling medical lines or catheters
- inject drugs.

Careful assessment of the patient will first ascertain whether an infection is suspected. In some patients, this will be easier to determine than in others. Getting the balance right between prompt treatment and accurate treatment can be a challenge in the realm of potential sepsis, especially in a time where antibiotic stewardship is so important. On suspecting infection or sepsis one must first ask, 'is this patient sick?' Tools such as NEWS, qSOFA and the red/amber sepsis criteria can be used to help quantify this →see Box 14.13.

In a sick patient (NEWS ≥7, any red flag criteria, ≥2 qSOFA criteria), it is prudent to start antibiotics within the first hour and then begin investigations to identify the

---

Box 14.13 Sepsis risk stratification tools

Quick sepsis organ failure assessment (qSOFA):

- Altered mental state (GCS ≤14)
- Respiratory rate >20 per minute
- Systolic blood pressure <100 mmHg

Two or more criteria is considered high risk

Amber flag sepsis criteria	Red flag sepsis criteria
• Relatives concerned about mental status • Acute deterioration in functional ability • Immunosuppressed • Trauma/surgery/ procedure in last 8 weeks • Respiratory rate 21–24 • Systolic BP 91–100 mmHg • Heart rate 91–130 or new dysrhythmia • Temperature <36° • Clinical signs of wound infection	• Objective evidence of new or altered mental state • Systolic BP ≤90 mmHg (or drop of >40 from normal) • Heart rate ≥130 per minute • Respiratory rate ≥25 per minute • Needs O_2 to keep SpO_2 ≥92% (88% in COPD) • Non-blanching rash/ mottled/ashen/cyanotic • Lactate ≥2 mmol/L • Recent chemotherapy • Not passed urine in 18 hours (<0.5 mL/kg/h if catheterised)

---

source and micro-organism. In less critically unwell patients (NEWS 5–6, amber flag criteria), it may be wiser to perform initial investigations (e.g. chest X-ray to differentiate pneumonia from pulmonary oedema) prior to choosing an antibiotic, preferably within 3 hours. In stable patients (NEWS 1–4, no red/amber flag criteria) use the first few hours to identify the correct diagnosis whilst closely monitoring the patient for deterioration.

In septic shock, the primary issues are vasodilation and increased vascular permeability, so the patient may feel warm to touch initially with bounding pulses and flushed skin. There may be a wide pulse pressure with a low diastolic pressure. Replacing fluids and filling the intravascular space may help somewhat, but much of the fluid bolus will leak into the interstitial space. Hence, vasopressors will often be needed to provide peripheral vasoconstriction.

Tx The traditional management of sepsis describes six key interventions (known as the 'Sepsis Six'):

- Oxygen (to keep SaO_2 >94%)
- Blood cultures and other microbiological tests (e.g. urine, sputum)
- IV antibiotics – aim for narrow spectrum (based on local guidelines) where the source of infection is known
- IV fluids – 10 mL/kg boluses of balanced crystalloid, up to 30 mL/kg. More if the patient also has significant hypovolaemia (e.g. diarrhoea, DKA)
- Lactate measurement (a serum lactate >4 mmol/L denotes very poor tissue perfusion)
- Fluid balance monitoring (this may require a catheter).

ICU referral should be made if there is an inadequate response to initial resuscitation. Norepinephrine is recommended a as first-line vasopressor agent for the treatment of septic shock and emerging research suggests that starting it early (i.e. before fluid boluses have finished) is associated with better outcomes. It can be given safely through a large peripheral cannula for the first few hours until central access is achieved. Aim for a mean arterial pressure (MAP) of 65 mmHg, which may need to be slightly higher for patients with chronic hypertension. IV hydrocortisone 50 mg should be given to patients on long term steroids or with known adrenal insufficiency.

Meningococcal sepsis → p. 355.
Neutropenic sepsis → p. 273

Cardiogenic shock

Cardiogenic shock may occur, secondary to structural or cardiomyopathic causes such acute coronary syndrome, severe aortic stenosis, acute valve rupture, myocarditis or decompensated chronic heart failure. Alternatively, it may result from the effects of the inability of the heart to deliver an effective stroke volume due to effects of an arrythmia or external toxins. Cardiogenic shock is 'forward failure' of the heart as opposed to the 'backward failure' of congestive cardiac failure, and both can co-exist.

The patient will usually have mottled, cool skin with a prolonged capillary refill time and thready pulses and listen for murmurs suggestive of valvular disease or papillary muscle rupture.

Investigations: There may be ECG changes or signs of heart failure on chest X-ray. Bedside echocardiography can assess for reduced left ventricular contractility, dilated inferior vena cava and B-lines of pulmonary oedema. The more advanced POCUS protocol named VExUS (venous congestion evaluation using ultrasound) can provide additional evidence.

Tx

- Ensure that the airway and breathing are satisfactory. Give oxygen to maintain sats above 94%. Non-invasive positive pressure ventilation (NIPPV), continuous positive airways pressure (CPAP) is indicated in severely dyspnoeic patients. Invasive ventilation is required in those with respiratory failure, reduced conscious level or physical exhaustion.
- Allow the patient to adopt whatever posture is most comfortable; this will usually be partially sitting up.
- Apply monitoring.
- Request a CXR, ECG, FBC, troponin, BNP and U&Es.
- Correct any bradycardia or tachyarrhythmia as per algorithms (→ *p. 174 and 178*)
- Refer to the cardiologist and ICU (considering whether the underlying cause is likely to be reversible).
- Insert a urinary catheter.
- Optimise blood pressure with noradrenaline
- Optimise contractility with dobutamine or milrinone. (*For a method of setting up an IV infusion of dobutamine → Box 14.14.*)

 Box 14.14 Intravenous infusion of dobutamine

- Remove 50 mL from 250 mL bag 0.9% saline, add 1 vial of dobutamine (250 mg in 50 mL) = 250 mg in 250 mL dobutamine solution (i.e. 1 mg/mL).
- This infusion can be given into a peripheral vein in the short term.
- A reasonable starting dose is 5 mcg/kg per min. The infusion rate in mL/h needed to give this dose can be calculated by multiplying the patient's body weight in kilogrammes by 0.3 (e.g. to give 5 mcg/kg per min to a 70-kg man: 70 kg × 0.3 = 21 mL/h).

- In rare cases, intra-aortic balloon pump (IABP) or veno-arterial extracorporeal membrane oxygenation (VA-ECMO) will be needed as a bridge to treatment or decision making.

Myocarditis

Although it can be subclinical, inflammation of the myocardium can lead to debilitating cardiomyopathy. The damage to the muscle tissue is thought to be caused by either toxins or an immunological reaction. A vast array of organisms and diseases have been associated with myocarditis. Enteroviruses (especially Coxsackie B virus) are the most common pathogens in the developed world. Covid-19, HIV, Lyme disease (→ *p. 268*), tuberculosis, rheumatoid arthritis and Kawasaki's disease (→ *p. 362*) are among the less common causes of myocarditis. The heart failure that follows Chagas' disease (caused by *Trypanosoma cruzi*) is an enormous problem in Central and South America.

Clinical presentations of myocarditis range from a mild febrile illness to overwhelming congestive cardiac failure. ECG and CXR changes are variable; echocardiography typically shows a globally dilated left ventricle. ESR, CRP, CK-MB and troponin may be raised. Treatment is supportive and symptomatic.

Endocarditis

Infective endocarditis is a serious condition with a mortality rate of 20% or more. Although it is primarily a disease of those with congenital or acquired structural heart disease, people who inject drugs (PWID) have a 30-fold higher incidence of endocarditis than the general population. Immune suppression and indwelling catheters are also risk factors. Infected vegetations occur on the endothelium of the heart, usually on areas of previous abnormality or damage. Left-sided infections are mostly found in patients with acquired valvular heart disease (e.g. rheumatic heart disease), but either side of the heart may be affected in those with congenital heart disease or prosthetic valves. The most common pathogens are *Streptococcus viridans*, *Staphylococcus aureus* and Enterococci. The HACEK organisms are less common and listed in Box 14.15. Most cases of right-sided endocarditis occur in PWID due to *S. aureus* infection of the tricuspid valve.

The symptoms of infective endocarditis are vague and may be the result of embolic phenomena. There is fatigue, weight loss and fever (above 38°C). Nausea, back pain and arthralgia may also occur. Cardiac murmurs are usually pre-existing. Septic emboli cause pulmonary, cerebral or systemic symptoms (e.g. pneumonia, headache,

> **Box 14.15 HACEK organisms of endocarditis**
>
> The HACEK organisms are gram negative bacteria commonly present in oral flora. They account for only around 3% of cases of endocarditis.
>
> - *Haemophilus* species
> - *Aggregatibacter* species
> - *Cardiobacterium hominis*
> - *Eikenella corrodens*
> - *Kingella* species

renal or splenic infarcts). Splinter haemorrhages, Janeway lesions and Osler nodes are classic signs of the disease.

> Modified Duke criteria are used to diagnose endocarditis using blood cultures and echocardiography.

Investigations: Three sets of blood cultures should be taken at different times (can be within 15–20 min in a critically unwell patient), including from any indwelling lines. CXR and ECG are usually non-specific. Echocardiography is used to detect endocardial involvement.

Tx Initial 'blind' antibiotic therapy is IV flucloxacillin and gentamicin. The flucloxacillin should be replaced with vancomycin and rifampicin if the patient has cardiac prostheses, is allergic to penicillin or if MRSA is thought to be a likely pathogen.

Prophylaxis against infective endocarditis

Antibiotics to prevent infective endocarditis are no longer recommended for adults and children with structural cardiac defects who are undergoing dental and non-dental interventional procedures.

Cardiac tamponade

This causes:

- hypotension
- raised jugular venous pressure (JVP) unless hypovolaemic
- muffled heart sounds
- pulsus paradoxus
- breathlessness.

The ECG findings in cardiac tamponade, in order of frequency, are tachycardia, low voltage QRS and electrical alternans (alternating larger and smaller QRS complexes). If the signs suggest a diagnosis of tamponade, then point of care ultrasound (POCUS) is a sensitive test to pick up pericardial effusion. However, there is not necessarily tamponade unless there are other features such as right ventricular collapse in diastole or plethoric inferior vena cava.

Underlying causes for pericardial effusion or haemorrhage include:

- trauma (→ *p. 80*)
- neoplasia
- bacterial/tuberculous/viral pericarditis
- thoracic aortic dissection
- renal failure.

Tx In a collapsed patient with a tamponade, attempt pericardiocentesis. This procedure may buy time but is not a definitive treatment so seek help immediately. It is recommended to perform 'controlled pericardial drainage' in the case of tamponade with aortic dissection, taking just 5–10 mL at a time, to maintain systolic blood pressure at 80–90 mmHg whilst arranging immediate operative management.

Hypertensive emergencies

A hypertensive emergency is a sudden increase in BP associated with end-organ damage such as:

- cerebral infarction
- cerebral haemorrhage
- acute pulmonary oedema
- acute coronary syndrome
- acute renal failure
- aortic dissection
- hypertensive encephalopathy.

Therefore, investigations may include ECG, chest X-ray, bloods for troponin, urea and creatinine, CT brain and CT aortogram.

Tx Aim to lower MAP by 25% in the first hour then to 160 mmHg systolic over 2–6 hours (see *Box 14.16* for calculating MAP). Exceptions to this are aortic dissection and severe pre-eclampsia where BP must be reduced quickly. Where cardiac ischaemia or pulmonary oedema is suspected, IV nitrates and beta-blockers are good choices. When lowering blood pressure in patients with acute intracerebral haemorrhage, the aim is to reach a systolic BP of 140 mmHg over 6 hours while ensuring there is not a drop of more than 60 mmHg per hour. Labetalol and nicardipine are reasonable choices. Phentolamine is the drug of choice in cases of

> **Box 14.16 Mean arterial pressure**
>
> Mean arterial pressure (MAP) is the average blood pressure over a single cardiac cycle. It is a product of the cardiac output and systemic vascular resistance. MAP of 60 mmHg is usually considered adequate to maintain organ perfusion in the average adult. It can be calculated using the following formula
>
> $$MAP = [(2 \times \text{diastolic pressure}) + \text{systolic pressure}] / 3$$

phaeochromocytoma. Benzodiazepines and then phentolamine are used for cocaine-induced hypertension. **Malignant hypertension** refers to the syndrome of:

- severe diastolic hypertension
- papilloedema
- retinal exudates and haemorrhages
- renal failure.

It occurs mainly in men in their third and fourth decades and pursues a rapidly downhill course to death from uraemia within a year unless properly treated. Patients with no symptoms of end-organ damage and normal fundi can be managed as outpatients by a GP.

Hypertensive encephalopathy is a rare condition in which transient neurological symptoms occur in the presence of a very high BP. The underlying acute focal cerebral ischaemia is caused by a mixture of cerebrovascular spasm, oedema and thrombosis. A CT scan is needed to rule out intracerebral haemorrhage. Treatment is with IV labetalol (IV bolus of 20 mg with repeat doses of 20–80 mg every 10 min – max 300 mg) or IV nicardipine (5 mg/hour infusion titrated up to max 15 mg/hour.)

Palpitations

Palpitations are the unpleasant awareness of one's own heart beating. Clarify with the patient what the rate and rhythm felt like and whether there was any pattern to the episodes. The underlying causes include the following:

- Sinus tachycardia
- Ectopic beats
- Paroxysmal dysrhythmias (→ *Chapter 11*)
- Chronic dysrhythmias (→ *Chapter 11*).

Sinus tachycardia may result from:

- anxiety or other emotion
- pyrexia
- anaemia

- drugs including caffeine
- hyperthyroidism.

A rapid onset and cessation of palpitations with polyuria in an otherwise normal individual are extremely suggestive of a paroxysmal dysrhythmia such as supraventricular tachycardia (SVT).

Investigations: FBC, electrolytes, glucose and thyroid function tests should be performed. An ECG is essential to demonstrate:

- the exact rhythm and rate
- congenital abnormalities of the cardiac conducting tissue such as Wolff–Parkinson–White syndrome
- unsuspected myocardial ischaemia and infarction.

Tx
Treatment of patients with a frank cardiac dysrhythmia → Chapter 11.

Patients with an abnormal ECG should be discussed with the acute medical team or cardiologist. Excessive and unexplained sinus tachycardia should also be investigated. Those with normal physical findings and a normal ECG can be discharged with advice to see their GP if symptoms are recurrent or persistent.

METABOLIC AND ENDOCRINE DISORDERS

Hypoglycaemia

The symptoms of low blood sugar are a common presentation of diabetes to an ED. Hypoglycaemia results from:

- too much insulin or oral hypoglycaemic (usually sulphonylureas) by accident or intent
- skipped meals
- alcohol intake
- excessive exercise
- change of routine, e.g. site of injection, type of insulin and new syringe size.

Initially, a hypoglycaemic patient is restless and agitated but, if untreated, rapidly becomes unresponsive or has a seizure. There is pallor, profuse sweating and a bounding pulse. Aggression can be such that the patient arrives in police custody and may be thought to be intoxicated. False localising neurological signs are sometimes seen, i.e. a stroke mimic.

Investigations: Venous or capillary blood should be taken for measurement of baseline glucose before treatment is instituted. In cases of unexplained hypoglycaemia, samples should also be sent for renal and liver function tests, insulin, C-peptide and paracetamol assay.

Tx Like hypoxia, hypoglycaemia rapidly leads to permanent brain damage. This can be avoided by prompt treatment with IV glucose into a large vein (150–200 mL of 20% solution for an adult). In a child, the dose is 0.2–0.5 mg/kg of glucose, which should be given as 10% dextrose (i.e. 2–5 mL/kg of 10% dextrose).

IM glucagon 1 mg (equal to 1 U) is an alternative treatment if venous access is delayed, although it is rather slow to work. The dose for children is 20 mcg/kg.

Conscious patients can have oral carbohydrate, e.g. sugary drink or glucose gel followed by a longer acting source, e.g. toast or biscuits.

When the patient has fully recovered, the reasons for the low blood sugar must be explored. The patient should be allowed home only if:

- he or she has been fully awake for a couple of hours and has had some food
- continuous supervision is available
- there has been an attempt to prevent a recurrence of the problem
- follow-up arrangements have been made.

Diabetic ketoacidosis

DKA in children → p. 357.

Diabetic ketoacidosis (DKA) is a life-threatening metabolic condition with three main components:

- hyperglycaemia (glucose >11 mmol/L or known diabetes),
- acidaemia (pH <7.3 or bicarbonate <15 mmol/L) and
- ketonaemia (>3 mmol/L or 2+ on urine dipstick).

Most of the cells of the body need insulin to allow them to take up glucose from the bloodstream. Ketoacidosis starts when this process is critically interrupted by absolute or relative deficiency of insulin. This is accompanied by an increase in counter-regulatory hormones (glucagon, cortisol, growth hormone and adrenaline) that stimulate hepatic gluconeogenesis and glycogenolysis. Two main problems result:

- The body cells have no glucose to metabolise and so are starving. They burn fat and then produce an excess of the ketoacids.
- Gross hyperglycaemia causes an osmotic diuresis, decreased tissue perfusion and circulatory collapse. There is dehydration and gross metabolic upset, failure of all body systems and eventually coma and death.

The patient looks ill and may have a decreased level of consciousness. The skin is dry, and there is tachycardia and hypotension. Kussmaul's respiration describes the characteristic deep, sighing breathing that may be mistaken for respiratory distress. There is frequently vomiting, abdominal pain and coffee ground haematemesis. Some patients present with only modest elevation of blood glucose, but with acidosis secondary to ketonaemia ('euglycaemic diabetic ketoacidosis'). The resolution of DKA in all cases depends on the suppression of ketogenesis.

Near patient testing for 3β-hydroxybutyrate (the predominant ketone in DKA) is now readily available.

Tx Hyperglycaemia is of less importance than the hyponatraemic dehydration and the cellular ketogenesis.

- The airway must be protected, and oxygen given to maintain adequate saturations.
- Resuscitate a shocked patient with a bolus of 500 mL 0.9% saline over 5–10 min then reassess. Patients who are still in shock after two boluses need urgent senior review and probably ICU admission. See Box 14.17 for typical deficits in DKA.
- When shock has improved start slow fluid replacement (→ *Box 14.18*)
- Full monitoring is essential.
- Blood glucose, ketones, bicarbonate and blood gases should be measured hourly initially (→ see *Box 14.19* for treatment targets).
- Hyperglycaemia is initially treated by rehydration. Soluble insulin is then given as a fixed rate infusion of 0.1 U/kg. An infusion of 10% glucose (dextrose) is introduced when the blood glucose falls to <14 mmol/L. The initial rate should be around 125 mL/h. The saline infusion should still be continued. It is wise to give glucose and insulin through the same cannula with a Y-connector attached, so that if a cannula kinks or displaces, the patient will not be getting one without the other.

Continue to give the patient's long acting insulin at the usual time

Serum potassium may be normal or high initially due to haemoconcentration. It will fall rapidly when the hypovolaemia and acidosis are corrected and will follow the glucose into the cells.

- Catheterisation allows a careful check on fluid balance. A strict recording of fluid input and output must be maintained.

 Box 14.17 Typical water and electrolyte deficits in DKA

Water	100 mL/kg
Sodium	7–10 mmol/kg
Chloride	3–5 mmol/kg
Potassium	3–5 mmol/kg
Phosphate	1 mmol/kg

Box 14.18 Fluid replacement in adults with DKA

Replace fluids in the first 12 hours as follows:

1 L saline over 60 min
1 L saline with potassium over 2 hours
1 L saline with potassium over 2 hours
1 L saline with potassium over 4 hours
1 L saline with potassium over 4 hours
Consider more cautious fluid replacement in people aged 18–25 years, elderly, pregnant, heart and renal failure.

Serum potassium level	Replacement using pre-made bags
>5.5	none
3.5–5.5	40 mmol/L
<3.5	Seek senior advice – may need central line replacement

Box 14.19 Treatment targets in DKA

- Reduction of the blood ketone concentration by 0.5 mmol/L per hour
- Increase of the venous bicarbonate by 3 mmol/L per hour
- Reduction of the (capillary) blood glucose by 3 mmol/L per hour
- Maintenance of the plasma potassium between 4.0 and 5.5 mmol/L

If the rate of ketone fall is not achieved, then the fixed rate insulin infusion should be increased (by 1 U/h increments hourly).

- The administration of prophylactic low-molecular-weight heparin (LMWH) should be considered.
- A cause for the development of the ketoacidosis must be sought. The condition usually develops over several days and is often precipitated by infection or other coexisting illness. Ask about insulin compliance and alcohol intake. Beware of missing the acute abdomen in a patient with DKA as abdominal pain is a frequent symptom that is often overlooked.

Consider ICU referral for the following patients

- Elderly and very young patients
- Heart or renal failure or other serious comorbidity
- Pregnant patients

- Ketones >6 mmol/L
- Bicarbonate <5 mmol/L
- Venous pH <7.1
- GCS <12
- Systolic BP <90 mmHg
- Oxygen saturations <92% on air
- Hyperkalaemia >5.5 mmol/L
- Anion gap >16 (anion gap = $(Na^+ + K^+) - (Cl^- + HCO_3^-)$)

The main causes of death in DKA are cerebral oedema, hypokalaemia, hypoglycaemia, acute respiratory distress syndrome (ARDS), sepsis and thromboembolism.

> There is no need to take arterial gases in a patient with DKA as the mean difference in pH between venous and arterial gases is 0.03. Painful arterial blood sampling can be a potential barrier to patients presenting early with DKA.

Hyperglycaemic hyperosmolar syndrome

A hyperosmolar state is usually seen in older patients who are not insulin dependent. In fact, many have no history of diabetes although they may have had polyuria and polydipsia for up to 2 weeks before presentation. As there is some insulin available to the body, ketoacidosis is not a feature of this condition. It is precipitated by infection or other illness in just the same way as DKA, but drugs, especially diuretics, may also play a part. Hyperosmolar coma has a very high mortality because of coexisting disease and late diagnosis.

There is profound dehydration (often 25% of body weight) with depression of consciousness and other neurological signs. There may be symptoms and signs of the precipitating disease, such as infection, myocardial infarction and stroke.

Investigations:

- Blood glucose, U&Es, haemoglobin, white cell count, lactate and haematocrit should be checked together with blood gases. Haemoconcentration and infection are likely findings.
- Serum osmolality is, of course, very high (>350 mmol/L) due to hyperglycaemia (>30 mmol/L) and hypernatraemia. Serum sodium is unreliable in the context of hyperglycaemia and lab levels will underestimate the actual concentration. The most common correction factor is 1.6 mmol/L decrease in serum sodium for every 5.6 mmol/L increase in glucose.
- Investigations for precipitating illness may include, ECG, chest X-ray, urine, sputum and blood cultures.

Tx Fluid resuscitation is essential with careful and frequent reassessment, especially in patients with comorbidities such as heart failure and renal failure. Insulin requirements are low, so insulin therapy should await fluid resuscitation. Patients usually require replacement of potassium and magnesium.

Patients with hyperosmolar coma are at high risk of thromboembolism, so they should be given prophylactic subcutaneous LMWH.

Thyrotoxicosis

Hyperthyroidism is a group of disorders including Grave's disease in which inappropriately high levels of circulating T4 hormone are seen, usually with very low thyroid stimulating hormone (TSH) levels. Thyrotoxicosis can mimic many other more common conditions such as sepsis, psychosis, heart failure or even meningitis. Hallmark features include fevers, tachycardia, hypertension, anxiety and tremulousness. Goitre is typically present, and the thyroid gland may be tender or nontender, depending on the underlying disease. About 25% of patients with Grave's disease will also have eye signs such as proptosis and diplopia.

Thyroid storm is the most severe form of thyrotoxicosis and is a medical emergency. There are no biochemical cut-offs that define thyroid storm, rather it is characterised by organ failure because of hyperthyroidism. This usually includes cardiac failure, and often severe vomiting and diarrhoea, acute kidney injury and electrolyte disturbance such as hyperglycaemia and hypercalcaemia. The patient may be restless, agitated or unconscious. Liver failure and jaundice are features suggesting very severe disease.

Tx Initial resuscitative management includes cooling, benzodiazepines for agitation and IV fluids. Once the diagnosis is confirmed, treatment should be started with expert help, with propylthiouracil, beta blockers, e.g. propranolol, steroids, e.g. hydrocortisone and then iodine.

Myxoedema coma

This is the most extreme form of hypothyroidism associated with mental state change. Chronic hypothyroidism can become decompensated due to infection, trauma, stroke or new medications e.g. lithium.

The patient will be hypothermic and confused or unresponsive, often with bradycardia, hypotension and non-pitting oedema of hands and feet. Look for other features of hypothyroidism, such a dry skin and sparse hair. TSH will be markedly high in most cases with a low T4.

Tx Good supportive care is important, with airway protection, treatment of infections and rewarming as priorities. Definitive management is with the replacement of thyroid hormones.

Adrenal crisis

Adrenocortical deficiency may be a consequence of primary adrenal insufficiency, a.k.a. Addison's disease, usually an autoimmune condition, that can also be caused by trauma, TB or other infiltrative conditions. Patients with Addison's disease are normally aware of how to increase their steroid doses when unwell and when to seek help for impending crisis. However, around 40% of patients with Addison's were diagnosed following a presentation with acute crisis.

Secondary adrenal insufficiency is caused by the longterm steroid therapy or pituitary disease. Remember to increase the steroid dose if a patient presents with acute illness who takes a maintenance dose every day.

An adrenal 'crisis' is often precipitated by acute physiological stress such as trauma or infection. It presents with severe hypotension which is often refractory to fluids. Other symptoms include vomiting, dehydration, weakness and delirium. Pigmentation and weight loss are features of the underlying disease.

Investigations: The plasma potassium and urea are usually high and the sodium is low (due to aldosterone deficiency). Blood glucose may be normal or low.

Tx
- Give oxygen as required to maintain the SaO_2 >94%.
- Take blood for routine tests and plasma cortisol levels.
- Start fluid resuscitation and if no response, start vasopressors.
- Give IV hydrocortisone 100 mg.
- Refer the patient to the acute medical team or ICU.

Hepatic encephalopathy

Hepatic failure is commonly caused by alcoholic cirrhosis or hepatitis (→p. 315) but can also be caused by other diseases and drugs. Acute hepatic encephalopathy can be precipitated by:

- An increased nitrogen load, such a GI bleed or infection
- Neurotransmitter alteration, due to alcohol, sedatives or hypoglycaemia
- Failure to break down toxic metabolites, due to constipation, renal failure.

The patient will usually be coagulopathic due to decreased synthesis of clotting factors, making spontaneous and traumatic intracranial bleeding an important differential diagnosis. Liver failure is also, paradoxically a thrombogenic state, making portal vein thrombosis and venous thromboembolism more likely. Ammonia levels will usually be high but measuring them is unlikely to change acute management, as a normal level does not rule out hepatic encephalopathy.

Clinical features include:

- hypoglycaemia
- hypothermia
- neurological changes and coma due to underlying cerebral oedema or encephalopathy
- renal failure (hepatorenal syndrome) and metabolic disturbance
- hypotension and pulmonary oedema
- asterixis (flapping tremor)
- jaundice and hepatic fetor.

Paracetamol poisoning may present late with:

- a vague, non-specific history
- a few days of malaise, anorexia, nausea and vomiting
- hypoglycaemic coma
- low levels of paracetamol detectable in the plasma.

Tx

- Protect and manage the airway
- Consider a CT scan of the head, particularly if trauma is suspected
- Careful fluid management with replacement of potassium and glucose
- Look for signs of GI haemorrhage, particularly in patients with a history of varices.
- Consider IV thiamine for treatment of Wernicke's
- Tap ascites, if present, to look for spontaneous bacterial peritonitis.
- Treat any suspected infections
- Avoid (or dose reduce) medications that are hepatotoxic or will accumulate, such as paracetamol, opiates, benzodiazepines and antiepileptics
- Start oral/NG lactulose
- Consider ICU referral for patients with a reduced conscious level
- Consider discussion with liver unit, where the cause is thought to be acute liver failure or paracetamol overdose.

Renal failure

Shock from any cause may result in a temporary 'prerenal failure' with anuria. Sustained hypotension leads to acute tubular necrosis and, in extreme cases, to acute cortical necrosis also → *Box 14.20*.

Acute renal failure is also seen in the following:

- **Acute-on-chronic failure**: precipitated by renal infection or dehydration
- **Primary renal disease**: acute glomerulonephritis or collagen vascular disease

> **Box 14.20 Causes of acute tubular necrosis**
>
> - Sustained hypotension – severe burns, diarrhoea
> - Massive haemorrhage
> - Septicaemia, especially when caused by Gram-negative organisms
> - Free circulating haemoglobin or myoglobin (→ *crush injuries on p. 262*)
> - Poisoning – NSAIDs, cytotoxics

- **Hepatorenal syndromes**: including Weil's disease (→ *p. 315*)
- **Postrenal obstruction.**

Oliguria is the cardinal sign (<300 mL in 24 hours) because the clinical features of severe uraemia are variable and non-specific:

- **Cardiovascular**: hypertension, heart failure, pericarditis
- **Neurological**: lethargy, weakness, confusion and eventually coma
- **Gastrointestinal**: anorexia, nausea, vomiting and hiccoughs
- **Dermatological**: pruritus, pallor, petechiae
- **Haematological**: anaemia, bleeding tendency, immunosuppression.

Other changes seen in acute renal failure are caused by hyperkalaemia and acidosis (→ *pp. 259 and 263*).

Investigations: The diagnosis is confirmed by the high blood urea and creatinine. Hyperkalaemia is common. Other investigations that should be performed are:

- FBC – low platelets
- Blood gases – acidosis
- CXR – pulmonary oedema or pleural effusions
- ECG – *For changes in hyperkalaemia → Box 14.21*
- Blood sugar
- Calcium studies
- Urine microscopy and culture – haematuria, casts and infection
- Bedside ultrasound can help detect patients with a potential obstructive cause by looking for bladder distension and hydronephrosis

The urinary sodium concentration is a useful investigation if there is any doubt about whether the oliguria is prerenal and amenable to fluid therapy or a result of acute tubular necrosis → *Box 14.22*.

Tx

- Record fluid balance carefully.
- Restore intravascular volume in prerenal failure.

> **Box 14.21 ECG changes in hyperkalaemia**
>
> - Tall, peaked (tented) T waves (early change)
> - Shortened Q–T interval (early change)
> - Widened QRS complex
> - Small or absent P waves
> - Increased P–R interval
> - Depressed ST segment
> - Ventricular dysrhythmias (fibrillation and asystole)
>
> Note that tall peaked T waves are higher than they are wide.

> **Box 14.22 Distinction between prerenal and renal uraemia**
>
> In volume depletion or hypoperfusion with a healthy kidney, the intact tubules can conserve sodium and concentrate the urine by the tubular reabsorption of sodium and water. In contrast, in acute tubular necrosis, the tubular function is impaired and the urinary sodium concentration rises.
>
> - Prerenal problem: urinary sodium ≤20 mmol/L
> - Acute tubular necrosis: urinary sodium ≥40 mmol/L

- Perform an aseptic catheterisation.
- Treat complications (e.g. LVF or hyperkalaemia).
- Arrange admission under acute medical or renal team.

Nephrotic syndrome: this may present with oedema. There is heavy proteinuria and hypoalbuminaemia. Various types of glomerulonephritis account for 80% of cases in adults, whereas there is usually minimal change glomerulonephritis in children.

Hyperkalaemia

High plasma potassium (>5.5 mmol/L) may be caused by the following:

- **Release from damaged cells**: burns, crush injury and rhabdomyolysis and transfusion
- **Abnormal movement out of cells**: acidosis, transfusion, hyperkalaemic periodic paralysis
- **Decreased excretion**: renal failure, Addison's disease, drugs such as potassium-sparing diuretics and NSAIDs

- **Poisoning**
- **Excessive intake**: rarely.

The effects of hyperkalaemia are:

- paraesthesia
- muscle weakness (flaccid paralysis)
- ventricular dysrhythmias (eventually asystole).

Investigations: The plasma potassium may be spuriously raised by haemolysis in the specimen tube. Blood gases should be taken to check for acidosis and an ECG looking for characteristic changes → *Box 14.21*.

Tx

Patients with severe elevation of the plasma potassium concentration (i.e. plasma potassium ≥6.5 mmol/L) and with toxic ECG changes: the first priority is to protect the patient from life-threatening cardiac dysrhythmias by giving:

- **Calcium**: under ECG monitoring, give 10 mL of 10% calcium chloride by slow IV injection over 2–5 min (10 mL of 10% calcium chloride contains 6.8 mmol calcium ions). This has an immediate effect that lasts for up to 1 hour. 30 mL of 10% calcium gluconate (equivalent to 6.9 mmol calcium ions) is an alternative. Calcium stabilises the myocardial cell membrane but does not affect the plasma potassium.

Then proceed as below to redistribute potassium and remove it from the body

- **Intravenous rehydration**: if the patient is hypovolaemic, then an important step is to increase circulating volume and thereby dilute circulating potassium concentration. Balanced crystalloid solutions such as Hartmann's solution are preferred (even though they contain potassium) as 0.9% saline causes hyperchloremia and metabolic acidosis, which may move potassium from the intracellular space into the interstitial fluid and plasma. The 4 and 5 mmol/L of K^+ in balanced crystalloids will be lower than the patient's plasma concentration so will have the net effect of trending potassium levels towards normal.
- **Salbutamol**: give salbutamol 10 mg by nebuliser (2.5–5.0 mg in children). Up to 20 mg may be required. IV salbutamol 0.5 mg (4 mcg/kg in children) is an alternative. Patients with known ischaemic heart disease may be safer with inhaled salbutamol. Via β_2 receptors in liver and muscle, salbutamol stimulates the Na^+/K^+ ATP pump to move potassium into cells. Within 30 min, the plasma potassium begins to fall (by up to 1.5 mmol/L after IV salbutamol and up to 1.0 mmol/L after the nebulised drug).
- **Insulin**: give 10 U soluble insulin in 50 g glucose intravenously over 15–30 min. Insulin stimulates the Na^+/K^+ ATP pump to increase the intracellular

uptake of potassium. This effect is independent of its hypoglycaemic action. Reduction in plasma potassium starts within 15 min and is maintained for 1–2 hours; a drop of around 1 mmol/L is to be expected. Close glucose monitoring is required, at least every 15 minutes for the first hour. In children (who increase their insulin production more rapidly than adults), IV glucose 0.5 g/kg may be given alone.

- **Bicarbonate**: may be useful if the patient has metabolic acidosis with pH <7.20. Give IV sodium bicarbonate (1 mmol/kg) over 5–15 min (→ *Box 14.25 on p. 264*). This acts within 15–30 min but has a limited effect on potassium levels when used alone.

Then proceed to remove excess potassium from the body.

Potassium can be eliminated from the kidneys, gut or directly from the blood:

- **Diuretics**: Patients who pass urine can be given loop diuretics, e.g. 40–80 mg furosemide to induce kaliuresis, as long as they are not volume deplete.
- **Sodium zirconium cyclosilicate**: Given orally, 10 g three times daily, binds potassium in the GI tract and can have an effect in 2–4 hours.
- **Renal replacement therapy**: Haemodialysis and haemofiltration are usually reserved for patients who fail to improve with the above treatments or those who are anuric.

Hypokalaemia

Low plasma potassium (<3.5 mmol/L) results from the following:

- **Abnormal movement into cells**: alkalosis, insulin, hypokalaemic periodic paralysis
- **Excessive loss from the GI tract**: diarrhoea, vomiting, high output stoma or fistula
- **Excessive renal loss**: Cushing's disease, diuretics, renal tubular acidosis, excess liquorice ingestion, hypomagnesaemia.
- **Other losses**: Sweat, burns, renal replacement therapy
- **Reduced intake**: malnutrition

The most common symptoms of hypokalaemia are tiredness and weakness. These may be the only symptoms and examination may be unremarkable. However, there may also be:

- paraesthesia and ascending paralysis
- arrythmias
- respiratory failure
- paralytic ileus.

Investigations: The blood gases should be checked. The ECG may show characteristic changes → *Box 14.23*.

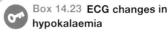

> **Box 14.23 ECG changes in hypokalaemia**
>
> - Flattening or inversion of the T wave
> - Depression of the ST segment
> - Prolongation of the Q–T interval
> - Ventricular dysrhythmias including VF

Tx Under ECG monitoring, IV potassium replacement can be commenced in symptomatic or at-risk patients. The rate can be up to 20 mmol/hour for an adult. Also check and replace magnesium if low. Many patients with no symptoms and normal ECGs will respond to oral supplements. Check digoxin levels if the patient is taking this medication as they are at particular risk of toxicity.

Hypercalcaemia

Older people may present with non-specific symptoms that are attributable to hypercalcaemia:

- Weakness and lethargy
- Confusion and other mental changes
- Anorexia, nausea and vomiting
- Constipation
- Polyuria and dehydration.

The ECG may show bradycardia and shortened QT interval. The most common causes are malignancy (lung, breast and kidney) and primary hyperparathyroidism.

Tx
- Monitoring, especially of the ECG
- Volume expansion with IV saline
- IV furosemide after volume repletion
- Admission for investigation and specific calcium-reducing therapy (bisphosphonates, calcitonin, etc.).

Hypocalcaemia and tetany

Hypocalcaemia gives rise to the state of increased neuromuscular excitability known as tetany. The features are:

- paraesthesia
- carpopedal spasm and muscular cramps
- stridor, caused by laryngospasm
- other signs of neuromuscular irritability (twitching, hyperreflexia, Trousseau's and Chvostek's signs)
- convulsions.

Tetany most commonly accompanies the calcium changes of hyperventilation (→ *p. 231*) but may also be seen in hypoparathyroidism, massive transfusion and a variety of other diseases. The ECG can show prolonged

QT interval which can lead to Torsades de Pointes. Hypocalcaemia and hypomagnesaemia often coexist.

Tx Patients with tetany should be carefully monitored and an ECG recorded. The initial dose of calcium in hypocalcaemic tetany is 2.25 mmol, which is present in 1 g calcium gluconate (i.e. 10 mL of 10% solution). This is given slowly intravenously and may be doubled if the response is unsatisfactory. It should be followed by an IV infusion of around 9 mmol/day.

> Volume for volume, a solution of calcium chloride contains three times as much ionised calcium as a similar strength solution of calcium gluconate. Calcium gluconate is often chosen for its less irritant effect on veins.

Hypomagnesaemia and magnesium therapy

Magnesium is an essential constituent of many enzyme systems, particularly those involved in energy generation. As magnesium is present in large amounts in the GI secretions, excessive losses in diarrhoea, stoma or fistula fluids are the most common causes of hypomagnesaemia; deficiency may also occur in people who are alcohol dependent and patients on diuretics. Hypomagnesaemia often causes secondary hypocalcaemia – with which it may be easily confused. Resistant tetany may result from a combination of the two. Symptomatic patients should be treated with a starting dose of 8 mmol (2 g) magnesium, diluted to 200 mL with saline and given intravenously over 15 min.

Other indications for treatment with magnesium in emergency medicine → Box 14.24.

> **Box 14.24 Indications for magnesium therapy in emergency medicine**
>
> 1 Control of some resistant ventricular dysrhythmias:
>   – VT secondary to hypokalaemia
>   – VT that is resistant to DC shock
>   – torsade de pointes (→ *p. 181*)
>   – some tachycardias that are secondary to the effects of drugs including digitalis, antiarrhythmics and occasionally tricyclics
> 2 Treatment of eclamptic fits (→ *p. 327*)
> 3 Treatment of asthma (→ *p. 213*)
> 4 Treatment of hypomagnesaemic tetany (→ *above*)

> The recommended starting dose of IV magnesium varies with the condition being treated. The total dose may be up to 16 mmol, followed by an infusion of 2.5 mmol/hour; 1 g magnesium sulphate contains approximately 4 mmol magnesium ions. Transient flushing – sometimes accompanied by hypotension – is to be expected in almost all patients.

Hyponatraemia

Hyponatraemia is a relatively common electrolyte disorder, especially in hospitalised elderly patients. It may occur in hypervolaemic, hypovolaemic and euvolaemic states. Low sodium levels lead to extracellular hypo-osmolarity and consequent movement of free water into the intracellular spaces. Causes of hyponatraemia include the following:

- Loss of body fluids (diarrhoea, vomiting, sweating, heat exhaustion and burns)
- Congestive heart failure
- Liver and kidney disease (including acute alcohol poisoning)
- Pulmonary and mediastinal disease
- CNS disease (including head injury)
- Endocrine disease (especially hypoadrenalism and hypothyroidism)
- Malignancies
- Polydipsia (including psychogenic polydipsia)
- Iatrogenic (too much IV dextrose)
- Feeding tap water or diluted milk to infants
- SIADH (syndrome of inappropriate antidiuretic hormone secretion)
- Antidepressant drugs, especially SSRIs
- Diuretic drugs
- Many other drugs (including MDMA [3,4-methylenedioxymethamfetamine]/'ecstasy').

The symptoms of low plasma sodium are vague and non-specific and mostly due to cerebral oedema. They include fatigue, irritability, anorexia, nausea, headache, weakness, cramps, confusion, hallucinations and convulsions. Hyponatraemia that develops over a short period (<48 hours) is more dangerous than a chronic fall in sodium levels. Rhabdomyolysis may occasionally occur (→ *p. 262*) and herniation of the brain stem is a risk with very low sodium levels.

Investigations: Plasma and urine sodium and osmolality should be measured. An acute drop in plasma sodium to <120 mmol/L is likely to be symptomatic with fits occurring at levels <110 mmol/L. The avid reabsorption of sodium in most cases of hyponatraemia leads to a urinary sodium concentration <20 mmol/L, whereas, with renal causes and SIADH, the urinary sodium is >20 mmol/L. SIADH causes inappropriately concentrated urine with an osmolality >100 mosmol/L. In most other cases of hyponatraemia, the urinary osmolality is <100 mosmol/kg.

A CT scan of the brain may be required to exclude other causes of cerebral swelling. Consider requesting thyroid function tests and serum cortisol levels.

Tx Sodium levels must be increased slowly to prevent the development of osmotic demyelination syndrome (→ *below*). The plasma sodium concentration should not increase by >10 mmol/L in 24 hours and should not normalise (or increase by >15–20 mmol/L) for at least 48 hours.

In the fitting patient, a bolus of hypertonic saline (e.g. 1.5–2.0 mL/kg of 2.7–3%) can be given over 5–10 min. If the patient continues to fit, a second bolus may be given. If hypertonic saline is unavailable, an alternative is sodium bicarbonate (e.g. 50 mL of 8.4%).

Isotonic crystalloid solutions can be infused as a resuscitation and maintenance fluids; in patients who appear hypovolaemic. Patients should be carefully monitored for signs of high urine output (>100 mL/h) and rapidly rising serum sodium (>6 mmol/L in 6 hours).

Hypervolaemic patients should be fluid restricted and given IV furosemide 20–40 mg to help excrete water.

SIADH is treated initially by water restriction. If this does not raise sodium levels sufficiently then demeclocycline (a tetracycline antibiotic) may be given to block the renal tubular effects of ADH. Tolvaptan (a vasopressin V$_2$-receptor antagonist) may also be used for this purpose. An endocrinologist should normally be involved in managing these patients.

Osmotic demyelination syndrome (also known as cerebral pontine myelinolysis) is more common after chronic hyponatraemic states and people who drink alcohol to excess seem to be particularly at risk. Symptoms start 1–3 days after treatment and include dysarthria, dysphagia, paresis, fits and reduced level of consciousness. MRI brain showing pontine demyelination is the gold standard test.

Rhabdomyolysis and myoglobinuria

Breakdown of muscle resulting in rhabdomyolysis and myoglobinuria may occur in several ways:

1 As a consequence of an acute crushing injury (e.g. trapped in a pit or under a lorry)
2 From other direct muscle injury, e.g. deep burns or compartment syndrome
3 After lying immobile for a long time on a hard surface. This is seen in:
   – elderly or debilitated people after a collapse (found on the floor)
   – alcohol-intoxicated patients
   – those who have been immobile or unconscious due to drug use or overdose
4 Following the excessive muscle activity caused by prolonged seizures, extreme exercise and some stimulant drugs (e.g. cocaine and ecstasy)
5 Myotoxic drugs such as statins may sometimes cause a dose-related myositis, which in rare cases leads to rhabdomyolysis
6 Heat related – heat stroke and neuroleptic malignant syndrome
7 Inflammatory causes such a polymyositis

The diagnosis should be suspected in any patient in the above categories, or in patients who complain of dark or tea coloured urine. Muscle pain and tenderness may be absent.

The main consequences are:

• metabolic and volume disturbance
• acute renal failure from myoglobinuria
• delirium and agitation

Investigations: The urine usually tests positive for blood, and the laboratory may find granular casts in it. A raised plasma creatinine kinase is also strongly suggestive of the diagnosis of rhabdomyolysis. Concentrations of creatinine kinase >5000 U/L are associated with a high incidence of acute renal failure. The serum myoglobin peaks at 4 hours and returns to normal within 12 hours of injury. As a result of this rapid clearance, myoglobin in the urine may easily be missed. Arterial blood gases, plasma electrolytes and calcium should also be measured.

Tx Initial resuscitation is with IV fluids, sometimes up to 10 L, to:

1 maintain normovolaemia (large quantities of fluid can be sequestered in damaged muscle)
2 ensure a steady urine output of >100 mL/h

Catheterisation is beneficial and there must be careful monitoring of clinical and biochemical parameters. Hyperkalaemia occurs in most cases and may need treatment. Calcium levels can be high or low during the development of the condition, so be wary when using calcium to treat hyperkalaemia. There is poor evidence for the benefit of sodium bicarbonate solution and mannitol. Dialysis may be required.

Fortunately, the prognosis for renal failure induced by myoglobinuria is excellent, with most survivors recovering fully within 3 months.

Inherited metabolic diseases

There are many rare conditions affecting the body's metabolism, including glycogen storage disorders and urea cycle disorders. Patients can present with hypoglycaemia, hyperammonemia and acid/base disturbance that frequently causes subtle symptoms, such as irritability or 'not right.' After assessing airway, breathing and circulation, the next priority is to check blood glucose, pH, electrolytes, ammonia and lactate. Aim for blood glucose of 6–10 mmol/L using 10% dextrose IV. Many patients have a written treatment plan for when they are unwell, otherwise, the British Inherited Metabolic Disease Group website has printable guidelines.

Acute porphyrias

Porphyrias are uncommon inherited disorders of haem biosynthesis, each of which is related to a specific enzyme deficiency. Transmission is autosomal dominant. The defective synthetic pathway results in the accumulation and increased excretion of porphyrins and their precursors. Of the seven types of porphyria, three are described as 'acute' and all produce similar clinical pictures:

1 Acute intermittent porphyria (the most common form).
2 Hereditary coproporphyria (there may be skin lesions).
3 Variegate porphyria (skin lesions are present).

Around 80% of sufferers are women aged 15–45 years. Patients are at risk of acute neurovisceral attacks, which may be life-threatening. Drugs, alcohol, infections, fasting or hormonal changes may trigger an attack. There is persistent and intense abdominal pain, often accompanied by lower back, buttock and thigh pain. Vomiting, constipation, tachycardia, fever and sweating may be present. The level of pain is out of keeping with the clinical signs. Neurological features include fits, local paresis, agitation and confusion.

Investigations: Radiological examination of the abdomen is normal. There may be hyponatraemia. With exposure to light for 10–30 min, the urine turns from reddish brown to black. The urinary PBG (porphobilinogen) is elevated (send in a plain tube protected from light).

Tx Attacks of acute porphyria require hospitalisation and urgent treatment to avoid life-threatening complications. Any neurological symptoms should provoke an ICU admission to anticipate possible respiratory paralysis. Immediate treatment includes the following:

- Analgesia with morphine or pethidine
- Prochlorperazine, ondansetron or cyclizine for nausea (not metoclopramide)

- Oral or IV carbohydrates as soon as possible: 500 g in 24 hours (this prevents the induction of ALA synthase)
- Encourage oral intake, but if unable, start IV fluids such as 0.9% saline containing 5% glucose.
- Chlorpromazine for psychiatric disturbance
- Consider treatment with haem arginate (human hemin) 3 mg/kg daily (up to maximum of 1 vial/250 mg daily) on four consecutive days. It is preferably given through a central line due to the significant risk of extravasation injury.

> Acute porphyrias are rare diseases, which are often misdiagnosed as other causes of abdominal pain. Drugs that are prescribed to alleviate symptoms may exacerbate the attack. A list of potentially unsafe drugs is available on the UK Porphyria Medicines Information Service website.

Metabolic acidosis

Metabolic acidosis may be due to the addition of an acid or the loss of base from the bloodstream. This is most commonly the result of tissue hypoxia and increased lactate production. Calculation of the anion gap ($\rightarrow$ Box 14.4) can identify causes where an additional unmeasured ion is present (high anion gap metabolic acidosis) such as:

- poisoning (e.g. salicylic acid, methanol, ethylene glycol and cyanide)
- renal failure (underexcretion of acids in advanced renal failure)
- ketosis (diabetic ketoacidosis, starvation and alcoholic ketosis)

Normal anion gap metabolic acidosis causes include:

- rapid saline infusion (hyperchloremic acidosis)
- GI losses (e.g. diarrhoea, fistulas)
- renal tubular acidosis
- Acetazolamide
- Addison's crisis

Metabolic acidosis leads to rapid 'Kussmaul' breathing, myocardial depression and hyperkalaemia. Other important tests include glucose, ketones, lactate, salicylates, ethanol, electrolytes, urea, creatinine and chloride. In the paediatric patient, consider inherited metabolic diseases (also known as inborn errors of metabolism) and check ammonia levels.

Correction of hypoxia and restoration of tissue perfusion is the mainstay of emergency treatment, followed by identification of the underlying cause. Bicarbonate therapy should not be used except in certain specific causes (→ Box 14.25).

For use of bicarbonate in tricyclic poisoning → p. 288.

> In a pure metabolic acidosis, the $PaCO_2$ in mmHg will be approximately the same as the last two digits of the arterial pH.

 Box 14.25 Bicarbonate therapy

Correction of an acidosis with IV sodium bicarbonate generates CO_2, which must be eliminated via the lungs:

$$HCO_3^- + H^+ = H_2O + CO_2$$

Thus adequate ventilation is a prerequisite for treatment.
Listed below are the main accepted uses of bicarbonate:

1 Hyperkalaemia with metabolic acidosis
2 Urinary alkalinisation for salicylate poisoning
3 Treatment of sodium channel blocker poisoning (e.g. tricyclic overdose)
4 Metabolic acidosis due to HCO_3 loss (e.g. renal tubular acidosis and fistula losses)

Metabolic alkalosis

Diagnosis and treatment of metabolic alkalosis → Box 14.26.
Respiratory causes of acid–base disorders → p. 211.

> The direction of the pH change (acidosis or alkalosis) indicates the primary disorder; overcompensation does not occur.

 Box 14.26 Differential diagnosis of metabolic alkalosis

Saline responsive (urinary chloride <10 mmol/L)

If the urinary chloride concentration is <10 mmol/L, the metabolic alkalosis is likely to be responsive to therapy with IV 0.9% saline.

The condition is characterised by sodium chloride and volume depletion, so both sodium and chloride are avidly reabsorbed by the kidney. This type of alkalosis usually results from:

• loss of gastric secretions (e.g. vomiting)
• diuretic therapy
• chloride diarrhoea

> Treatment will involve antiemetics, proton pump inhibitors (to reduce loss of acid from stomach) and stopping diuretics.

Saline resistant (urinary chloride ≥20 mmol/L)

If the urinary chloride concentration exceeds 20 mmol/L, the metabolic alkalosis is probably resistant to simple infusion of saline. The underlying metabolic disturbance is excessive hydrogen ion secretion by the kidney. This occurs in hyperadrenal states and severe hypokalaemia. Chloride excretion remains unaffected. Causes include the following:

• Primary aldosteronism
• Cushing's disease
• ACTH-producing tumours
• Steroid therapy
• Severe potassium depletion
• Milk alkali syndrome (excessive intake of calcium-containing antacids causing hypercalcaemia and renal failure)

ZOONOSES AND DISEASES RELATED TO TRAVEL

When assessing an unwell returned traveller or recent arrival to the UK, it is important to ascertain where exactly the patient has been and when. The two serious syndromes of illness to be aware of are the febrile patient with acute respiratory distress and the febrile patient with extensive bruising or bleeding. These symptoms should prompt the clinician to consider High Consequence Infectious Diseases (HCID) such as viral haemorrhagic fever → *Box 14.27,* and to isolate the affected patient. The UK Health Security Agency website has useful information on endemic countries and algorithms for suspected cases.

Remember to ask about sexual activity in patients returning with a febrile illness. Offer HIV testing if appropriate.

 Box 14.27 **High consequence infectious diseases**

Contact transmission	Airborne transmission
• Argentine haemorrhagic fever	• Andes virus infection
• Bolivian haemorrhagic fever	• Avian influenza A H7N9, H5N1, H7N7
• Crimean Congo haemorrhagic fever	• Middle Eastern respiratory syndrome (MERS)
• Ebola virus disease	• Monkeypox
• Lassa fever	• Nipah virus infection
• Lujo virus disease	• Pneumonic plague (Yersinia pestis)
• Marburg virus disease	• Severe acute respiratory syndrome (SARS)
• Severe fever with thrombocytopaenia syndrome	

Malaria

Malaria is the world's most important parasitic disease. It is a protozoal infection that is transmitted to humans by the bite of an infected female anopheles mosquito. Five species of the parasite are infectious to humans: *Plasmodium falciparum, P. vivax, P. ovale, P. knowlesi* and *P. malariae*. Half the world's population live in areas where malaria is transmitted. 250 million people contract the disease each year and 600 thousand die from it, invariably from *P. falciparum* malaria. In some parts of the world (mainly Africa), malaria is endemic, and as most adults develop partial immunity, the disease mainly affects children, pregnant women and travellers. In other areas (such as Asia and Central America), disease transmission occurs in epidemics, usually around rainy seasons, when mosquitos can lay their eggs on stagnant water.

The incubation period is typically 1–3 weeks, but relapses can occur for many years in untreated *P. vivax* and *P. ovale*. The initial features last for 2–3 days – malaise, anorexia, fever and headache. There is then an abrupt onset of rigors and sweating, with or without the following:

• nausea, vomiting and diarrhoea
• tachycardia

• splenomegaly and occasionally splenic rupture
• jaundice.

The fever may become periodic as the erythrocytic phases of the parasite's life cycle become synchronous; every 48 hours or 'tertian' for *P. vivax* and *P. ovale* infection and every 72 hours or 'quartan' for infection with *P. malariae*.

The addition of acute neurological findings (disorientation, fits or coma) indicates cerebral malaria, a complication of *P. falciparum* infection. Blackwater fever, where malaria causes haemoglobinuria and renal failure, is another potentially fatal variant of this infection. Severe anaemia and hypoglycaemia are common lab findings in severe infection. Respiratory distress is sometimes a feature.

Investigations: The diagnosis is confirmed by microscopic examination of blood films but this may require several films. There are also rapid antigen tests commercially available. The blood film will allow an estimation of the parasitaemia level, i.e. the percentage of erythrocytes containing parasites. >4% *P. falciparum* parasitaemia is considered severe.

Tx In patients who are very unwell start an IV infusion. Measure the blood sugar and correct any hypoglycaemia. A specialist in infectious diseases should be contacted for advice in all cases. IV Artesunate is the first-line drug in severe (invariably *P. falciparum*) infection, with Quinine as second line. Supplementary broad-spectrum antibiotics are often recommended for patients with severe disease due to the frequency of concomitant Gr- bacteraemia seen in African children with *P. falciparum*. Uncomplicated *P. falciparum* can be treated with oral artemether and lumefantrine.

Admission is usually required only for infection with *P. falciparum*; other forms of malaria can be treated in the community (with chloroquine or artemether/lumefantrine). For *P. vivax* and *P. ovale* infection, the patient must also be treated with primaquine to kill dormant hypnozoites and prevent relapses. They will need screening for G6PD deficiency first as primaquine can cause haemolysis in these individuals.

Malaria is not contagious and so the patient does not have to be isolated.

Rabies

Any bite from an animal outside the UK carries a potential risk of rabies. Within the UK, bats can transmit EBLV2 (European bat Lyssavirus type 2), which is closely related to the classic rabies virus. Most cases of rabies occur within a few days of the bite but occasionally symptoms are delayed for weeks or even months. It is said that the more peripheral the wound, the longer the incubation period is likely to be because it takes time for the virus to migrate to the CNS.

> An unprovoked attack may suggest a rabid animal, but an animal that is known to be alive and well several days after the bite is unlikely to be rabid.

Rabies flourishes in dirty, contused wounds. The earliest signs are a failure of wound healing and paraesthesia or anaesthesia at the site of the injury. Eventually, florid CNS signs, including hydrophobia, develop. Symptomatic rabies has a 100% case fatality rate.

*For features that suggest the development of rabies →
Box 14.28.*

Tx OF BITES FROM POTENTIALLY RABID ANIMALS
- Clean, debride and dress the wound.
- Give antitetanus therapy.
- Discuss the patient with a specialist in virology or infectious diseases. Rabies vaccine with or without human rabies immunoglobulin should be given as soon as possible.

> **Box 14.28 Features of an animal bite that are suggestive of rabies infection**
>
> - Bite occurred outside the UK or from a bat within the UK
> - Animal dead or whereabouts unknown
> - Dirty wound; wound not healing well; paraesthesia
> - Accompanying CNS symptoms or signs

Poliomyelitis

This highly infectious disease is still prevalent in many parts of the world, although the last 'non-imported' case in the UK was in 1984. The polio virus is spread by droplet infection and faecal–oral contamination with an incubation period of 3–21 days. An initial flu-like illness is followed by pyrexia, headache, vomiting and neck stiffness accompanied by muscle pain and tenderness. Symptoms may subside after 48 hours but in susceptible patients (around 1 in 75 adults and 1 in 1000 children) a flaccid paralytic phase will ensue as the muscle pain continues and weakness develops. This is a result of the involvement of the anterior horn cells and the onset of an irreversible motor neuropathy. Signs are asymmetrical and may include the brain stem and bladder as well as the limbs.

Tx Patients must be isolated and discussed with a specialist immediately.

Haemorrhagic fevers

These deadly viral diseases have short incubation periods and are unlikely diagnoses if the patient has been out of an endemic area for more than 3 weeks.

- **Lassa fever**: Nigeria and other west African countries
- **Marburg fever**: Democratic Republic of Congo and surrounding countries
- **Ebola fever**: As for Marburg, plus outbreaks in Sierra Leone and Liberia.
- **Crimean Congo haemorrhagic fever**: throughout Africa

The haemorrhagic fever starts abruptly as a flu-like illness with malaise, shivering and pyrexia. Other features that quickly develop are:

- severe headache, backache and other myalgia
- pharyngitis
- anorexia, nausea and vomiting
- abdominal pain and diarrhoea (watery stools often containing blood and mucus)
- maculopapular rash
- chest pain and pleural effusions
- spontaneous bleeding.

Tx Seek advice from a consultant specialising in infectious diseases *before* taking blood samples. Barrier nurse the patient in the interim. Patients are not infectious until they become very ill, but transmission may occur through contact with infected body fluids.

Travellers' diarrhoea and vomiting

This has many different infectious causes:

- **Viral infections**, especially Norovirus
- **E. coli** and *Campylobacter*
- **Staphylococcal toxins**: abrupt onset of violent symptoms within a few hours of a meal
- **Bacillus cereus toxins**: diarrhoea 12–24 hours after eating recooked rice
- **Shigella**: bacillary dysentery with pyrexia, abdominal pain and bloody diarrhoea
- *Salmonella* **spp. (including paratyphi A and C)**: abdominal pain and pyrexia
- **Entamoeba histolytica**: amoebic dysentery (chronic diarrhoea)
- **Giardia**: gradual onset diarrhoea with foul smelling greasy stools

- **Other protozoan** – *Cryptosporidium* and *Cyclospora*
- **Helminths** – *Strongyloides*

Tx
- Commence rehydration with IV fluids or oral rehydration solution.
- Take blood for FBC, U&Es and glucose.
- Send stool for microscopy, including ova, cysts and parasites and culture. Be sure to inform microbiology staff of the patient's travel history.
- Prevent spread of infection – advise the patient about hand hygiene.

Mild cases can be managed with loperamide, and for patients at high risk of severe illness or those visiting high-risk areas (Asia, the Middle East, Africa and Latin America), azithromycin (500 mg once daily for 1–3 days). Food poisoning, infectious bloody diarrhoea and suspected *Escherichia coli* O157 infection are all notifiable diseases.

Diarrhoea and vomiting in children → p. 362.
Gastroenteritis → p. 321.
Notifiable diseases → p. 407.
Scombroid fish poisoning → p. 299.

Other infections in travellers

Cholera

Infection with the causative organism of cholera – *Vibrio cholerae* – causes profound diarrhoea ('rice-water' stools) and the rapid development of life-threatening dehydration. This is accompanied by hyponatraemia and hypokalaemia. Rehydration is the key treatment.

Typhoid fever

Infection with *Salmonella typhi* causes a non-specific, but high fever for the first week of the illness. During the second week, more specific signs develop:

- Abdominal pain and diarrhoea
- Relative bradycardia, considering the high pyrexia
- 'Rose spots'
- Splenomegaly.

Salmonella paratyphi infection causes a similar but usually less severe illness. Typhoid fever is diagnosed on blood or stool culture and is treated with ciprofloxacin, azithromycin or ceftriaxone. High rates of fluoroquinolone resistance are reported in South Asia.

Sandfly fever

This disease is a viral infection, transmitted by the bite of the sandfly in the Mediterranean and Middle Eastern areas. There is a sudden onset of fever, headache,

facial flushing and myalgias lasting 2–3 days with complete recovery.

Dengue fever

This is a mosquito-borne infection from a member of the *flavivirus* genus of which there are four serotypes. It is endemic throughout most of the tropics. Dengue fever is usually a mild, self-limiting febrile illness with:

- Cough, sore throat, coryza
- Headache and photophobia
- Nausea and vomiting
- Back pain and arthralgias
- Generalised mobiliform or maculopapular rash

Repeat infection with dengue usually causes a much more severe illness, such as Dengue haemorrhagic fever (DHF) and Dengue shock syndrome (DSS), although some primary infections can lead to these complications. They range from mild capillary leak and thrombocytopaenia to severe bleeding and multiorgan failure.

Diagnosis is confirmed with viral antigen testing and treatment is supportive.

Yellow fever

Yellow fever is a dangerous viral infection, which is transmitted by mosquitoes in the central belt of Africa and South America. Travellers to these areas should be vaccinated. Disease occurs after 3–6 days incubation and is followed by profound illness:

- Pyrexia
- Headache, nausea, vomiting and photophobia
- Jaundice
- Hypotension
- Purpura and bleeding.

Chikungunya fever

Chikungunya is a viral infection transmitted by mosquito bite. It has spread significantly in recent decades and is now a global health problem. Chikungunya is rarely fatal. Symptoms include fever, severe joint and muscle pains, headaches and skin rash which resolve in 1–2 weeks. Joint pain may persist for several months or years, hence the name, which translates as 'that which bends up' from the Makonde language of Tanzania. There is no vaccine against Chikungunya virus and no specific treatment for it.

Rickettsial illness

Rickettsial infections occur worldwide and caused by Gr-bacteria transmitted from an ectoparasite such as a louse, mite, flea or tick. The genus *Rickettsia* is divided into the spotted fever group (SFG), where patients present with fever and spots, and the typhus group (TG). Doxycycline is the drug of choice for treatment of both.

Rocky mountain spotted fever is caused by *Rickettsia rickettsi* and is usually confined to dogs and rodents. It occurs in the western and southern states of the USA and in South America. After an incubation period of 7 days, there may be an eschar at the site of a tick bite with regional lymphadenopathy. A blotchy rash appears on day 3 or 4 and gradually becomes petechial. Untreated, the course of the disease may be mild or rapidly fatal.

Louse-borne or epidemic typhus is caused by *Rickettsia prowazeki* and is transmitted by the infected faeces from a human louse, usually inoculated by scratching. After 2 weeks' incubation, there is an onset of rigours, frontal headaches and pain in the back and limbs. Chest infection and confusion develop, with a rash appearing on days 4–6. At first, this rash is morbilliform, but it soon becomes petechial and mottled. During the second week, symptoms may increase in severity and overwhelming septicaemia, pneumonia or renal failure may lead to death.

Monkeypox

Monkeypox is a sporadic zoonosis of Western and Central Africa identified in 1970, which has seen transmission within the UK since 2022. The smallpox vaccine previously provided some protection, but susceptibility to monkeypox has risen since the eradication of smallpox and cessation of vaccination. Case fatality rates seem to be higher in cases prior to 1996 compared with the more recent epidemics. Severe cases are more common among people with underlying immunodeficiencies and young children. There are two main strains: the Congo strain, which is more severe, and the West African strain, which has a lower case fatality rate. Viral transmission is by close physical contact and the incubation period ranges from 5 to 21 days.

The prodrome of fever, headache and cervical lymphadenopathy precedes the evolution of a macular, vesicular and then scabbed rash. Complications (which are rare) include pneumonia, keratitis, septicaemia and encephalitis. The rash of monkeypox usually appears and progresses all at once, rather than the appearance of lesions of different ages seen in chicken pox. Lymphadenopathy is more marked compared to chicken pox and the rash is most dense on the face and limbs rather than the torso.

Zika virus disease

Zika virus was first discovered in Africa and has been occasionally noted in countries in Africa and Asia since then. In 2015/16, the largest known outbreak of Zika affected the whole of Central and South America, the Caribbean and some parts of North America.

Infection is from a mosquito bite or very occasionally through sexual contact. Incubation is 3–14 days and symptoms include fever, rash, itching, headache and red eyes. Most people have very mild, or no symptoms. Becoming infected with Zika during pregnancy can lead to Congenital Zika Syndrome, a condition with severe consequences for the baby.

Helminth infections

Parasitic infections are rare in the returned traveller. Consider helminth infection in a patient with a travel history and acute eosinophilia and discuss with an infectious disease specialist.

Strongyloides stercoralis is an intestinal worm that infects humans through contact with soil that contains their larvae, in endemic areas. It is asymptomatic in 60% of cases with the rest suffering predominantly gastrointestinal symptoms. Unlike other helminths, strongyloides infection can be lifelong and poses a risk of hyperinfection syndrome if the patient later becomes immunosuppressed.

Cutaneous larva migrans is one of the most common parasitic infestations affecting travellers returning from beach destinations in the Caribbean, Mexico, Brazil and Southeast Asia. It is a self-limiting condition caused by migrating larvae of hookworm species, which presents with extremely itchy, serpiginous, raised, tracks on the skin. Although usually self-limiting, oral anthelmintic treatment (e.g. ivermectin or albendazole) speeds up the resolution of symptoms.

Infectious hepatitis → p. 315.
Covid-19 and Influenza see → pp. 223 and 224.
Weil's disease (leptospirosis) → p. 315.

Zoonoses (human infections of animal origin)

Lyme disease

Visits to parks or woods where there may have been deer, or sometimes other animals, may lead to infection by *Borrelia burgdorferi*, a tick-born spirochaete. There is:

- a papule at the site of the bite that develops into erythema migrans – a spreading target shaped lesion with central sparing.
- fever, headache and fatigue
- polyarthritis and lymphadenopathy

Complications include:

- meningitis
- atrioventricular block → *p. 172*
- keratitis and uveitis

- Bell's palsy
- post-Lyme syndrome – chronic arthritis and neuro-logical symptoms

Diagnosis is made clinically if the classic rash is present, otherwise antibody testing is available with follow-up and repeat testing if negative but still symptomatic at 4–6 weeks. Treatment for uncomplicated disease is with doxycycline or amoxicillin. More severe illness will require admission for admission and IV antibiotics. Be aware that a Jarisch–Herxheimer reaction may cause initial worsening of symptoms but does not usually warrant stopping antibiotics. Post-Lyme, or chronic Lyme syndrome, do not require antibiotics.

The safest way to remove ticks is with a pair of fine-tipped tweezers or a tick removal tool, pulling it out firmly holding the head, so as to not pull the body off the head.

Brucellosis

Brucellosis is a highly transmissible zoonosis, which is caused by bacteria of the genus *Brucella*. It affects a wide variety of mammals. Human infections arise through direct contact with infected animals or their milk, by either ingestion or inhalation. High risk countries include Portugal, Spain, Greece, Turkey and North Africa.

After an incubation period of 5–30 days, there is fever, malaise, headache and joint pains. The disease is rarely fatal but causes debilitation for many weeks. Brucellosis is treated with a combination of doxycycline and rifampicin for at least 6 weeks.

West Nile fever

Despite its name, West Nile fever is endemic in southern Europe, Africa and North America. The causative flavivi-rus (WNV) is transmitted to humans from its primary hosts; birds and horses, by mosquitoes and the incuba-tion period is usually 3–15 days. Around 80% of those infected with WNV have no symptoms at all but 20% have a mild flu-like illness (fever, headache and muscle pains), sometimes with swollen lymph glands or a rash on the trunk. However, a small proportion (about 1 in 150 peo-ple infected) develop more severe disease – usually an encephalitis or meningitis. These people may have head-aches, fever, stiff neck, sore eyes, disorientation, muscle weakness, convulsions and coma; numbness and paraly-sis may also occur. People over the age of 50 are more likely to develop this serious form of West Nile fever.

Glanders

This zoonosis is caused by the bacterium *Burkholderia mallei* and is primarily a disease of donkeys, mules and horses, mainly seen in the tropics. Human infection is rare but may be rapidly fatal. Glanders is spread to humans by inhalation or directly into wounds so unsurprisingly, those who work with these animals are most at risk. There is an incubation period of 10–14 days before symptoms appear. There is a high fever, malaise and muscle pains. Abscesses of the skin, nasal passages or lungs may be followed by septicaemia. Cases should be isolated.

Melioidosis

The causative organism of melioidosis, *Burkholderia pseudomallei*, is found in the soil and water of tropical regions such as Thailand, India and northern Australia. It may enter the body through wounds or by inhalation, but most patients will have had an episode of gross con-tamination, e.g. near drowning. Features include fever, headache, muscle pains, pneumonia and septicaemia. Untreated severe disease is nearly always fatal. Cases should be isolated.

Plague

Bubonic plague presents with pyrexia, malaise and discharging buboes (swollen, hard lymph nodes) in the groin or axilla. *Yersinia pestis* is transmitted by flea bites from a rodent reservoir, but if inhaled, causes a very contagious pneumonia (pneumonic plague). Democratic Republic of Congo, Madagascar and Peru are the three most endemic countries.

Anthrax

Infection by the organism *Bacillus anthracis* occurs most often in wild and domestic animals in Asia, Africa and parts of Europe; humans are rarely infected. The organism can exist as spores that allow survival in the environment for many years. (*Cutaneous form of anthrax → p. 425*).

Inhalational anthrax presents with a flu-like illness that progresses to severe respiratory difficulties and shock. Signs on CXR include pleural effusions, mediastinal widening and pulmonary infiltrates. The disease is often biphasic, with a prodrome of general malaise for 2–3 days, followed by a day or two of apparent remission before the full-blown picture develops. Swabs, sputum samples, blood cultures and EDTA blood for polymerase chain reac-tion (PCR) should be taken before starting treatment for *B. anthracis* with ciprofloxacin, clindamycin and a penicillin.

Anthrax should be considered in those handling imported animal products and in people who inject drugs with any severe soft-tissue or systemic infection. The source has occasionally been contaminated heroin. Anthrax immunisation is indicated for those with a high risk of occupational exposure.

Anthrax is a notifiable disease

Cutaneous anthrax → p. 425.
Q fever → p. 223.
Tularaemia → p. 425.

HAEMATOLOGICAL CONDITIONS

Indications for transfusion of different blood components → Box 14.29.

Use of prothrombin complex concentrate → Box 14.30 on p. 272.

Sickle cell disease

Sickle cell disease is hereditary and occurs predominantly in African and African–Caribbean patients. It is also seen to a lesser extent in those from the Middle East, India and Mediterranean countries.

Polymerisation of abnormal haemoglobin S leads to deformity of the red cells, with a consequent increase in blood viscosity and blockage of capillaries. This 'sickling'

is usually precipitated by hypoxia, dehydration or infection, although there are many other causes.

Patients with sickle cell disease frequently live with high levels of pain and are often under-treated with analgesia in hospital. They are at high risk of becoming seriously unwell and should be seen as a priority in ED. Clinical presentations of sickling include the following 'crises':

- **Severe bone pain**: can be due to avascular necrosis, vaso-occlusion or infection
- **Abdominal pain and vomiting**: hepatic and splenic sequestration causes pain in the right and left upper quadrants. Splenic sequestration is more common in young children, characterised by enlarging spleen and hypotension.
- **Acute chest syndrome**: fever, chest pain, dyspnoea and haemoptysis

---

 Box 14.29 Indications for transfusion of blood components in emergency medicine

The codes given are those assigned to the indication by the National Blood Service of the UK.

Red cell concentrates
R1 Acute blood loss with haemodynamic instability
R2 Hb ≤70 g/L stable patient
R3 Hb ≤80 g/L stable patient and acute coronary syndrome

Cryoprecipitate
2 pooled units will increase fibrinogen by approximately 1 g/L in adults

C1 Clinically significant bleeding and fibrinogen
C2 Fibrinogen <1 g/L and pre-procedure, with a risk of bleeding
C3 Bleeding associated with thrombolytic therapy
C4 Inherited hypofibrinogenaemia – fibrinogen concentrate not available

Fresh frozen plasma (FFP)
Dose = 15–20 mL/kg (equivalent to 4 U for an adult)

F1 Major haemorrhage: in trauma setting, transfuse 1 : 1 ratio with red cells, other settings give at least 1 unit to every 2 units of red cells.
F2 PT ratio /INR >1.5 with bleeding
F3 PT ratio/INR >1.5 pre-procedure
F4 Liver disease with PT ratio/INR >2 and pre-procedure

Platelet concentrates
Dose = 15 mL/kg (equivalent to one therapeutic dose for an adult)

P1 Reversible bone marrow failure – Plt $<10 \times 10^9$/L
P2 Plt 10–20 $\times 10^*9$/L with sepsis/haemostatic abnormality, or other additional risk factor for bleeding
P3 To prevent bleeding associated with invasive procedures
   P3a Plt >20 $\times 10^*9$/L – central venous line
   P3b Plt >40 $\times 10^*9$/L – lumbar puncture/ spinal anaesthesia
   P3c Plt >50 $\times 10^*9$/L – pre-percutaneous liver biopsy/major surgery
   P3d Plt >80 $\times 10^*9$/L – epidural anaesthesia
   P3e Plt >100 $\times 10^*9$/L – critical site surgery e.g. CNS/eye
P4 Therapeutic use to stop bleeding
   P4a Major haemorrhage – Plt <50 $\times 10^*9$/L
   P4b Empirically in major haemorrhage pack
   P4c Critical site bleeding, e.g. CNS – Plt <100 $\times 10^*9$/L
   P4d Clinically significant bleeding – Plt <30 $\times 10^*9$/L
P5a DIC pre-procedure or with bleeding
P5b Immune thrombocytopenia (emergency treatment pre-procedure/severe bleeding)
P6a Consider if critical bleeding on anti-platelet medication

- **CNS**: stroke and cerebral venous sinus thrombosis
- **Visual loss**: retinal infarction
- *Priapism* → *p. 340*
- **Infection**: the leading cause of death – note that loss of splenic function predisposes to pneumococcal infection
- *Rhabdomyolysis* (→ *p. 262*)
- **Hyper-haemolytic crisis**: characterised by acute drop in Hb with high bilirubin and reticulocyte counts
- **Aplastic crisis**: commonly secondary to Parvovirus B19 infection. Patients are pale and tachycardic due to failure of erythropoiesis. Reticulocyte count will be low.

Investigations: A full blood count, reticulocytes, urea and electrolytes and liver function tests should be carried out. Haemoglobin is normally low in patients with sickle cell disease and will be very low in a crisis.

Chest X-ray is needed for patients with chest signs, looking for infiltrates in acute chest crisis and consolidation.

CT brain scan is indicated in the presence of neurological signs.

Tx

- Give a high concentration of oxygen.
- Commence rehydration with IV fluids. Blood transfusion dilutes HbS but may increase blood viscosity.
- Give adequate analgesia, usually morphine, within 30 min of arrival, patient controlled analgesia (PCA) is often needed.
- Keep the patient warm
- Consider IV antibiotics if infection is suspected as the trigger
- Blood transfusion may be required where haemoglobin concentration drops below 5 g/dL with associated aplasia – discuss with a haematologist.
- Exchange transfusion may be required in patients with stroke, severe chest syndrome, multiorgan failure or treatment-resistant priapism.

Acquired haemophilia

Acquired haemophilia is a rare condition where patients produce inhibitors to clotting factors. It is most frequently seen in elderly patients without any underlying disease but also occurs:

- as a feature of autoimmune diseases
- as a drug reaction
- in some malignancies and lymphoproliferative disorders
- in pregnant and postpartum patients.

The haemophilia may present with a rapid onset of bleeding into the muscles, soft tissues or retroperitoneum or may complicate a situation in which there is already severe bleeding. Sometimes, the incidental finding of prolongation of the activated partial thromboplastin time (APTT) is the first sign of the condition.

Patients may require recombinant human coagulation factor VIIa, recombinant porcine factor VIII or activated prothrombin complex concentrate if acutely bleeding. Consult a Haematologist.

Low platelets

There are many causes of thrombocytopenia (a platelet count $<150 \times 10^9$/L):

1 **Decreased production**: bone-marrow failure due to disease, cytotoxic therapy or irradiation, acute leukaemias, uraemia
2 **Decreased survival**: usually immunological causation such as idiopathic thrombocytopenic purpura (ITP) or drugs
3 **Increased consumption**: DIC, thrombotic thrombocytopenic purpura (TTP), large haemangiomas, some infections
4 **Sequestration**: hypersplenism and hypothermia
5 **Excessive loss**: massive haemorrhage and consumption coagulopathy
6 **Dilution**: massive transfusion of stored blood.

Platelet transfusions are used for the prevention and treatment of bleeding associated with thrombocytopenia or platelet function defects. Serious spontaneous haemorrhage due to thrombocytopenia alone is unlikely to occur at platelet counts $>10 \times 10^9$/L. Massive haemorrhage, DIC, bone marrow failure and acute leukaemias are all indications for platelet therapy, as is post-transfusion purpura (PTP). In ITP, TTP and heparin-induced thrombocytopenia (HIT) platelet transfusion is contraindicated unless there is life-threatening bleeding.

TTP: Pentad of thrombocytopaenia, fever, haemolytic anaemia, neurological abnormalities and renal dysfunction. Treatment is with plasma exchange.

HIT: Acute thrombocytopaemia usually 5–10 days after starting heparin. Condition improves when heparin is stopped.

ITP: Relatively common and usually benign condition. Treatment is with steroids and sometimes intravenous immunoglobulin (IVIG).

Haemolytic uraemic syndrome

Haemolytic uraemic syndrome (HUS) is a systemic disease with three main components:

1 Haemolytic anaemia
2 Acute renal failure
3 Thrombocytopenia.

HUS is caused by the effects of a circulating toxin that binds to endothelium, particularly in the renal, gastro-intestinal and central nervous systems. Thrombin and fibrin are deposited in the damaged microvasculature and erythrocytes are then injured (and subsequently haemolysed) as they pass through the partially occluded blood vessels. Platelets are sequestered but coagulation is relatively unaffected.

Typical (infection-induced) HUS is caused by a toxin from *E. coli* O157:H7 called Shiga toxin. Contaminated food products, water and direct contact with farm animals or infected people are possible routes of transmission. Other bacteria and some viruses (including HIV) may also be associated with HUS and the atypical form of the disease (10% of cases) may be induced by certain drugs, systemic lupus, cancer and pregnancy. The disease (which is notifiable) occurs as both sporadic cases and larger outbreaks. It is most common at the extremes of age (especially children under 3 years), in summer months and in rural communities.

E. coli O157:H7 may cause a haemorrhagic colitis but only around 15% of cases progress to HUS (after 5-14 days) and many infected adults remain asymptomatic. Initial profuse diarrhoea becomes bloody after a couple of days with fever, vomiting and abdominal pain. In the UK, HUS is the most common cause of acute renal failure in children.

Investigations:

- FBC and blood film (looking for anaemia, haemolysis and a low platelet count)
- Blood chemistry (to show renal involvement)
- Stool sample (for culture and phage typing of *E. coli*).

Tx The treatment of bloody diarrhoea and HUS is supportive, with no evidence for specific treatments. Antibiotics are not beneficial and anti-diarrhoeal drugs should be avoided. Fluid and electrolyte losses may be high due to both diarrhoea and capillary leakage. The case fatality rate is 2-5% with most deaths occurring in children and elderly people. Around half of children with HUS require dialysis.

Reversal of oral anticoagulant drugs

The main adverse effect of drugs such as warfarin and direct oral anticoagulants (DOACs) is haemorrhage.

With warfarin, bruising and bleeding increase significantly with INRs >5 (therapeutic INRs are between 2 and 4). Vitamin K$_1$ (phytomena-dione) can be used to reverse the effects caused by over-anticoagulation of warfarin, the dose being dependent on the INR result and the presence of bleeding.

- **INR 6.0–8.0 with minor or no bleeding:** stop oral anticoagulants and recheck the INR every 2 days to ensure that it is falling. Recommence anticoagulants when the INR is <5. There is no indication for vitamin K.
- **INR >8.0 with minor or no bleeding:** stop oral anticoagulants and recheck the INR every 2 days to ensure that it is falling. Recommence anticoagulants when the INR is <5. If the patient has risk factors for bleeding (age >70 years, previous history of bleeding including epistaxis), give oral vitamin K 0.5–2.5 mg stat. Recheck the INR after 24 hours and repeat the vitamin K if necessary.
- **Major bleeding:** stop oral anticoagulant drugs. The anticoagulation can be rapidly and effectively reversed with prothrombin complex concentrate (→ *Box 14.30*) and IV vitamin K$_1$ 5 mg stat.

DOACs: No standard clotting screen exists for assessing the degree of anticoagulation from these drugs. It is therefore advisable to contact a Haematologist when

Box 14.30 Prothrombin complex concentrate

Prothrombin complex concentrate (PCC) is a human-activated coagulation factor concentrate containing the vitamin K-dependent factors, II, VII, XI and X and also protein S and protein C. It is indicated for the treatment of bleeding and for perioperative prophylaxis in acquired deficiency of PCC factors due to vitamin K antagonists or autoantibodies.

In emergency medicine, it is used primarily for patients who require rapid reversal of warfarin therapy, especially in cases of intracranial haemorrhage or other major haemorrhage (instead of the less effective FFP). It is issued from the blood transfusion laboratory under brand names Octaplex® and Beriplex®. The concomitant administration of IV vitamin K (5 mg) should always be considered because warfarin activity can last longer than the effect of PCC. The dose is usually between 20 and 50 units/kg, according to the patient's INR and weight in kilogrammes (dosing can vary between organisations):

Initial INR	<3.0	3.0–5.0	>5.0
Approximate dose	40 mL (1000 IU)	80 mL (2000 IU)	120 mL (3000 IU)

The single dose should not exceed 3000 IU (120 mL or six vials of PCC) in 24 hours. The main risk is that of thromboembolism but allergic reactions may also infrequently occur.

there is life-threatening bleeding in a patient on these medications.

- Dabigatran is a direct factor thrombin inhibitor, aPTT is the most useful test to assess its anticoagulation effects. Idarucizumab is a specific reversal agent for dabigatran in adults when rapid reversal is required. The dose is 5 mg IV, repeated after 5–10 min.
- Apixaban and rivaroxaban are direct inhibitors of activated factor X (factor Xa). Andexanet alfa is a recombinant form of human factor Xa licenced for the reversal of apixaban and rivaroxaban. It is recommended by NICE for uncontrolled GI haemorrhage or as part of a clinical trial for other bleeding, until the full guideline is produced. Prothrombin complex concentrate at 50 units/kg is considered a suitable alternative until more research data is available and is the only reversal treatment available for major haemorrhage in patients on edoxaban.

Neutropenic sepsis

Certain categories of patients are at a high risk of developing neutropenia (a neutrophil count $<1.0 \times 10^9/L$) and consequent life-threatening sepsis:

- Patients who have received recent cytotoxic chemotherapy
- Patients who have an acute haematological malignancy (such as acute lymphoblastic or myelobastic leukaemia)
- Patients with an absolute neutrophil count of $\leq 0.5 \times 10^9/L$ for any reason.

In such patients, all febrile episodes must be taken very seriously and treated urgently with antibiotics. For this purpose, fever is defined as a temperature of 38°C or more measured by the patient themselves or medical staff at any point. However, fever may not be present, and the possibility of infection should be considered in all neutropenic patients who are unwell. Shock, acute respiratory distress and multiple organ failure are possible extreme presentations of neutropenic sepsis.

> There is a particularly high risk of neutropenia around one week after receiving chemotherapy.

Over 50% of febrile neutropenic patients prove to have an infection and many have a bacteraemia. This is usually due to Gram-positive cocci or Gram-negative bacilli such as *E. coli*, *Klebsiella* spp. or *Pseudomonas aeruginosa*. Acute respiratory viral infections and fungal infections may also be associated with severe illness in the immunocompromised host. Infections in neutropenic patients typically take between 2 and 7 days to respond to antimicrobial therapy.

Investigations:
- Blood cultures, including from any indwelling lines
- FBC, blood chemistry, LFTs, glucose, CRP, plasma lactate and coagulation screen
- CXR and MSU (midstream urine).

Tx
- A broad-spectrum antibacterial (such as IV piperacillin with tazobactam) should be given as soon as the diagnosis is suspected, and cultures have been obtained. Many EDs have systems to instigate this from the point of triage.
- IV teicoplanin or vancomycin should be added for catheter-related infections or if methicillin-resistant *S. aureus* (MRSA) is likely. Discuss with the microbiology team whether a 'line lock' should be employed (instilling a concentrated dose of antibiotic into the line and leaving it for a set duration).
- A stat dose of recombinant human granulocyte colony-stimulating factor (lenograstim or filgrastim) can also be given subcutaneously to stimulate the production of neutrophils.
- Admission should be arranged to a side room with strict barrier nursing.
- Liaise with oncology and haematology teams.

DERMATOLOGICAL CONDITIONS

Acute generalised pustular psoriasis (of von Zumbusch) is an explosive, eruptive form of psoriasis accompanied by fever and toxicity. The patient (who is often middle-aged) initially has red, tender skin and feels ill. Clusters of superficial, sterile pustules (2–3 mm in diameter) appear within hours. They are widely distributed over the body but concentrated in the flexures, genital regions and fingertips. Within 24 hours, the pustules coalesce, dry and desquamate. The underlying skin is smooth and erythematous but new crops of pustules may appear over a period of days or weeks. There is a neutrophilia and a raised CRP. Albumin, calcium and zinc levels are low and renal tubular necrosis may occur. This is a life-threatening condition and the patient must be admitted to hospital for skin care and IV rehydration.

Bullous pemphigoid is a blistering skin disease that usually affects older people. The blisters are due to an immune reaction within the skin and cause intense itching. Crops of tense, fluid-filled bullae develop which are filled with clear, cloudy or bloodstained fluid. The eruption may be very widespread and, in severe episodes, there may be blisters over the entire skin surface and in the mouth. In such cases, hospital admission may be required so that the blisters and raw areas can be carefully dressed. IV fluids and steroids are usually given and antibiotics may be required for secondary bacterial infection.

Eczema herpeticum can affect any age group but most commonly children with atopic eczema. It is a complication of the first or a recurrent episode of *herpex simplex* 1 or 2. Widespread, itchy and painful blisters occur on both previously normal and eczema affected skin. The patient is unwell with fever and lymphadenopathy. Admission is needed for antivirals such as acyclovir.

Erythroderma is intense redness of the skin, covering at least 90% of the body surface area. It usually occurs in those with pre-existing inflammatory skin disease such as psoriasis. There will often be desquamation of the skin, itching and lymphadenopathy. Treatment is with emollients and cool, moist dressings, stopping trigger medications and sometimes corticosteroids. Severe cases need admission to ICU or a burns unit due to the risk of complications such as electrolyte balance, dehydration, secondary bacterial infection and hypothermia.

Stevens-Johnson syndrome and toxic epidermal necrolysis are variants of the same condition, where severe mucocutaneous reactions are caused by medications, such as NSAIDs and anti-epileptics. A painful rash starts on the trunk and spreads to the face and limbs in hours to days. It starts as macules which develop to blisters and then desquamation of the epidermis. There are mouth ulcers and irritated eyes. Again, treatment is supportive, in hospital or intensive care. The offending drug should be stopped and adequate analgesia provided.

Necrotising soft tissue infections

There is a large spectrum of clinical conditions in which there is a spreading necrosis of soft tissue ranging from relatively localised pyodermas to fulminating gas gangrene. Anaerobic streptococci, staphylococci, *Bacteroides* spp., enterococci and clostridia are the most commonly implicated organisms. People who inject drugs have an above-average risk of such infections, especially those who inject subcutaneously ('skin-popping'). The possibility of anthrax infection (→ *pp. 269 and 425*) should also be considered in an injecting drug user with a necrotising soft-tissue infection.

Necrotising fasciitis Spreading necrosis of the fascial plane is usually polymicrobial in nature with cultures yielding a mixture of four or more species of both anaerobic and aerobic bacteria. Group-A haemolytic streptococcus is the most common single organism isolate. Although rare, the condition has a mortality rate of around 25%. It is more common in males and in people aged >60 years. Patients often have an underlying condition that predisposes to infection such as diabetes, peripheral vascular disease, alcoholism or injecting drug use. Fournier's gangrene of the scrotum (which tracks abdominally via Scarpa's fascia) is an eponymous variant of the same condition.

Necrotising fasciitis can affect any part of the body. It usually follows a trivial injury such as an insect bite or a small abrasion. There can be a delay of up to a week from the beginning of the early symptoms after which there is severe and rapid progression over minutes to hours. The patient is pyrexic, tachycardic and looks unwell with a seemingly disproportionate amount of pain. The tenderness often occurs beyond the area of erythema and oedema, due to spreading infection 'below the surface.' As the condition develops, the area becomes dusky and haemorrhagic with bullae formation. Overwhelming sepsis can progress rapidly to shock and multiorgan failure.

Gas gangrene Fulminating necrosis of muscle occurs when damaged or devitalised tissue becomes contaminated with the anaerobic bacteria *Clostridium perfringens* from soil. As the bacteria multiply, they produce toxins which digest muscle and subcutaneous tissues. The destructive processes liberate free gas and other noxious metabolites.

In this situation, clostridia have a short incubation period; contaminated wounds begin to putrefy around 1–3 days after injury. The surrounding tissues crepitate because of the free gas and emit a foul odour. The patient has a high fever, hypotension and usually a toxic delirium. The condition progresses rapidly to systemic sepsis and organ failure.

Investigations: Diagnosis of soft-tissue necrosis is almost entirely clinical. However, around 50% of patients with necrotising fasciitis (and many more with gas gangrene) have air in the soft tissues on plain radiography. Almost all patients have an elevated white cell count and urea. In the later stages, there is metabolic acidosis and coagulopathy.

Tx Resuscitation with IV fluids and administration of broad-spectrum IV antibiotics (e.g. a beta-lactam, metronidazole and clindamycin) is required. Call for surgical input as soon as the diagnosis is suspected. Extensive surgical debridement of affected areas must not be delayed.

Hereditary and other non-allergic angio-oedemas

Allergic angio-oedema and anaphylaxis → p. 306.

There are several types of angio-oedema that do not respond to treatment with antihistamines, corticosteroids or epinephrine. These include:

- **Hereditary angio-oedema (HAE):** this affects 1 in 50 000 people. There is an inherited mutation in the

C1-inhibitor gene, leading to a reduced level of C1 esterase inhibitor or a C1 inhibitor protein that does not work properly. The lack of this physiological regulator results in an overproduction of bradykinin and consequent leaky blood vessels (→ *Figure 14.2*). The absence of a family history does not rule out the diagnosis of HAE; in up to 25% of cases a spontaneous mutation is responsible. The frequency, severity and duration of attacks are variable, but most patients have a first attack before the age of 20. There are many possible triggers including concurrent illnesses, surgery, emotional stress, hormonal changes and specific foods. Many patients experience prodromal symptoms of some sort.

- **Drug-induced angio-oedema**: ACE inhibitors are the most frequent culprit (→ *Figure 14.2*).
- **Acquired angio-oedema**: this can develop during serious illnesses such as malignancies or autoimmune disorders.
- **Idiopathic angio-oedema**.

At least the first three of these angio-oedemas are mediated by excess bradykinin production (→ *Figure 14.2*). There may be swelling of the face, lips, tongue, pharynx and larynx. Throat tightness, drooling, hoarse voice and stridor can occur. The oedema may cause airway obstruction and shock (due to fluid redistribution). In HAE, recurrent colicky abdominal pain

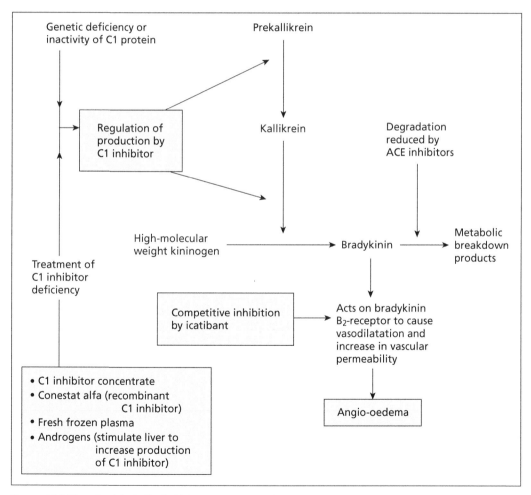

Figure 14.2 The role of the kallikrein–kinin system in the pathogenesis and treatment of non-allergic angio-oedemas. ACE, angiotensin-converting enzyme.

(sometimes with vomiting and diarrhoea) may be repeatedly misdiagnosed.

Bradykinin mediated, compared with histamine mediated angioedema, is associated with no urticaria or itching and a slower onset (24–26 hours). It is more likely to be asymmetrical.

Tx Airway obstruction can kill rapidly, ensure advanced airway care can be provided, including fibreoptic intubation and emergency cricothyroidotomy.

Icatibant is a specific and selective competitive bradykinin B_2-receptor antagonist that has been used for the emergency treatment of HAE. In theory it displaces bradykinin from its receptor and thus reduces the oedema and shortens the duration of attacks. Unfortunately, despite a biologically plausible mechanism, there is a lack of evidence for its effectiveness for this indication.

C1 inhibitor concentrate (Berinert® or Cinryze®) may be administered intravenously in an acute attack. Recombinant C1 inhibitor (Conestat alfa), is available as an alternative to the plasma-derived concentrate for where religious reasons may prohibit human blood-derived products. It is contraindicated in patients with allergy to rabbits. Two units of FFP can be used if C1 inhibitor concentrate is not available.

A kallikrein inhibitor (ecallentide) may be available in the UK in the future.

15

Poisoning

Jodie Wilkinson
Royal Oldham Hospital, Oldham, UK

GENERAL PRINCIPLES IN POISONING

Poisoning may be the result of:

1 Deliberate self-poisoning (self-harm)
2 Therapeutic overdose (accidental)
3 Recreational substance use
4 Environmental contamination (deliberate or accidental).

> Bizarre symptoms and signs or unusual combinations of clinical features should always suggest the possibility of poisoning.

Initial assessment and management

ABCs → Chapter 1.

The first priority should be to carry out an ABCDE assessment and to provide any immediate supportive or stabilisation treatments.

A. Administer a high concentration of oxygen by mask and protect the airway if necessary.

B. Measure oxygen saturations and respiratory rate, perform an arterial blood gas and assess the level of respiratory support required (opioid and sedative drugs may depress the protective reflexes of the airway more than might normally be expected for a given level of consciousness).
C. Perform an ECG, assess heart rate, QRS width, QTc prolongation and treat any arrhythmias – this may require treatment of any metabolic acidosis. Check the patient's BP and assess if haemodynamic support is required. Obtain venous access and give intravenous fluids if appropriate.
D. Assess level of consciousness, pupil size and reactivity and control any seizures with benzodiazepines.
E. Measure the patient's core temperature and blood glucose level.

The early involvement of senior ED colleagues or anaesthetic support is advised for those patients requiring immediate intervention or for those patients at risk of deterioration.

As some of these patients will not be able to provide any history due to their clinical condition, the initial assessment should also look for signs of a specific toxidrome. A toxidrome describes a constellation of signs and symptoms that consistently result from exposure to particular toxins. The presence of a toxidrome may help guide subsequent management → *see Table 15.1*.

The RCEM Lecture Notes: Emergency Medicine, Fifth Edition. Edited by Catherine Williams and Amy Nickson.
© 2024 John Wiley & Sons Ltd. Published 2024 by John Wiley & Sons Ltd.
Companion website: www.wiley.com/go/LNEM5

Table 15.1 Toxidromes and their associated drugs, signs and symptoms

Toxidrome	Drug causes of this toxidrome	Signs and symptoms
Sympathomimetic	• caffeine • cocaine • amphetamines • Ritalin • LSD • theophylline • MDMA	• tachycardia • dysrhythmias • hypertension • delusions • paranoia • diaphoresis • seizures • hyperthermia • mydriasis
Anticholinergic	• Anticholinergics – atropine, glycopyrrolate • Antihistamines • Antipsychotics – chlorpromazine, clozapine, olanzapine, quetiapine • Antispasmodics – oxybutynin • Cyclic antidepressants – amitriptyline, nortriptyline • Mydriatics – cyclopentolate, tropicamide • Others – carbamazepine, class 1A antiarrhythmics, certain plants – belladonna	• confusion • dry mouth • urinary retention • mydriasis • flushed skin • tachycardia • absent bowel sounds • hyperthermia
Cholinergic	• organophosphates • certain mushrooms • pesticides • Novichok	• defecation • urination • miosis • bradycardia • emesis • lacrimation • sweating • bronchospasm • bronchorrhoea • hypertension • muscle fasiculations • paralysis
Opioid	• morphine • codeine • tramadol • methadone • fentanyl • heroin • oxycodone	• pin pint pupils • respiratory depression • decreased bowel sounds • reduced level of consciousness

Further assessment and management

Ask about what they have taken

- Nature of substance taken
- Amount – if uncertain it is safest to assume the maximum possible
- Type of preparation taken – slow-release preparations may cause delayed or protracted poisoning

- Other substances (e.g. alcohol) also taken
- Route of poisoning (e.g. oral, IV)
- Time taken.

Ask questions that will help assess their risk level of further self-harm (if relevant)

- Description of the event
- Intended result of poisoning

- Previous episodes of poisoning
- Psychiatric history
- The presence of any ongoing suicidal ideation.

→ *Chapter 19 Page*

When the substance taken is unknown

- Obtain as much history and background information as possible
- Examine the patient and their clothing and possessions
- Consider trauma or co-existent disease
- Instigate immediate treatments and supportive treatments as indicated by the patient's condition.

Specific actions to undertake in the poisoning patient

- Measure the plasma urea and electrolytes (U&ES) and glucose.
- Consider the need to measure the blood gases, plasma osmolality and plasma chloride. The osmolar gap and the anion gap can then be calculated → *p. 235*.
- Measure or screen for plasma salicylate and paracetamol levels 4 hours after the estimated time of ingestion, this should be done irrespective of the history of substance taken in deliberate poisoning.
- Seek specific poisons advice (*Sources of advice → p. 282*).
- Consider the need for gastric decontamination (→ *later*).
- Consider the need for specific supportive measures (→ *p. 281*).
- Consider the need for specific toxicology levels (e.g. lithium, iron, theophylline, methanol, ethylene glycol, digoxin and carboxyhaemoglobin).
- Consider the need for specific therapies (→ *below*).
- Give IV saline (at least 10 mL/kg) unless there is a specific contraindication.
- Catheterise the bladder and measure the urine output if appropriate.

Biochemical abnormalities in poisoning

A metabolic acidosis with an increased anion gap (and a normal chloride concentration) indicates retention of non-volatile organic acids such as may be present in renal failure, ketoacidosis and lactic acidosis, or following the ingestion of substances such as methanol, ethylene glycol, salicylate and iron. In the absence of circulatory failure, diabetes, alcoholism, uraemia, or another cause of elevated lactate, an increased anion gap strongly suggests poisoning with one or more of these substances.

An increased osmolar gap indicates that one or more substances are present in high molar concentrations. Most drugs, including salicylates, are not identified this way because they are dissociated or do not attain high enough serum concentrations on a molar basis. The ingested substances best able to increase the osmolar gap are those that have a low molecular weight and are present in high mass units – such as the lower alcohols and glycols. Poisoning with methanol or ethylene glycol commonly causes severe metabolic acidosis and elevation of both the anion and osmolar gaps → *p. 235*. The metabolic changes associated with certain poisonings are summarised in → *Table 15.2*.

Table 15.2 Biochemical abnormalities and their associated drugs

Clinical features	Example agent(s)
Hypernatraemia	Sodium salts
	MDMA (rarely)
Hyponatraemia	MDMA (commonly)
	SSRIs
	Levamisole (adulterant in cocaine)
	Diuretics (chronic)
Hyperkalaemia	Digoxin
	ACE inhibitors
	Potassium-sparing diuretics
Hypokalaemia	Theophylline
	Salbutamol
	Digoxin
	Diuretics (chronic)
	Insulin
	Sulphonylureas
	Paracetamol
Hyperglycaemia	Theophylline
	Salicylates
	Calcium channel antagonists
Hypoglycaemia	Insulin
	Sulponylureas
	Ethanol
	Salicylates
	Sodium valproate
Hypocalcaemia	Ethylene glycol
	Hydrofluoric acid
Increased anion gap	Ethanol
	Ethylene glycol
	Iron salts
	Isoniazid
	Methanol
	Metformin
	Paraldehyde
	Salicylates

(Continued)

Table 15.2 (Continued)

Clinical features	Example agent(s)
Increased osmolar gap	Ethanol
	Ethylene glycol
	Acetone
	Hyperosmolar IV solutions, e.g. mannitol
Metabolic acidosis	Carbon monoxide
	Cyanide
	Ethylene glycol
	Gamma hydroxybutyrate (GHB)
	Iron
	Isoniazid
	MDMA
	Metformin
	Methanol
	Paracetamol
	Acetazolamide
	Salicylates
	Sodium valproate
	Theophylline
	Tricyclic antidepressants
Respiratory acidosis	Sedative agents, e.g.
	Barbiturates
	Benzodiazepines
	Gamma hydroxybutyrate (GHB)
	Ethanol
	Opiates
	Tricyclic antidepressant
Metabolic alkalosis	Bicarbonate
Respiratory alkalosis	Salicylates
	Theophylline
	MDMA

Calculation of the anion gap → p. 235.
Calculation of the osmolar gap → p. 235.
Metabolic acidosis → p. 263.

Gastric decontamination

Controversy still surrounds the efficacy of the different modes of gastric decontamination although none are currently a mainstay of modern treatment. All methods aim to reduce the absorption of residual toxins from the gastrointestinal (GI) tract. The risks of each form of decontamination must be carefully weighed against the likely benefits. Any form of gastric decontamination is of doubtful value if more than 1 hour has passed since the ingestion of poisons.

Activated charcoal

Single-dose activated charcoal should be given if the patient has ingested a potentially toxic amount of a poison, which is known to be absorbed by charcoal, within the previous hour. It should only be given if the patient has an intact or protected airway. The initial dose of activated charcoal is 50 g for adults and 1 g/kg for children.

Activated charcoal will not absorb:

- iron, lithium and other metallic compounds
- cyanides
- strong acids and alkalis
- alcohols
- petroleum distillates
- malathion and DDT.

Repeated administration of charcoal should be considered only if a patient has ingested a life-threatening amount of carbamazepine, dapsone, digoxin, phenobarbital, quinine or theophylline.

If multiple doses are needed, then the dose can be repeated every 4 hours; however, if vomiting is a problem then 12.5 g hourly or 25 g every 2 hours in adults and smaller amounts every 2 hours in children may be better tolerated.

Charcoal may induce vomiting or constipation and rarely small bowel obstruction. If a patient develops delayed bowel motility, then they should receive no further doses of charcoal and evidence of ileus should be looked for regularly in these patients, especially in those receiving atropine.

Many patients find activated charcoal unpalatable – mixing with cola improves tolerability and concordance.

Gastric lavage

At present, there is no evidence showing that gastric lavage should be used routinely in the management of poisoning. In the rare instances in which gastric lavage is indicated, it should only be performed by individuals with the correct training and expertise, and usually only on the advice of a poisons centre.

Whole bowel irrigation

Whole bowel irrigation can be considered for potentially toxic ingestions of sustained-release or enteric-coated drugs particularly for those patients presenting later than 2 hours after the ingestion when activated charcoal is less effective. It can be used for patients who have ingested substantial amounts of iron, lithium, potassium or for body packers (→ *see page 401*), where the mortality is high and there is a lack of other potentially effective options for gastrointestinal decontamination.

It should only be considered where the airway is protected and is contraindicated in patients with bowel obstruction, perforation or ileus, and in those with hemodynamic instability. It should be used cautiously in debilitated patients and in patients with medical conditions that might be further compromised by its use. The concurrent administration of activated charcoal and whole-body irrigation might lead to a decrease in the effectiveness of the charcoal.

Supportive treatment

Treatment of respiratory depression

There are four main factors:

1 **Airway protection**: positioning and suctioning
2 **Airway maintenance**: positioning and adjuncts
3 **Support of breathing**: assisted ventilation
4 **Reversal of specific opioid-induced respiratory depression**: naloxone.

Treatment of circulatory depression

This involves the following:

• Maintenance of adequate oxygen supply to the heart → *before*
• Maintenance of normovolaemia – IV fluids
• Correction of cardiac dysrhythmias – may need specialist advice to avoid dangerous interactions (e.g. prolongation of the Q–T interval → *p. 181*)
• Correction of bradycardia – atropine initially; may need an isoprenaline or adrenaline infusion or cardiac pacing (→ *p. 172*)
• Treatment of hypotension or hypertension
• Maintenance of cardiac contractility – inotropes such as dobutamine (→ *p. 252*). Specialist monitoring is necessary to optimise cardiac output in this situation.

Treatment of hyperthermia

Hyperthermia may result from the following:

1 Stimulant drugs (e.g. amphetamines)
2 Excessive exercise and dehydration
3 Idiopathic reactions to drugs (e.g. neuroleptic malignant syndrome [→ *p. 308*] and malignant hyperthermia)

4 A combination of the above (e.g. amphetamines and convulsions → *p. 243*).

Treatment must be promptly instituted to prevent the development of multi-organ failure. Cooling measures include:

• removal of clothing
• mist and fan techniques
• placement of ice packs in the axillae and groins
• external cooling devices
• infusion of cooled IV fluids
• cold fluid lavage (gastric, bladder and peritoneal)
• intravascular cooling techniques

Drugs that may be used in some situations to promote cooling include the following:

• **Diazepam**: muscle relaxant and sedative
• **Dantrolene**: muscle relaxant. Dantrolene is used for the treatment of malignant hyperthermia and as such is kept in all operating theatres. Its use should be discussed with an intensivist. An initial dose of 1 mg/kg is given intravenously over 10 min, repeated if necessary every 15 min to a maximum of 10 mg/kg in 24 hours.

Convulsions → p. 243.
Hyperpyrexia and hyperthermia → p. 249.

Antidotes

The majority of antidotes should be available either within the ED or the hospital. Antivenom and the less frequently required antidotes will need to be discussed with the National poisons service.

When using antidotes it is important to be aware of:

• The short half-life of some antidotes – naloxone and flumazenil have a shorter therapeutic half-life than the opiates and benzodiazepines they are the treatment for, meaning symptoms are likely to recur
• Consider the length of infusion and the hospital supplies – for example, a glucagon infusion will require fifty vials of 1 mg glucagon in order to reconstitute, flumazenil will be kept only in certain areas of the hospital and an ethanol infusion may be needed for several days which may exhaust your hospital's supplies.
• Antidotes can precipitate withdrawal in patients with dependence – e.g. naloxone and flumazenil
• They can be dangerous in themselves – dicobalt edetate can cause significant hypotension, flumazenil can cause convulsions in epileptics and arrhythmias in patients on cardiotoxic drugs
• They may not act against any toxic metabolites already present, e.g. in ethanol glycol poisonings

Poisons information services

Specific poisons information may be obtained from the following:

1 The internet (TOXBASE, the primary clinical toxicology database of the UK National Poisons Information Service is available on the internet to registered users)
2 Telephone enquiries to the UK National Poisons Information Service (NPIS)
3 Textbooks, including the front of the *British National Formulary*
4 Databases (e.g. tablet, plant and fungi identification charts).

POISONING WITH COMMON MEDICINES

The frequency with which poisoning with a drug occurs usually reflects its availability in a society.

Treatment of toxicity caused by local anaesthetic agents → p. 412.

Paracetamol (acetaminophen)

Paracetamol is a common drug involved in self-poisoning in the UK; this reflects its widespread usage and over-the-counter availability. It is also a common ingredient in compound tablets, combined with opiates, caffeine and many other drugs. The only early features of isolated paracetamol poisoning are nausea and vomiting, which usually settle within 24 hours. Malaise beyond this time, especially if accompanied by right subcostal pain and tenderness, usually indicates the development of hepatocellular necrosis, the major toxic effect of paracetamol poisoning. Late presentations of paracetamol overdose are characterised by liver failure with cerebral oedema, coagulopathy, jaundice and hypoglycaemia occurring. An acute kidney injury due to renal tubular necrosis may also be a feature.

A significant paracetamol overdose for adults is when more than 150 mg/kg or 12 g is taken in any 24-hour period. Rarely toxicity can also occur with ingestions of between 75 and 150 mg/kg within a 24-hour period. Children rarely ingest large quantities of paracetamol and so deaths attributable to this drug before the teenage years (and especially age <6 years) are extremely unusual.

Investigation and treatment depend on the time since ingestion and where this is unknown or uncertain the patient should be managed as a staggered paracetamol overdose.

Paracetamol overdose ingested over a period of 1 hour or less – presenting less than 8 hours after acute ingestion

A venous blood sample should be taken for measurement of plasma paracetamol 4 hours from the last ingestion of paracetamol; also U&Es, creatinine, bicarbonate, LFTs, INR and FBC should also be checked. The risk of liver damage should be assessed by plotting the patient's plasma concentration on the plasma paracetamol concentration/time from ingestion graph (→ *Figure 15.1*). Acetylcysteine should be given if the plasma paracetamol concentration is above the at-risk line or if the patient has biochemical test suggesting acute liver injury (e.g. ALT above the upper limit of normal); even if the plasma paracetamol concentration is below the at-risk line.

Paracetamol overdose ingested over a period of 1 hour or less – presenting 8–24 hours after acute ingestion

Venous blood samples should be taken at presentation; however, acetylcysteine should be given immediately if more than 150 mg/kg of paracetamol has been taken or if the biochemical tests suggest an acute liver injury. Otherwise, the results of the blood tests should be obtained, and the plasma paracetamol concentration should be plotted onto the nomogram to assess if acetylcysteine should be given.

If the patient presents more than 12–15 hours after overdose, then the concentration of paracetamol requiring treatment with acetylcysteine may be close to the limit of detection of the paracetamol assay, which varies between laboratories. In this situation, acetylcysteine should be given irrespective of the plasma paracetamol concentration.

Paracetamol overdose ingested over a period of 1 hour or less – presenting 24 hours after acute ingestion

Acetylcysteine treatment should be commenced immediately if the patient is jaundiced or has hepatic tenderness. If neither of these features are present then blood samples should be taken for paracetamol concentration,

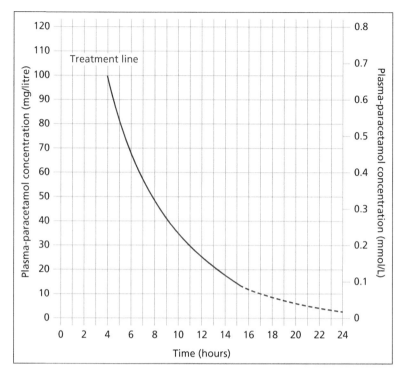

Figure 15.1 Paracetamol treatment nomogram.

U&Es, LFTs, bicarbonate, FBC and INR. Treatment with acetylcysteine should be started if:

- ALT is above the upper limit of normal
- INR is greater than 1.3 (in the absence of another cause, e.g. warfarin)
- Paracetamol concentration is detectable.

If the patient is asymptomatic, has presented more than 7 days after the last dose of paracetamol was ingested and has no history of chronic kidney disease or liver disease then they will not require further medical assessment.

Clinically significant hepatotoxicity is unlikely if at least 4 hours or more after the most recent paracetamol ingestion:

- the paracetamol concentration is less than 10 mg/L, **AND**
- the INR is 1.3 or less, **AND**
- the patient has no clinical features suggesting liver damage.

Acetylcysteine can be discontinued in patients not considered to be at risk of clinically significant liver damage.

Staggered paracetamol overdose (non-therapeutic ingestions of excessive paracetamol over a period of more than 1 hour)

Treatment with acetylcysteine should be commenced without delay in all patients who present following a staggered overdose. Blood tests to check paracetamol concentration, U&Es, creatinine, bicarbonate, LFTs, FBC and INR should be done at least 4 hours after the last paracetamol ingestion.

Therapeutic excess (ingestion of excessive paracetamol with intent to treat pain or fever and without self-harm intent)

In this situation, the patient has ingested paracetamol at a dose greater than the licenced daily dose and more than or equal to 75 mg/kg/24 hours, for the treatment of pain or fever without any self-harm intent. This usually occurs over more than 24 hours but may occur over less than 24 hours. Therapeutic excess can involve the use of excessive doses of the same paracetamol product or inadvertent use of more than one paracetamol-containing product at the same time.

The risks of developing toxicity depend on the maximum dose that has been taken in any 24-hour period:

- Serious toxicity may occur in patients ingesting more than 150 mg/kg in any 24-hour period.
- Rarely, toxicity can occur with ingestions between 75 and 150 mg/kg within any 24-hour period in some patients.
- Doses consistently less than 75 mg/kg in any 24-hour period are very unlikely to be toxic, although risk may be increased if this dose is repeatedly ingested over two or more days
- Ingestion of a licenced dose is not considered an overdose (e.g. in adults 4 g in a 24-hour period).

In patients with clinical features of hepatic injury such as jaundice or hepatic tenderness then urgent treatment with acetylcysteine is indicated. In other patients, the management is determined by the maximum dose of paracetamol ingested in any 24-hour period. If the maximum dose is more than 75 mg/kg within any 24-hour period, then check the paracetamol concentration, LFTs, INR U&Es, bicarbonate and FBC at least 4 hours after the last paracetamol ingestion. Acetylcysteine should be commenced if the patient is symptomatic, or blood tests show a risk of hepatotoxicity. Clinically significant hepatotoxicity is unlikely if at least 4 hours or more after the most recent paracetamol ingestion:

- the paracetamol concentration is less than 10 mg/L
- the ALT is within the normal range
- the INR is 1.3 or less
- the patient has no clinical features suggesting liver damage.

If the maximum dose is more than the licenced 24-hour dose for that patient (e.g. 4 g in an adult) but less than 75 mg/kg/24 hours over the preceding 2 or more days, then the risk of hepatoxicity is small. However, blood tests should be checked if there is any doubt about the doses taken or there any other factors present that may increase the risk of hepatotoxicity. The factors that increase the risk of hepatotoxicity are:

- long-term treatment with carbamazepine, phenobarbital, phenytoin, primidone, rifampicin, St John's Wort or other drugs than induce liver enzymes
- regular consumption of ethanol in excess of recommended amounts
- likely glutathione depletion, e.g. eating disorders, cystic fibrosis, HIV, starvation and, cachexia

If the maximum dose taken is consistently less than the licenced 24-hour dose for that patient (e.g. 4 g in an adult) and consistently less than 75 mg/kg for that patient over the preceding 24-hour period then further assessment is not needed, provided a reliable history has been obtained and the patient is well.

Overdose with intravenous paracetamol

The paracetamol treatment nomogram cannot be applied to patients with an overdose secondary to intravenous paracetamol. Plasma paracetamol concentrations taken more than 4 hours after intravenous injection will usually be lower than predicted if the same dose had been taken orally. As intravenous paracetamol is often given to patients who are unable to take oral intake, this group of patients is also at risk of having a poor nutritional state. As a consequence of these two factors, a lower treatment threshold of 60 mg/kg should be used in these cases.

In the case of a single acute overdose, acetylcysteine should be given if more than 60 mg/kg has been administered. Where there has been repeated excess dosing give acetylcysteine if more than 60 mg/kg in 24 hours has been given.

If there is uncertainty about the dose given, then the paracetamol nomogram may be used based on a blood sample taken 4 hours after the last dose. Usually treatment would be commenced if the 4-hour plasma paracetamol concentration was 100 mg/L or above; however, in this situation you that figure should be halved, i.e. start treatment at above 50 mg/L at 4 hours.

Tx

Two n-acetylcysteine regimes are currently used in the UK → *Box 15.1*

The total dose of *N*-acetylcysteine given is the same in both regimens; however, there is a lower peak plasma *N*-acetylcysteine concentration in the SNAP protocol due to the different rate and duration of treatment. As a result, there is a significantly lower risk of anaphylactoid reactions, and this regimen should be considered for patients who have had a previous anaphylactoid reaction to *N*-acetylcysteine.

Anaphylactoid reactions occur in up to 30% of patients treated with the standard acetylcysteine regime, usually during or soon after the first infusion as a result of large amounts of *N*-acetylcysteine being given rapidly. Adverse reactions are more likely in women, atopic individuals and in patients with lower paracetamol concentrations. If a reaction occurs then the infusion should be stopped, antihistamines given and once the reaction has settled the infusion then can be restarted at half the previous rate.

In pregnant patients the toxic dose as well as the *N*-acetylcysteine dose in both regimes should be calculated using the patient's pre-pregnancy weight.

Box 15.1 **Treatment with N-acetylcysteine**

Standard 21-hour regimen

- 150 mg/kg in 200 mL of 5% glucose over 15 minutes
- 50 mg/kg in 500 mL of 5% glucose over 4 hours
- 100 mg/kg in 1000 mL of 5% glucose over 16 hours

Bloods should be checked just before or at the end of the 16-hour infusion. Acetylcysteine may be stopped if the following criteria are met:

- INR is 1.3 or less **AND**
- ALT is within the normal range

If the ALT is above the normal range (with an INR of 1.3 or less) acetylcysteine may still be stopped if:

- ALT is less than two times the upper limit of normal **AND**
- The increase in ALT value is not more than a doubling of the admission value

Acetylcysteine should be continued and the 16-hour infusion repeated if any of the following criteria are met:

- The ALT is more than two times the upper limit of normal **OR**
- The ALT has doubled or more since the admission measurement and is above the upper limit of normal **OR**
- The INR is greater than 1.3 and the ALT is above the upper limit of normal

Modified 12-hour regimen (SNAP protocol)

- 100 mg/kg in 200 mL of 5% glucose over 2 hours
- 200 mg/kg in 1000 mL of 5% glucose over 10 hours

In the SNAP regimen bloods are repeated just before the end of the 2nd treatment bag. If the blood results show an INR of 1.3 or less, the ALT is in the normal range, the paracetamol concentration is less than 10 mg/L and the patient is asymptomatic then no further treatment with acetylcysteine is required. The second bag will need to be repeated if:

- The ALT is increased above the normal range **OR**
- The INR is greater than 1.3
- The paracetamol concentration is greater than 10 m/L

In obese patients the toxic dose and n-acetylcysteine dose for both regimens should be calculated using a maximum weight of 110 kg rather than the patient's actual weight.

Children under 40 kg are treated with the same doses and regimen as adults but the quantity of intravenous fluid given is modified in order to avoid causing fluid overload; the full infusion information is available from Toxbase or the NPIS.

If intravenous access is not possible then N-acetylcysteine can be given as an oral therapy, but the taste is unpleasant and requires masking with fruit juice or cola. Methionine is another oral antidote that can be used in paracetamol overdose; however, the UK product licence has expired and should this treatment be required it would need to be discussed with the NPIS.

If the patient's paracetamol concentration is very high (greater than 700 mg/L) in association with a reduced level of consciousness or an elevated lactate, then haemodialysis is indicated in addition to N-acetylcysteine. If a patient is on haemodialysis, then the dose of N-acetylcysteine should be doubled.

Mechanism of action of antidotes in paracetamol toxicity → Figure 15.2.

Patients with signs of liver damage should be discussed early on with a specialised liver unit and transplantation should be considered for patients who met the modified King's college criteria:

- pH < 7.3
- INR > 6 (PT > 100 seconds)
- Creatinine > 300 mmol/L
- Grade III or IV encephalopathy
- Lactate concentration > 3.5 after early resuscitation (4 hours) or > 3.0 after 12 hours of fluid resuscitation.

Salicylates

Aspirin

Nausea, vomiting, tinnitus, deafness and dizziness are common in mild poisoning, and this is usually associated with a peak salicylate concentration of less than 300 mg/L. A salicylate concentration of 300–700 mg/L counts as a moderate poisoning and features would include sweating, hyperventilation and respiratory alkalosis due to stimulation of the respiratory centre in the medulla. In severe poisoning, where the salicylate concentration is more than 700 mg/L, cardiac arrhythmias, pulmonary oedema, coma, cerebral oedema, renal failure and hyperpyrexia can occur. Due to disruption of the Krebs cycle, there is an accumulation of lactate and pyruvic acid and this leads to the development of a high anion gap metabolic acidosis.

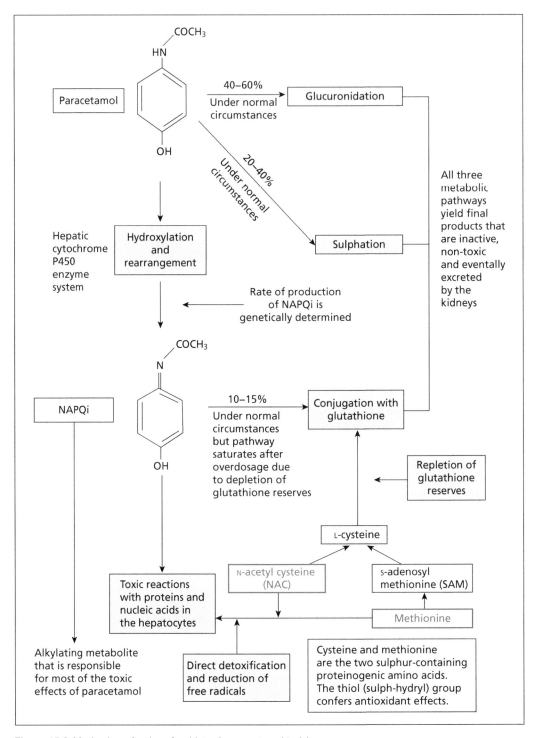

Figure 15.2 Mechanism of action of antidotes in paracetamol toxicity.

Tx

Plasma salicylate levels should be measured 2 hours after ingestion if symptomatic and at 4 hours after ingestion if asymptomatic. Repeated salicylate levels every 2 hours are indicated in all patients who are symptomatic and if the plasma concentration is over 200 mg/L until the patient's symptoms have improved, or the concentration begins to fall.

In salicylate poisoning, there may be a benefit to a second dose of charcoal in patients who have taken an enteric preparation or where the plasma concentration continues to rise; gastric lavage may be considered if a life-threatening overdose has occurred.

The mainstay of treatment is intravenous fluids, potassium replacement, correction of any acidosis, urine alkalinization (by administration of sodium bicarbonate) and dialysis for severe poisoning. There is risk of significant decompensation when these patients are intubated due to the loss of the compensatory respiratory drive and wherever possible correction of hypokalaemia and urine alkalinisation should be instigated first.

Other NSAIDs

Ibuprofen is of low toxicity and poisoning with <100 mg/kg does not require any treatment; symptoms can be expected when more than 400 mg/kg has been taken.

Mefenamic acid is associated with a dose-dependent risk of CNS toxicity in overdose manifested by convulsions and reduced level of consciousness.

Salbutamol

This β_2-receptor agonist causes predictable adrenergic side effects and metabolic changes:

- Tremor
- Tachycardia
- Agitation and headache
- Hypokalaemia, hypophosphataemia and hypomagnesaemia
- Hyperglycaemia – delayed hypoglycaemia can also occur
- Elevated lactate with or without metabolic acidosis
- ECG abnormalities – QT prolongation, ST changes, atrial fibrillation, ventricular tachycardia, supraventricular tachycardia and myocardial infarction
- Convulsions
- Rhabdomyolysis
- Acute pulmonary oedema.

Tx

Consider activated charcoal for all patients, especially if a controlled-release preparation has been taken.

Monitor the heart rate, BP and ECG continuously.

Measure the U&Es and glucose.

Admit for observation, monitoring and symptomatic treatment.

β Blockers

The effects of poisoning vary considerably according to the specific drug. Sotalol in particular may cause bizarre dysrhythmias (*For torsade de pointes and prolongation of the Q–T interval by sotalol → p. 181*). Beta blockers which are more lipid soluble (carvedilol, labetalol, metoprolol and propranolol) are more likely to cross the blood brain barrier causing drowsiness, confusion, convulsions, hallucinations, dilated pupils and in severe cases coma. In comparison, hydrophilic beta blockers (atenolol, bisoprolol, esmolol and sotalol) have few CNS effects.

In overdose, most β blockers can cause:

- severe bronchospasm
- bradycardia, hypotension and syncope
- pulmonary oedema and cardiogenic shock.

Tx

- Apply supportive measures and consider activated charcoal in recent ingestions and for modified-release preparations.
- Give nebulised salbutamol for wheezing.
- Administer IV atropine for bradycardia (0.5–1.2 mg for an adult or 0.02 mg/kg for a child). Repeat doses may be necessary.
- Dobutamine or isoprenaline for resistant bradycardia or bradycardia associated with hypotension.
- Establish transvenous pacing for intractable bradycardia.
- Give IV glucagon for hypotension, heart failure or cardiogenic shock. This is given as a bolus of 5–10 mg for an adult; 50–150mcg/kg for a child followed by an infusion.
- High-dose insulin therapy with dextrose infusion has been shown to improve myocardial contractility and improve systemic perfusion; it is particularly useful in the presence of acidosis.

Calcium channel blockers

Poisoning with calcium channel blockers causes gastrointestinal upset, dizziness, confusion and coma. Metabolic acidosis, hyperkalaemia and hypocalcaemia can also occur; hyperglycaemia is common and may be a marker of severe poisoning.

Bradycardia, AV block, junctional escape rhythms, atrio-ventricular conduction block and asystole may all be features. Hypotension in this situation may be delayed or prolonged and is caused by either cardiac depression (verapamil and diltiazem) or profound vasodilatation (nifedipine), although the selectivity of calcium antagonists tends to disappear when taken in overdose.

Tx

Activated charcoal is effective if given within 1 hour of ingestion or after modified-release preparations (when repeated doses may also be considered). IV calcium may be used to treat hypotension either as boluses or an infusion → *page 261*. As in beta blocker toxicity bradycardia is treated with atropine and dobutamine or isoporenaline if it is associated with hypotension; high-dose insulin and dextrose infusions can also be given. Adrenaline, noradrenaline infusions and dopamine can also be used for resistant hypotension.

Digoxin

Digoxin toxicity can be classified as chronic or acute. Acute toxicity causes initial nausea and vomiting, followed by hyperkalaemia and arrhythmias (atrial tachycardia, VT, VF, conduction delays) and shock at 6–12 hours post ingestion.

Chronic toxicity is common in elderly patients and those with renal impairment and symptoms can appear over days to weeks. Symptoms include anorexia, GI upset, confusion, drowsiness and yellow halos in vision.

Ix   digoxin levels taken at least 6 hours after the last dose are useful in the generally unwell patient who is taking digoxin. 12-lead ECG and 3-lead monitoring is essential. The 'digoxin effect' on ECG (downsloping ST depression with a characteristic 'reverse tick' or 'Salvador Dali sagging' appearance) is caused by taking digoxin but does not represent toxicity.

Tx   Hyperkalaemia and arrythmias are managed in the usual way, but arrhythmias may be refractory. Digoxin-specific antibody (DigiFab) is the definitive treatment for severe bradyarrhythmias and for life threatening ventricular arrhythmias. – discuss cases with NPIS.

Diabetes medications

Insulin taken in overdose can be rapidly fatal, and prolonged periods of profound hypoglycaemia may result in catastrophic neurological damage. Treatment is with IV glucose (dextrose) – initial bolus of 50 mL 50% glucose, followed by infusion of 10% at 100 mL per hour. Doses higher than 100 mL per hour can lead to hyponatraemia, so if control of blood sugar is difficult, a central line may be needed to give a 20–50% glucose infusion.

Metformin induces cellular hypoxia and inhibits mitochondrial function. When taken in overdose it is usually benign, but doses over 10 g can cause a profound lactic acidosis. Severe poisoning is also more likely to occur in patients over the age of 60, in those who have type 2 diabetes or if taken alongside anti-hypertensives or par-

acetamol. Haemodialysis is indicated for those patients with a severe lactic acidosis unresponsive to fluid resuscitation or administration of sodium bicarbonate.

Sulfonylureas can cause profound hypoglycaemia, usually 4–6 hours post ingestion. Treatment is with IV glucose and octreotide.

Warfarin

Warfarin inhibits vitamin K, which is needed for the synthesis of clotting factors II, VII, IX and X. Peak effects of overdose are seen at 72 hours, and so patients need prophylactic treatment with vitamin K and observation for regular INR measurements. For bleeding on warfarin, see *page 272*.

Tricyclic and related antidepressants

Tricyclic antidepressants (TCAs) have a narrow therapeutic index, and studies have shown that the poisoning with TCAs is associated with significantly higher fatality rates when compared to poisoning with other antidepressants. Severe toxicity occurs from sodium channel blockade and may cause arrhythmias, cardiovascular collapse, convulsions and coma.

Arrhythmias are the commonest cause of death, and the ECG signs of severe toxicity are:

- QRS complex >100 ms
- QTc interval > 480 ms
- R-wave amplitude aVR >3 mm
- Heart rate > 120 beats per minute.

A QRS duration of greater than 160 ms in the context of a TCA overdose suggests severe cardiotoxicity with a very high risk of arrhythmia, although arrhythmias can occur with lesser degrees of QRS prolongation.

The other features seen are those of anti-cholinergic toxicity: sinus tachycardia, confusion, drowsiness, hot dry skin, dry mouth and tongue, dilated pupils, urinary retention and ileus. Ataxia, nystagmus, divergent squint, hallucinations, myoclonus and hyperreflexia with extensor plantar reflexes may occur, although if the patient is in a coma all reflexes including brainstem reflexes may be abolished.

Tx

Sodium bicarbonate is the treatment for the metabolic acidosis and cardiotoxicity associated with TCA overdose and 50–100 mL of 8.4% sodium bicarbonate should be prescribed if the patient has the following conditions even in the absence of acidosis:

- QRS complex >120 ms
- Hypotension unresponsive to fluids.

If the QRS prolongation persists, then further boluses of sodium bicarbonate should be given especially if there is persistent acidosis, aiming to achieve a pH of 7.5–7.55.

The patient's electrolytes must be monitored because of the risk of hypokalaemia and sometimes hypernatraemia from the administration of substantial amounts of sodium bicarbonate.

Drugs that exacerbate sodium channel blockade (class Ia – quinidine, disopyramide, procainamide; class Ib – phenytoin and class Ic – flecainide) should be avoided after poisoning with sodium channel blocking drugs and in the presence of increased QRS width.

Due to the significant CNS effects of TCA poisoning, these patients require an airway assessment; if airway protection is required, they will need admission to the intensive care unit.

Bicarbonate therapy (general information) → *p. 264.*

Selective serotonin reuptake inhibitors

Selective serotonin reuptake inhibitor (SSRI)-type drugs inhibit the reuptake of serotonin (5-hydroxytryptamine or 5HT). Some related compounds (serotonin–noradrenaline reuptake inhibitors or SNRIs) also inhibit the reuptake of noradrenaline. These drugs are widely prescribed for the treatment of depression and consequently self-poisoning with them is common. SSRIs in overdose cause:

- sweating and dizziness
- drowsiness, convulsions and coma
- hypoglycaemia, hypokalaemia, hyponatraemia, metabolic acidosis and hypoglycaemia
- tachycardia, hypotension or hypertension, prolongation of the QTc interval and the QRS complex may also occur with consequent ventricular dysrhythmias; torsade de pointes is a particular risk → *p. 181.*

Serotonin toxicity may occur if taken with other serotonergic agents.

Serotonin syndrome (which may be a feature of SSRI poisoning) → *p. 308.*

Tx

Activated charcoal may be given if a significant amount of an SSRI has been ingested within the previous hour. Otherwise, treatment is supportive with correction of any metabolic abnormalities a priority due to the risk of cardiac complications. Patients with a long QT will require treatment with magnesium sulphate to reduce the risk of torsade de pointes.

Theophylline

Theophylline toxicity results from adenosine antagonism and catecholamine release, causing sympathomimetic effects.

The normal therapeutic serum theophylline concentration range is 5–15 mcg/mL with toxicity likely to occur above this concentration. After acute ingestion, life-threatening features occur when the serum theophylline concentration exceeds 80 mcg/mL and at the lower concentration of 40 mcg/mL in chronic toxicity. If a theophylline level is not readily available, then a low serum potassium (<3.0 mmol/L) is a useful surrogate marker of theophylline toxicity in acute overdose patients. Features of toxicity may also be delayed for up to 24 hours after acute overdose with sustained-release preparations.

Mild/moderate toxicity:

- Nausea, vomiting, epigastric pain, haematemesis and pancreatitis.
- Sinus tachycardia, sustained complex atrial or ventricular ectopics, hypotension
- Anxiety, insomnia, agitation, restlessness, confusion and hallucinations

Metabolic features are common and include hypokalaemia, hyperglycaemia, hypophosphataemia, hypomagnesaemia and hypercalcaemia. Metabolic acidosis is common with acute overdose, but respiratory alkalosis may also occur.

Severe toxicity is characterised by cardiac arrhythmias and convulsions, which may occur in the absence of milder symptoms. Hypotension, myocardial ischaemia and infarction, respiratory failure, acute lung injury, skeletal muscle excitation (e.g. myoclonus, fasciculations), hyperthermia, rhabdomyolysis, acute compartment syndrome and renal failure may occur.

In chronic poisoning, gastrointestinal symptoms and metabolic changes are less common than with acute poisoning. Hyponatraemia secondary to SIADH has been reported. Severe effects, such as convulsions and hemodynamically significant dysrhythmias, are more common with chronic overdoses than with acute overdoses.

Tx

1 Consider activated charcoal and in severe poisoning multiple doses of activated charcoal can be given.
2 Supportive treatment with correction of any metabolic abnormalities.
3 Sinus tachycardia or supraventricular tachycardia can be treated with intravenous beta blockers or verapamil. Propanolol may be effective at treating the metabolic complications such as hypokalaemia associated with theophylline overdose.

Haemodialysis can be used to improve elimination of theophylline and the indications for haemodialysis are:

- Acute exposure: theophylline concentration >100 mg/L (555 micromol/L).
- Chronic exposure: theophylline concentration >60 mg/L (333 micromol/L).
- Theophylline concentration >50 mg/L (278 micromol/L) if the patient is either less than 6 months of age or older than 60 years of age.

Table 15.3 Therapeutic and toxic levels of common drugs

Drug	Lower level (mg/L)	Upper level (mg/L)	Possible toxicity (mg/L)	Severe toxicity (mg/L)
Theophylline	10	20	20	60
Phenytoin	8	15	20	40
Carbamazepine	4	10	25	40

- The presence of convulsions, life-threatening dysrhythmias, or shock.
- Rising theophylline concentration despite optimal therapy and clinical deterioration despite optimal care.
- Gastrointestinal decontamination cannot be administered.

Plasma levels → Table 15.3

Lithium

An acute overdose in someone who is lithium naïve usually results in mild toxicity compared to an acute on chronic overdose, which can lead to serious toxicity as extravascular tissues are already saturated with lithium. The most common cause of lithium toxicity is chronic accumulation, which can be due to dehydration, infection, administration of too high a dose, impaired renal function or concomitant administration of drug which impairs renal clearing of lithium. Chronic accumulation is the aetiology that carries the greatest risk of causing neurotoxicity.

The symptoms of acute overdose of lithium may be delayed for up to 24 hours, particularly in lithium-naïve patients. In cases of mild poisoning, there is polyuria, dizziness, altered taste and a fine resting tremor. Mild and severe cases are characterised by CNS symptoms such as fasciculation, myoclonic twitches, choreoathetoid movements, ataxia, convulsions and cerebellar signs. In severe cases, the neuropsychiatric features can be irreversible. ECG changes, hypernatraemia, hypotension and renal failure can also occur in severe cases.

Tx Lithium levels should be measured immediately in patients on lithium and at 6 hours after the overdose in patients who are lithium naïve. In both instances, repeat levels are required in a further 6 hours and for longer periods if symptomatic. Haemodiaylsis is the treatment of choice in severe poisoning and may prevent irreversible neurotoxicity.

Phenytoin

The average lethal dose of phenytoin for adults is between 2 and 5 g, but there is a marked variation among individuals with respect to the toxic effects of a given serum level of phenytoin. The initial symptoms are predominantly neurological with nystagmus, ataxia and dysarthria but later on there may be:

- coma
- fixed pupils
- hypotension
- respiratory depression.

Tx
The agent is cardiotoxic and sodium bicarbonate should be given in the presence of hypotension or a prolonged QRS.

Plasma levels → Table 15.3

Carbamazepine

Carbamazepine causes toxicity due to anticholinergic activity and sodium channel blockade in the heart and CNS. Overdose will lead to cerebellar signs and in severe cases convulsions, coma, respiratory depression and cardiovascular features.

Tx Carbamazepine overdose is an indication for repeated doses of activated charcoal otherwise treatment is supportive and symptomatic.

Plasma levels → Table 15.3

Benzodiazepines

The main toxic effect of benzodiazepines is CNS depression, and this effect is potentiated if they are taken together with alcohol or other CNS depressants. Benzodiazepines exert their action on specific BZ receptors, which are closely associated with γ-aminobutyric acid (GABA) receptors. GABA is an inhibitory neurotransmitter that is widely distributed throughout the brain and spinal cord. Potentiation of GABA transmission thus causes a generalised depression of CNS activity and results in:

- reduced level of consciousness
- flaccidity
- ataxia and dysarthria
- hypotension
- hypothermia.

Flumazenil is a specific benzodiazepine antagonist that is an effective treatment in patients with an isolated benzodiazepine poisoning. It may be used for patients who develop either respiratory depression become comatose or who otherwise would require mechanical ventilation.

However, it should be given with caution in benzodiazepine-dependent patients where it may cause a withdrawal syndrome, in mixed overdoses or when the drug taken is unknown. It is also contraindicated in the following situations:

- When patients have co-ingested medicines that may cause convulsions, for example a benzodiazepine and a tricyclic antidepressant.
- In a patient prone to seizures
- In the presence of features suggestive of tricyclic antidepressant ingestion, including a wide QRS interval with large pupils.
- In a patient post-cardiac arrest.
- As a diagnostic test.

Consequently it is rarely of use other than in therapeutic/iatrogenic overdose. For comparison of benzodiazepine half-lives → *see Table 15.4.*

Flumazenil has a half-life of 52 min with a duration of action of 1–2 hours; this is much shorter than the half-life of the benzodiazepines commonly encountered in overdose cases. Patients treated with flumazenil therefore need to be kept under observation for 4 hours in case toxicity recurs.

Phenothiazines (e.g. prochlorperazine, chlorpromazine) and other major tranquillisers

These drugs cause:

- drowsiness and confusion
- hypotension

Table 15.4 Comparison of benzodiazepines

Drug	Half-life (h)	Equivalent dose (mg)
Diazepam	20–50	5
Chlordiazepoxide	6–30	15
Nitrazepam	24	5
Lorazepam	12	0.5
Temazepam	8	10
Oxazepam	6–8	15

- hypothermia
- sinus tachycardia and cardiac dysrhythmias
- convulsions and coma (with large doses).

Extrapyramidal effects including acute dystonic reactions may occur but are not dose related. Neuroleptic malignant syndrome, although related to long-term use of major tranquillisers, is not usually a feature of poisoning → *p. 308.*

Tx Acute dystonic reactions usually respond to antimuscarinic agents such as procyclidine; diazepam can be used as an alternative if antimuscarinics are unavailable. Otherwise treatment is supportive.

POISONING WITH RECREATIONAL AND ILLEGAL DRUGS

It is important to be aware that illegal drugs can be adulterated with other drugs, their purity can vary greatly and there may be co-ingestion of other drugs occurring.

Misuse of Drugs Act 1971 and the Misuse of Drugs Regulations 2001 → *p. 394.*

Opioid poisoning

Opioid poisoning is an increasing problem in many parts of the world and in the United States it is deemed a public health emergency. Opioid poisoning can occur by both the oral and parenteral routes. The drugs involved can be illegal drugs or prescription medications including combination analgesics, where narcotic effects may be accompanied by paracetamol poisoning (→ *p. 282*). Signs of acute poisoning with opioids include:

- a depressed level of consciousness
- respiratory depression (usually the respiratory rate is most affected)
- pinpoint pupils.

Opioids can cause histamine release leading to pruritus and urticarial and there is a risk of serotonin syndrome if they are taken in conjunction with other serotonergic agents.

The metabolism of certain opioids such as tramadol and codeine is affected by polymorphism in the gene for the enzyme CYP2D6 responsible for their metabolism. As a result, some individuals are predisposed to be more extensive metabolisers of these drugs into morphine. This results in more morphine being produced and therefore leads to a greater risk of toxicity. In the presence of renal failure, the risk of toxicity is also significantly increased for overdoses involving morphine, codeine, pethidine and diamorphine because of reduced elimination of either the opioid or its metabolite.

Tx Naloxone is an opioid antagonist used in the treatment of opioid poisoning, and it can be used as a diagnostic test in suspected cases. Naloxone is given as boluses initially; however, the aim of treatment is not to restore the patient to full consciousness but to reverse the respiratory depression and to restore and maintain the patient's airway protective reflexes. The duration of action of naloxone is significantly shorter than that of all the opioid analgesics and if repeated boluses are required following the initial one, then an intravenous infusion of naloxone is necessary. The hourly infusion rate is started at 60% of the dose needed initially to reverse the respiratory depression and is then titrated to the desired clinical effect.

Stimulant drugs

Many substances can lead to stimulant type clinical features in overdose. This includes drugs of misuse such as amphetamines, MDMA, cocaine and new psychoactive substances, as well as prescription medications such as methylphenidate.

The clinical features of stimulant toxicity include tremor, sweating, dilated pupils, agitation, convulsions and hallucinations. Cardiovascular features are common with chest pain, dyspnoea and arrhythmias, both atrial and ventricular occurring. In severe cases, hyperthermia, stroke, myocardial infarction, hyponatraemia, rhabdomyolysis, DIC, pulmonary oedema, hepatic and renal failure may occur. Persistent convulsions, coma, focal neurological signs or hyperthermia above 39° are poor prognostic signs.

Tx Treatment for all stimulant drugs is mainly supportive with the focus on intravenous volume replacement, seizure control, arrhythmia management and correction of any underlying acidosis. Agitation is the main clinical challenge, and benzodiazepines are the drug of choice for this situation – high doses may be required. Hyperthermia is a predictor of mortality and should be managed as a priority → Page 249. Critical care should be involved in the management of all patients with severe features.

Amphetamines

The toxicity of amphetamines is due to enhanced dopamine, norepinephrine and serotonin neurotransmission. In addition to the features of stimulant toxicity amphetamines cause psychostimulation with euphoria, increased alertness, intensified emotions and self-esteem.

MDMA (ecstasy)

MDMA leads to the release of serotonin, noradrenaline and dopamine in the CNS which is the cause of its toxicity.

Four patterns of severe clinical toxicity can occur:

- Hyperpyrexial toxicity (severe serotonin toxicity) – severe pyrexia accompanied by metabolic acidosis, disseminated intravascular coagulation, neuromuscular hyperactivity, rhabdomyolysis and multi-organ failure.
- Hepatic toxicity – an acute hepatitis that may progress to fulminant hepatic failure
- Cerebral toxicity – characterised by agitation, psychosis, convulsions, cerebral oedema, hyponatraemia and fluid overload.
- Cardiovascular toxicity – tachycardia, arrhythmias, hypertension and heart failure.

Cocaine

In addition to increasing the level of neurotransmitters in the brain, cocaine also has sodium and potassium channel-blocking effects, causes vasoconstriction and increases sympathetic activity. As with other stimulant drugs, the purity of cocaine is varied; however, crack cocaine consists of crystals of relatively pure cocaine.

While the treatment is similar for all stimulant drugs, cocaine use is associated with some clinical complications that require specific management.

Cocaine is the most cardiotoxic of all these drugs and its use can lead to coronary artery vasospasm and myocardial infarction; this complication can occur with any route of cocaine administration. In patients with cocaine-associated chest pain, conventional acute coronary syndrome management can be initiated with GTN, buccal nitrate, morphine and anti-platelets. Benzodiazepines should also be given early as they can relieve chest pain. Chest pain not responsive to these measures can be treated with a GTN or labetalol infusion, and these patients should be discussed with the local PCI centre. Arrhythmias are common following cocaine use – benzodiazepines should be used for sinus arrhythmias and as a first-line treatment for narrow complex tachyarrhythmias. Ventricular tachycardias should be treated with sodium bicarbonate (or lidocaine IV as second line). Beta-blockers should be avoided as this can lead to unopposed alpha-adrenergic stimulation which can worsen any hypertension or vasospasm that is present.

Methaemoglobinaemia can occur when cocaine is adulterated with drugs such as local anaesthetics. This may require treatment with methylene blue depending on the MetHb level and the patient's symptoms.

Gamma-hydroxybutyrate

Gamma-hydroxybutyrate (GHB) and its analogues (GBL, GVL, GHV and 1,4 BD) are potent CNS sedatives that are easily synthesised and can be made from commercially available solvents such as nail polish removers. GHB may cause a rapid onset of coma and respiratory depression such that 10% of patients presenting to an ED after its ingestion require endotracheal intubation. Concurrent ethanol, benzodiazepine, antipsychotic and other CNS depressant usage exacerbates the effects of GHB. Treatment is largely supportive. One of the hallmarks of GHB intoxication is a rapid recovery to full consciousness after profound coma.

Ketamine

Ketamine is primarily a central nervous system NMDA receptor antagonist that disrupts electrophysiological signalling leading to a dissociative anaesthesia, amnesia and analgesia. Other features include delusions, hallucinations, respiratory depression and a dose-dependent reduction in consciousness. Chronic users of ketamine can develop chronic cystitis, neuropsychological impairment and chronic abdominal pain. Treatment is supportive.

Lysergic acid diethylamide (LSD)

The potent hallucinogen lysergic acid diethylamide (LSD) initially causes excitement and euphoria; however, this is followed by confusion, agitation, tachycardia and hallucinations, which can be auditory, visual or tactile in nature. The main focus of treatment is to control any agitation or psychosis that is present by using benzodiazepines or antipsychotics. Sedation may be required in severe cases. Otherwise, treatment is symptomatic and supportive with patients usually recovering within a few hours. Occasionally, hallucinations can persist for up to 48 hours and psychotic states for 3–4 days. Patients may also have flashback hallucinations weeks or months after their last dose of LSD.

Cannabis (marijuana or 'weed')

Cannabis causes anxiety and excitement followed by euphoria and calmness before progressing to drowsiness and sleep. It is unusual for patients to present to an ED, but in severe cases, ataxia, fasticulations and atrial fibrillation have been reported. Patients who have used cannabis for a long time may develop a cannabinoid hyperemesis syndrome with a cyclical pattern of hyperemesis occurring every few weeks or months. This resolves with abstention from cannabis. In an acute setting, treatment is with intramuscular haloperidol.

Mushroom poisoning

Poisonous mushrooms can be divided according to the toxin they contain. The most dangerous fungi in the British Isles is the Death cap mushrooms (*Amanita phalloides*) which contains amatoxins as well as phallotoxins, virotoxins and toxophallin. Amatoxins are not destroyed by freezing, drying or cooking and the fatal dose of amatoxins is very low; just one single mushroom can contain a lethal adult dose. Amatoxins irreversibly bind to RNA polymerase II causing transcription arrest in metabolically active cells in the liver and kidneys.

Following ingestion, there is usually a latent period of more than 6 hours (often 8–12 hours) before severe gastrointestinal features including vomiting, abdominal pain and diarrhoea develop. The latent period may rarely be shorter, or in some cases absent, after very large ingestions or when a mixture of different mushrooms have been eaten. The shorter the interval between ingestion and the onset of diarrhoea, the worse the prognosis. An interval of less than 8 hours after ingestion appears to indicate a poor prognosis.

As a consequence of fluid losses during the gastrointestinal phase, patients can develop oliguria, hypotension, acid base disturbances and renal failure. The first signs or hepatic centrilobular necrosis usually develop 24–48 hours following ingestion. The initial signs can range from an asymptomatic increase in transaminase activity to full liver failure. Elevated cardiac enzymes and cardiogenic shock can occur. Renal failure occurring during this phase is usually the result of direct toxic damage and this can be irreversible.

Tx Gastric lavage should be considered in adults who present within the first hour after ingestion. Amatoxin poisoning is an indication for multiple-dose activated charcoal as this can interrupt their enterohepatic circulation and increase elimination; it can be of value up to 3 days post-ingestion.

Penicillins reduce the uptake of amatoxins into the liver in experimental models and a continuous infusion of benzylpenicillin can be given or ceftazidime if the patient is penicillin allergic. There is also some evidence for the use of *N*-acetylcysteine in these cases and the same regime that is used in cases of paracetamol poisoning can be given. Extracorporeal elimination techniques can be considered but are unlikely to be of benefit in removing amatoxins after 24–48 hours post-ingestion. These patients should be referred early to a specialised liver unit particularly those patients with a short latent period as transplantation may be needed.

The other poisonous mushroom toxidromes that can occur are:

- **Gyromitrin toxin**: initial GI symptoms progressing to liver toxicity with haemolysis and methamoglbinaemia as well as seizures, coma and respiratory failure
- **Muscarine toxin**: cholinergic features
- **Coprine toxin**: only toxic if consumed with ethanol. Features include flushing of the face, neck and chest, vomiting, tachycardia, headache and hypotension
- **Psilocybin toxin**: This is the toxin found in magic mushrooms and consumption leads to hallucinogenic effects within an hour of ingestion. In addition, dilated pupils impaired judgement, euphoria, ataxia and drowsiness can occur.
- **Muscimol toxin**: Drowsiness, confusion, ataxia, hallucinations, myoclonus and seizures.
- **Orellanine toxin**: Loin pain, anuria, renal dysfunction and renal failure developing 7–21 days after exposure.

Solvent abuse

Toluene is the most common solvent but others include benzene and xylene found in plastic cement and butane; a component of lighter fuel. Butane appears to be one of the most dangerous because sudden death may result from a cardiac dysrhythmia.

Following exposure to toluene, there is an initial feeling of euphoria and hallucinations; this is then superseded by confusion, drowsiness, ataxia, respiratory failure and convulsions. Cardiovascular features are more common in chronic exposure but arrhythmias and myocardial infarction can be a consequence.

When chronic abuse occurs there are three major patterns of presentation:

- Muscle weakness due to hypokalaemic paralysis
- Gastrointestinal complaints – abdominal pain and haematemesis
- Neuropsychiatric disorders – bizarre behaviour, acute paranoid psychosis, confusion, visual and auditory hallucinations, peripheral neuropathy, cerebellar signs and memory loss.

New psychoactive substances

These are synthesised drugs and made to replace illegal drugs such as cannabis, cocaine and ecstasy that first began to appear around 2008. While many of these drugs were once legal, in the UK, the Psychoactive Substances Act 2016 makes it illegal to produce, supply or import them for human consumption – including for personal use. They are often bought from the internet as "research substances - not for human consumption". They include the following:

- **Synthetic cannabinoids, e.g. 'Spice'**: were designed to mimic cannabis, but are far more potent and unpredictable. They can cause trance-like states, anxiety, psychosis, seizures and palpitations.
- **Stimulant types, e.g. 'mephedrone'**: cause similar effects as amfetamines and cocaine
- **Hallucinogenics**: Bromo-dragonfly is a benzodifuran derivative that can cause prolonged hallucinogenic effects for 2–3 days. It can cause vasoconstriction in limbs and coronary arteries.

Alcohol (ethanol)

Alcohol is freely available in most societies and is associated with many social problems (→ *Chapter 20*). It is frequently taken as a component of self-poisoning. The ethanol dose that causes intoxication is dependent on an individual's tolerance to ethanol so although blood ethanol concentrations can be used as a guide for toxicity these are best used in combination with clinical assessment. Alcohol naïve patients will have severe symptoms at much lower serum alcohol concentrations.

Features of mild ethanol toxicity include disinhibition, emotional lability, euphoria, decreased reaction time, fine motor incoordination, diminished judgement and dysarthria. In moderate toxicity patients can be aggressive, disorientated, confused and develop ataxia and vasodilation. Diplopia, hypothermia, hypoglycaemia, convulsions, respiratory depression and coma are present in severe cases.

Ethyl alcohol is metabolised in the liver to carbon dioxide and water via acetaldehyde and acetate. This breakdown normally occurs at a constant rate (about 10–15 g/h) irrespective of the amount of alcohol present in the body (zero-order kinetics). Above a level of about 100 mg/dL, liver metabolism is unable to cope and further alcohol intake may cause a very rapid increase in blood concentrations. Similarly, at very high blood levels (probably >300 mg/dL) alcohol concentration decreases more quickly than can be explained by zero-order kinetics alone.

Recognition of alcohol-related attendances to the ED provides an important opportunity to introduce preventative measures. Evidence shows that each attendance to ED as a result of hazardous drinking creates an opportunity to provide information and support. Every ED clinician should be able to deliver health advice regarding alcohol consumption and offer referral to specialist services.

Alcohol withdrawal states → p. 379.
Medicolegal aspects of alcohol abuse (including driving) → p. 394.

POISONING WITH SUBSTANCES FOUND AT HOME AND AT WORK

Iron

In normal circumstances, iron is absorbed by the mucosal cells of the duodenum and jejunum and transported in the blood bound to transferrin. After an acute overdose, the intestinal barrier is overwhelmed and the transferrin is saturated. Unbound iron then causes cardiovascular, hepatic, CNS and metabolic damage.

Oral iron preparations are ferrous salts and contain differing amounts of elemental iron (e.g. 200 mg ferrous sulphate contains 60 mg pure iron). Toxicity is dependent on the amount of elemental iron ingested → Table 15.5.

The early features of iron poisoning, which occur at 1–6 hours post-ingestion, result from corrosive damage and haemodynamic effects (vascular dilatation and capillary leakage). There may be:

- nausea and vomiting (vomitus may have a metallic odour)
- abdominal pain and diarrhoea
- haematemesis and rectal bleeding.

This can be followed by a latent phase with apparent resolution of the initial symptoms, it is important not to misinterpret this as a clinical recovery; there is usually a persisting acidosis.

The serious features that occur after twelve hours are mostly the result of intracellular poisoning and include:

- coma and convulsions
- circulatory collapse and pulmonary oedema
- profound metabolic acidosis
- liver failure with hypoglycaemia and coagulopathy
- renal failure
- further GI haemorrhage.

Patients can be affected by delayed sequelae 2–5 weeks after the overdose with gastric scarring causing strictures or pyloric stenosis.

Table 15.5 **Toxicity of elemental iron.**

Ingested dose elemental iron (mg/kg/body weight)	Likely toxicity
More than 20	Features likely
More than 75	Severe features possible
	Fatalities may occur
More than 150	Severe or fatal poisoning possible

Investigations

An iron concentration should be requested; however, iron can cause haemolysis at high concentrations making it difficult to obtain or interpret. After 6 hours, the peak concentration may have been passed and interpretation may be difficult; the use of desferrioxamine will also preclude interpretation of subsequent iron concentrations.

An abdominal X-ray may be helpful to confirm the presence of iron tablets if the history is uncertain. It is highly unlikely a significant overdose was taken if more than 6 hours have passed since ingestion and no symptoms have developed.

Patients who have ingested 20 mg/kg or more of elemental iron or in those who are symptomatic but without severe features need their iron concentrations measured at four and 6 hours post ingestion to obtain a peak concentration; management depends on this peak concentration.

In cases of severe poisoning desferrioxamine which chelates trivalent iron should be given as soon as possible, without waiting for the serum iron concentration. Whole bowel irrigation should also be considered particularly for large ingestions of modified release products, and an abdominal X-ray may be helpful in confirming the presence of iron tablets beforehand.

Vitamins

These are usually not harmful in an isolated acute ingestion, but the estimated amount taken should be checked against known poisons information. Some compound preparations may contain iron and other substances.

Oral contraceptives

These are not harmful although nausea and vomiting may occur. Female patients should be warned about the slight possibility of withdrawal bleeding.

Methanol and ethylene glycol

Substances such as methanol (methyl alcohol or wood alcohol) and ethylene glycol (antifreeze) cause features of intoxication in the early stages. As these substances are metabolised patients develop a high osmolar gap which falls thereafter and is followed by a severe high anion gap metabolic acidosis, due to the production of toxic metabolites.

Although comparatively rare, this type of poisoning should be suspected in the following circumstances:

- Where there is a distinct latent period between ingestion and the development of toxic features.

- The presence of an unexplained metabolic acidosis (or hyperventilation).
- An inexplicably raised anion or osmolar gap (with a normal serum chloride).

Ethylene glycol

The toxicity of ethylene glycol is the result of its metabolism to glycolic, glyoxlic and oxalic acids; these cause extensive cellular damage to various tissues particularly the kidneys. Glycolic acid is largely responsible for the metabolic acidosis seen in severe cases. The lethal dose of ethylene glycol is approximately 100 g of ethylene glycol (90 mL of pure ethylene glycol). It is rapidly absorbed from the GI tract, reaching peak blood concentrations between 1 and 4 hours after ingestion. Approximately 80% of ethylene glycol is metabolised in the liver and 20% is excreted unchanged by the kidneys. The elimination half-life of ethylene glycol is approximately 3 hours, but this is prolonged to around 18 hours after inhibition of alcohol dehydrogenase.

Three stages of ethylene glycol poisoning are classically described: a neurological stage, followed by a cardiopulmonary stage and, finally, a renal stage. In many cases, however, there is a considerable overlap between these three phases:

1 **Neurological features (1–12 hours after ingestion)**: symptoms similar to those of ethanol intoxication may be observed. Nausea and vomiting can occur. As metabolism progresses, acidosis and CNS features are seen. The latter include hypotonia, hyporeflexia, nystagmus, ataxia, ophthalmoplegia, myoclonic jerks, seizures, cranial nerve palsies, convulsions and coma.
2 **Cardiopulmonary features (12–24 hours after ingestion)**: tachycardia and mild hypertension frequently occur. In serious cases, severe metabolic acidosis with compensatory hyperventilation, pulmonary oedema and cardiac failure can develop.
3 **Renal features (24–72 hours after ingestion)**: the symptoms of the third stage can include oliguria, flank pain, acute tubular necrosis, renal failure and electrolyte disturbances including hypocalcaemia, hyperkalaemia and hypomagnesaemia.

The presence of hyperkalaemia, a severe metabolic acidosis, convulsions and coma signifies a poor prognosis. Recovery of renal function is often complete but may require several months of haemodialysis. Serious damage to the liver is rare.

Methanol

Although methanol itself is only mildly intoxicating, it is converted in the liver to highly toxic metabolites. The lethal dose of pure methanol is estimated to be around 1–2 mL/kg but both permanent blindness and death have been reported with as little as 0.1 mL/kg (i.e. 6–10 mL in adults). Methanol is rapidly absorbed from the gut, skin and lungs with peak serum concentrations occurring within 30–60 min after oral ingestion. It distributes throughout the body water and is then slowly metabolised by the liver, following zero-order kinetics. First, methanol is slowly oxidised by the enzyme alcohol dehydrogenase to yield formaldehyde. This is then further oxidised by formaldehyde dehydrogenase to create formic acid (this second step occurs rapidly so that little formaldehyde accumulates in the serum). Finally, the formic acid is metabolised to carbon dioxide and water. It is the accumulation of formic acid that is responsible for the resulting metabolic acidosis. Formic acid also inhibits cellular respiration with consequent lactic acidosis and directly damages the retina and the optic nerve.

The initial symptoms of methanol poisoning mimic those of ethanol with ataxia, nystagmus, drowsiness and dysarthria occurring within thirty minutes of ingestion. This is then followed by a latent period of 12–24 hours before metabolic toxicity becomes apparent with a high anion gap metabolic acidosis. This acidosis, in association with visual symptoms, is the hallmark of methanol poisoning. Patients usually describe blurred or double vision, changes in colour perception, photophobia and the appearance of an 'apparent snowfield'. There may be visual field loss and partial blindness with pupillary dilatation and loss of pupillary reflexes. Further features include respiratory changes, amnesia, acute pancreatitis, confusion, agitation, extrapyramidal features, electrolyte disturbances and profound hypotension. Poor outcomes are associated with coma, seizures, persistent acidosis, bradycardia and renal failure.

Tx

The mainstay of treatment is to minimise any further metabolism of ethylene glycol and methanol and thereby prevent the formation of toxic metabolites; this is achieved by the early administration of fomepizole or ethanol. Both antidotes act against alcohol dehydrogenase – the enzyme that catalyses the oxidation of ethanol and methanol and the preliminary step in the metabolism of these drugs to their toxic metabolites. Fomepizole is a competitive inhibitor of alcohol dehydrogenase and ethanol has a much greater affinity for alcohol dehydrogenase then ethylene glycol or methanol and therefore competitively inhibits the metabolism. Fomepizole is the preferred antidote as it does not cause inebriation, does not require monitoring of blood concentration and is associated with less complications. Fomepizole is also preferred in patients who have liver dysfunction, a depressed level of consciousness, pregnant women, children and in those who have taken disulfiram or metronidazole as ethanol may cause hypotension or flushing in this situation.

In cases of ingestion, an antidote should be started before laboratory confirmation if there is a suspicion that more than 10g of methanol or ethylene glycol has been ingested (>0.1g/kg in a child) or there is evidence of toxic exposure, with either a high anion gap metabolic acidosis or an osmolar gap greater than 10nosmols/kg. Treatment may be needed for several days and should be continued till the concentration of ethylene glycol or methanol is undetectable or till the concentration of either is less than 50mg/L and the acidosis and systemic toxicity have resolved.

Haemodialysis is the other mainstay of treatment as it can remove methanol, ethylene glycol and their respective metabolites. It also significantly reduces the half-life of both substances and will help correct any metabolic abnormalities.

The other specific treatment that should be given in methanol poisoning is folinic acid because folate dependent systems are responsible for the oxidation of formic acid to water and carbon dioxide.

All other treatment is supportive; however, calcium should not be given for hypocalcaemia (unless a prolonged QT or persistent seizures) because it may increase precipitation of calcium oxalate crystals in the tissues.

Mechanism of action of antidotes in poisoning with methanol and ethylene glycol → Figure 15.3.

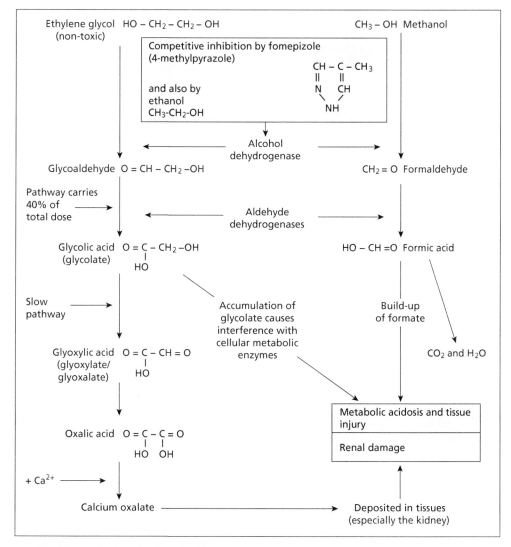

Figure 15.3 The mechanism of action of antidotes in poisoning with methanol and ethylene glycol.

Household substances

Children may be suspected of ingesting an enormous variety of domestic substances. Most of these are harmless but some are not and so caution is always advisable. Treatment consists of milk and the recommendations of a poisons information service.

Cleaning materials

Most are harmless. Two notable exceptions are bleach and dishwasher products for machines. These can burn the mouth and damage the oesophagus. Emesis is therefore contraindicated. Patients should be given milk and observed in hospital.

Turpentine

This can refer to turpentine, the essential oil, which is highly toxic and can be lethal. Its abbreviated name, 'turps', usually refers to a white spirit substitute that can cause CNS depression and pulmonary toxicity.

Plants and garden substances

Earth, faecal material, insects and worms generally present little risk. The possibility of ingesting ova, cysts and parasites is probably quite small. Berries and seeds are commonly ingested. Some such as laburnum seeds may cause GI upset and drowsiness. Deadly nightshade may be mistaken for elderberry and lead to atropine poisoning.

Tx
If the ingested plant material is presented; it may be identified with the aid of a guidebook or online resource. Most ingestions of this type, including those where the material is unidentified, should be treated by an appropriate period of observation.

Button battery ingestion

Button battery ingestion is a true emergency even if asymptomatic. The primary risk occurs if the button battery becomes impacted in the oesophagus. This usually occurs at the level of the aortic arch and is more common with larger batteries (and smaller children). Hydroxide formation at the negative electrode of the battery leads to tissue hydrolysis. This can cause severe tissue damage in as little as 2 hours, and perforation into vascular structures can occur with catastrophic consequences (this may occur even weeks after the battery has been removed).

Suspect button battery ingestion with all possible 'coin' ingestions unless these were directly witnessed by a reliable adult. If the battery has passed into the stomach or beyond the risk is low.

Tx Perform an urgent chest and abdominal X-ray for all potential ingestions. Look for the 'double rim' sign to differentiate it from a coin.

If X-ray shows button battery in the oesophagus:

- Urgently refer for removal by endoscopy. Discussion with regional retrieval teams may be required.
- Administer honey orally (10 mL every 10 min) unless the battery has been *in situ* >12 hours. Sucralfate can also be used to reduce mucosal damage if available.
- If battery is in the stomach or beyond (and only one has been ingested):
  - If patient is symptomatic refer for immediate endoscopy
  - If patient is asymptomatic they may be discharged with instructions to return if symptoms develop, to inspect stools for passage of the battery and to return for repeat X-ray if not passed within 10 days
- In a child <6 years who has ingested a large battery (>15 mm) repeat X-ray at day 4 and refer for removal if still in the stomach.
- If multiple batteries have been ingested, admit for observation and repeat X-ray at 2 days post ingestion.

Magnet ingestion

Ingestion of more than one magnet, or a magnet with another metallic object can result in bowel perforation and fistulae as the two attract through the bowel wall causing pressure necrosis. Rare earth metal (neodymium) magnets pose a particular risk and are often small and brightly coloured, making them attractive to small children.

- Obtain a chest and abdominal X-ray to locate the magnet
- Consider a lateral X-ray if only one magnet is seen, to ensure a multiple ingestion is not overlooked
- Note that rare earth metal magnets are often marketed in ball-bearing shape – assume a 'string' of balls to be multiple magnets until proven otherwise. They may appear to be stuck together, but the bowel trapped between is not visible on X-ray.
- Prompt referral to the paediatric surgical team of all symptomatic patients and those who have ingested multiple magnets or co-ingested a battery or other metallic object

Patients may be suitable for discharge if the following criteria are met:

- Confirmed single magnet ingestion
- Tolerating oral intake
- Accidental ingestion
- Caregiver able to closely observe

Advise the patient to avoid clothing with metallic fastenings and proximity to external metallic objects (e.g. buckles).

Repeat X-rays should be obtained after 6–12 hours of neodymium magnet ingestion to confirm progress through the GI tract. These should be reviewed by a radiologist and if no movement has taken place, referral to paediatric surgery is necessary.

Envenoming

As a result of international travel and pet ownership, there is a potential wide variety of animal bite and stings that patients can be exposed to. In all cases, wounds should be cleaned, dressed, tetanus prophylaxis confirmed and prophylactic antibiotics considered. Advice can be obtained from your local infectious diseases centre or from the NPIS. Marine animals and snakes are the two main envenoming situations to be aware of.

Marine envenoming encompasses

- **Venomous sea creatures:** these inject a toxin directly via spines or stinging cells (nematocysts); the most common UK examples of these two types of venomous sea creatures are weever fish and jellyfish, respectively.
- **Ingestion of *Scombroid fish:*** If not completely fresh, fish of the family *Scombridae* (which includes mackerel and tuna) may be decomposed by bacteria to produce histamine from histadine in fish muscle. Similar processes may occur in both tinned and fresh fish of other non-scombroid species such as herring. Around 30 min to several hours after eating the fish patients experience features that resemble histamine reactions. This can be mistaken for an allergic reaction. Treatment is with antihistamines if required and symptoms usually resolve within 12 hours.
- **Shellfish poisoning:** four patterns of shellfish poisoning can occur; paralytic, neurotoxic, amnesic or diarrhoetic shellfish poisoning. None of these are commonly found in shellfish found in UK waters.

Jellyfish, weever fish, caterpillar, wasp and bee stings in the British Isles → p. 419.

Adder bites

There are three species of snake that are native to the UK; however, the European Viper or adder (*Vipera berus*) is the only poisonous one. It has a grey/brown body with a distinctive zigzag pattern along its back. As it hibernates in the winter bites are rare at this time of year.

Non-venomous bites from *V. berus* or the two non-venomous snakes found in the UK should be treated symptomatically with antibiotics if required, tetanus status checked and consideration of a retained tooth fragment if there is local inflammation. Retained snake tooth fragments are visible on X-rays.

Local *V. berus* envenoming occurs within 30 min of being bitten and initially causes local swelling. This then progresses to pain, tenderness, erythema, swelling and regional lymph node enlargement. In severe cases, the whole limb can become swollen and bruised with involvement of the trunk (and in children the whole body). Fluid resuscitation may be required due to massive extravasation into the affected limb. Secondary bacterial infection, necrosis and compartment syndrome are extremely rare; however, the effects can mimic compartment syndrome and intra-compartmental measurements should be carried out if there are any concerns.

Systemic *V. berus* envenoming is less common than local envenoming and the main features are:

- **Acute kidney injury**: particularly in paediatric patients
- **Increased kidney permeability**: leading to haemoconcentration, widespread swelling, focal angiooedema, pulmonary oedema and cerebral oedema
- **GI effects**: gastric dilation, ileus and acute pancreatitis
- **Bleeding diathesis** although this is very uncommon. Bleeding from the gums, nose and into the GI, GU and lungs may occur. Heparin should not be given to any envenomed patient as this may make any bleeding worse.
- **Cardiac effects**: tachy or brady-dysrhythmias, heart block, global ECG changes suggesting ischaemia and myocardial infarctions due to hypotension.
- **Coma and convulsions** secondary to cardiovascular shock and profound hypotension.
- **Haematomological:** anaemia, thrombocytopenia and very high white cell counts which indicate systemic envenoming.

Acute anaphylaxis can develop within minutes of the bite due to a direct effect of *V. berus* venom on the body. In people who have previously been sensitised, e.g. snake handlers, then anaphylaxis can occur via IgE-mediated hypersensitisation.

Tx Initial management involves immobilising the affected limb and avoiding interference with the bite. Washing or sucking the bite site, applying tourniquets, ligatures or compression bandages should all be avoided. Adrenaline, hydrocortisone and chlorpenamine should be given for anaphylaxis or angioedema.

The indications for antivenom are:

- Early anaphylaxis-like reactions
- Hypotension persisting for more than 10 min
- Systemic features including abdominal pain and vomiting

- Definite leukocytosis
- ECG abnormalities
- Metabolic acidosis
- Elevated CK
- Marked local envenoming even in the absence of systemic signs, i.e. swelling beyond the next major joint from the site of the bite.
- Any other evidence of systemic envenomation, e.g. spontaneous bleeding.

Antivenom should rapidly stop progression of swelling and erythema in local envenoming and quickly improve cardiovascular status in those with systemic envenoming. The sooner antivenom is given the greater the likelihood of effectiveness; however, there can still be benefit if given up to 24 hours after being bitten. Patients envenomed by *V. berus* can deteriorate rapidly and even after antivenom administration patients should be reviewed regularly. Look particularly for changes in the bitten limb and the patient's blood pressure. If there is progression of the swelling or sustained systemic effects, then a repeat dose of antivenom should be given. The dose for both adults and children is 8 mL (diluted in isotonic saline) by IV infusion over 30 min. It is not dosed on the patient's weight or age as it is based on the amount of venom injected during a *V. berus* envenomation. If there is little improvement, this may be repeated after 1–2 hours. The antivenom itself may cause an anaphylactic reaction and serum sickness can occur 1–2 weeks after antivenom is given; this manifests as fever, urticarial, arthralgia and albuminuria.

Carbon monoxide

This under-recognised condition hospitalises more than 200 people and causes about 40 deaths every year in the UK. Carbon monoxide is a colourless, tasteless, non-irritating gas produced by incomplete combustion of any carbon-containing material (including gas, oil, wood and coal) and so is a sinister and insidious enemy. The main causes of poisoning with carbon monoxide in the UK are as follows:

1 *Deliberate self-harm* (45%)
2 *Faulty domestic heating and cooking apparatus* (33%)
3 *Smoke inhalation in fires* (20%) (cyanide and other toxic fumes may also be released during the combustion of common materials such as polyurethane foam in furniture → *p. 303*).

Think of carbon monoxide poisoning if a patient has:

- a history of smoke inhalation (→ *p. 141*)
- unexplained neurological symptoms, including headache
- an unexplained metabolic acidosis

and if:

- more than one patient presents from the same site
- there are known to be animals that are unwell or have died
- the patient gets better when away from home
- the patient comes from a community that uses traditional cooking methods
- the patient reports that there are black, sooty marks on the walls around stoves, boilers or fires or that their gas appliances burn with yellow rather than blue flames.

Carbon monoxide causes tissue hypoxia by the following methods:

1 Binding to haemoglobin (to form carboxyhaemoglobin or COHb) and thus preventing the carriage of oxygen (its affinity for haemoglobin is 240 times greater than that of oxygen)
2 Moving the oxyhaemoglobin dissociation curve to the left
3 Binding to cellular proteins (such as cytochrome oxidases) which are essential for oxidation.

Tissues with a high requirement for oxygen, such as nervous tissue and myocardium, are most severely affected.

Symptoms and signs: Symptoms vary widely and include malaise, headache, nausea and myalgia (→ *Table 15.6*). A collection of these vague symptoms may mimic influenza or food poisoning. However, there may also be overt neurological, cardiovascular and biochemical findings such as:

- confusion, coma and psychological changes
- dizziness, syncope and ataxia
- dysphasia, dyskinesia, paresis and cortical blindness
- hypotension, angina, dysrhythmias, left ventricular failure, pulmonary oedema and myocardial infarction
- renal failure
- metabolic acidosis, hypokalaemia and leukocytosis
- rhabdomyolysis (very rarely).

Table 15.6 Common symptoms of carbon monoxide poisoning

Symptom	Approximate frequency (%)
Headache	90
Nausea and vomiting	50
Vertigo	50
Alteration in consciousness	30
Subjective weakness	20

These problems may persist or reoccur and are not well correlated to the COHb level. This is probably because the half-life of carbon monoxide bound to intracellular myoglobin and respiratory enzymes is up to 48 hours, as opposed to 5 hours in the blood as COHb. Binding to mitochondrial cytochrome A_3 is thought to be particularly important in the causation of carbon monoxide toxicity. Neurological damage seems to be the result of free radical generation and lipid peroxidation.

Patients with coexisting medical problems (heart disease, respiratory disease and anaemia) and children are usually the worst affected and may experience symptoms at lower levels of COHb. Carbon monoxide has a special affinity for foetal haemoglobin and so babies and pregnant women present a special risk.

The severity of poisoning is related to:

- the concentration of carbon monoxide inhaled – an initial level above 30% is likely to be associated with severe poisoning
- the length of exposure
- the level of activity during the exposure.

> A cherry-red skin colour occurs only when COHb concentrations exceed about 20% and is rarely seen in living patients.

Investigations: Investigations may include:

- **blood gases**: metabolic acidosis with normal oxygen tension
- **ECG and troponin measurement**: ischaemia
- **foetal cardiotocograph (FCTG):** foetal hypoxia
- **plasma electrolytes, glucose and osmolality**: to exclude other causes of poisoning
- **COHb levels** ($\rightarrow$ Box 15.2).

> Laboratory measurement of arterial blood gases looks at the oxygen dissolved in the plasma rather than the oxygen bound to haemoglobin and so the PaO_2 level in CO poisoning may be surprisingly near to normal. Traditional pulse oximeters will also give a false normal value because they cannot differentiate between oxyhaemoglobin and carboxyhaemoglobin. However, pulse CO-oximeters are now available.

Tx

Treatment consists of high-concentration oxygen therapy for 120 min, given via an endotracheal tube or tight-fitting mask (the half-life of COHb is reduced to around

Box 15.2 The effects of increasing carboxyhaemoglobin levels

- COHb should be <5% of total haemoglobin in a non-smoker and <10–13% in a smoker
- COHb >10% causes mild headache and dyspnoea on vigorous exertion
- COHb >20% causes severe headache, dyspnoea on mild exertion and sometimes early neurological symptoms and signs
- COHb >30% causes severe headache, irritability, fatigue, dimness of vision and other neurological symptoms and signs
- COHb >40% causes severe headache, tachycardia, lethargy, confusion, collapse and sometimes coma
- COHb >60% causes coma, convulsions and cardiovascular collapse
- COHb >70% is very rapidly fatal

80 min when breathing 100% oxygen). Hyperbaric oxygen therapy is not currently recommended. All unresponsive patients should be intubated and ventilated. Acidosis will resolve with oxygenation and should not be treated with bicarbonate.

Cyanide $\rightarrow$ *p. 303.*
Methaemoglobinaemia $\rightarrow$ *p. 302.*

POISONING WITH HARMFUL AGENTS THAT HAVE BEEN RELEASED INTO THE ENVIRONMENT

Chemical and biological agents

Chemical agents

Chemical and biological agents are still used intentionally during armed conflicts, terrorism incidents and political assassinations. In the former cases, the release of these agents may be overt and clearly identifiable; however, in the latter two situations, the release may be covert or there may be no prior warning. Release of these agents in the context of a major incident will lead to exposed patients presenting at hospitals distant from the incident site.

The main types of agents used for such purposes:

- Nerve agents, e.g. sarin, VX
- Vesicating or blistering agents, e.g. mustard gas

- Irritants and asphyxiants such as chlorine, phosgene, ammonia and ammonium nitrate
- Cyanides
- Lacrimating or riot control agents, e.g. pepper gas, CS
- Biotoxins, e.g. ricin, abrin
- Incapacitating agents such as anticholinergic agents.

Tx All cases should be discussed with a specialist, initially a public health consultant or a poisons unit adviser.

Ammonium nitrate → p. 303.
Botulinum toxin → p. 246.
Chemical accidents and decontamination → p. 151.
Chlorine, phosgene, ammonia and sulphur dioxide →
p. 303.
Cyanide → p. 303.
Organophosphate and carbamate insecticides and nerve
gases → p. 304.
Ricin and abrin → p. 304.
Strychnine and brucine (see tetanus) → p. 245.

Incapacitating sprays and aerosols

Patients may present who have been assaulted with a variety of irritant powder aerosols, e.g. pepper spray, CS (tear gas) or CN (mace). There is profound irritation of the eyes, skin, mucous membranes and respiratory tract.

Tx Hospital treatment is rarely needed as the effects of these agents are usually self-limiting, resolving within 15–30 min of cessation of exposure. Most patients require irrigation to the face and eyes only; a weak alkaline solution (or soap and water) can be used for the skin. Continuing discomfort of the eyes merits examination with fluorescein to exclude chemical damage. Severe dermatitis can be treated with topical steroids. Good ventilation of the treatment areas is essential to protect staff and other patients.

Methaemoglobinaemia (MetHb)

Exposure to toxic fumes or drugs may oxidise the iron of haem to its ferric (Fe^{3+}) form, and the resulting methaemoglobin (met-Hb) cannot carry oxygen. Common precipitating drugs include nitrite derivatives, e.g. amyl nitrite ('poppers'), nitroprusside, dapsone, sulfonamides, local anaesthetics, topical anaesthetics and antimalarials. The inability of met-Hb to carry oxygen leads to the characteristic presentation of methaemoglobinaemia which is persistent cyanosis despite adequate oxygenation.

Methaemoglobinaemia should be suspected if:

- The cyanosis fails to respond to oxygen therapy.
- The PaO_2 is normal in the presence of a decreased measured oxygen saturation on blood gas analysis.
- The arterial blood is chocolate brown in colour and remains dark on aeration (the urine may also be discoloured brown or black).

Methaemoglobin levels can be checked by taking a blood gas sample and the concentration of MetHb determines what clinical effects are likely:

0–10%	Features unlikely
10–30%	Mild effects – fatigue, dizziness, headaches, blue-grey 'apparent' central cyanosis
30–50%	Moderate effects – weakness, tachypnoea, tachycardia
50–70%	Severe effects – coma, convulsions, acidosis, arrhythmias, respiratory depression
>70%	Potentially fatal

Treatment is with methylthioninium chloride (methylene blue) 1–2 mg/kg given in an infusion of 5% dextrose over 5 min. This should be given to all patients with life-threatening features even if point-of-care testing is not available, and in those with a MetHb concentration of 30% or more. It should also be considered in those patients who are more susceptible to hypoxia, e.g. heart failure, pulmonary disease, even if the concentration is less than 30%.

Methylene blue may be ineffective in the following circumstances:

- The patient has glucose-6-phosphate dehydrogenase deficiency. This deficiency results in a low concentration of NADPH, which is required for methylene blue to work.
- The agent the patient has been exposed to causes haemolysis as well as methaemoglobinaemia, reducing the effectiveness of therapy.
- The poisoning agent involved may continue to induce methaemoglobin formation (e.g. dapsone).
- Chlorate poisoning – chlorate may inactivate glucose-6-phosphate dehydrogenase.
- The patient has hereditary methaemoglobinaemia. Such conditions are very rare.
- Some agents, e.g. sulfonamides, that cause methaemoglobinaemia also cause sulphaemoglobinaemia. No mechanism for the reconversion of sulphaemoglobinaemia exists and methylthioninium chloride is ineffective. However, sulphaemoglobinaemia seldom occurs in concentrations large enough to result in hypoxia.

Exchange transfusion should be considered where treatment with methylene blue is ineffective.

Noxious vapours and gases

Occupational poisoning may occur with gases such as sulphur dioxide, chlorine, ammonia and phosgene. In most cases, there is immediate dyspnoea, choking, coughing, watering eyes and incapacity. However, pulmonary oedema may develop up to 36 hours after a severe exposure, especially following exertion.

Tx Most patients will require inpatient observation. Symptomatic treatment may include:

- oxygen therapy
- nebulised steroids (e.g. budesonide 2 mg repeated as necessary)
- cough suppressants
- continuous positive airway pressure (CPAP)
- ventilation with positive end-expiratory pressure (PEEP)
- correction of methaemoglobinaemia (→ *above*).

Ammonium nitrate → *below.*
Carbon monoxide → *p. 300.*
Cyanide → *p. 303.*

Hydrogen sulphide

Hydrogen sulphide is a colourless, flammable gas that has a characteristic odour of rotten eggs. It is a by-product of certain industrialised processes but can also be made by mixing domestic cleaning fluid (an acid source) is mixed with a sulphur-containing substance; which has led to it being used as a method of suicide particularly in some parts of the world.

It directly inhibits ion channels and cellular enzymes causing a disruption of the electron transport chain and anaerobic metabolism. Inhalation of a high concentration leads rapidly to collapse, respiratory paralysis, cyanosis, convulsions, coma, arrhythmias and death within minutes. Acute exposures can also cause long-term neurological impairment including extrapyramidal signs and severe eye damage.

Ammonium nitrate

Ammonium nitrate is an acidifying salt with diuretic effects. It is used to manufacture of explosives, fertilisers and ice packs. It is well absorbed if ingested and is reduced to nitrates by bacteria in the gastrointestinal tract. Toxicity following exposure is due to the vasodilatory properties of nitrate and the formation of methaemoglobinaemia. Symptoms range from blurred vision, dyspnoea, throat irritation, headache and dizziness in mild cases; to hypoxia, arrhythmias, convulsions and respiratory depression in severe cases.

Methaemoglobinaemia should be treated if present otherwise treatment is supportive.

Cyanide

Cyanide poisoning can be a consequence of smoke inhalation, exposure in industries that use cyanide, e.g. metal processing, photography or ingestion of cyanide compounds. Cyanide is also present naturally in the kernels and stones of many fruits including cherries, apricots and peaches.

Cyanide ions act on the mitochondrial enzyme cytochrome C oxidase and prevents it transporting any electrons to oxygen thus disrupting aerobic cellular respiration and stopping adenosine triphosphate (ATP) production.

Blood cyanide concentrations will give a guide to toxicity with mild toxicity less than 1 mg/L, moderate toxicity 1–3 mg/L and severe toxicity occurring with more that 3 mg/L. Unfortunately, cyanide assays are only performed at a small number of laboratories and the results are unlikely to be rapidly available. In the absence of a cyanide concentration, the following features suggest possible cyanide poisoning:

- Lactate more than 7 mmol/L
- Elevated anion gap metabolic acidosis
- An increased venous oxygen concentration, relative to that expected given the inspired and arterial oxygen concentrations.

The initial features of cyanide toxicity include headache, dizziness, nausea, drowsiness, tachycardia and palpitations. In cases of moderate toxicity, there is confusion, loss of consciousness, vomiting and hypotension. Severe cases are characterised by deep coma, fixed unreactive pupils, cardiovascular collapse, respiratory depression and profound bradycardia or AV dissociation. Cherry red skin and a bitter almond odour on the patient's breath are characteristic but only present in a small number of cases. Cyanosis is often a late sign and may not be present in all cases.

Tx
Treatment should be initiated in all patients with suspected moderate or severe poisoning while awaiting the results of cyanide concentrations.

There are several possible antidote regimens for the treatment of severe, life-threatening cyanide poisoning:

1 Hydroxocobalamin – 70 mg/kg in a child or 5 g for an adult by IV infusion over 15 min; this can be repeated, if necessary depending on the severity of the poisoning and the patient's symptoms. In this situation, vitamin B_{12} acts as a chelating agent.

2 Sodium thiosulphate – 400mg/kg for children and 12.5g for adults; this dose can be repeated. Sodium thiosulphate acts as a substrate for the enzyme rhodanase which catalyses the conversion of cyanide to the relatively non-toxic thiocyanate. It can be given as an adjunct to hydroxocobalamin. Due to its slow onset of action, it is less effective as a solo agent in severe cyanide poisoning.

3 Dicobalt edetate is a very effective cyanide antidote, however, production was discontinued in 2019 by the manufacturer. If it is available then the case should be discussed with the NPIS prior to use. In the absence of cyanide poisoning, it is potentially toxic as it can induce cobalt toxicity.

A reduction in lactate or cyanide concentration and improved haemodynamic status are all indicators of a response to treatment.

Cholinesterase inhibitors (nerve agents)

Nerve agents are related chemically to organophosphorus insecticides and have a similar mechanism of toxicity, but they have a much higher acute human toxicity. They act on the enzyme acetylcholinesterase (AChE) leading to the accumulation of acetylcholine. The acetylcholine binds to nicotinic and muscarinic receptors and this causes enhancement and prolongation of cholinergic effects and a depolarization blockade. Recovery of the enzyme function is dependent on re-synthesis of AChE which can take several weeks; this is because these agents also make the enzyme resistant to breakdown and reactivation.

The weaponized substances in this group include sarin, Novichok and VX. Nerve agents are absorbed through intact skin as well as through the lungs and the gut. Off-gassing from casualties may cause symptoms in emergency personnel.

The symptoms are the direct result of the two receptors affected:

- **Muscarinic (parasympathetic) effects**: miosis, lacrimation and rhinorrhoea; hypersalivation and sweating; bronchospasm and bronchorrhoea; vomiting and diarrhoea; bradycardia
- **Nicotinic (motor and postganglionic sympathetic) effects**: muscle fasciculation and flaccid paralysis; hypertension and tachycardia

Death is usually due to respiratory arrest.

Tx
The diagnosis can be confirmed by obtaining baseline samples for measurement of red cell acetylcholinesterase activity or plasma cholinesterase activity.

Resuscitation and stabilisation of patients affected by nerve agents should be done before any decontamination is carried out. Atropine antagonises the muscarinic effects of acetylcholine and should be given if the patient develops increased secretions, bronchorrhoea, bronchospasm, hypotension or bradycardia (especially hypersecretion and bradycardia). The IV dose is 2–4 mg and this should be doubled every 5 min until secretions are minimal, the patient's lungs are clear, the heart rate is above 80 and the blood pressure is adequate. An atropine infusion may be required.

Pralidoxime chloride should be given to all patients who require atropine as this antidote can restore the activity of AChE after the enzyme has been inhibited by organophosphates. It is given a 30 mg/kg intravenous loading dose followed by a continuous infusion. In cases of overdose or poisoning pralidoxime can be obtained from one of the pralidoxime holding centres. In the setting of major incident, it will need to be obtained via the NHS England regional on call manager for the area affected. Early intubation should be considered as there is a trend towards worse outcomes in patients not intubated before pralidoxime administration.

Ricin and abrin

Ricin is a toxin that is extracted from the beans of the castor oil plant which inhibits protein synthesis by damaging ribosomes, leading to cell death. Accidental poisoning has followed the ingestion of castor oil seeds and as few as three seeds have killed an adult. When ingested gastrointestinal symptoms occur within a few hours with vomiting, abdominal pain and gastrointestinal bleeding as the main symptoms. Other features include:

- Miosis, mydriasis and blurred vision
- Fluid and electrolyte losses which can lead to the patient being shocked
- Intravascular haemolysis
- Renal and liver failure
- Pulmonary oedema and ARDS
- Seizures

Ricin can also be injected causing severe local lymphoid necrosis and splenitis in addition to the features above. When inhaled it causes an allergic syndrome with conjunctivitis, coryzal symptoms, urticarial, wheeze and potentially necrotising interstitial and alveolar inflammation with oedema and pneumonia. In cases of inhalation, the toxic effects do not affect any other organ systems.

Abrin is a similar toxin that is found in the Jequirity bean, the seed of the plant *Abrus precatorious*. The features of poisoning with abrin are similar to those with ricin, but abrin is significantly more potent.

Tx Patients should be removed from the source of an aerosol exposure and decontaminated (by personnel with full respiratory and body protection) following resuscitation. Contaminated clothing should be removed and open wounds decontaminated first.

There is no antidote for ricin or abrin and so treatment is supportive.

Biological agents

There are certain infectious diseases that have the potential for military or terrorist use. This is either because they are known to have been the subject of attempted weaponization or because they have characteristics that make deliberate release a dangerous possibility. Such infectious organisms are invariably able to survive for long periods away from their natural host and can potentially be distributed as an aerosol for subsequent inhalation by intended victims. Many of these infections are zoonoses. The main diseases listed by Public Health England are as follows:

Anthrax → pp. 269 and 425.
Botulism → p. 246.
Brucellosis → p. 269.
Glanders and melioidosis → p. 269.
Plague → p. 269.
Q fever → p. 223.
Smallpox.
Tularaemia → p. 425.
Viral haemorrhagic fevers → p. 266.

In instances where there has been a deliberate release of a bacterial agent then Public Health England may recommend early prophylactic antibiotics. In the initial treatment phase, this will likely involve a relatively large group of patients receiving antibiotics as simplicity and speed of initiation is critical. The number of people requiring antibiotics will decrease in the next stage, the extended treatment phase, as the more information becomes available and the at-risk group become more easily identifiable. The first-line prophylactic agent is ciprofloxacin followed by doxycycline and amoxicillin or co-amoxiclav.

The recommended prophylaxis periods are:

- Anthrax up to 60 days – a shorter period may be recommended
- Tularaemia 14 days
- Plague 7 days

FURTHER CONSIDERATIONS IN POISONING

Mental state and psychiatric assessment

All patients should have a mental health triage by an ED nurse on arrival and their medical review should include a risk assessment of suicide and further self-harm. All patients should be seen by a member of the mental health team while in the ED, although this may have to delayed if the patient is not medically fit to be assessed (→ p. 378).

Child abuse

Poisoning in childhood is usually the result of accidental ingestion with babies and toddlers particularly at risk. However, there are circumstances where isolated poisoning in a child may suggest the possibility of child abuse. This should be considered when accidental poisoning is not consistent with the child's developmental age, the history is inconsistent, there is a past history of poisoning or poisoning from illicit drugs or unusual poisoning from household substances is suspected.

Safeguarding and non-accidental injury→ p. 369.

Heavy metal poisoning

Heavy metals such as cadmium, arsenic, mercury and lead are the most usual suspects in chronic poisoning. Heavy metal poisoning can occur as the result of industrial exposure, air or water pollution, foods, medicines or the ingestion of lead based paints. Suspicion of chronic poisoning merits medical referral for detailed investigation. Antidotes for heavy metals include dimercaprol, penicillamine, sodium calcium edetate and dimercaptosuccinic acid (DMSA).

Mercury. Fish and shellfish are the main sources of mercury exposure to humans; it is also found in dental amalgams, thermometers, sphygmomanometers, fluorescent lamps and in some illegal skin-lightening creams. It is poorly absorbed from the skin and GI tract and inhalation is the main route of exposure (e.g. vacuuming up a broken thermometer). Elemental iron is oxidised by the body to mercuric iron which then reacts with organic compounds on structural proteins, receptors, enzymes, DNA and RNA rendering them inactive.

Acute inhalation can lead to a spectrum of respiratory problems from flu-like symptoms all the way to pulmonary oedema and ARDS. Hypersalivation, tremor, ataxia, peripheral neuropathy, thrombocytopenia, acute tubular necrosis, hallucinations and memory loss can also occur. In those patients chronically exposed to mercury vapour, faint, diffuse grey-coloured pigments are present on the oral mucosa. All patients exposed should have blood and urine mercury concentrations measured and a decision to institute chelation therapy should be made after consultation with the NPIS.

Lead. Poisoning usually results from long-term occupational exposure (ingestion or inhalation) in professions such as plumbers, lead miners, shipbuilders, construction workers, pottery manufacturers and demolition workers. In addition, some hobbies (painting, soldering, target shooting and pottery), the ingestion of lead weights, gunshot wounds and exposure to some traditional remedies and cosmetics may all be associated with lead poisoning. Elemental lead is less well absorbed than soluble lead salts, which are highly toxic. Lead poisoning causes a metallic taste, severe abdominal pain, diarrhoea with black stools, vomiting, hypotension, muscle weakness, cramps, fatigue, abnormal liver function tests, acute interstitial nephritis and encephalopathy in its acute form. Chronic features include anorexia, abdominal pain, constipation, headaches, irritability, fatigue, insomnia, depression, peripheral neuropathy, renal dysfunction and anaemia.

In patient with a retained lead shot or slug this should be removed if it is associated with a joint or an increased blood lead concentration. Measurement of the lead concentration will then determine if chelation or only monitoring of concentrations is required.

Following a potentially life-threatening ingestion of lead, gastric lavage should be considered within the first hour. A plain abdominal radiograph can be used to both confirm recent ingestion of elemental lead and to confirm effective decontamination. Chelation should be considered if a raised blood lead concentration is present. The lead should be removed endoscopically or surgically if it fails to progress though the GI tract, and the patient develops GI symptoms or if the blood lead concentration is raised.

Iron poisoning → p. 295.

Forensic aspects

If there is a suspicion of criminal poisoning, the police should be contacted. If samples such as blood or urine are required, then these samples should be obtained by a police doctor or an emergency physician trained in taking samples forensically; this is to ensure a chain of evidence can be provided for any subsequent legal proceedings. This includes drug assisted sexual assault (→ p. 294).

ATYPICAL REACTIONS TO DRUGS AND OTHER SUBSTANCES

Allergic reactions

Anaphylaxis is common and affects 1 in 300 of the European population. Drugs, foods, stinging insects and latex are the most common triggers. A significant number of cases are idiopathic. Fatal anaphylactic reactions usually occur very soon after contact with the trigger. A fatal food reaction can cause a respiratory arrest within 30–35 min, and death caused by an intravenous medication is most common within 5 min.

> Biphasic reactions, where a second wave of symptoms appears 4–8 hours after the initial remission, are seen in a small proportion of patients with anaphylaxis. Patients should be observed for 6–12 hours, and the risk and symptoms of biphasic reaction discussed on discharge. Steroid treatment is no longer recommended following an episode of anaphylaxis.

There is not a consistent clinical manifestation to patients with anaphylaxis and a range of possible presentations is possible combining elements of the following:

Airway (upper airway obstruction)
There is airway swelling, e.g. throat and tongue swelling, laryngeal oedema and the patient may have stridor, a hoarse voice, difficulty in breathing and swallowing and a feeling that the throat is 'closing up'.

Breathing (bronchospasm)
The patient may have dyspnoea, wheeze and can be confused or cyanosed due to hypoxia.

Circulation (shock)
The circulatory collapse is a result of direct myocardial depression, vasodilatation and maldistribution of fluid. The patient may be shocked, tachycardic, hypotensive and can have a decreased level of consciousness. Anaphylaxis can cause ECG and myocardial ischaemia even in the presence of normal coronary arteries.

Skin and mucosal changes
This is often the first sign of anaphylaxis and the changes can affect the skin, mucosa or both. Erythema, urticaria and angioedema are the clinical signs to expect, however, in order to signify anaphylaxis they need to be an associated airway, breathing or circulation problem.

Tx
- Remove the trigger if possible, e.g. stop an IV antibiotic infusion
- Call for senior help
- Administer IM adrenaline 0.5 mg (0.5 mL of 1 : 1000). This can be repeated at 5 min intervals according to the patient's response.
- IV adrenaline can be given by clinicians experienced in the use and titration of vasopressors. It is given as boluses of 50 mcg (0.5 mL of 1 : 10 000) → *see Box 15.3.*
- If repeated adrenaline doses are needed, then an IV infusion should be commenced.

Box 15.3 **Adrenaline for anaphylaxis**

- 1 in 1000 adrenaline contains 1 mg (1000 mcg)/mL; it is usually supplied as a 1-mL (i.e. 1-mg) ampoule
- 1 in 10 000 adrenaline contains 0.1 mg (100 mcg)/mL; it is usually supplied as a 10-mL (i.e. 1-mg) ampoule
- Dosing:
  - **Adult and child >12 years:** 500 mcg IM (0.5 mL of 1 : 1000)
  - **Child 6–12 years:** 300 mcg IM (0.3 mL of 1 : 1000)
  - **Child 6 months–6 years:** 150 mcg IM (0.15 mL of 1 : 1000)
  - **Child <6 months:** 100–150 mcg IM (0.1–0.15 mL of 1 : 1000)

- Other vasopressors and inotropes (noradrenaline, vasopressin, glucagon, metaraminol) can be used for prolonged shock.
- Consider nebulised adrenaline (5 mg) and early tracheal intubation
- Consider bronchodilator therapy with salbutamol (nebuliser or IV), ipratropium (inhaled), aminophylline (IV) or magnesium (IV). It is important to remember IV magnesium is a vasodilator and can make hypotension worse.
- Give an IV fluid challenge (500–1000 mL)
- Antihistamines are considered a third-line intervention and are not a priority in the early phase of treatment, Non-sedating antihistamines may be preferable to chlorphenamine and may be given following initial stabilisation.

Mast cell tryptase

Patients who have had a suspected anaphylactic reaction should have samples taken for mast cell tryptase analysis. An initial sample should be taken as soon as feasible after resuscitation has been started and second sample at 1–2 hours after the start of symptoms.

All patients who have suffered a suspected anaphylactic reaction should be given clear instructions on when to return to hospital, be prescribed an adrenaline auto-injector and be trained in its use and have a follow-up plan in place with their general practitioner and an allergy clinic.

Hereditary angio-oedema (C1 inhibitor deficiency): A congenital deficiency of C1 inhibitor causes episodes of soft-tissue swelling that may either arise spontaneously or be precipitated by factors such as trauma or illness. There may be swelling of the lips, tongue mouth and pharynx as well as oedema of the face and abdominal symptoms. This hereditary angio-oedema (HAE) is resistant to standard therapy for allergic reactions.

Hereditary angio-oedema (HAE)/C1 (esterase) inhibitor deficiency → p. 274.

Acute dystonic reactions

Dystonia refers to sustained muscle contractions leading to twisting and repetitive movements or abnormal postures which can affect any part of the body. Acute dystonic reactions are a recognised extrapyramidal side effect of several medications:

- **Antipsychotic:** all current available antipsychotics have the potential to cause dystonic reactions
- **Antiemetic drugs**, e.g. metoclopramide, proclorperazine
- **Antibiotics**, e.g. erythromycin
- **Antimalarials**, e.g. chloroquine
- **Anticonvulsants**, e.g. carbamazepine
- **H2 receptor antagonists**, e.g. rantidine
- **Recreational drugs**, e.g. cocaine

Young adults and children are most commonly affected and the reaction usually occurs within a few hours of taking the causative medication but the onset can be delayed by a few days.

The presentation is varied but includes:

- **Laryngeal dystonia:** a rare but potentially life-threatening variant characterised by throat pain, dyspnea, stridor and dysphonia.
- **Oculogyric crisis:** rotatory eye movements or deviated gaze
- **Blepharospasm and other facial spasms:** spasm of the eyelids (unable to open eyes) or other facial muscles
- **Buccolingual crisis:** protruding or pulling sensation of the tongue
- **Torticollis, antecollis or retrocollis:** twisting of the neck, or the head forced forwards or backwards
- **Torticopelvic crisis:** abdominal rigidity and pain
- **Scoliosis or lordosis:** lateral flexion of the spine or extension.
- **Opisthotonic crisis:** spasm of the entire body characterised by back arching, flexion of the upper limbs and extension of the lower limbs.

Tx

Symptoms should be relieved within 5–30 min of an IM or IV administration of a centrally acting anticholinergic (e.g. procyclidine 5–10 mg or benzatropine 1–2 mg). Benzodiazepines (e.g. diazepam 5–10 mg) are also effective. It must be remembered that the antidote is unlikely to last as long as the causative substance and subsequent oral doses may be needed for 2–3 days.

Oculogyric crises may look very similar to the spasms of both tetanus and strychnine poisoning.

Tetanus and strychnine poisoning → p. 245.

Neuroleptic malignant syndrome

This rare, idiosyncratic reaction is most commonly seen soon after starting antipsychotic (neuroleptic) drugs such as haloperidol and chlorpromazine; it can also occur with atypical antipsychotics such as olanzapine and quetiapine. The syndrome most commonly occurs 3–9 days after starting the medication but can occur in patients who have been taking the medication for a long time. Although it is thought to be idiosyncratic in nature higher doses, rapid increase in dose and intravenous use of neuroleptics appear to predispose to developing neuroleptic malignant syndrome. Typical features of neuroleptic malignant syndrome include:

- muscular rigidity
- hyperthermia
- autonomic instability – pallor, raised BP and tachycardia
- altered mental status

About 12–20% of patients with this syndrome will die, usually as a result of rhabdomyolysis, multiple organ failure, hyperprexia and disseminated intravascular coagulation.

Tx
- Give oxygen.
- Start fluid resuscitation
- Begin cooling measures (→ p. 249).
- Send blood for electrolytes, glucose, blood gases and creatinine kinase assay.
- Give an antimuscarinic drug to reduce rigidity (e.g. IV procyclidine 5–10 mg).
- Consider correcting any acidosis with bicarbonate (→ p. 264).
- Consider arranging admission to a high dependency unit (HDU) or ICU.
- Discontinue antipsychotic medication

Pharmalogical treatment options include diazepam, dopamine agonists such as bromocriptine and muscle relaxants such as dantrolene.

Serotonin syndrome

Serotonin syndrome is a disorder of serotonin excess caused by the ingestion of two or more drugs that increase the effect of serotonin on serotonergic synapses. It can be secondary to an acute overdose or as a result of

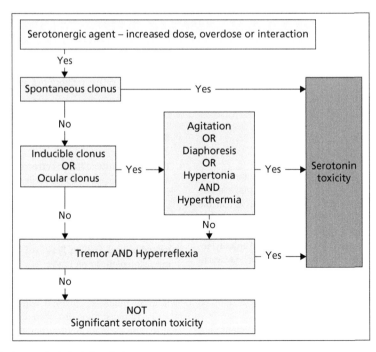

Figure 15.4 Hunter serotonin toxicity criteria.

taking prescribed medications. Medications that can be involved include, SSRIs, SNRIs, MAOIs, TCAs, 5HT3 antagonists, tramadol, triptans and stimulant drugs.

Symptoms begin within minutes to hours after exposure and there are three main groups of symptoms:

1 **Mental changes (seen in 40% of patients)**: agitation, confusion, hallucinations, drowsiness and coma
2 **Neuromuscular hyperactivity (seen in 50% of patients)**: tremor, shivering, hyperreflexia and myoclonus
3 **Autonomic instability (seen in 50% of patients)**: tachycardia, fever, hypertension or hypotension. Flushing diarrhoea and vomiting can also occur.

In severe cases, fits, hyperthermia, rhabdomyolysis, renal failure and coagulopathies may also develop.

There is a spectrum of toxicity from mild symptoms such as a tremor to severe with multi organ failure and hyperprexia occurring. Diagnosis is based on the Hunter Serotonin Toxicity Criteria → *Figure 15.4.*

Tx Most mild cases resolve spontaneously within 24 hours. Serotoninergic drugs should be stopped and electrolytes and creatinine kinase monitored in all patients. Supportive therapy includes anticonvulsants, IV fluids and cooling measures. Standard treatment of serotonin toxicity is benzodiazepines and in serious cases cyproheptadine and chlorpromazine can be given. Treatment of malignant hyperthermia with dantrolene (→ *p. 281*) may be required.

Poisoning with SSRIs → p. 289.

16

Abdominal pain and GI problems

Catherine Williams

Emergency Medicine Consultant, Royal Bolton Hospital, Bolton, UK
Health Education North West, Manchester, UK

Abdominal pain and gastrointestinal problems are a common cause for emergency department (ED) attendance. The differential diagnosis spans the full scope of acuity, from catastrophic to trivial, and encompasses surgical, medical, urological and gynaecological diagnoses.

ELDERLY PATIENTS

WITH ABDOMINAL PAIN

Beware the elderly patient with abdominal pain – statistically this cohort are at high risk of adverse outcomes. 20–30% will require surgery, and overall mortality rate is between 5% and 10%. Signs and symptoms may be subtle, and this may be compounded by cognitive impairment. Inflammatory response is often blunted due to age or medication (e.g. steroids), and vital signs may be influenced by medication (e.g. beta-blockers). Have a low threshold for referral and admission in this group.

Abdominal injury → p. 81.
Children with abdominal pain → p. 362.
Perineal problems → Chapter 17.

Immediate assessment and management

If the patient is distressed and in severe pain or otherwise clearly unwell:

- Give high-concentration oxygen.
- Start an infusion of crystalloid solution.

- Monitor pulse, BP, SaO_2 and temperature.
- Consider 12-lead ECG.
- Give intravenous (IV) analgesia with an antiemetic.
- Pass a urinary catheter if there is a distended bladder or any suggestion of fluid depletion.
- Consider inserting a nasogastric tube if there is abdominal distension.
- Seek surgical advice.

Causes of collapse with abdominal pain → Box 16.1.

A leaking abdominal aortic aneurysm is common, but the symptoms and signs are often minimal initially. The diagnosis should always be considered in patients who either have collapsed or have trunk/flank pain. Beware the elderly patient with 'renal colic'.

Further assessment

Ask about

- Site and speed of onset of the pain
- Character and duration of the pain
- Exacerbating and relieving factors
- Radiation of the pain
- Accompanying features such as nausea and vomiting
- General health, family and past history, drugs and allergies

The RCEM Lecture Notes: Emergency Medicine, Fifth Edition. Edited by Catherine Williams and Amy Nickson.
© 2024 John Wiley & Sons Ltd. Published 2024 by John Wiley & Sons Ltd.
Companion website: www.wiley.com/go/LNEM5

Box 16.1 **Causes of collapse with abdominal pain**

- Acute blood loss from the upper gastrointestinal tract (oesophageal varices and peptic ulceration)
- Perforation of a peptic ulcer, sigmoid diverticulum or the appendix
- Acute pancreatitis
- Leaking aortic aneurysm
- Mesenteric infarction
- Intra-abdominal sepsis with septic shock
- Ruptured ectopic pregnancy
- Hypovolaemia from any abdominal cause
- Diabetic ketoacidosis
- Cardiorespiratory pathology (e.g. myocardial infarction [MI] or pulmonary embolism [PE])

- Drug or alcohol use
- Travel abroad.
- Consider the patient's reason for attendance. If there is a long history why did the patient choose today to present – has something changed?

Look for

- Abdominal tenderness and guarding
- Rebound or percussion tenderness
- Rigidity
- Bowel sounds
- Loin tenderness
- Hernias
- Perineal signs (→ *Boxes 16.2 and 16.3*)
- Chest disease.

Sudden deterioration in a patient with abdominal symptoms is often caused by acute blood loss, frequently from the upper GI tract or an aortic aneurysm. Rectal examination or the introduction of a nasogastric tube can be diagnostic.

 Box 16.2 **Rectal examination**

This can provide information about:

- perianal pathology
- sphincter tone

- the rectal contents (empty, consistency of stool and presence of blood or melaena)
- the rectal wall (age >50 years carcinoma is common)
- pelvic masses or tenderness, including the appendix
- the prostate gland

If the presenting symptoms and signs could not be expected to be associated with any of the abnormalities in this list, then there is no indication to undertake a rectal examination.

 Box 16.3 **Vaginal examination**

This is a very invasive procedure, particularly for young or nulliparous women. Any necessary examination should be carried out only once, and by an individual trained to interpret the result. Do not consider undertaking any intimate examination unless you have:

- appropriate training
- an experienced chaperone
- privacy
- the confidence of the patient
- reason to believe that the findings of the examination will influence management

Before the examination
- Explain the need for the procedure and what it will entail (including any potential pain or discomfort).
- Give the patient an opportunity to ask questions.
- Obtain the patient's permission.
- Give the patient privacy to undress and later to dress; use sheets to protect the patient's dignity.

During the examination
- Do not make any irrelevant, personal or ambiguous comments.
- Encourage questions.
- Stop immediately if the patient becomes distressed or requests that you terminate the examination.
- Allow the patient to dress before discussing examination findings and next steps.

PAIN AND BLEEDING IN THE OESOPHAGUS AND UPPER ABDOMEN

Oesophageal pain

Oesophagitis is caused by reflux of gastric contents. It is sometimes associated with a hiatus hernia. The patient is often overweight and experiences burning retrosternal pain on lying flat and bending down. The pain is relieved by antacids and sitting up. Severity of symptoms does not correlate well with endoscopic findings.

> Oesophageal spasm is rare and should not be diagnosed in the ED. Myocardial pain is almost identical and is very common. Pain described as 'indigestion' does not reduce the likelihood of myocardial ischaemia.

Investigations: Consider MI → *p. 185*. A normal ECG does not exclude an MI and troponin assay is likely to be necessary.

Tx Once MI has been confidently excluded, if:

- the history is indicative of oesophagitis;
- the examination and ECG are normal;
- the patient responds to antacid;

then the patient can be discharged, and referral can be made to the GP for ongoing management. Lifestyle advice may include weight reduction, small regular meals, stopping smoking, antacids and alginates. A course of a proton pump inhibitor (e.g. omeprazole 20 mg daily for 4 weeks) will give rapid relief of symptoms and promote healing.

In patients with symptoms of dysphagia or aged over 55 years with weight loss, upper abdominal pain, reflux or dyspepsia, the differential diagnosis includes upper GI malignancy and prompt onward referral (via the 2-week wait system in the UK) must be made to expedite investigation.

Oesophageal pain and bleeding after vomiting

Oesophageal injury may be caused by repeated vomiting, often after excessive alcohol consumption. A small tear of the mucosa may cause bleeding (Mallory–Weiss syndrome). This may be a result of alcohol excess, gastroenteritis, cyclical vomiting, bulimia nervosa or hyperemesis gravidarum. This is the cause of up to 15% of upper GI bleeds and is usually self-limiting.

Occasionally intense vomiting may result in an oesophageal perforation. This uncommon transmural injury is characterised by diffuse, intense, retrosternal pain (Boerhaave's syndrome). Mediastinitis may then follow and is potentially fatal.

Investigations: If oesophageal perforation (Boerhaave's syndrome) is suspected, a plain chest X-ray may reveal air in the mediastinum or a pleural effusion. CT with oral and intravenous contrast can confirm the diagnosis.

Tx In cases of Mallory–Weiss tear, antiemetics and rehydration are the mainstay of treatment. Endoscopy (OGD) may be necessary to confirm the diagnosis; however in a low-risk patient, with small volume bleeding, in whom symptoms have resolved, this can be considered as an outpatient. → *Glasgow Blatchford Score Box 16.4*

Box 16.4 Glasgow Blatchford score

Risk marker on admission		Score	
Blood urea (mmol/L)	6.5–8.0	2	
	8.0–10.0	3	
	10.0–25.0	4	
	>25	6	
Haemoglobin (g/dl)	12–12.9	Men	Women
		1	–
	10–11.9	3	1
	<10	6	6
Systolic blood pressure (mmHg)			
	100–109	1	
	90–99	2	
	<90	3	
Other factors			
Pulse >100/min		1	
Melena		1	
Syncope		2	
Cardiac disease		2	
Hepatic disease		2	

>Low risk = Score of 0. Any score >0 is high risk for needing intervention (transfusion, endoscopy or surgery)

If oesophageal perforation is suspected, the patient should be kept nil by mouth and IV fluids prescribed. Analgesia, systemic antibiotics and antifungals are required, and the patient should be referred to a specialist centre for further management.

Bleeding from oesophageal varices → p. 314.

Dyspepsia and gastritis

Epigastric pain and tenderness are often seen in young adults, especially after alcohol ingestion. Vomiting may also occur, especially with a gastric ulcer. Some cases will settle with minimal therapy, whereas others will subsequently prove to result from peptic ulceration. The non-endoscopic diagnosis of gastritis is dependent on the history and the magnitude and duration of the symptoms and signs. Management depends on the severity and duration of the symptoms and signs. The differentiation between gastric and duodenal ulceration is of little clinical importance in the ED.

Tx In the ED, the key task is to rule out alternative diagnoses such as MI, perforated viscus, pancreatitis or biliary disease. Most patients with a recent onset of dyspepsia will settle quickly with antacids. A course of a proton pump inhibitor (e.g. omeprazole 20 mg daily) is also effective. Patients in severe pain will require analgesia and possibly admission for investigation, including barium meal or gastroscopy. The eradication of *Helicobacter pylori* is now one of the main aims of long-term therapy.

Patients aged over 55 years with weight loss and upper abdominal pain, reflux, or dyspepsia should be referred for prompt investigation to rule out gastric carcinoma.

There are three other serious acute presentations of peptic ulceration, none of which necessarily follow episodes of dyspepsia:

1 *Gastrointestinal haemorrhage → below*
2 *Perforation and peritonitis → p. 316*
3 *Pyloric stenosis → p. 365*

Gastrointestinal haemorrhage

The patient with a GI bleed may present with any combination of:

- haematemesis
- melaena
- passage of bright-red blood per rectum (usually lower GI bleeding)
- hypotension, shock and collapse
- subacute symptoms (fatigue from anaemia, etc.).

Upper GI bleeding (proximal to the ligament of Treitz) is typically bright-red haematemesis, 'coffee-ground' vomitus or melaena. However, brisk upper GI bleeding may present with red rectal bleeding due to rapid transit.

Peptic ulceration is by far the most common cause of serious GI haemorrhage (more than half of all cases), but bleeding may also be seen in:

- gastritis and gastric erosions (e.g. after alcohol or non-steroidal anti-inflammatory drugs [NSAIDs])
- oesophagitis
- Mallory–Weiss syndrome (oesophageal tear after vomiting) → p. 312
- oesophageal or gastric varices → p. 314
- diverticulitis (copious melaena or bright-red blood)
- neoplastic and clotting disorders (variable presentations)
- minor conditions of the rectum (e.g. haemorrhoids → p. 325).

Severe bleeding from the small intestine is rare.

For patients admitted to hospital with upper GI bleeding, overall mortality is around 1 in 10; most deaths occur in older people.

High-risk factors in patients with GI bleeding → Box 16.4.

Tx
- Protect the airway and give oxygen.
- Site two large-bore cannulae and send blood for crossmatch, clotting screen, full blood count (FBC), glucose, urea and electrolytes (U&Es), and liver function tests (LFTs). *Management of major haemorrhage → Figure 1.1 on p. 6.*
- Monitor vital functions and resuscitate with blood products.
- Discuss the patient with the admitting teams (often both medical and surgical liaison is appropriate).
- Correct clotting abnormalities (In patients taking warfarin give prothrombin complex concentrate [PCC]. Give fresh frozen plasma [FFP] in other patients with prolonged prothrombin time→ p. 258). Consider acquired haemophilia → p. 271.
- Give platelet transfusion in patients who are actively bleeding with a platelet count <50 × 10⁹/L.
- Tranexamic acid has not been shown to be effective in GI bleeding, and it may have adverse effects, so it is not recommended

- In suspected gastroduodenal bleeding, defer use of intravenous PPI until endoscopy has been carried out. In any patient with risk factors for varices, treat promptly as variceal bleed → *below*.
- Endoscopic assessment (which should be performed within 24 hours of admission) usually precedes any decision to operate and may be life-saving in very severe bleeds.
- Patients who are stable, with a Glasgow Blatchford score of 0 may be considered for outpatient management (→ *Box 16.4*)

Variceal haemorrhage

Haemorrhage from oesophageal (or gastric) varices is a devastating complication of portal hypertension that usually occurs in patients with chronic liver disease. The mortality rate is between 10% and 20% in the 6 weeks following the episode. Raised pressure in the portal vein usually develops as a consequence of increased intra-hepatic vascular resistance and increased blood flow through the portal system. Venous collaterals enlarge, in an attempt to decompress the portal system. These varices occur mainly at the portosystemic anastomoses in the gastro-oesophageal junction and the rectum. Post-hepatic causes of portal hypertension include the Budd–Chiari syndrome (hepatic venous obstruction) and constrictive pericarditis.

> In diseases such as cirrhosis, collagen replaces the normal hepatic matrix and impedes intrahepatic blood flow. Thus, 90% of patients with cirrhosis will develop gastro-oesophageal varices within 10 years.

The diagnosis should be suspected in patients with hae-matemesis or melaena who have a history or signs of chronic liver disease or a history of alcohol excess. Unexplained thrombocytopenia may be due to portal hypertension.

Tx
The treatment is that detailed above for GI bleeding with special attention to potential coagulopathy and throm-bocytopenia. For patients with massive bleeding, activate the major haemorrhage pathway and transfuse accordingly. *Management of major haemorrhage → Figure 1.1 on p. 6.* Otherwise, fluid repletion should be cautious, avoiding hypertension and transfusing to a haemoglobin of between 70 and 80 g/dL in haemody-namically stable patients (over-transfusion increases

portal venous pressure). There is no evidence that saline infusions are harmful in the presence of peripheral oedema or ascites.

- Prophylactic broad-spectrum antibiotics have been shown to reduce mortality (e.g. IV piperacillin with tazobactam or ciprofloxacin).
- Involve gastroenterology and intensive care teams early.
- In patients with massive bleeding, endoscopy should rapidly follow initial resuscitation. For stable patients, endoscopy should be undertaken within 24 hours.
- Vasoactive drug therapy controls bleeding by reducing portal venous pressure. This is achieved by vasocon-striction of the splanchnic bed, which reduces the blood flow into the portal circulation. Several drugs may be used:
  - Vasopressin (20 U IV over 15 min) induces vasocon-striction in almost all vascular beds. This causes inevitable side effects including myocardial and cerebral ischaemia. For this reason, nitrates are usually administered concurrently. However, the use of vasopressin has been largely superseded by terlipressin.
  - Terlipressin (2 mg IV) is a synthetic analogue of vasopressin. It is a prodrug with a slower onset of action, a longer half-life and fewer side effects than the parent drug. It is still relatively contraindicated in the presence of severe coronary heart disease, peripheral vascular disease or pregnancy.
  - Somatostatin (250 mcg IV bolus followed by an infusion of 250 mcg/h) induces vasoconstriction in the splanchnic vascular bed. It is seldom used in the UK.
  - Octreotide (50 mcg IV bolus followed by an infusion of 50 mcg/h) is an analogue of somatostatin. It is useful for patients who have contraindications to terlipressin or if terlipressin and somatostatin are unavailable.

Placement of a Sengstaken–Blakemore tube may be required as a temporising measure in continuing severe haemorrhage and is effective in up to 90% of patients. Variceal tamponade with a Sengstaken–Blakemore tube is most appropriate and safest for patients under general anaesthesia with airway protection. This device has two balloons and two aspiration ports (gastric and oesopha-geal in both cases). Inflation (with around 200 mL of air) and gentle traction on the gastric balloon alone is usually adequate to control bleeding. Inflating the oesophageal balloon may cause damage, especially post-sclerotherapy. However, if fresh blood continues to be aspirated from the oesophageal port, then the oesophageal balloon may be inflated to a pressure of 40 mmHg.

There are several ways of stopping variceal bleeding more definitively:

- Endoscopy (preferably under general anaesthetic [GA]) should take place within 12 hours of the onset of bleeding or much sooner in severe cases. Variceal band ligation is the preferred method to achieve haemostasis, or gastric varices may be injected with cyanoacrylate glue.
- An intrahepatic portosystemic shunt (TIPSS procedure) can be inserted via the transjugular route by an interventional radiologist. This decompresses the portal vein by creating an artificial shunt through the liver. This may be an option if bleeding cannot be controlled endoscopically.
- Surgical interventions include oesophageal transection or creation of a splenorenal shunt.

Hepatitis

Hepatitis is caused by the following:

- Viruses with an enteric mode of transmission (hepatitis A and E) → *below*
- Viruses with a parenteral mode of transmission (hepatitis B, C and D) (*immunisation against hepatitis B → p. 332*)
- Weil's disease (leptospirosis) → *below*
- Drugs.

Leptospirosis or Weil's disease: this uncommon infection occurs after mucosal contact with water that has been infected by rats' urine. It is sometimes fatal and should always be considered when a pyrexia and abdominal pain is found in people who may have been in contact with contaminated water.

After an incubation period of about 10 days (range 4-21 days), there is a rapid onset of fever, headache and myalgia. A purpuric rash sometimes develops, and jaundice is common.

Infectious hepatitis: Hepatitis A is by far the most common cause of hepatitis. Transmission is by the faecal–oral route, and the incubation period is 6 days to 6 weeks. Most cases occur in childhood and are asymptomatic or with only mild symptoms. Infection in adulthood is more likely to be symptomatic, but only a third develop jaundice. Outbreaks may occur in primary schools and in other institutions.

Hepatitis causes a variable degree of:

- anorexia and malaise
- nausea and vomiting
- abdominal pain and right upper quadrant tenderness
- jaundice
- dark urine and pale stools
- pyrexia

- urticaria
- hepatomegaly and splenomegaly.

Ix: Acute hepatitis is characterised by raised alanine aminotransferase which may be as much as 100 times normal limits. Leucopenia is common. Anaemia and thrombocytopenia may be present. There may be bilirubin and urobilinogen in the urine. Hepatitis viral titres confirm the diagnosis.

Tx Admission is required for patients who:

- are significantly jaundiced.
- are clearly very unwell.
- have an uncertain diagnosis.

Those with hepatitis A (young, short duration of symptoms and limited signs) can be treated at home and followed up by the GP. Strict hygiene must be observed with a light diet and no alcohol.

Biliary disease

Biliary pain is usually associated with gallstones, is almost inevitably recurrent and may be precipitated by a fatty meal, often eaten some hours previously.

Biliary colic: this is caused by the passage of a gallstone through the bile ducts and presents as sudden, constant (not colicky), epigastric and right hypochondrial pain radiating to the back. There may be tenderness in the right upper quadrant; nausea and vomiting are common. Symptoms may be transitory or last for several hours, with the pain disappearing as suddenly as it started. Impaction of a stone in the common bile duct is uncommon but is associated with more prolonged symptoms and the gradual appearance of obstructive jaundice. Prolonged obstruction of the cystic duct leads to acute cholecystitis.

Acute cholecystitis: acute inflammation of the gallbladder with or without intermittent obstruction at its neck causes:

- constant right upper quadrant pain, often referred to the back
- localised tenderness
- nausea and vomiting
- fever and malaise
- a palpable gallbladder with a positive Murphy's sign (sometimes).

The condition is differentiated from biliary colic by its less abrupt onset, longer duration, more profuse vomiting and the presence of a fever. In more chronic cases, dyspepsia may be the presenting symptom. Pain is worse after a large, fat-laden meal, and heartburn and belching are common. If these are the only symptoms, then further investigation can be pursued on an outpatient basis.

Rarely, in elderly or diabetic patients, perforation of the gallbladder may occur with subsequent biliary peritonitis. **Cholangitis:** infection of the biliary ducts is more commonly seen in elderly patients and is characterised by upper abdominal pain, fever and the development of obstructive jaundice (Charcot's triad). Hypotension and other signs of severe sepsis are common. Suppuration may lead to hepatic abscesses. *Escherichia coli* is the most common pathogen. The mortality rate is high (33%).

Ix: Early ultrasound examination visualises the gallstones and the swollen gallbladder and/or bile ducts. Abdominal radiographs are not indicated but may show air in the biliary tree in cholangitis if taken for other reasons. Inflammatory markers (white cell count [WCC] and C-reactive protein [CRP]) may be raised in acute cholecystitis and cholangitis, although 50% of patients with infection of the biliary ducts have a normal or reduced WCC. The plasma amylase may be mildly raised.

Tx Analgesia, IV fluids and admission are required. In the presence of a features of infection, antibiotics (a cephalosporin, ciprofloxacin or gentamicin) should be prescribed. Patients with cholangitis may have severe sepsis (→ p. 250), and IV piperacillin with tazobactam is appropriate antibacterial therapy.

Pancreatitis

The main predisposing factors are:

- biliary disease (gallstones)
- excess alcohol consumption

The pain is typically sudden-onset epigastric or upper abdominal pain, which often radiates to the back. It is usually accompanied by vomiting and may be relieved by sitting forward. There is epigastric tenderness and guarding, and there may be decreased bowel sounds (due to ileus). Pyrexia is uncommon, but tachycardia is usual. In severe cases (10–20%), the patient may become hypovolaemic and required aggressive fluid resuscitation.

Ix:
- A serum amylase >3× the upper limit of normal is considered diagnostic. Lower levels may be caused by other intra-abdominal conditions or by a MI.
- The sodium, potassium and calcium are usually low.
- The plasma WCC is invariably raised.
- The serum bilirubin may be raised.
- There may be hypoxia and an effusion on CXR.
- ECG may show non-specific abnormalities which may mimic myocardial ischaemia.

Tx
- Treat with prompt fluid resuscitation, parenteral analgesia and antiemetics.

- Keep the patient nil by mouth.
- Consider antibiotics if there is a strong clinical suspicion of infection (e.g. fever).
- Correct hypokalaemia, hypomagnesaemia and hypocalacemia.
- Admission to high dependency or intensive care may be required depending on disease severity.

> Hypomagnesaemia is common in patients with chronic alcohol excess or malnutrition.

Spontaneous bacterial peritonitis

Patients with cirrhotic liver disease may develop spontaneous bacterial peritonitis due to translocation of bacteria into the ascitic fluid from the gut (most commonly *E. Coli* and enterococci). Symptoms may include abdominal pain, diffuse tenderness, vomiting, altered mental status and signs of sepsis. Patients may also have mild symptoms or even be asymptomatic. It is consequently recommended that *all* patients with ascites who are requiring hospital admission should undergo diagnostic paracentesis. Samples should be sent for ascitic cell count, biochemistry and culture. Patients presenting with signs of systemic inflammation, GI bleeding, hepatic encephalopathy (→ p 257), abdominal pain or tenderness, should be given immediate empirical antibiotic treatment while awaiting ascitic fluid analysis. An ascitic WBC count of >250/mm^3 is considered diagnostic.

PAIN AND BLEEDING IN THE CENTRAL AND LOWER ABDOMEN

Peritonitis

Generalised peritonitis usually occurs secondary to a perforated viscus following:

- peptic ulceration
- appendicitis
- diverticular disease
- neoplastic or inflammatory bowel disease
- trauma
- iatrogenic injury.

It results in:

- severe abdominal pain
- a rigid (board-like) abdomen
- hypotension and shock.

The pain of perforation classically begins suddenly. Pain may subsequently ease slightly, but peritoneal irritation results in abdominal guarding or rigidity on examination. The patient may be tachycardic but is not usually 'shocked' initially. Symptoms may increase later as bacterial peritonitis develops, and the patient may develop signs of sepsis. The physiological response of immuno-suppressed or elderly patients is often dampened, meaning that clinical signs such as guarding or rigidity are reduced. *Abdominal pain in the elderly →p. 310*

Ix: An erect chest X-ray will show gas under the diaphragm in many cases; however, the sensitivity of erect chest X-ray (around 80%) is inadequate to rule out perforation. Abdominal X-ray is not indicated. A CT scan of the abdomen is helpful, before laparotomy, to confirm the diagnosis and elucidate the cause of the peritonitis.

Tx Fluid resuscitation, analgesia and surgical referral are required. Antibiotics may be given: piperacillin with tazobactam (or a cephalosporin and metronidazole) are reasonable first-line choices.

Leaking abdominal aortic aneurysm

Leaking aortic aneurysm is most often seen in an older (>50 years) patient who has generalised vascular disease. Symptoms and signs are variable but include the following:

- Back pain (sometimes with a previous episode a few days before)
- Generalised abdominal pain with vague tenderness and fullness (pain may radiate to the groin)
- Hypotension
- Pallor and sweating
- Sudden collapse.

Classic features are often absent; an expansile, pulsatile mass may not be detected, and the femoral pulses may be present and not delayed with respect to the radial ones. Pain may not be severe. Patients with contained rupture into the retroperitoneal space may be haemodynamically stable initially, with back pain as the predominant feature. All patients over 50 years presenting with abdominal, back or loin pain, or unexplained collapse should have this diagnosis ruled out promptly with point-of-care ultrasound (POCUS). → *Figure 16.1 and 16.2*

Only about 50% of patients with a ruptured aortic aneurysm reach hospital alive. A further 10% are unsuitable for surgery. For the remainder, the surgical mortality rate is about 40%.

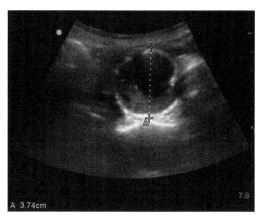

Figure 16.1 POCUS measurement of aortic lumen diameter.

Ix: Routine blood tests including clotting studies should be ordered. On admission, 60% of patients with a ruptured aortic aneurysm have coagulopathy, 40% have low platelets and 30% have impaired renal function.

The ECG often shows ischaemic changes because a majority of this group of patients have coronary heart disease and the pre-existing coronary ischaemia is worsened by hypotension. (Atherosclerosis of other vascular beds is also common.)

There is no indication for a plain abdominal radiograph. However, if performed in cases where the diagnosis is not yet established, it may show the lumbar vertebrae notched by a chronically expanding aorta and an enlarged, calcified vessel wall.

Ultrasonography will demonstrate an enlarged aorta. Aortic diameter >3 cm is considered aneurysmal. Risk of rupture increases with aortic diameter, but aneurysmal rupture can occur at any size. Point of care ultrasound is used to identify the presence of an aneurysm rather than detect rupture, as contained rupture into the retroperitoneum may not be detectable on POCUS. Identification of aneurysm in a symptomatic patient should prompt urgent discussion with a vascular surgeon. CT with contrast will demonstrate the position, size and extent of the aneurysm and enable surgical planning. The decision to proceed to CT versus emergency surgery must be made in conjunction with the vascular surgeon.

Tx
- Give oxygen.
- Monitor pulse, BP, SaO_2 and ECG.
- Place two large-bore cannulae.
- Volume replacement in the ED should be carefully controlled. The objective is to maintain adequate cerebral and coronary perfusion without increasing blood loss and a permissive hypotension strategy is

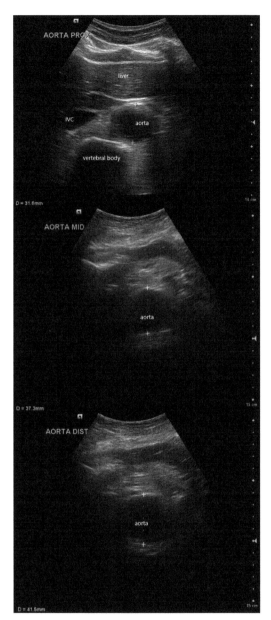

Figure 16.2 POCUS examination identifying aorta and other anatomical features.

recommended preoperatively. Fluids should be given until large pulses are palpable, aiming to keep systolic BP around 70–90 mmHg but no higher.
- Call for surgical and anaesthetic help. Prompt transfer to a vascular centre is essential if on a different site. Further investigation and treatment must not delay transfer.

- Blood products are likely to be required, but cross-matching must not delay transfer, and blood products are not usually transferred with the patient unless transfusion is already in progress.
- If in a vascular centre, cross-match 6 units of packed red blood cells and order a similar number of units of both FFP and platelets (median transfusion requirements are 6–10 units).
- Send blood for FBC, clotting studies, U&Es and glucose.
- Obtain an ECG and a CXR.
- Give IV analgesia as required, with careful dose titration.
- Pass a urinary catheter and measure the urine output.

Other intra-abdominal bleeding

- Ruptured ectopic pregnancy → *p. 331.*
- The diseased and enlarged spleen may bleed dramatically after trivial injury or even spontaneously (e.g. during malaria or glandular fever).
- Patients with haemophilia and those on anticoagulant therapy may bleed spontaneously. Consider acquired haemophilia → *p. 271.*

Management of major haemorrhage → Figure 1.1 on p. 6.

Mesenteric vascular disease

Problems with the blood supply of the bowel are difficult to diagnose, as clinical signs are limited and non-specific. These diagnoses should be thought of in older patients (usually >60 years) with other evidence of cardiovascular disease, who are disproportionately unwell and distressed for their clinical signs.

Mesenteric infarction: this usually involves the superior mesenteric vessels and is approximately equally split between cases of embolism and thrombosis. Symptoms are caused by infarcted, dying bowel in the abdominal cavity and are compounded by fluid loss into the bowel and perforation. Once the condition has developed, the patient is hypotensive and looks very ill. The pain is diffuse, severe and poorly localised. There is generalised abdominal tenderness and guarding with shifting dullness. Bowel sounds are decreased, and there may be some abdominal distension. Vomiting is an early feature, and bloody diarrhoea may be passed per rectum. The mortality rate is very high (>50%).

Mesenteric angina: recurrent bouts of severe abdominal pain in elderly patients may be a result of ischaemia of the bowel. The pain may be followed by episodes of obstruction or bloody diarrhoea (ischaemic colitis).

Mesenteric venous thrombosis: venous occlusion gives rise to a similar clinical picture to infarction but is even more insidious in onset and in symptoms and signs.

Investigations: Lactate is likely to be significantly elevated and to continue to climb on repeated testing. The haemoglobin and amylase are often raised, with a high WCC. An elevated D-dimer, although not at all specific, is a very sensitive indicator of ischaemic bowel, so a normal D-dimer makes the diagnosis less likely.

Plain radiographs are not indicated as they lack both sensitivity and specificity for this diagnosis. ECG should be performed to rule out coexisting myocardial ischaemia and to look for a source of emboli (e.g. atrial fibrillation). CT may demonstrate perforation, peritonitis or infarction.

Tx
- Administer oxygen to target oxygen saturations at 94–98%.
- Obtain IV access and administer analgesia and IV crystalloid.
- Prompt referral to surgical and intensive care colleagues is recommended.
- Give IV antibiotics (piperacillin and tazobactam is a reasonable choice).
- In patients who are unlikely to benefit from invasive treatment, the option of a palliative approach should be discussed with the multi-disciplinary team.

Appendicitis

Appendicitis may occur at any age but is most common between the ages of 15 and 30 years and is uncommon under the age of 2 years. The usual features are:

- abdominal pain (initially periumbilical or epigastric, later radiating to the right iliac fossa)
- localised tenderness
- nausea and anorexia
- mild leucocytosis.

Pyrexia and tachycardia are unusual. The right iliac fossa is usually the most tender and guarded part of the abdomen, but symptoms and signs may vary from the classic description:

- **Retrocaecal appendix**: pain may be elicited by right hip extension or be greatest in the right hypochrondrium.
- **Pelvic appendix**: rectal examination reveals tenderness high up on the right. There may be diarrhoea.
- **Gangrenous or perforated appendix**: signs of generalised peritonitis (→ *p. 316*). Occasionally, an appendix mass will have developed.

Ix: The diagnosis is made on the basis of history and examination; special investigations are not indicated in

> **Box 16.5 The differential diagnosis of acute appendicitis**
>
> - Urinary tract infection
> - Mesenteric adenitis
> - Ovulation pain (Mittelschmerz)
> - Salpingitis
> - Ovarian cyst torsion
> - Constipation
> - Pancreatitis
> - Psoas haematoma (in patients with haemophilia)
> - Perforated Meckel's diverticulum
> - Non-specific abdominal pain

the ED unless alternative diagnoses are being considered (→ *Box 16.5*).

Tx The patient should be referred for surgical admission.

Diverticular disease

This usually occurs in patients aged >50 years. There are three common acute presentations:

1 Inflammation (diverticulitis) causes periumbilical pain radiating to the left iliac fossa. There is localised tenderness and guarding in the left lower quadrant and a mass may be palpable. The patient may be pyrexial.
2 Perforation may occur without previous symptoms, producing acute peritonitis → *p. 316*.
3 Copious bleeding per rectum may occasionally cause profound shock → *p. 324*.
4 Complicated diverticulitis may result in intestinal obstruction, fistulae to bladder or vagina, perforation or intraabdominal abscess.

Tx Patients with acute diverticulitis who are systemically well may be managed conservatively with analgesia and advice to return if symptoms worsen. In patients with signs of systemic illness who do not require admission, consider oral antibiotic treatment (co-amoxiclav is an appropriate choice). Patients requiring hospital admission should be treated with intravenous antibiotics and referred for surgical admission. In cases where complicated diverticulitis is suspected, a contrast CT scan within 24 hours is recommended to confirm diagnosis and help plan treatment.

Inflammatory bowel disease

Ulcerative colitis: Ulcerative colitis is characterised by relapsing and remitting colonic mucosal inflammation. The patient with known ulcerative colitis may present to the ED with an acute flare of the disease, sometimes as the index presentation. Acute severe ulcerative colitis is a potentially life-threatening condition characterised by frequent and bloody stools (6/day), fever, tachycardia (>90 bpm), anaemia (<105 g/L) and elevated inflammatory markers (CRP >30). Truelove and Witts score can be used to assess attack severity.

Crohn's disease: this may rarely present as undiagnosed abdominal pain to the ED. There is usually a long history of recurrent diarrhoea and colic leading to anaemia and the development of an abdominal mass. The cicatrised small bowel may obstruct or perforate. If the patient presents with acute pain in the right iliac fossa, the previous history of diarrhoea may help to distinguish the condition from appendicitis. In patients with established Crohn's disease, presentations may include abdominal pain, abscesses and intestinal obstruction.

Ix: Check blood tests including FBC, U&E, LFT, CRP, ESR and magnesium. Stool culture and *Clostridium difficile* assay should be requested. Imaging with either plain abdominal X-ray or CT is recommended in acute severe ulcerative colitis. Assessment with flexible sigmoidoscopy will usually be necessary.

Tx: Replace fluid losses and correct electrolyte disturbances. Acute severe ulcerative colitis should be treated with high dose IV corticosteroids (100 mg hydrocortisone 6 hourly, or 60 mg methylprednisolone daily). Patients with IBD have a 2–3× risk of venous thromboembolism compared to other inpatients, and so prophylactic LMWH should be given, even in the context of rectal bleeding.

Joint involvement of both gastroenterology and surgical specialists may be required.

Intestinal obstruction

The basic causes of intestinal obstruction are as follows:

- **Blocked lumen:** food, foreign body, faeces and very rarely a gallstone
- **Thickened wall:** carcinoma, Crohn's disease and tuberculosis
- **Altered geometry:** intussusception and volvulus
- **External compression:** herniae, inflammatory bands and adhesions
- **Absent peristalsis:** paralytic ileus and mesenteric infarction.

The early features of intestinal obstruction can easily be mistaken for mild gastroenteritis. Small-bowel obstruction in the femoral hernia of an obese patient may be overlooked.

Paralytic ileus: this occurs after major abdominal surgery but is most often seen in the ED in association with retroperitoneal haematomas, spinal and head injuries, and electrolyte disturbances.

Small-bowel obstruction: this usually begins with periumbilical, intermittent and colicky pain. Vomiting is an early feature of jejunal obstruction but is delayed by a few hours in ileal obstruction. The patient usually presents at an early stage of the obstructive process; visible peristalsis may occasionally be seen in the slim patient, and bowel sounds may be increased. Central abdominal distension is occasionally evident. After the large bowel has been evacuated, there is 'absolute constipation' (no faeces or flatus per rectum). The patient will eventually become dehydrated and oliguric if there is a delay to presentation or treatment.

Large-bowel obstruction: this usually presents as an acute-on-chronic problem. Increasing constipation is the first symptom, and abdominal distension is marked before the colicky pains become significant. The caecum becomes enlarged and tender unless the ileocaecal valve is incompetent. Vomiting is a late feature. Dehydration and major electrolyte abnormalities are often present by the time the patient is seen in the ED.

Strangulated bowel: when the blood supply to obstructed bowel is impaired, e.g. by the neck of a hernial sac, strangulation quickly ensues. Pain may be sudden in onset and become more generalised. Rarely, these signs of impending necrosis and perforation are present without early evidence of obstruction if only part of the bowel wall is captured in a hernial sac (Richter's hernia).

Investigations: In the presence of obstructed bowel, an abdominal X-ray may show dilated segments of intestine and fluid levels (although there are many causes of fluid levels). It is not always easy to differentiate between small- and large-bowel obstruction → *Figure 16.3.* A CT scan is better at confirming presence of obstruction than a plain X-ray, and it may demonstrate the cause of the obstruction or reveal an alternative diagnosis. FBC, U&Es and glucose can be surprisingly normal or alternatively reveal gross dehydration and metabolic disturbance.

Tx
- Administer IV fluids. Fluid loss can be considerable, especially in small-bowel obstruction.
- Give analgesia.
- Consider the need for a nasogastric tube.
- Measure urinary output (may need a catheter).
- Refer to the admitting surgical team. Management depends on underlying cause; small-bowel obstruction often settles with conservative management, whereas large bowel obstruction usually requires surgical intervention.

Intussusception in children → p. 363.

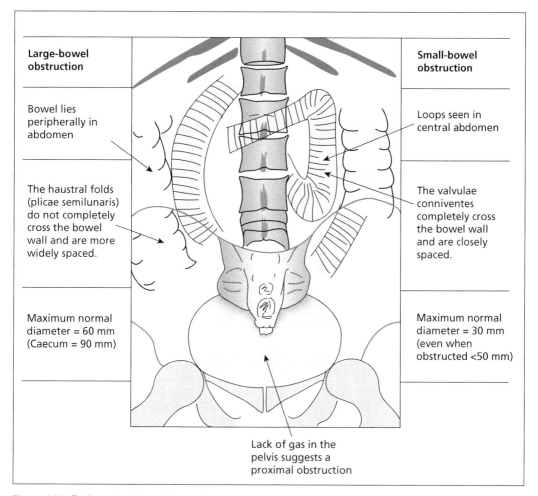

Large-bowel obstruction		Small-bowel obstruction
Bowel lies peripherally in abdomen		Loops seen in central abdomen
The haustral folds (plicae semilunaris) do not completely cross the bowel wall and are more widely spaced.		The valvulae conniventes completely cross the bowel wall and are closely spaced.
Maximum normal diameter = 60 mm (Caecum = 90 mm)		Maximum normal diameter = 30 mm (even when obstructed <50 mm)

Lack of gas in the pelvis suggests a proximal obstruction

Figure 16.3 Radiographs in bowel obstruction.

Gastroenteritis

Diarrhoea and vomiting in children → p. 362.

Gastroenteritis usually refers to a combination of diarrhoea with nausea or vomiting. Colicky central abdominal pain may also be present. The severity of the illness may vary from mild and inconvenient to severe and life-threatening. In high income countries, 'D&V' is the most common reason for missing work, whereas, in lower and middle income countries, it remains a leading cause of death. Acute gastroenteritis is usually caused by infectious agents (or their toxins). Viruses are responsible for 50–70% of cases in the UK, whilst a wide assortment of bacteria cause a further 15–20% and parasites are found in around 10%. These microbes produce GI upset by several different mechanisms: adherence to enterocytes, mucosal invasion, enterotoxin production and cytotoxin production (sometimes pre-formed before ingestion). All mechanisms result in increased fluid secretion and/or decreased absorption in the bowel. The increased luminal fluid content cannot be adequately reabsorbed, leading to dehydration and the loss of electrolytes and nutrients.

The history and examination are directed towards ensuring that the patient is not seriously ill and excluding other causes of GI upset such as:

- appendicitis → *p. 319*
- pelvic abscess
- infective and travellers' diarrhoea → *p. 266*
- metabolic disturbance
- recent antibiotic therapy
- recent surgery

- athlete's diarrhoea (up to a third of athletes have a history of GI upset; the cause is usually not clearly defined, although gut ischaemia has been implicated).

Ix: Further work-up is required only in patients who:

- appear seriously ill or dehydrated
- have a high fever, bloody stools, severe abdominal pain or persistent diarrhoea
- are immunocompromised
- are suspected of being part of a wider epidemic of gastroenteritis.

Tx Treatment in the ED is directed towards the following:

- Rehydration (oral or IV as required)
- Treatment of symptoms (especially fever and pain)
- Prevention of the spread of infection.

Oral rehydration is very successful, even for severe gastroenteritis. Small amounts of fluid can be given frequently, even while the patient is still vomiting. However, oral rehydration does not reduce the volume or the duration of the diarrhoea. A light diet should be reintroduced as soon as possible. Milk can be given safely. Despite the possibility of post-infective lactose intolerance, lactase deficiency is relatively uncommon, and most adults and children can tolerate non-human milk without any difficulty throughout a bout of acute gastroenteritis.

World Health Organisation (WHO)-recommended oral rehydration solution → Box 16.6.

Antiemetics may be useful in the treatment of nausea and vomiting. Antidiarrhoeals (antimotility agents) have traditionally been discouraged because of concerns about causing bacteraemia. However, they may have a role in the symptomatic treatment of mild-to-moderate symptoms in adults. Patients who are clearly ill or significantly dehydrated will require admission
Norovirus is also known as Norwalk or winter vomiting virus and is the most common cause of gastroenteritis in the UK. The infection spreads rapidly in hospitals,

other large institutions and cruise ships, with a short incubation period of between 12 and 48 hours. Norovirus infection is usually diagnosed by the history. Some of the early symptoms include nausea, a sudden onset of vomiting, moderate diarrhoea, headache, fever, chills and myalgia. Uncontrollable vomiting is a classic sign, and vomiting almost always predominates over diarrhoea. Spontaneous resolution occurs within 36–48 hours. Strict hygiene is essential to prevent spread.
Rotavirus causes epidemics of gastroenteritis in children's schools and nurseries.

Diarrhoea and vomiting in children → p. 362.
Scombroid fish poisoning → p. 299.
Travellers' diarrhoea and vomiting → p. 266.

Notifiable diseases: food poisoning, infectious bloody diarrhoea and suspected *Escherichia coli* O157 infection are all notifiable diseases.

Acute bloody diarrhoea in children → p. 362.
Haemolytic uraemic syndrome → pp. 362 and 271.
Notifiable diseases → p. 407.

Non-specific abdominal pain

Some patients have abdominal pain for which no obvious diagnosis can be found. Non-specific abdominal pain should be diagnosed only in an adult aged <50 years, whose minimal symptoms and signs settle quickly. If discharged, the patient should be given safety netting advice, and instruction to seek further medical advice if symptoms recur or persist.

Cyclical vomiting syndrome

This disorder may start in childhood or adolescence. Patients may present with intense episodes of nausea, vomiting and abdominal pain, lasting hours to days. The underlying aetiology is poorly understood but is believed to be closely related to migraine. A total of five attacks following this pattern (or 3 in 6 months) with full recovery in between and no other identified cause is required for diagnosis. Management is supportive, including IV fluid rehydration, analgesia and antiemetic. A less stimulating environment may be beneficial. Triptans may abort the episode if given early; however, evidence remains very limited.

Cannabinoid hyperemesis syndrome

Severe and recurrent bouts of vomiting may occur in patients with a history of regular (daily) or long-term use of cannabis. Underlying pathophysiology is not fully

Box 16.6 WHO-recommended oral rehydration solution

Na$^+$ 90 mmol/L; K$^+$ 20 mmol/L; Cl$^-$ 80 mmol/L; Glucose 20 g/L; Osmolarity = 310 mmol/L; CHO:Na$^+$ ratio = 1.2:1

The dose in severe diarrhoea is 250 mL (approximately 8 oz) every 15 min until fluid balance is clinically restored and then 1.5 L of oral fluid per litre of stool.

elucidated and may be related to splanchnic congestion and delayed gastric emptying. Dehydration and abdominal pain may ensue. Patients often compulsively take hot showers or baths to ease the nausea. Early research suggests that capsaicin cream may be effective in reducing symptoms. Intramuscular haloperidol has been shown to be effective in terminating an episode. The only effective long-term treatment is discontinuation of cannabis use.

Gynaecological causes of abdominal pain → *Chapter 17*

Pelvic inflammatory disease → p. 333
Ovarian cysts, torsion and rupture → p. 334
Bleeding PV → p. 332.
Ectopic pregnancy → p. 331.
Threatened and incomplete miscarriage → p. 330.

Non-surgical causes of abdominal pain

Many conditions may present with abdominal pain as a feature. They include the following:

- **Cardiac pain**: myocardial ischaemia may present as acute upper abdominal pain. Right ventricular failure, leading to hepatic engorgement, may be associated with right hypochondrial pain → *p. 185*.
- **Diaphragmatic irritation**: pleurisy caused by a chest infection or pulmonary embolus may present with hypochondrial pain, worse on deep inspiration. There is usually referred shoulder-tip pain in addition.
- **Pneumonia**: patients with pneumonia (particularly lower lobe) may present with abdominal pain → *p. 220*.
- **Alcohol withdrawal**: This may cause surprisingly severe epigastric pain and tenderness → *p. 379*.
- *Poisoning → Chapter 15.*
- **Diabetes**: generalised abdominal pain associated with hyperglycaemia → *p. 255*.
- **Acute porphyria**: recurrent attacks of generalised or right-sided abdominal pain → *p. 263*.
- **Hereditary angioedema (HAE):** recurrent attacks of colicky abdominal pain, sometimes accompanied by diarrhoea and vomiting → *p. 274*.
- *Migraine → p. 239, epilepsy → pp. 243 and 356 and lead poisoning → p. 305.* All may present with acute central abdominal pain.
- **Herpes zoster**: unilateral pain extending round either flank in the distribution of a cutaneous nerve. The herpetic eruption appears 24–48 hours after the onset of pain → *p. 441*.
- **Collapsed vertebra**: usually the result of osteoporosis but may be caused by a secondary neoplastic lesion or tuberculosis. Pain may be generalised and not evidently arising from the spine.

- **Muscle injury**: rupture of part of the rectus abdominis or avulsion of the origin of the external oblique produces severe abdominal pain. It is exacerbated by attempting to sit up with the arms folded over the chest.
- *Sickle cell crisis → p. 270.*

> A patient who has presented with acute abdominal pain should not be discharged unless the diagnosis is confidently recognised as non-serious or the patient has been discussed with and assessed by a senior colleague.

PAIN FROM THE GENITOURINARY TRACT

Ureteric ('renal') colic

In the UK, renal calculi have a lifetime incidence of around 12% in men and 4% in women, and these figures are doubled in those with a positive family history. The peak age for a first attack of ureteric colic is between the age of 35 and 45 years. It presents as severe and sudden bouts of pain radiating from the loin, around the flank, into the groin. Pain may radiate to the labia in women, or testicles in men. Vomiting and sweating are usual, and patients are often restless and struggle to lie still. The calculus is frequently held up proximal to the ureteric orifice in the base of the bladder at the trigone. The sensory nerve supply of the latter is identical to that of the external urethral meatus because they share a common embryological origin. Hence, trigonal pain is interpreted as arising from the tip of the external meatus. The patient may strain to pass small quantities of urine as the stone irritates the detrusor muscle at the vesicoureteric junction. Renal and ureteric pain may also be caused by infections such as pyelonephritis and conditions such as renal carcinoma and renal infarction. It can be mistaken for the pain of a leaking aortic or iliac aneurysm and also that of biliary colic and peritonitis.

Ix: Around 85% of patients with ureteric colic have haematuria (usually microscopic). Urine should be tested for blood with reagent sticks and then sent for microscopy and culture. Blood tests should include serum calcium and uric acid levels as well as standard FBC and U&Es.

A plain abdominal X-ray may be requested to show the course of the ureters in the abdomen and pelvis (a 'KUB' or kidney–ureter–bladder radiograph). However, although nearly 90% of stones are radio-opaque; in reality, a plain film has a low sensitivity as a first diagnostic investigation and has largely been superseded by CT. A non-contrast CT scan (CT-KUB) is both sensitive (96%) and specific (97%) for stones. As it has the added ability to rule out aneurysms and renal infarcts, it is the investigation of choice for patients aged >60 years. Intravenous urography (IVU) has a similar sensitivity and specificity for calculi and also has the advantage of demonstrating renal function. An ultrasound scan can be used to rule out an aneurysm but will image only larger stones (>5 mm) in the proximal or distal (not mid) ureters.

> The absence of haematuria and/or lack of positive findings on a KUB radiograph does not rule out the possibility of pain due to renal calculi.

Tx Analgesia must be given as soon as possible. NSAIDs (e.g. rectal diclofenac 150 mg) are effective for lesser degrees of pain and should be added to IV opiates and antiemetics for more severe pain. Many patients will require admission for further analgesia and investigation, including those with the following:

- Pain that has not completely settled
- Fever or other signs of sepsis
- Recurrent attacks of ureteric colic
- A raised creatinine level
- Stones >6 mm in diameter (too large to pass).

Other patients can be followed up in a urology outpatient clinic.

Stones elsewhere in the urinary tract: bladder stones are rare in the UK. Stones in the renal pelvis are common but usually present to the outpatient clinic or are entirely asymptomatic. (They may cause chronic, dull pain and loin tenderness with intermittent infection or haematuria.)

Urinary tract infection

The symptoms of urinary tract infection (UTI) vary according to the site of infection and the age and sex of the patient. Pyelitis causes unilateral loin pain, tenderness and fever. Cystitis gives dysuria, frequency and urgency with or without haematuria. Both may cause some lower abdominal pain and tenderness. Some patients with UTI will be generally unwell, with evidence of systemic infection but few localising signs (especially infants and elderly people). Beware of attributing significant abdominal pain to lower UTI in older patients – it is rarely the cause.

Investigation and treatment of UTI → p. 335.

Acute retention of urine

This causes severe abdominal pain, usually accompanied by a history of inability to pass urine. The enlarged bladder is easily palpable, although it may be overlooked in the obese patient. An ultrasound bladder scan may be useful (but is not essential) to confirm bladder volume prior to catheterisation.

Causes and treatment → p. 338.

Pain from the testis and epididymis

Scrotal pain is usually referred to the lower abdomen. Always examine the perineum of a patient with abdominal pain.

PERINEAL PROBLEMS

Perianal abscess

Abscesses arising from the glands of the anal canal present as extremely painful swellings around the anus. Deeper infection in the ischiorectal fossa may cause a more diffuse swelling of the buttock. The patient should be referred to the surgical team for drainage under general anaesthesia. It is totally inappropriate to attempt incision under local anaesthesia in the ED.

Pilonidal abscess

This presents as a tender, red swelling in the upper part of the natal cleft. The underlying pilonidal sinus may not be visible. Inpatient care is necessary for this condition.
Gluteal abscesses may extend deep into the buttock and are also generally best treated in theatre.

Foreign bodies in the rectum

Rectal foreign bodies may be difficult to remove because of spasm of the sphincters. Removal under general anaesthesia is often needed.

Rectal bleeding

The loss of a significant amount of blood from the rectum should be treated in the same manner as any other bleeding, i.e. resuscitation, crossmatch of blood and immediate specialist referral → p. 313.

Lesser amounts of bleeding, in an apparently well patient, can be referred back to the GP for investigation and referral as appropriate. Remember to consider the possibility of sexually acquired proctitis such as lymphogranuloma venereum (LGV) (→ *p. 337*)

Haemorrhoids

Haemorrhoids or piles are enlarged cushions of anal mucosa accompanied by varicosities of the neighbouring (superior haemorrhoidal) veins. They may cause:

- bright-red blood with and after the motions
- pain on defecation and consequent constipation
- perianal irritation
- a prolapse of mucosal tissue (on straining – second-degree piles; or constant – third-degree piles).

Tx If the bleeding has stopped and abdominal and rectal examination is unremarkable, then further investigation can be undertaken by the GP. Extreme pain such as that caused by a strangulated pile or suppurative, ulcerated lesions should be referred to the duty surgeon.

Thrombosed external pile

This is a perianal haematoma caused by the rupture of a tributary of the inferior haemorrhoidal vein. There is pain and a dark-blue swelling at the anal margin. If it discharges or begins to resolve spontaneously, then no further treatment is needed. If not, incision may be required either in the ED under local anaesthetic or in some cases by a surgeon in theatre.

Anal fissure

A tear at the anal margin may cause severe pain with defecation. It may be associated with a tag of anal epithelium known as a sentinel pile. Multiple fissures are a feature of Crohn's disease. Treatment is within the province of a general surgeon.

Perianal irritation

Pruritis ani is the predominant symptom of a perianal dermatitis. A build-up of moisture and small particles of faeces reduces the efficacy of the normal skin barrier in a manner similar to that which causes nappy rash. Scratching and secondary bacterial infection then compound the damage.

Tx
- The perianal skin must be kept clean and dry.
- Scratching and chemical irritants should be avoided.
- After every bowel action, the area must be cleaned by bathing or by using shower jets, a bidet or medicated wipes. Strong soap and abrasive methods of cleaning are not suitable.
- The area should be gently dried after cleaning with a soft towel or a hairdryer.
- Talcum powder, ointments and creams should not be used.

17

Obstetric, gynaecological and genitourinary problems

Amy Nickson

Emergency Medicine Consultant, Royal Bolton Hospital, Bolton, UK
Sexual Offences Examiner, Lancashire SAFE Centre, Preston, UK

OBSTETRIC PROBLEMS

The abdomen in pregnancy → Figure 17.1.

Precipitant delivery

In the UK, most pregnant women have planned maternity care and so have made clear arrangements for the delivery of their baby. However, occasionally women arrive at the emergency department (ED) in the second stage of labour (i.e. after the cervix is fully dilated). Delivery of the baby may be imminent, and assistance must be given (→ *Boxes 17.1 and 17.2 and Figure 17.2*).

Antepartum haemorrhage

This is vaginal bleeding occurring after 24 weeks' gestation and can be caused by placental abruption, placenta praevia, or other less common lesions. The bleeding of

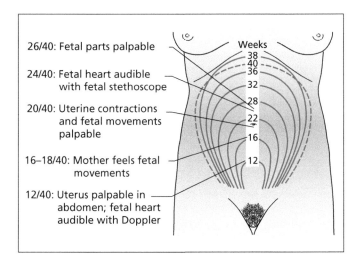

26/40: Fetal parts palpable

24/40: Fetal heart audible with fetal stethoscope

20/40: Uterine contractions and fetal movements palpable

16–18/40: Mother feels fetal movements

12/40: Uterus palpable in abdomen; fetal heart audible with Doppler

Weeks
38
40
36
32
28
22
16
12

Figure 17.1 Examination of the abdomen during pregnancy.

The RCEM Lecture Notes: Emergency Medicine, Fifth Edition. Edited by Catherine Williams and Amy Nickson.
© 2024 John Wiley & Sons Ltd. Published 2024 by John Wiley & Sons Ltd.
Companion website: www.wiley.com/go/LNEM5

Box 17.1 **Precipitant delivery**

- Reassure the patient and take her to a private room.
- Summon help (obstetrician, midwife, and paediatrician).
- Request a delivery pack, warm towels and turn on the neonatal resuscitation trolley heater.
- Try to ascertain the gestational age of the baby and, briefly, the obstetric history of the mother.
- Examine the abdomen to discover the foetal lie.
- Allow the patient to adopt any position that she chooses and administer Entonox if required.
- If liquor is draining, check the colour. Meconium staining indicates foetal distress.
- If the patient is 'pushing', look to see if the presenting part is visible at the vulva. If it is, put on gown and gloves and place towels around the delivery area.
- If umbilical cord is presenting, this is **cord prolapse** which is an emergency. Place mum in a 'head down tilt' on her left side and do not handle the cord except to gentle place into the vagina if protruding and call for help.
- As the head is delivered, encourage the mother to pant rather than push. If a **breech** appears, support the body gently **without** traction.

- Check for the cord around the baby's neck and free it if necessary.
- Allow the baby's head to turn laterally as the shoulders rotate. With the next contraction the body will be expelled. Deliver it by lifting the baby up and on to the mother's abdomen.
- If the body does not deliver or the head appears to retract, there is **shoulder dystocia**. Lie mum flat with her knees to her chest and discourage pushing. In a 'CPR grip', apply downwards pressure just above the pubic bone directed towards the side the baby is facing. A rocking motion can be applied if this is not successful. This is a serious emergency with high mortality for the infant if not delivered within 5 min. Call for urgent help.
- Tie or clamp the cord in two places at least 10 cm from the umbilicus and cut between the ties. If the baby is born in a good condition, this can be delayed 1–3 min to allow cord blood to return to baby.
- *For resuscitation of the baby → Box 17.2.*
- Administer 500 mcg/1 mL IM Syntometrine® to mum (kept in fridge). A rush of blood and lengthening of the cord represent detachment of the placenta which can be gently delivered (do not pull it hard).

placenta praevia is usually painless and starts around week 32 of gestation as the lower uterine segment is beginning to form. With abruption, severe blood loss and shock may occur in the absence of significant external bleeding (concealed haemorrhage). There may be pain and a hard, 'wooden' uterus. Abruption can be caused by abdominal trauma.

Tx The patient requires resuscitation with blood products and immediate referral to the obstetric service.

Digital vaginal examination should not be performed until an ultrasound rules out placenta praevia.

Postpartum haemorrhage (PPH)

Bleeding may occur soon after delivery or later in the puerperium. Bleeding after delivery is usually caused by uterine atony, a tear or a retained placenta. It is usually the later bleeds (secondary PPH) that are seen in the ED.

The most common causes are retained products of conception and infection.

Consider the '4Ts':

- **Tone**: uterine atony.
- **Trauma**: lacerations of the uterus, cervix or vagina.
- **Tissue**: retained placenta or clots.
- **Thrombin**: pre-existing or acquired coagulopathy

Tx Should include, depending on severity of bleeding; transfusion of red blood cells and FFP 1:1 ratio, IM Syntometrine (oxytocin 5 U and ergometrine 0.5 mg in 1 mL, contraindicated in hypertension), IV Syntocinon 5 IU by slow IV injection, IV tranexamic acid 1 g, bimanual compression of the uterus (in primary PPH). Bleeding >1000 mL is a major haemorrhage and requires immediate obstetric assistance.

Eclampsia

Women who are in late pregnancy or postpartum may occasionally present to an ED with eclamptic fits.

Box 17.2 Resuscitation of the newborn

Resuscitation Council (UK) algorithm for life support of the newborn infant → Figure 17.2.
Summon paediatric/neonatology help.
The assessment of the newborn depends primarily on three factors:
1 Colour
2 Respiratory effort
3 Heart rate

The Apgar score requires assessment of muscle tone and reflex irritability (grimace) in addition to these three parameters.
A pink, crying baby needs no active resuscitation. The baby should be dried, wrapped up and given to the mother.
A blue baby who is gasping or apnoeic and has a heart rate >60 beats/min is in a state of primary apnoea. This will often respond to:

• warmth and stimulation
• airway opening manoeuvres
• inflation breaths using a bag and mask

A pale, apnoeic, floppy baby with a slow heart rate is in terminal apnoea. He or she needs:

• pharyngeal suctioning if meconium seen in the mouth
• ventilation breaths for 60 seconds
• cardiac compression if the heart rate remains <60 beats/min (three compressions after each inflation with a compression rate of 120/min)
• intubation if there is a skilled operator present (clumsy attempts may result in vagal bradycardia and laryngospasm) (endotracheal [ET] tube size = 3 mm after 28 weeks' gestation) adrenaline via the IV or umbilical vein routes (the weight of a full-term neonate is usually about 3.5 kg and the dose of adrenaline = 10–30 mcg/kg)

Tx

• Summon senior anaesthetic and obstetric help.
• Manage the airway and breathing.
• Control the fitting with IV magnesium sulphate (→ *below*).

Magnesium therapy: Magnesium sulphate is the standard treatment for the control of eclamptic seizures. An IV injection of 4 g is given over 5–10 min, followed by an IV infusion of 1 g/h for at least 24 hours. If fits recur, then a further 2-4 g is given intravenously over 5 min.

Further information about magnesium → p. 261.

Pre-eclampsia: Symptoms include headache, swelling of the hands and feet and blurred vision after 20 weeks of pregnancy with raised BP and proteinuria. Admission for monitoring and antihypertensives is recommended if BP is >140/90. The patient should have bloods taken to look for signs of HELLP syndrome (haemolysis, elevated liver enzymes and low platelets). Signs of severe disease include BP >160/110, severe headache, epigastric pain, clonus or deranged bloods. First-line treatment for severe pre-eclampsia is oral or IV labetalol.

Major trauma in pregnancy

Management of major trauma in pregnancy → p. 32.

When patients in late pregnancy are supine, the uterus may compress the inferior vena cava. This impairs the venous return to the heart and causes a profound fall in cardiac output. To avoid this problem, women in the last trimester of pregnancy should be tilted into a left semi-lateral position or have the uterus manually displaced to the left.

Women who may have suffered abdominal trauma and who are rhesus D negative will require anti-D immunoglobulin.

Pregnant women are at increased risk of intimate partner violence. Remember to ask any pregnant patients with injuries if these were deliberate and if they feel safe at home.

Other presentations in pregnancy

Sepsis, pyelonephritis and pulmonary embolism are all common reasons for pregnant patients to be admitted to hospital. It is recommended that all acutely unwell patients in the 2nd and 3rd trimesters be seen by an obstetric team prior to discharge, or soon after admission, with anything but the most minor of ailments. Remember

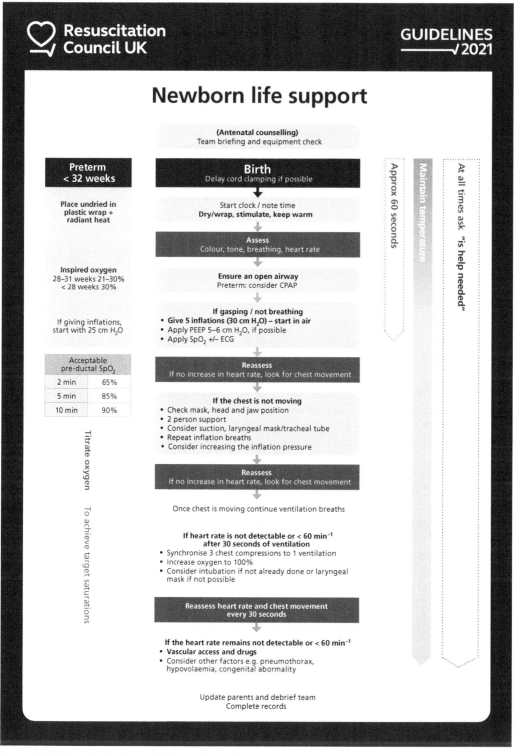

Figure 17.2 Resuscitation Council (UK) algorithm for life support of the newborn infant. Reproduced with the kind permission of the Resuscitation Council (UK).

to use observation charts modified for pregnancy, such as maternal early warning score charts (MEWS).

Chickenpox - any pregnant patient who has had contact with chickenpox and has not had previous infection or is unsure should be referred to the maternity team for antibody status testing and consideration of varicella zoster immunoglobulin (VZIG).

Reduced foetal movements – any patient who has felt established foetal movements and now has a change in this pattern of movements should be referred for foetal wellbeing checks by the maternity team.

Cholestasis of pregnancy – 1% of pregnancies are complicated by intense pruritus and raised serum bile acids. LFTs are usually normal. Treatment is usually with ursodeoxycholic acid (but the evidence base for this is poor) and induction of labour at 37/40.

Pelvic girdle pain – affects one in five pregnant women, causing pain in the pelvis, hips and thighs. Simple measures include paracetamol and advice about posture and movement. More severe cases may require mobility that aids up until delivery. The patient should talk to their midwife about further support within the local service.

Pulmonary embolism in pregnancy → p. 230

GYNAECOLOGICAL PROBLEMS

Guidance about intimate examinations → pp. 311 and 407.
Treatment of suspected rape or sexual abuse → p. 394.

Hyperemesis gravidarum

Hyperemesis gravidarum (HG) is a severe form of nausea and vomiting in pregnancy characterised by >5% pre-pregnancy weight loss, dehydration and electrolyte disturbance. Around 75% of all pregnant women experience some degree of nausea and vomiting, but hyperemesis occurs in only 0.5-2% of pregnancies and may affect the wellbeing of both the mother and the foetus. The peak incidence is at 8-12 weeks of pregnancy and symptoms usually resolve by week 20 in all but 10% of patients. HG is associated with rising human chorionic gonadotrophin (hCG) levels and conditions with higher levels, such as multiple pregnancy and gestational trophoblastic disease. Pregnancy-Unique Quantification of Emesis (PUQE) score is validated to classify the severity of a patient's symptoms (→ *see Box 17.3*).

Tx Rehydration with IV fluids is usually required. Safe and effective antiemetics include cyclizine, prochlorperazine and metoclopramide. Adjunctive therapy can include proton pump inhibitors (PPIs) if acid reflux is problematic, thiamine supplements if malnourished and electrolyte replacement.

Vaginal bleeding in early pregnancy

Vaginal bleeding in early pregnancy is common but does not always represent a miscarriage. It is estimated that around one in five pregnancies end in miscarriage,

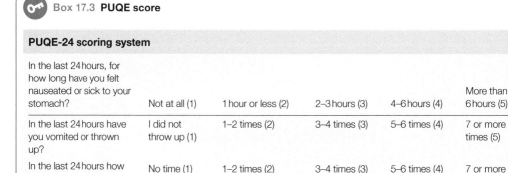

Box 17.3 PUQE score

PUQE-24 scoring system

In the last 24 hours, for how long have you felt nauseated or sick to your stomach?	Not at all (1)	1 hour or less (2)	2–3 hours (3)	4–6 hours (4)	More than 6 hours (5)
In the last 24 hours have you vomited or thrown up?	I did not throw up (1)	1–2 times (2)	3–4 times (3)	5–6 times (4)	7 or more times (5)
In the last 24 hours how many times have you had retching or dry heaves without bringing anything up?	No time (1)	1–2 times (2)	3–4 times (3)	5–6 times (4)	7 or more times (5)

Total score indicating severity of symptoms is the sum of replies to each of the three questions: mild ≤6; moderate 7–12; severe 13–15.

usually prior to 12 weeks. The ED will be a stressful and chaotic place for a patient worrying about losing her pregnancy and so effort should be made to provide dignified and compassionate care. Healthcare professionals often underestimate the psychological impact of early pregnancy loss and fail to provide the necessary support to help women navigate this difficult time.

It is unusual for patients in early pregnancy to be seriously unwell due to miscarriage, although haemorrhagic shock can occur if bleeding is severe, and cervical shock, causing hypotension, bradycardia and severe pain, can occur if products are lodged in the cervical os.

Tx Severe bleeding necessitates resuscitation with blood products and an oxytocic (e.g. Syntometrine 1 mL IM), if it is certain that the bleeding is due to miscarriage. Remember, young and healthy patients often do not show physiological signs of shock until very late! Removal of tissue from the os can be performed with sponge-holding forceps via a speculum which should immediately improve cervical shock.

It is recommended that women >6 weeks pregnant be seen by an early pregnancy service for an ultrasound scan within 24 hours, but those with heavy bleeding (using a sanitary pad or more every hour) or suspected ectopic pregnancy should be seen more quickly. Patients who are <6 weeks pregnant can be managed conservatively, as it would not be possible to visualise the pregnancy at this point with ultrasound. They should be advised to take a home pregnancy test in 2 weeks and return if they develop heavy bleeding or symptoms of ectopic.

Patients who are rhesus D antibody (RhD) negative with a gestation of 12 weeks or more must be protected from developing anti-D antibodies to foetal RhD-positive cells, which may have leaked into the maternal circulation. This is achieved by the administration of anti-D immunoglobulin within 72 hours of the onset of vaginal bleeding. The dose is 250 IU by deep IM injection for patients with a gestation of <20 weeks and 500 IU for those with a gestation of ≥20 weeks.

Ectopic pregnancy

Sites for ectopic pregnancies → Figure 17.3.

Ectopic pregnancy continues to be a cause of maternal death, often in women not known to be pregnant, presenting to hospital in shock or cardiac arrest where ectopic was not considered as a diagnosis. The diagnosis must be considered in any woman of child-bearing age with abdominal pain, collapse or shock.

UK incidence, 1 in 200 pregnancies, almost all in the fallopian tubes.

Pregnancy in isthmus of tube ruptures early (4–8 weeks' gestation) and causes sudden, acute lower abdominal pain and guarding with shock.

Pregnancy in ampulla of tube does not cause symptoms until 8–12 weeks' gestation. Blood leaking into the peritoneal cavity then causes intermittent pains over several days.

There may be any of the following:

- A history of amenorrhoea (perhaps only for a couple of weeks and not by any means essential for the diagnosis)
- Vaginal bleeding (may be minimal and is absent in about 25% of cases)
- Tenderness in the lower abdomen and adnexae
- Shoulder tip pain (referred pain due to blood irritating the diaphragm)
- Dysuria or diarrhoea (due to peritoneal irritation from internal bleeding)

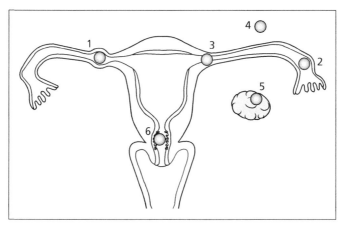

Figure 17.3 Sites for ectopic pregnancies: (1) fallopian tube – isthmic; (2) fallopian tube – ampullary; (3) cornual; (4) abdominal; (5) ovarian; (6) cervical.

Investigations: Serum or urine βhCG tests will be the first line if there is uncertainty about whether the patient is pregnant. Point-of-care ultrasound scan (POCUS) can be used to look for abdominal free fluid, suggesting ruptured ectopic. Consider ectopic pregnancy in any female patient of childbearing age who presents in shock. Stable patients will likely undergo transvaginal ultrasound scan and serial βhCG tests.

Tx
- Establish IV access and cross-match blood.
- Refer the patient to a gynaecologist.

Most ectopic pregnancies will be treated with either methotrexate or surgery, depending on the size of the pregnancy and whether it has ruptured.

Other vaginal bleeding

Heavy menstrual bleeding in a patient who is well and not severely anaemic can be managed in primary care, but a short course of oral NSAIDs or tranexamic acid can help reduce the amount of blood loss.

Severe bleeding may need admission for urgent gynaecological assessment. Post-menopausal bleeding or bleeding associated with a mass will require a 2 week wait referral for suspected cancer.

Emergency contraception

Two main methods are currently used for emergency postcoital contraception:

1 Hormonal therapy → *below*
2 Immediate insertion of a copper-containing intrauterine contraceptive device (Cu-IUD)

The Cu-IUD is the most effective method of emergency contraception (<0.1% pregnancy rate) and can be inserted within 5 days of unprotected sexual intercourse or ovulation, whichever is latest. It works by inhibiting fertilisation of the ova or inhibiting implantation if fertilisation has already occurred.

Oral emergency contraception, ulipristal acetate 30 mg, should be given as soon as possible, up to 5 days after unprotected sex, and is likely to be the more practical choice for the ED. It works by delaying ovulation so is unlikely to be effective if ovulation has already taken place. The pregnancy rate after ulipristal is 1–2% and has been shown to be more effective than levonorgestrel. The patient should use barrier contraception for the next 5 days as ulipristal is a progesterone receptor blocker which can impair the effectiveness of other progesterone containing contraception. Oral emergency contraception is thought to be less effective in patients with very high BMI and those on enzyme-inducing drugs, so

consider seeking specialist advice. Ulipristal is contraindicated in patients with severe asthma managed with oral steroids.

These factors should be borne in mind when counselling patients about emergency contraception whilst also remembering to discuss sexually transmitted diseases → *see below*.

Post-exposure prophylaxis for blood borne viruses

Post exposure prophylaxis (PEP) is the administration of antiviral therapy after possible sexual exposure or needle stick injury exposure to HIV, in addition to consideration of hepatitis B immunisation → *see Box 17.4*. Patients benefit from time taken to carefully explain the risks posed by their exposure and the reason why PEP may or may not be indicated. It can be useful to discuss the risk of transmission following blood exposure → *see Table 17.1*.

Risk of HIV transmission
= Risk that the source is HIV positive
 × Risk of exposure

 Box 17.4 Hepatitis B immunisation

- An accelerated course of hepatitis B vaccine should be initiated in patients who have received significant exposure and are unvaccinated (Day 0, 1 month, 2 months and 12 months post-exposure). Half dose is used for age 15 years and under. Those who have received exposure from a source with confirmed HBV should also be given hepatitis B immunoglobulin (HBIG).
- For patients who are partially vaccinated, a further dose of hepatitis B vaccine should be given and the vaccination course completed.
- Fully vaccinated patients who have received exposure from HBV positive or unknown status source should be offered a booster.
- HBIG should be offered in addition to HBV vaccine to patients who have received exposure from a positive or unknown status source and are known vaccine non-responders (AntiHBs <10 IU/mL 1–2 months post-vaccination).
- The dose of HBIG varies with age:
  - **Age 0–4 years:** 200 IU (2 mL)
  - **Age 5–9 years:** 300 IU (3 mL)
  - **Adults and children aged 10 years and above:** 500 IU (5 mL).

Table 17.1 Estimated risks of seroconversion after blood exposure

Infection	Route	Risk (%)
HIV (known HIV+ and not on antiretrovirals)	Mucocutaneous	<0.1
HIV (known HIV+ and not on antiretrovirals)	Percutaneous	0.3
HCV (detectable RNA)	Percutaneous	1–3
HBV (HBeAg+)	Percutaneous	30 (for non-immune individual)

Co-factors affecting the risk of HIV transmission include coexisting sexually transmitted infections, high HIV viral load, breeches in mucosal membranes, bleeding, trauma, and the type of sexual activity.

The use of PEP is recommended only when the individual presents within 72 hours of potential exposure, and then the drugs should be administered as soon as possible. Such exposure includes the following:

- Receptive anal sex with a partner of unknown HIV status or known HIV* (routinely offer)
- Receptive vaginal sex with a partner with known HIV* (routinely offer)
- Insertive vaginal sex with a partner with known HIV* (consider PEP)
- Insertive anal sex with a partner with unknown HIV status or known HIV* (consider PEP)
- Needlestick injury or splash into mucosa of blood from a person known to have HIV*

*with known detectable viral load or unknown viral load (people living with HIV who have undetectable viral load can NOT pass on the virus).

PEP is not routinely recommended for semen/bodily fluid splash injuries or human bites. Bodily fluids that are not considered infectious are vomit, saliva, tears, urine and faeces (unless any of these are visibly blood stained.)

The HIV risk from a needlestick from an unknown source in the community is minimal and so patients can be reassured.

The first-line regimen is tenofovir disoproxil 245 mg/emtricitabine 200 mg fixed dose combination plus raltegravir 1200 mg once daily for 28 days. This is better tolerated than previously recommended combinations, and so routine prescription of antiemetics and antidiarrhoeal treatment is not required.

In all cases of occupational exposure, send blood from the patient ('receiver') to the laboratory for storage and possible later testing (in the unlikely event of seroconversion, and this sample can be used to prove if the disease was occupationally acquired). Where the source patient ('donor') is known, the incident should be explained to them, and consent should be sought for testing for HIV, HBV and HCV if status not already known. If the donor patient is unable to consent, the decision should be made as to whether blood borne virus testing is in that person's best interest.

Consider discussing all cases for possible PEP after sexual exposure with a specialist genitourinary physician. All patients who have received PEP should be followed up at a specialist clinic (GUM for sexual contacts and occupational health for needlestick injuries).

Pelvic inflammatory disease

PID encompasses endometritis, salpingitis, parametritis, oophoritis, tubo-ovarian abcess and pelvic peritonitis as a result of infection ascending from the cervix. In the UK, around one-quarter of cases are accounted for by *Neisseria gonorrhoea* and *Chlamydia trachomatis* infection. The remainder of cases are caused by a range of bacteria usually found in the vagina. The risk is slightly higher in the 6 weeks following insertion of an IUD.

The presenting symptom is usually bilateral lower abdominal pain, although unilateral discomfort may be seen. The history may also reveal deep dyspareunia, abnormal vaginal bleeding (postcoital, intermenstrual and menorrhagia) and vaginal discharge. Signs include fever, abdominal tenderness and cervical motion tenderness. There may be tenderness of the uterus and in the adnexae.

Investigations: FBC and CRP should be taken but are non-specific and may only be elevated in severe disease. Send a mid-stream urine specimen for culture and perform a pregnancy test. Testing for gonococcus and chlamydia is necessary and may be via a self-taken vulvo-vaginal swab.

Tx A delay in treatment increases the risk of sequalae such as ectopic pregnancy, infertility and pelvic pain, and empirical antibiotic treatment is recommended prior to the results of microbiological testing (→ *Box 17.5*). Patients who are pregnant, have severe disease (pyrexia or signs of peritonism), or suspected tubo-ovarian abscess should be admitted for parenteral therapy.

 Box 17.5 Antibiotic regimen for PID

- Intramuscular ceftriaxone 1000 mg single-dose plus
- Oral doxycycline 100 mg BD for 14 days plus
- Oral metronidazole 400 mg BD for 14 days

Or

- Oral ofloxacin 400 mg BD for 14 days
- Oral metronidazole 400 mg BD for 14 days

Follow-up with sexual health is recommended for contact tracing and completion of treatment. Patients should be advised to avoid intercourse until they and their partner have completed screening and treatment.

Ovarian cyst

Torsion or rupture of an ovarian cyst typically presents with sudden onset intense lower abdominal pain. In the case of a large cyst with significant bleed into the peritoneum, the patient may complain of shoulder tip pain. There is often a palpable lower abdominal mass. However, presentation may be non-specific and easily mistaken for appendicitis or other cause – a high index of suspicion is required. Ovarian torsion presents with a sudden onset of severe unilateral pain (right more commonly than left) and vomiting, in any age group. 20–25% occur in pregnancy. It is also associated with ovarian masses and cysts. Ultrasound can show twisting of vessels 'whirlpool sign', ovarian oedema and reduced blood flow on colour Doppler but is not a 'rule out' test. Prompt laparoscopy with detorsion is the preferred treatment to preserve ovarian function.

Tx Perform a pregnancy test and take bloods for FBC and CRP. Refer promptly to the gynaecology team for urgent laparoscopy (do not wait for ultrasound results if this is delayed).

Endometriosis

Gives rise to recurrent or chronic abdominal pain, which is often cyclical. Pain may worsen after sexual intercourse, and defaecation may be painful. Gold standard investigation is laparoscopy. Prescribe analgesia – paracetamol and NSAID in combination are recommended. Referral to the general practitioner for ongoing management (such as oral contraceptives) and onward referral if symptoms are not controlled.

Ovarian hyperstimulation syndrome

OHSS is a complication of fertility treatments such as in vitro fertilisation (IVF), whereby the presence of multiple luteinised ovarian cysts causes high levels of oestrogens and progesterone and vasoactive substances that increase membrane permeability. Up to 1/3 of IVF patients experience some form of OHSS, but more serious cases require admission to hospital and occasionally ICU. Patients may present to ED with symptoms, including bloating, nausea and vomiting and then breathlessness. Clinical features are of ascites, hydrothorax, oliguria, hypoproteinaemia and acute respiratory distress syndrome in critical cases.

Tx Manage fluid and electrolyte replacement, and provide VTE prophylaxis and refer to the gynaecology team. Ascitic and chest drains are occasionally needed. Avoid nephrotoxics and NSAIDs.

Mid-cycle pain

Ovulation may sometimes be associated with unilateral pelvic or abdominal pain called Mittelschmerz.

Vaginal discharge

A slight discharge is normal in women of reproductive age. It may be increased by the oral contraceptive pill. Candidiasis (thrush) causes a creamy discharge with itching. Bacterial vaginosis (BV) causes a fishy, watery grey discharge with no itching.

Tx treat based on symptoms unless the patient is pregnant, has risk factors for STI, and has abdominal pain or recurrent symptoms:

- Fluconazole PO or clotrimazole PV for candidiasis
- Metronidazole oral for BV

Consider PID in patients with vaginal discharge and abdominal pain. Other patients should be referred to their GP or genitourinary medicine (GUM) clinic for vaginal examination, swabs and cervical smear.

Vaginal foreign bodies

Women may present with retained vaginal foreign bodies, most commonly tampons or condoms. The posterior fornix is the site where such objects are often lodged.

Tx The foreign body should be visualised with the aid of a Cusco's speculum and removed with sponge-holding forceps. A digital examination must also be performed if the object is not found. It is worth noting that occasional cases of missed intravesical foreign body have been described.

Women who have had a retained vaginal foreign body for some days may be at risk of toxic shock syndrome.

Uterovaginal prolapse

The sensation of dragging and heaviness in the pelvis and a palpable mass in the vagina may be alarming enough to prompt a presentation to ED. Uterovaginal prolapse can usually be identified as a soft tissue mass within the vagina or seen at the introitus. The patient will need to be referred for ongoing management by a gynaecologist as an outpatient.

Labial abscess

An abscess may form in the Bartholin's gland, which is situated in the posterior third of the labia majora. The whole labium is swollen, inflamed and extremely tender. The patient must be referred to the gynaecologist on call for drainage and marsupialisation.

Breast conditions

Mastitis is inflammation or infection of the breast tissue that usually (but not always) occurs during lactation. A complication of mastitis is a breast abscess, most frequently caused by *Staphylococcus aureus*. Redness, swelling and heat of the overlying skin, a fever or failure to improve with oral antibiotics should prompt referral to the breast surgeon for investigation and management of a possible abscess.

Breastfeeding patients should be encouraged to continue breastfeeding to prevent milk stasis, whilst applying a warm compress to the breast.

Refer urgently to breast clinic any patients with breast lump, skin changes or new inverted nipple.

GENITOURINARY PROBLEMS

Urinary tract infection

Urinary tract infection (UTI) is more common in women than in men; when it occurs in men there is often an underlying anatomical or pathological abnormality. Infection of the lower urinary tract is characterised by the classic symptoms of dysuria, frequency and urgency. Haematuria and proteinuria may be present, but physical signs are usually minimal. Suprapubic pain and tenderness are sometimes seen. A patient with pyelonephritis is usually systemically unwell with pyrexia, loin pain, rigours and tenderness over the affected kidney.

> In children and elderly people, UTI may cause general malaise with non-specific features such as pyrexia, vomiting, abdominal pain and confusion.

Tx
- Test the urine with dipstick and if positive for leucocytes or nitrites send an MSU to the laboratory.
- Commence antibiotic therapy in symptomatic patients with positive dipstick → *below*.
- Give advice on seeking help if symptoms do not resolve or if symptoms of pyelonephritis appear.

But note the following:

- In men, UTI is often secondary to sexually transmitted infection and so genitourinary clinic follow-up should be arranged.
- Elderly patients frequently have asymptomatic bacteriuria. A positive dipstick or culture does not always mean their illness is due to a UTI. Dipstick testing is **not** recommended in the over 65 seconds, but a midstream urine sample may be sent for culture if the patient has symptoms suggestive of a UTI.
- Urinary catheters are always colonised with bacteria, and pyuria has no relation to the presence of infection. Do not use urinary dipstick testing in these patients.
- UTI in a pregnant patient requires more aggressive management as pyelonephritis is associated with perinatal complications. Consider antibiotics and obstetric follow-up for asymptomatic patients with nitrites in the urine.

Antibiotics for UTI: the most common organism found in UTI is *Escherichia coli*. Other causative bacteria include Gram-negative bacilli of the *Proteus* and *Klebsiella* genera and enterococci. *Staphylococcus saprophyticus* is a common cause of UTI in sexually active young women.

For non-pregnant women, a 3-day course of trimethoprim or nitrofurantoin is recommended, or 7 days for men. Trimethoprim should not be used in pregnancy. Upper UTI can be treated with antibiotics such as co-amoxiclav, ceftriaxone or gentamicin. Consult local guidelines for second line management and treatment of UTI in catheterised patients.

Consider an NSAID as an alternative to an antibiotic in a non-pregnant woman under 65 years of age with suspected uncomplicated UTI depending on the severity of their symptoms. This is essentially a self-limiting condition, and antibiotic treatment may be associated with side effects.

UTI in children

Can present with a more generalised febrile illness, especially in the under 3 seconds. Alternatively, and in older children, there may be an obvious urinary problem such as dysuria, frequency, urgency, haematuria, enuresis or incontinence. The prevalence of UTI in children with undifferentiated febrile illness is approximately 5%.

Risk factors include age <1 year, female sex, previous UTI, voiding dysfunction, and vesicoureteric reflux. Infants and children with vesicoureteric reflux are more likely to have recurrent UTIs which may lead to renal damage and chronic renal failure.

Consider UTI in patients with unexplained fever or symptoms suggestive of UTI such as dysuria, frequency, abdominal pain and vomiting. Loin pain or tenderness (especially with fever) is suggestive of an upper UTI (pyelonephritis).

Investigation Collect a clean catch urine specimen. 'Urine bag' specimens and cotton wool balls in the nappy are not recommended due to high rates of contamination. Stimulation of the suprapubic area with gauze soaked in cool water can stimulate micturition and speed up the process. Test the urine with a dipstick test and send to the laboratory for microscopy and culture.

Consider a urine dipstick in a child with unexplained fever, although under 3 months of age a urine dipstick is not recommended. Instead send for microscopy (white cell count and gram stain). Start antibiotics if nitrites are positive but consider another source of infection if just leucocytes are positive, whilst waiting for culture results. In this, case urinary leucocytes can be due to systemic infection or inflammation outside of the urinary tract (e.g. appendicitis).

Tx Infants under 3 months with UTI should be referred for paediatric admission. Over 3 months of age, patients with suspected upper UTI who are well enough for discharge should be treated with oral cefalexin. Patients with lower UTI may be treated with trimethoprim or nitrofurantoin.

Children with recurrent or atypical UTIs (non-*E. coli*, sepsis, failure to respond to treatment, abdominal mass and poor urine flow) should be investigated with renal tract ultrasound. Follow-up with a DMSA (dimercaptosuccinic acid scintigraphy) scan may also be required for children under 3 years with recurrent or atypical UTI, or older children with recurrent UTI.

Haematuria in the absence of signs of infection

Patients with mild haematuria may be referred back to their GP. Those over 45 years of age warrant investigation for bladder cancer. Severe haematuria merits admission, especially in patients on anticoagulant. Beware of clots causing urinary retention (→*see below.*)

Prostatitis

Bacterial infection of the prostate gland can occur with *E. coli*, *Enterococcus* and *Proteus* species. The patient has the following:

- The features of prostatism – frequency, hesitancy and poor stream – possibly leading to retention
- Pain on ejaculation, lower abdominal, rectal and perineal pain
- Pyrexia, leucocytosis and a very tender prostate gland on rectal examination.

Tx Acute prostatitis is treated with either ciprofloxacin or trimethoprim for 14 days. Arrange follow-up for 48 hours' time to check response to treatment and review urine culture. Advise about the risk of retention and signs of tendonitis (if taking a fluoroquinolone). Consider admission for patients with severe symptoms, immunosuppression or signs of sepsis. Consider GUM referral for those at risk of STI.

Testicular swelling and pain

> A male patient aged <25 years with testicular pain must be assumed to have a torsion until proved otherwise.

Testicular torsion causes pain that is unilateral and usually, but not always, sudden in onset. It may radiate to the lower abdomen. There may have been previous episodes of the same pain. The testis is swollen and tender with a small hydrocele. Absent cremasteric reflex, a high riding testicle and patient who is vomiting are all extremely suggestive of torsion. In children, the presenting complaint may just be abdominal pain and vomiting, and unless the testes are examined the diagnosis will be missed.

Epididymo-orchitis may be seen in older men after a UTI, or younger men with sexually transmitted infection. The testis and cord are painful, tender and swollen, and the patient is pyrexial. Orchitis may also occur as a feature of mumps → *p. 442.*

Investigations: An ultrasound scan of the scrotum can distinguish testicular swelling from paratesticular lesions and can demonstrate free fluid and tumours but should not delay urological review for scrotal exploration.

Tx Patients with acute testicular pain or swelling should be seen by the urological surgeon on call.

Sexually transmitted infections

Most suspected STIs should be managed by the genitourinary medicine department, who have the expertise and diagnostics needed, as well as partner notification provisions. The common STIs occurring in young, sexually active people, are *Neisseria gonorrhoeae* and *C. trachomatis*. Gonorrhoea is asymptomatic in 10% of men and 50% of women, and Chlamydia is asymptomatic in 50% of men and 70% of women. Hence, many cases are detected through contact tracing and asymptomatic screening.

Early disseminated gonococcal infection presents as a triad of tenosynovitis, migratory polyarthritis and dermatitis and can lead to septic arthritis, endocarditis or even meningitis.

Chlamydia is the most common cause of pelvic inflammatory disease (PID) but is also responsible for some cases of reactive arthritis, presenting with a triad of arthritis, uveitis and cervicitis/urethritis. Lymphogranuloma venereum (LGV) is caused by L1, L2 and L3 serovars of *C. trachomatis* and leads to inguinal lymphadenopathy, genital ulcer and haemorrhagic proctitis. It is more common in men who have sex with men.

Fitz-Hugh-Curtis syndrome is a complication of both Chlamydia and Gonorrhoea and presents with acute right upper quadrant abdominal pain. Hence, it is important to ask a sexual history in patients presenting with a myriad of symptoms. The embarrassment about asking the questions more often comes from the doctor rather than the patient!

Ulcers, warts or herpetic lesions of the genitalia may present to the ED, especially if they make urination painful or difficult. Ulcers are most frequently due to herpes simplex or syphilis. Referral should be made to the GUM clinic. Petroleum jelly can be used on the area if there is irritation from clothes or skin rubbing, and NSAIDs and lignocaine gel can be used for more painful lesions.

Penile discharge is also invariably a symptom of sexually transmitted infection. It may be accompanied by dysuria and inguinal lymphadenopathy. Referral should again be made to GUM.

Human immunodeficiency virus (HIV)

HIV is a single-stranded RNA retrovirus which uses the CD4 receptor to enter and destroy lymphocytes, leading to severe immunosuppression over the course of around 10 years from the transmission of infection. Globally, 37.7 million people were living with HIV at the end of 2020. Modes of transmission include:

- Unprotected sexual intercourse with an infected person
- Injection of infected blood
- An infected mother to her baby before or during birth or by breast-feeding.

HIV infection can be encountered in any patient although it is most common in:

- Homosexual and bisexual men
- People who inject drugs
- People from sub-Saharan Africa (or sexual contacts of people from sub-Saharan Africa).

An acutely unwell patient with HIV may not be immuno-suppressed if they have been started on and are compliant with antiretroviral medications, and most HIV patients live a normal, healthy life. The patients most at risk of serious illness are those where doctors have failed to suspect and diagnose the condition.

The most common presentations of a patient with undiagnosed HIV to ED are with illness caused by seroconversion or an opportunistic infection (→ *Box 17.6*).

HIV testing should occur in ED where an indicator condition occurs; that is one where the prevalence of undiagnosed HIV in people with the condition is thought to be >1/1000. These conditions are listed in RCEM and British HIV Society guidelines and include

- STIs
- Herpes zoster
- Unexplained lymphadenopathy
- Mononucleosis-like illness (frequently seen during seroconversion)
- Community acquired pneumonia
- Peripheral or mono-neuropathy
- Unexplained oral candidiasis

> Before an HIV test, lengthy counselling is not required (unless a patient requests or needs it). The minimum requirement is just to ensure informed patient consent to the test.

Box 17.6 Opportunistic infections in AIDS

- Pneumonia, classically caused by *Pneumocystis jirovecii* (formerly called *Pneumocystis carinii*)
- Tuberculosis (pulmonary, or extra pulmonary, e.g. TB meningitis or miliary TB)
- Meningitis and encephalitis (headache, fever, fits and coma – toxoplasmosis, cryptococcal, *Streptococcus pneumoniae* and meningococcal)
- Bacteraemia (particularly non-typhoid salmonella, *S. pneumoniae* and mycobacteria)
- Gastrointestinal upset (anorexia, weight loss and diarrhoea – cryptosporidium, cytomegalovirus, salmonellae or atypical mycobacteria)
- Hepatitis
- Fungal infections
- Skin infections

Pneumocystis jirovecii pneumonia typically presents with a sub-acute history of increasing breathlessness and dry cough. CXR classically shows bilateral symmetrical peri-hilar infiltrates which could be mistaken for Covid-19 pneumonitis.

Investigations: CD4 count and viral load blood tests can be usual to assess severity of HIV disease, but the results will not be available immediately.

Tx A patient with newly diagnosed HIV or severe disease (CD4 <200) who presents acutely unwell should be referred to infectious diseases specialists. All HIV-positive patients with unexplained fever, neurological signs or any suggestion of significant infection should be admitted for investigation. Do not start anti-retrovirals without specialist input.

Pneumonia → p. 220.
Post-exposure prophylaxis → p. 332.
TB → p. 225.

Syphilis

Syphilis is on the increase in the UK. Acquired syphilis is divided into early (primary, secondary and early latent infection) and late (>2 years after infection) stages:

- *Primary syphilis* presents as a painless ulcer usually (but not always) in the anogenital area with regional lymphadenopathy. This ulcer heals in a few weeks and may go unnoticed. The incubation period of the underlying treponemal infection is usually 3–4 weeks (range 9–90 days).
- *Secondary syphilis* causes a widespread, polymorphic rash on the trunk (typically with involvement of the palms and soles as well). There is lymphadenopathy, mucocutaneous ulcers (especially in the mouth), headache and vague malaise.
- *Early latent syphilis* is characterised by positive treponemal serology with no symptoms.
- *Late syphilis* can present as neurosyphilis with headache, altered behaviour, difficulty coordinating, paralysis, sensory deficits and dementia.

Around a third of diagnosed patients are found to have primary syphilis, another third secondary syphilis and the remainder early latent syphilis.

> Moist primary and secondary syphilitic lesions are highly infectious!

Ix: Patients from high-risk groups presenting with genital or oral ulceration, non-itchy rashes or lymphadenopathy should be tested for syphilis. The diagnosis is confirmed by positive serology.

Tx Patients with positive serological tests or with suspicious ulcers on their genitalia should be referred urgently to a genitourinary (GU) clinic.

HIV post-exposure prophylaxis after sexual exposure (PEPSE) → p. 332.
Pelvic inflammatory disease (gonococcal or chlamydial infection) → p. 333.

Post-coital bleeding

Post-coital bleeding may occur in both sexes. Women with this symptom can be referred back to their GP for speculum examination and cervical smear. Occasionally very heavy post-coital bleeding will require gynaecology review. Sensitively ask if there was any genital trauma or non-consensual sex.

Men are usually found to have torn the frenulum of the foreskin. A small blood vessel may be bleeding profusely. It should be cauterised with silver nitrate.

Retention of urine

Acute retention of urine causes extreme distress. There is lower abdominal pain and an inability to micturate, although the patient may be unaware of the latter problem if obtunded. Painless retention should raise alarm bells for neurological pathology such as acute spinal cord compression

In male patients, retention is most often caused by obstruction of the urethra by an enlarged prostate gland, but a variety of other conditions may also cause it, including:

- urethral stricture (congenital or acquired)
- urinary tract malignancy
- urinary tract infection or bleeding ('clot retention')
- severe constipation or faecal impaction
- drugs (e.g. anticholinergics, tricyclics)
- neurological problems.

Tx Treatment consists of careful, aseptic catheterisation and controlled drainage of urine with treatment of the underlying cause as appropriate. Patients should only be discharged if there is a pathway in place for follow-up and removal of the catheter.

If transurethral catheterisation proves impossible or is contraindicated (e.g. in cases of traumatic injury to the lower urinary tract (*Chapter 6 Page 86*)), then suprapubic catheterisation will be required. This requires considerable experience to avoid complications such as bladder or bowel perforation.

In an emergency situation, with reduced specialist support, it may be appropriate to consider bladder aspiration with a fine needle as an interim measure.

Balanitis

Infection of the prepuce and glans may occur, especially in younger boys with an unretractable foreskin.

Tx Severe infection or difficulty with micturition merits referral. Other patients require:

- a local swab to be sent to the laboratory
- soak the penis in warm salty water 2–3 times per day, and avoid using soap of fragranced products on the area
- prescribe topical hydrocortisone/imidazole if simple hygiene measures were not effective
- referral to the GP or GUM for follow-up.

Some patients will go on to require circumcision.

Paraphimosis

Retraction of a tight foreskin can impair the venous return from the glans causing distal engorgement and extreme swelling.

Tx Reduction may be attempted in the ED. Analgesia and lubrication are obtained by the application of lidocaine gel or, if experienced, a dorsal penile nerve block (→ *Figure 17.4 and Box 17.7*). The thumb is placed on the

Box 17.7 **Dorsal penile nerve block**

- Insert a small needle at the base of the penis at 10 and 2 o'clock.
- You should feel a pop when passing through the superficial fascia.
- Aspirate to ensure you are not in a blood vessel.
- Inject 1–2 mL lignocaine (without adrenaline) on each side.

This nerve block also works well for zipper entrapments.

glans and gentle, but increasing pressure applied as the foreskin is drawn over it with the index and middle fingers. If this is unsuccessful, the patient should be referred to a urological surgeon. Reduction under anaesthetic may be required and occasionally, in adults, a dorsal slit is needed.

'Fracture' of the penis

Trauma to the erect penis during intercourse may sometimes rupture one of the engorged corpora cavernosa. This is known as a 'fracture' of the penis. The patient presents with a history of increasing perineal discomfort and bruising after intercourse. The penis, scrotum and

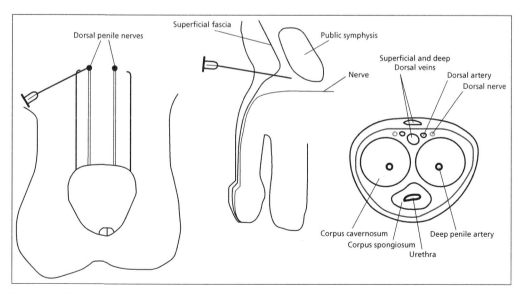

Figure 17.4 Dorsal penile nerve block.

suprapubic area are found to be very swollen and bruised without any other external sign of injury. Patients with this condition should be referred immediately to a urologist for exploration of the damaged area. If left untreated, impotency can result.

Iatrogenic priapism

This is defined as persistent erection of the penis, without sexual stimulation or desire. Causes include:

- Veno-occlusion/ischaemic – often due to sickle cell disease. This has the worse prognosis for future sexual function.
- Non-ischaemic – usually due to trauma or cavernosal injection causing bleeding into the

Tx First establish whether the priapism is ischaemic or non-ischaemic by sampling blood from the corpus cavernosum with a small gauge needle and testing on the blood gas analyser. Ischaemic blood will be black, acidotic, hypoxic and hypercarbic.

Non-ischaemic priapism will usually resolve spontaneously but will need admission under the urology team until it does.

For ischaemic priapism, attempt aspiration and phenylephrine, alongside referral to the urologist. Involve a haematologist if the patient has sickle cell disease.

- Draw up 10 mg of the α agonist phenylephrine into a syringe, diluted with saline to 20 mL (500 μg/mL).
- Insert a 19 G butterfly needle into either corpus cavernosum (3 or 9 o'clock position).
- Withdraw 20–40 mL blood using a syringe. This will usually relieve the pain.
- Inject 0.5 mL (250 μg) aliquots of the phenylephrine solution (via the same needle) every 10 min up to maximum 1 mg, while monitoring the patient's BP.
- If there is little improvement, the patient will require shunt surgery.
- Provide broad spectrum antibiotics.

18

Children's problems in the emergency department

Catherine Williams

Emergency Medicine Consultant, Royal Bolton Hospital, Bolton, UK
Health Education North West, Manchester, UK

Patients aged <16 years account for about 25% of the attendances at a typical emergency department (ED) in the UK, with a disproportionate number of such children aged <5 years. Experiences of hospitals gained in childhood may influence patients throughout their lives.

IN THE UK IN 2021 (BASED ON MOST RECENT DATA)

- Around 10% of children have a mental health problem
- More than 1 million children have a disability
- 67 per 10 000 children are in care
- 15.6% of children are from low-income families
- Over 80% of all illnesses in childhood are managed by the family
- Around 25–30% of calls to NHS 111 involve children
- ED attendances for children aged 0–4 years are 655 per 1000 children/year
- Infant mortality rate (<1 year) is 3.9/100 000
- Child mortality rate (1–17 years) is 10.8/100 000

Assessment of the ill or injured child: the differences between adults and children

Children differ from adults not only in terms of their size but also their anatomy, physiology, and psychological response to illness and treatment. Nevertheless, many of the principles of assessment and emergency treatment are similar to those applicable to an adult.

The size of children

Children range in weight from the 2 and 3 kg neonate to an 80 kg adolescent. The variable age and hence size of children affects physiological measurements, drug doses and equipment sizes.

Every effort should be made to obtain an accurate weight on your patient. In almost all cases, other than need for immediate resuscitation or severe injury it should be possible to weigh the child, and departments managing children should ensure they have appropriate equipment to enable this to be done reliably.

The RCEM Lecture Notes: Emergency Medicine, Fifth Edition. Edited by Catherine Williams and Amy Nickson.
© 2024 John Wiley & Sons Ltd. Published 2024 by John Wiley & Sons Ltd.
Companion website: www.wiley.com/go/LNEM5

> **Box 18.1 Estimating the weight of a child**
>
> Average birthweight of a full-term infant = 3.5 kg
> Between the ages of 1 and 12 years the approximate weight of a child in kilograms can be calculated by the following formulae:
>
> 0 – 12 months: Weight in kg
> $$= (0.5 \times \text{Age in months}) + 4$$
> 1– 5 years: Weight in kg
> $$= (2 \times \text{Age in years}) + 8$$
> 6 – 12 years: Weight in kg
> $$= (3 \times \text{Age in years}) + 7$$
>
> For convenience, the Advanced Life Support Group have also produced a quick reference table including estimates of weight and resuscitation drug doses.

In an emergency, alternative methods may be necessary. Options include:

- Parents/caregivers records
- Age-based calculation
- Length based calculation (e.g. Broselow tape).

Estimating a child's weight from their age → Box 18.1.

The anatomy and physiology of children

Children differ from adults in their body proportions. They also have a more elastic skeleton. This leads to a different pattern of injury and an airway that requires different techniques to manage. As a result of the elastic chest wall, children are far less likely to have rib fractures, although they may have severe underlying damage to the lung, liver or spleen (*also → Chapter 6*).

Children are generally able to compensate for acute illness more effectively than adults in the initial phase of illness, but may later decompensate rapidly.

The fast metabolism and low reserves of children explain why they get ill, hypoxic, hypoglycaemic and hypothermic very quickly. However, their general health and high capacity for repair make for a speedy recovery.

Consent and capacity in children → Chapter 20

IMMEDIATE ASSESSMENT AND MANAGEMENT

Cardiac arrest protocols for children → Chapter 11.
Principles of immediate assessment → Chapter 1.
Resuscitation of the newborn infant → p. 328.

> The skills required for the resuscitation of infants and children are best learned on an advanced paediatric life support course.
>
> A structured approach should be used, encompassing the same ABCDE approach as used in adult practice.

A – Airway

Checking for responsiveness

The presence of a response is usually immediately obvious. If it is not, then gentle shaking may establish verbal communication with an older child. The young child will respond by eye movement, cry or body posture.

> Always consider the possibility of an inhaled foreign body in children who are unresponsive or dyspnoeic.

The child's airway

Children are more at risk of airway obstruction than an adult. Their airways are narrower, shorter and more anterior. The narrowest point is the subglottis, creating a funnel shape which is prone to foreign body aspiration – and toddlers are particularly prone to putting things in their mouths.

Airway positioning in children and adolescents is the same 'sniffing the morning air' position as in adults; however, infants require a neutral position with face horizontal, parallel with the ceiling. Infants have a large occiput leading to neck flexion when supine. This can make airway positioning more challenging – using a folded towel or blanket under the shoulders can help.

Choking protocols → p. 207.
Management of other laryngotracheal obstruction in children → p. 208.

> Do not examine the throat with any instrument in children with stridor or suspected partial airway obstruction. Doing so may convert the problem to complete obstruction. In general, a hands off approach in such children until skilled help arrives is advisable.

The need for aids to maintain the airway is assessed on the same criteria in the child as in the adult. However, the soft tissues of the airway are more easily traumatised in children, and the gag reflex may be more sensitive, so airway adjuncts should be used with care.

Artificial airway and endotracheal tube sizes → Box 18.2.

Box 18.2 **Artificial airway and endotracheal tube sizes**

Oropharyngeal airway size = approximately the distance from the centre of the lips to the angle of the jaw.
Nasopharyngeal airway size = approximately the distance from the tip of the nose to the tragus of the ear.

Endotracheal tube size
Internal diameter (in mm) = (Age/4) + 4 [neonate 3 to 3.5 mm tube]
Oral tube length (in cm) = (Age/2) + 12
Nasal tube length (in cm) = (Age/2) + 15

Endotracheal intubation of infants

Intubation of infants should (other than possibly in cardiac arrest) be undertaken by senior staff with appropriate experience. The technique for intubation differs in infants as the relatively large floppy epiglottis needs to be lifted out of the way with a straight-bladed laryngoscope. Historically, the endotracheal tubes used in infants have been uncuffed, due to concerns about the risk of pressure injury to the tracheal mucosa. With modern endotracheal tubes and appropriate checking of cuff pressures, these concerns have diminished, and cuffed tubes are now recommended in most situations.

B – Breathing

The oxygen saturation shown by the pulse oximeter should be close to 100% in a normal healthy child breathing air.

Normal respiratory rates in children → Table 18.1.

Very slow respiratory rates in children suggest imminent respiratory arrest or poisoning with narcotic drugs (e.g. methadone).

Table 18.1 Normal respiratory rates and pulse rates in children

Age (years)	Respiratory rate (breaths/min)	Heart rate (beats/min)
>1	30–40	110–160
1–5	25–30	95–140
5–12	20–25	80–120
>12	15–20	60–100

Note that the heart rate is roughly four times the respiratory rate at all ages.

Oxygen therapy

Oxygen should be titrated to oxygen saturation, and in most cases, a range of 94–98% will be appropriate. Lower oxygen saturations may be tolerated in some cases, for example, stable infants with bronchiolitis appear to benefit from targeting saturations >92%. Oxygen should be delivered at the lowest concentration required to achieve target saturations – hyperoxia is increasingly recognised to have potentially deleterious effects. It is usually counterproductive to make an unwilling child wear an oxygen mask. Nasal speculum oxygen is usually better tolerated. In some cases 'wafting' oxygen via a mask held by a parent may be best in the short term.

C – Circulation

Checking for a central pulse

The brachial or femoral pulses should be used in infants rather than the carotid pulse. The absence of a central pulse or a rate <60 beats/min in infants indicates the need to commence chest compressions and treat as a cardiorespiratory arrest (→ *p. 169*).

In a child with ventricular fibrillation and no obvious precipitating factors, consider poisoning with tricyclic antidepressants.

Cardiac arrest and dysrhythmia protocols → Chapter 11 on p. 157.

Cardiovascular parameters

Normal heart rates in children → Table 18.1.

- Blood pressure varies with age. It can be difficult to measure in young, moving children. It is essential to ensure that the cuff is appropriately sized. Hypotension is a late sign of circulatory collapse in a child. Increasing cardiac output and then vasoconstriction will maintain blood pressure until late in the clinical course.

Check blood pressure cuff size is correct before acting on an unexpected blood pressure reading.

- A useful formula is:

  Expected systolic BP (in mm Hg)
  = 80 + (Age in years × 2)

- Blood volume is approximately 85–90 mL/kg in neonates, 75–80 mL/kg in infants and 70–75 mL/kg in children.

Important signs of circulatory disturbance in children

Diarrhoea or vomiting may lead to significant dehydration in a small child. Infection leading to sepsis may cause fluid maldistribution and circulatory collapse.

- Central capillary refill is a useful assessment of circulation – this should be checked on sternum or forehead, not peripheries which may be affected by environmental factors.
- Heart rate is a useful measure but may be influenced by fever, pain and distress. An unexplained or disproportionate tachycardia should be assumed to be due to circulatory compromise.
- Clinical signs of dehydration all have limitations. Reduced skin turgor is a very late sign. Dry mucous membranes may be obscured if sips of water have been taken.
- In infants, a depressed anterior fontanelle is a useful, if late, sign of severe fluid loss.
- Wet nappies, or their absence is a useful measure in infants and young children, this should be confirmed with the parent/caregiver. Weighing nappies may be useful in some circumstances.
- Infants with cardiac failure or fluid overload may develop oedema, which will be best appreciated in the dependent areas of the groin and sacrum. They may also develop hepatic congestion and hepatomegaly, appreciable on abdominal examination. This is a useful sign to check repeatedly during the administration of resuscitation fluid.

Venous access

The need for and site of intravenous access should be considered carefully. While in adult practice, 'routine' blood tests are often performed, in paediatrics, a blood test is a major, and potentially traumatic event for most children and so should only be used where a normal or abnormal result will change management.

Where clinical condition allows, it is recommended to use local anaesthetic cream to reduce pain during cannulation – this will make the procedure less distressing for the child and parent, easier for the clinical team and reduce difficulty encountered on subsequent attempts. Every effort should be made to maximise the chance of first-time success with careful preparation and positioning of the child – the best position in a young non-critically ill child is likely to be on the parent/caregiver's knee, with site of cannulation positioned out of site (e.g. behind the parent's back), and active distraction attempts. Adjuncts such as infrared vein finders or cold lights are helpful to identify sites for venous access.

In a critically ill child in whom intravenous access has not been rapidly obtained (maximum of two attempts), there should be a low threshold for obtaining intraosseous access (→ *Box 18.3*).

 Box 18.3 Intraosseous cannulation

- This is recommended in children if intravenous (IV) access cannot be achieved rapidly. It is a safe technique and so every ED should have the equipment and expertise. The intraosseous (IO) route can be used for both volume resuscitation and drug therapy.
- Mark the anteromedial tibia 2–3 cm below the tibial tuberosity or the anterolateral femur about 3 cm above the lateral femoral condyle
- Prepare the skin and insert local anaesthetic in a conscious child
- The use of an Intraosseous drill makes this procedure straightforward; however, the use of a manual needle may be of value in neonates and small infants.
- Attach the IO needle to the drill and insert the needle at 90° to skin until it rests firmly against the bone.
- Depress the trigger until a 'give' is felt as the needle enters the marrow cavity. The hub of the needle should not abut the skin, but stand a little proud.
- Remove the trochar and use a 5-mL syringe to aspirate and confirm the cannula's position. Blood samples may be taken – these are useful for point of care glucose and cultures, but cannot be used for full blood count or crossmatching. Theoretically, they can be used for biochemistry but can damage lab equipment so discuss with the hospital lab before sending.
- Volumes of blood/marrow obtained are likely to be small – this does not mean the IO line is misplaced.
- Fix the needle in position
- Connect an extension tube and three-way tap
- Give drugs or fluid in boluses from a syringe. This may require significant pressure and a standard drip or pump will not run adequately
- Check the site regularly (e.g. compress the calf if a tibial IO is in place) to ensure extravasation is not occurring- this can lead to raised compartment pressures if not noticed.

Fluid replacement

- Bolus fluid therapy = 10 mL/kg, repeated as necessary after further assessment up to 40–60 mL/kg in the first hour.
- In children with trauma, any evidence of uncontrolled bleeding should be sought and brought under control urgently. If there is evidence of bleeding, administration of blood products should be considered, along with prompt administration of tranexamic acid. In the absence of bleeding, fluid replacement with 10 mL/kg aliquots of crystalloid is appropriate.
- Maintenance fluid therapy:
  - 4 mL/kg per hour for the first 10 kg
  - 2 mL/kg per hour for the next 10 kg
  - 1 mL/kg per hour for subsequent weight.
  For example, a 25-kg child needs:

$$(4\,mL/kg \times 10\,kg) + (2\,mL/kg \times 10\,kg) + (1\,mL/kg \times 5\,kg)$$
$$= (40) + (20) + (5)\,mL/h = 65\,mL/h.$$

> As routine maintenance and replacement fluid, children should be given isotonic crystalloid.

> The palm and adducted fingers of a child's hand are approximately equal to 1% of their body surface area and can be used to make a quick estimate of the fluid replacement required for a burn (→ p. 142).

D – Disability

> Always consider hypoglycaemia as a cause for a reduced level of consciousness in children.

Level of consciousness

AVPU scoring (→ p. 8) is as useful for children as for adults. The standard, adult Glasgow Coma Scale (GCS) is suitable for children of school age but special variants of the GCS are more appropriate in children aged <4 years (→ Box 18.4). Even sleepy children should be fairly easy to rouse.

Other signs

- Agitation or an odd cry or affect may be the first signs of cerebral irritation.
- Check the fontanelle (if still open) for suggestion of raised pressure, however, be aware the fontanelle of a healthy infant will bulge with straining or crying.

> **⚷ Box 18.4 The Children's coma scale**
>
> | Response elicited | Score |
> |---|---|
> | *Best eye response* | |
> | Open spontaneously | 4 |
> | Open to speech | 3 |
> | Open to pain | 2 |
> | No response | 1 |
> | *Best motor response* | |
> | Moves normally and spontaneously or obeys commands | 6 |
> | Localises pain | 5 |
> | Withdraws in response to pain | 4 |
> | Flexes abnormally to pain (decorticate movements) | 3 |
> | Extends abnormally to pain (decerebrate movements) | 2 |
> | No response | 1 |
> | *Best verbal response* | |
> | Smiles, follows sounds and objects, interacts | 5 |
> | Cries consolably or interacts inappropriately | 4 |
> | Cries with inconsistent relief or moans | 3 |
> | Cries inconsolably or is irritable | 2 |
> | No response | 1 |

- Examine for tone and power in the limbs, looking particularly for posturing, asymmetry and abnormal movements. Always check pupillary reaction in a child with altered level of consciousness.
- Neonatal seizures may appear differently to the typical tonic–clonic seizure observed in older children and adults.

E – Exposure and environment

Comfort, warmth and the proximity of the parent or familiar caregiver are extremely important to children. Attention to these details early on can radically change the well-being and demeanour (and hence ease of assessment) of a child. Clothing may have to be removed to facilitate assessment. Exposure must be balanced with keeping the child warm and maintaining their dignity. Infants in particular can cool quickly in a resuscitation room, and use of hats, warming pads or a Resuscitaire® can be used to maintain body temperature.

F – Fits

Anticonvulsant therapy for children → p. 356.

'Febrile convulsions' are a common cause of seizures in young children and the temperature may rise before, during or after the seizure. In all children with seizures consider:

- hypoglycaemia
- meningitis
- poisoning
- cerebral oedema.

G – Glucose

Children are particularly prone to hypoglycaemia due to their low glycogen reserves and high metabolic rate. It is essential to check glucose in any unwell child, particularly those presenting with a reduced level of consciousness, abdominal pain or unexplained tachypnoea. Hypoglycaemia should be corrected with 2–5 mL/kg of 10% dextrose solution (0.2–0.5 g/kg of glucose) through a large vein. Intramuscular (IM) glucagon (20 mcg/kg) is an alternative if venous access is delayed. Symptomatic hypoglycaemia below a threshold of 2.6 should prompt a screen for metabolic disease.

H – History

The initial AMPLE history (→ p. 10) should be obtained from the child or from the carers.

I – Immediate needs of the child

Some immediate needs will have been assessed as part of the 'environment'. These include the provision of warmth, the removal of wet clothing and the need to ensure psychological support from the parent/caregiver. Unless requiring active resuscitation, the best position for a young child is almost always on the knee of a parent/caregiver (who may sit on the examination trolley to facilitate interventions). A position of comfort is also mandatory; it may be life-saving in conditions such as epiglottitis.

Analgesia

Appropriate analgesia must be provided promptly. Not only will this relieve distress, but it will also gain trust, facilitate a better examination and turn a fraught situation into a calm one. Provision of analgesia will not mask physical signs, and this should never be used as a reason to withhold it.

Limb splintage: simple limb support with troughs and pillows, or use of a sling can be very helpful in children

with limb injuries and help reduce pain and distress. Distal circulation should be assessed before and after positioning limbs in the same way in children as in adults.

Covering wounds promptly with dressings will be helpful in reducing distress caused by the appearance of the injury

Cervical collars and blocks: conscious children often do not tolerate these well. If immobilisation is distressing a child significantly, its removal is preferable. The use of manual inline stabilisation is better tolerated. A child who is struggling or distressed due to immobilisation is likely to move the neck more than a calm child lying still without immobilisation.

Ask yourself

Does this child need:

- drugs to relieve pain? (→ *Boxes 18.5 and 18.6*)
- splintage?
- freedom from splintage?

Box 18.5 Opiate analgesics for children

Children aged >12 months

Morphine injection	0.1–0.2 mg/kg
Fentanyl injection	Increments of 0.5 mcg/kg
Diamorphine intranasal spray	0.1 mg/kg
Oral morphine solution	0.2–0.4 mg/kg

Infants aged between 3 and 12 months
They should be given half the above doses of morphine

Infants aged <3 months
They are especially sensitive to opioids and so should be given a quarter of the usual paediatric dose

Box 18.6 Antipyretic analgesics for children

Should be given to relieve distress rather than with the sole aim of bringing down the temperature

Paracetamol suspension
10–15 mg/kg every 4–6 hours; paracetamol may also be given rectally as a suppository (loading dose = 15–20 mg/kg).

Ibuprofen suspension
5 mg/kg up to four times a day

FURTHER ASSESSMENT OF THE CHILD

This will be greatly facilitated by a gentle approach and a child-friendly environment.

Additional features in a paediatric history

Perinatal history

A clear perinatal and birth history is especially important when treating infants and younger children. This should include details about the birth and whether there was any need for resuscitation or neonatal intensive care (NICU). Maternal health and medication history is important in the neonatal period. If your patient is still in the neonatal period, ask about risk factors for neonatal sepsis (prolonged rupture of membranes, maternal pyrexia) and any treatment given at the time.

Siblings and family history

Understanding the family circumstances is essential in any paediatric history, and it should become routine to ask about siblings, family make-up and who lives at home with the child. Remember the adult with the child may not be the full-time caregiver. Previous health problems encountered by siblings will have a great impact on the family's response to this episode – particularly if they have experienced loss of a child.

Consanguinity may be important when considering genetic conditions, and this should form a routine part of history taking.

Development

Establish whether the parents/caregivers have any concerns regarding the child's development and ask about developmental milestones relevant to the age of the child. In the school-age child, this can include questions about play, schoolwork, activities and relationships.

Immunisations

It is important to understand which immunisations your patient has received and reasons for any missed immunisations where relevant. Remember that different countries have different immunisation schedules. Current UK schedule of immunisation in the UK → *Table 18.7 on p. 368.*

Communication with children

A visit to the emergency department and an assessment by a healthcare professional can be a frightening experience for children of all ages. Engaging and communicating with your child patient is essential, and communication needs to be pitched at their level in a manner that is non-threatening. In an infant, this may be as simple as smiling, blowing bubbles or showing an interest in a toy. Adjust your language according to the terms used by parent and child when referring to body parts. Children can be surprisingly sophisticated in their language and understanding – do not underestimate their ability to tell their own story. Asking the child for their account first before corroborating key facts with the parent/carer can be an effective strategy.

Children with complex needs and/or learning difficulties may require different communication strategies. Care givers will be experts in communicating with the child in an effective manner so follow their lead. Never assume that the child cannot communicate or understand – non-verbal children are often able to communicate their needs using Makaton (or similar sign language), facial expressions or vocalisations, which the parent/caregiver will usually be able to interpret.

Do not hesitate to use translation services where necessary – many children may be more adept at English than their parents and should not be put in the position of translator during the consultation.

Examination may need to be opportunistic and adapted to the child. In young children in particular, playing with them can often yield far more information than a clumsy attempt at a 'formal examination' in a resistant child. Many departments have play therapists who are highly skilled in working with children and young people, and experienced paediatric nursing support is invaluable.

The needs of the adolescent

Adolescence is an important developmental phase, during which the patient transitions from being a child to being an adult. Emergency department attendances of this group are rapidly rising, and their particular biopsychosocial needs are distinct.

It should be routine to offer to see an adolescent patient independently of their parents/caregivers. This is an important part of transition to adult care and gives the patient a vital opportunity to discuss potentially embarrassing topics in private.

Use of the HEEADSSS assessment provides a framework for exploring the biopsychosocial needs of the adolescent patient – it is important this is carried out empathetically, as a conversation rather than a checklist to be completed!

HEEEADDS assessment → *Box 18.7*
Consent and capacity in children→ *Chapter 20*

 Box 18.7 HEEADSSS assessment

- HOME: Who is at home? What are the relationships like?
- EDUCATION: School attendance? Stress of exams? Bullying? Friends?
- EATING: Stress from eating habits, weight or body shape changes?
- ACTIVITIES: Do you have any hobbies? Internet use? Meeting with friends?
- DRUGS?: Do you use drugs or alcohol? Do friends or family?
- SEXUALITY?: Previous or current relationships? Sexual orientation? Gender uncertainty/discomfort?
- SUICIDE?: Low mood? Stress? Current or previous thoughts of self-harm?
- SAFETY: Risk-taking behaviour? Violence or bullying at school or home?

The needs of the parents

It is essential to understand, empathise with and directly address parental concerns, even if you do not share them following your assessment. Parent/caregivers are the experts in their child and will often pick up subtle signs of deterioration that healthcare professionals may overlook. Several early warning score systems now include 'parental concern' as a key component as a result.

To enact your management plan, you will need the understanding, cooperation and often active participation of the parent/caregivers (especially if you are contemplating discharge or outpatient management). Take the time to ensure that they understand and are happy with the proposed treatment.

Whenever possible (almost always) the parent/caregiver should be allowed to remain with their child, including during cardiopulmonary resuscitation. If conscious, their presence will calm and reassure your patient. Witnessing resuscitation attempts is believed to be beneficial to the bereavement process in the event of an unsuccessful resuscitation.

Continuing assessment

Assessment must continue during initial treatment and transportation. Children may change their physiological status very rapidly. It is particularly important to assess the effect of any interventions.

Monitoring must be appropriate to the child's condition and should not replace careful observation. It needs to be considered in terms of both usefulness of information obtained and acceptability to the child. In a conscious child, this probably means that:

- pulse oximetry is better than
- ECG monitoring, which is better than
- BP monitoring.

Consideration of other children in the vicinity

In many situations, such as severe infections, fires, poisoning and abuse, other children may have been exposed to the same agents as the patient. In such cases, it is appropriate to assess the risk to these children also.

RESPIRATORY PROBLEMS

Also → *Chapter 13*.

Respiratory disorders are responsible for around a third of all paediatric admissions to hospital in the UK.

Stridor

Angio-oedema → *pp. 274 and 306*.
Foreign body obstruction → *p. 1*.

Stridor is a harsh respiratory noise, which is loudest in inspiration and usually indicates obstruction of the extrathoracic airways. It can be caused by:

- epiglottitis (supraglottitis)
- laryngotracheobronchitis (croup)
- bacterial tracheitis
- foreign body obstruction
- angio-oedema
- thermal, chemical or other damage to the airways
- other rarer causes of obstruction (e.g. diphtheria, quinsy, glandular fever).

Accompanying features, including the degree of respiratory distress, depend on the cause of the stridor. They may include:

- hoarseness or inability to speak
- coughing
- drooling
- sternal and subcostal recession (this is a good indicator of the degree of obstruction whereas the intensity of the stridor is not)
- tachypnoea and tachycardia
- indicators of hypoxia such as cyanosis, agitation or drowsiness.

Do not put anything, including a spatula or a thermometer, in the mouth of a child with stridor – it may precipitate complete respiratory obstruction.

Differences between epiglottitis and croup

Epiglottitis is fortunately now rare in children in the UK thanks to vaccination against *H. Influenzae*. Croup, however, remains prevalent and is a common cause of ED attendance. Despite its name, the swelling of epiglottitis usually involves more than just the bright-red, cherry-like epiglottis. It is, in fact, a complete 'top of the larynx-itis'. This is different from the 'bottom of the larynx-itis' caused by croup. Spasmodic or recurrent croup is a variant form of the disease, which is more common in atopic children and is thought to have an allergic component.

Differences between the two most common infectious causes of stridor → Table 18.2.

Table 18.2 Differences between epiglottitis and croup

	Epiglottitis	Croup
Age of child	1–6 years	6 months–5 years
Onset of symptoms	Hours	Days
Runny nose	No	Yes
Cough	Slight	Characteristic barking
Speech	Difficult	Hoarse
Stridor	Soft	Harsh
Able to drink	No	Yes
Drooling	Yes	No
Pyrexia	>38.5°C	<38.5°C
Appearance	Pale and toxic	Variable
Respiratory distress	Severe	Variable
Site affected	Supraglottis	Lower larynx and trachea
Causative organism	*Haemophilus influenzae* b	Parainfluenza and other viruses
Decreased incidence (since Hib vaccine)	Yes – now rare in the UK	No – still common
Need for observation	Yes	Yes
Need for intubation	Yes	Sometimes (5%)
Need for antibiotics	Yes	No
Helped by steroids	No	Yes

XR There is no place for radiographs in the management of stridor.

Tx

- Leave the child in the position of comfort, usually sitting up and probably on the parent/caregiver's knee or with them close by.
- Avoid interventions that may precipitate crying; oxygen may sometimes be tolerated but attempts at IV access will not.
- Ask for paediatric help.

If significant respiratory distress accompanies the stridor, then:

- Nebulised adrenaline may reduce the swelling and buy time for other treatment to take effect. For young children, 0.5 mL/kg of a 1 in 1000 solution of adrenaline is appropriate (up to a maximum of 5 mL). The benefit of the adrenaline only lasts for 30 min and so, in suspected croup, it should be followed immediately by nebulised or oral steroids → *later*.
- Occasionally, airway obstruction will be so significant that intubation is necessary. In these circumstances, intubation is also likely to be difficult, and so a senior anaesthetist must be present. Gaseous induction is usually felt to be the safest option, which in many hospitals will necessitate a prompt transfer to theatre. Intubation should of course be attempted if respiratory arrest occurs.

Croup

A croup score can be used to describe the clinical severity of the illness. It is calculated by scoring five features → *Table 18.3*.

Two alternative steroid treatments have been shown to lead to marked clinical improvement in croup. Treatment is recommended even in mild cases if the diagnosis is suspected.

- Oral dexamethasone (0.15 mg/kg).
- Nebulised budesonide 2 mg (4 mL) stat or 1 mg (2 mL) repeated after 30 min if required
- Oral prednisolone (1 mg/kg) is also used by some units.

Bacterial tracheitis

Fortunately rare, infection of the airway with staphylococci, streptococci or *Haemophilus influenzae* may cause bacterial tracheitis (pseudomembranous croup). The trachea contains copious purulent secretions with mucosal oedema and necrosis, features that can lead to severe airway obstruction. An affected child is unwell and toxic with a high pyrexia and stridulous breathing. Early review by anaesthesia/intensive

Table 18.3 Westley croup score

Clinical sign	Degree	Score
Stridor	None	0
	Heard at rest on auscultation	1
	Heard at rest without auscultation	2
Chest wall retractions	None	0
	Mild	1
	Moderate	2
	Severe	3
Air entry	Normal	0
	Decreased	1
	Severely decreased	2
Cyanosis	None	0
	With agitation	4
	At rest	5
Consciousness level	Normal	0
	Altered	5

Maximum score = 17, mild <4, moderate 4–6, severe >6.

care is recommended as three-quarters of such children ultimately require intubation. Antibiotic therapy should be a combination of cefotaxime and flucloxacillin (→ Table 18.4).

Bronchiolitis

Bronchiolitis is the most common serious respiratory infection of childhood, affecting 10% of all children at some time. It is a disease of infants; 90% of attacks occur in children aged <9 months and it is rare over the age of 2 years. Bronchiolitis is usually caused by respiratory syncytial virus and may occur in epidemics, usually in the winter.

Mucus plugging and mucosal oedema lead to narrowing and obstruction of the smallest airways (in contrast to the bronchoconstriction seen in preschool wheeze and asthma). Initial fever and upper respiratory tract symptoms progress to dry coughing and signs of dyspnoea:

- Poor feeding
- Tachypnoea with intercostal recession
- Hyperinflated lungs and thus easily palpable liver
- Fine inspiratory crepitations and expiratory wheezes
- Mild hypoxia on pulse oximetry
- Tachycardia.

Some infants with severe bronchiolitis (around 2%) will require ventilation, usually because of exhaustion. Signs of imminent deterioration include:

- pallor
- extreme tachypnoea (>60 breaths/min)
- exhaustion
- apnoeic spells
- significant hypoxia.

Some babies can be predicted to have a stormier course including those with a history of:

- heart disease
- failure to thrive
- prematurity.

XR Chest X-ray is not generally useful in typical cases, however, if performed to rule out another cause, may show hyperinflated lungs and, in about a third of infants, areas of segmental collapse or consolidation (this should not be assumed to be due to bacterial infection or lead to reflex antibiotic treatment).

TX Most babies can be managed at home. Those who are feeding adequately (>50% normal) with an SaO_2 >94% on air and who appear to be otherwise stable, with appropriate home circumstances can usually be discharged with safety netting and support of community healthcare teams. Some babies will require admission for

Table 18.4 Doses of common antibiotics for children

	1–5 years	<12 years	Adult
Oral			
Amoxicillin (mg)	125 three times daily	125–250 three times daily	250–500 three times daily
Clarithromycin (mg)	125 twice daily	187.5–250 twice daily	250–500 twice daily
Trimethoprim (mg)	50 twice daily	100 twice daily	200 twice daily
Flucloxacillin (mg)	125 four times daily	125–250 four times daily	250–500 four times daily
Parenteral			
Cefotaxime	50–80 mg/kg three times daily	1–2 g three times daily	1–2 g three times daily
Benzylpenicillin (mg)	300 (0.5 MU) four times daily	600 (1 MU) four times daily	1200 (2 MU) four times daily

observation, monitoring and therapy with humidified oxygen. The threshold for admission should be lower in infants under 6 weeks of age, those with a history of cardiac disease, or babies who were born prematurely. Symptoms usually peak at around 5–7 days and so the point in the disease course should also be considered. The symptoms usually settle over 10–14 days.

Treatment is supportive. Antibiotics, antivirals, bronchodilators, steroids, adrenaline and hypertonic saline have all proven ineffective.

High-flow nasal cannula is a method of providing warmed humidified oxygen at a rate closer to the patient's peak inspiratory flow rate, along with a little positive pressure. This is an option (as is nasal CPAP) in patients who remain hypoxic on standard oxygen therapy. Evidence around the indications and best use continues to evolve, but it is probably not helpful to commence HFNC as first-line treatment or in the emergency department.

'Viral Wheeze' in pre-schoolers

Attacks of wheezing in pre-school age children are very often due to viral infection. The differential diagnosis includes bronchiolitis, pneumonia, aspiration pneumonitis, cystic fibrosis, tracheomalacia and other congenital conditions. Prematurity and low birth weight are risk factors for recurrent wheezing.

These children share many of the clinical features of children with asthma, but the main differentiating feature is an absence of symptoms outside of periods of viral infection, and they are less likely to suffer from atopy.

Bronchodilator therapy delivered in 'bursts' using a metered dose inhalers coupled to spacer devices fitted with facemasks is first-line treatment. A starting dose should be up to 10 puffs of salbutamol delivered one at a time according to response. Nebulised or IV therapy for asthma may be indicated in more severe cases.

Oral steroids have not been shown to be effective in children well enough to be discharged from the emergency department but may reduce length of stay in patients requiring admission. Many children with recurrent episodes of viral-induced wheezing in infancy do not go on to develop chronic asthma, so they do not need regular prophylactic medication.

The parents of these children should be advised about the relationship between exposure to cigarette smoke and attendances with wheeze in childhood.

Asthma in children

This section is mostly concerned with asthma in young children. Asthma in adults and older children → p. 213.

One in 11 children in the UK is receiving treatment for asthma, and it remains one of the most common reasons for admission to a paediatric ward. Diagnosis is based on presentation with respiratory symptoms such as cough, wheeze or breathlessness; however, many children will present with these symptoms without having underlying asthma. Features such as symptom variability, episodic symptoms, recorded episodes of wheeze and a personal history of atopy make the diagnosis more likely.

Asthma attacks are often precipitated by a viral infection, allergen exposure, exercise, cold air or emotion. Asthma is characterised by reversible airways obstruction. The clinical signs and symptoms resulting from this obstruction include:

- **Increased work of breathing**: wheezing, tachypnoea, recession and use of accessory muscles
- **Reduced efficacy of breathing**: poor air entry and lung hyperexpansion
- **Failure of gas exchange**: tachycardia, agitation and eventually drowsiness and cyanosis.

It is important to note that clinical signs, in particular volume of wheeze, correlate poorly with the severity of airway obstruction; some very ill children do not appear to be distressed especially if they are becoming exhausted. **Severe attacks** are characterised by the following:

- Child too breathless to talk or too breathless to feed (cannot complete sentences in one breath)
- Respiratory rate >40/min in children aged 2–5 years or >30/min in children aged >5 years (usually with marked recession and use of accessory muscles)
- Pulse rate >140/min in children aged 2–5 years or >125/min in children aged >5 years
- Arterial O_2 saturation (SaO_2) <92% on air, but any reduction in SaO_2 from the normal of ≥97% must be given serious consideration.

Life-threatening features include:

- fatigue or exhaustion
- agitation, drowsiness, confusion or a depressed level of consciousness
- cyanosis
- a silent chest
- poor respiratory efforts
- bradycardia or hypotension (bradycardia is often a preterminal sign)
- SaO_2 <92% on air.

It is very useful to know what has happened during previous attacks, particularly whether they have required admission, intravenous therapy, intubation and HDU/ICU level care.

Investigations: Measurement of peak expiratory flow rate (PEFR) can usually be performed on children aged >5 years provided that they are not too breathless or too distressed to cooperate. This is especially useful if the child and parent are familiar with performing peak flows and know their normal values. *Predicted PEFRs in children → Figure 18.1.*

Investigations, including chest radiograph (CXR) and blood tests, are not generally indicated in recurrent attacks of asthma, unless there is a possible history of foreign body inhalation or severe systemic upset.

Tx

- Maintain oxygen saturations at 94–98% using either mask or nasal cannula.
- Inhaled beta agonist – usually salbutamol although terbutaline is an alternative.
  - If the child is not requiring oxygen, it is best to deliver this using a metered dose inhaler via a spacer with facemask. Administer 1 puff every 30–60 seconds up to 10 puff (according to response), allowing up to 10 breaths for each puff to optimise drug delivery.
  - *Nebulised salbutamol 5 mg (or terbutaline 10 mg)* (salbutamol 2.5 mg or terbutaline 5 mg if the child is aged <5 years) via oxygen-driven nebuliser. The oxygen flow rate should be around 5 L/min to produce small particles without excess loss of drug from around the facemask.

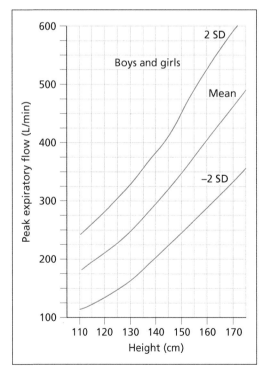

  - If symptoms do not respond to initial beta-agonist treatment, add *ipratropium bromide (250 mcg)* mixed with the beta-agonist nebuliser solution.
- *Soluble prednisolone* 1–2 mg/kg orally (up to a maximum of 40 mg). Children who are already receiving maintenance steroid tablets should be given prednisolone 2 mg/kg (up to a maximum of 60 mg). If the child is unable to swallow liquids or is vomiting, give IV hydrocortisone 4 mg/kg. This should be repeated every 6 hours or followed by a continuous infusion of hydrocortisone 1 mg/kg per hour.

If the patient is not responding to initial therapy or if they are deteriorating despite treatment ensure that senior staff are involved. With life-threatening features or in a deteriorating situation request the presence of an anaesthetist or paediatric intensive care (PICU) consultant, so that intubation and ventilation can be performed if the child does not improve. (Induction of anaesthesia may be performed with bronchodilating agents such as ketamine.) Children whose SpO_2 remains <92% on air after initial treatment should also be considered for PICU/HDU referral.

Remember that a patient who is becoming quieter and more compliant may actually be deteriorating and becoming exhausted, and that volume of wheeze is not a reliable indicator of degree of bronchospasm as it is so dependent on air flow.

Second line treatments

- *Nebulised ipratropium bromide* 250 mcg (125 mcg if the child is aged <2 years). This may be repeated after every 20–30 min for children who are responding poorly to β_2 agonists.
- *Continuous nebulised β_2 agonists* ('back to back nebs')
- *IV salbutamol* 15 mcg/kg given over 10 min. This is an alternative to repeated salbutamol or terbutaline nebulisers for children aged >2 years. It is followed by a salbutamol infusion at a rate of 1–5 mcg/kg per min. ECG and electrolytes must be monitored to detect dysrhythmias and hypokalaemia
- *Magnesium sulphate* 25–40 mg/kg given intravenously over 20 min (maximum dose 2 g; single dose only). *Further information on magnesium → p. 250.*
- *Aminophylline* 5 mg/kg given intravenously over 20 min under ECG monitoring, followed by a maintenance infusion of 1 mg/kg per hour in 5% dextrose. The infusion rate is reduced to 800 mcg/kg per hour for children between the ages of 10 and 16 years and to 500–700 mcg/kg per hour for adults. The initial loading dose should not be given to patients who are already receiving oral theophyllines.

Signs of clinical improvement include:

- Improved activity levels or responsiveness: urge to eat, drink or play

Figure 18.1 Predicted peak expiratory flow rates in children.

- Falling pulse rate
- Rising peak flow rate.

Potential discharge

Patients who have responded well to treatment may be suitable for discharge, but this needs careful consideration. The clinical effects of salbutamol last somewhere between 3 and 5 hours and so it is usual practice to observe the child for a period of time (usually at least 3–4 hours) after treatment to ensure that they remain stable. Patients should not be discharged unless their SaO$_2$ is >94% on air, and the PEFR is >75% of the predicted value. All children with features of severe asthma should be admitted. For discharge planning, the following are usually required:

- A period of observation (e.g. 4 hours) in an assessment area (whether this is in ED or on a ward depends on local policy)
- Oral (soluble) prednisolone for 3–5 days (1–2 mg/kg per day in either one morning or two divided doses up to a maximum of 40 mg/day)
- Follow-up in an asthma clinic for reassessment and a review of current therapy.
- An assessment of inhaler technique (all children should use a spacer device)
- A personalised Asthma Plan including
  - Instructions on stepping down bronchodilator therapy
  - Requirement for inhaled steroid treatment
  - Details of any oral steroid treatment
  - Safety netting guidance

Further information about the discharge of a patient with asthma → p. 216.

Pneumonia

Pneumonia occurs in 29 per 10 000 children under 5 years of age and becomes still less common in older children. Children with congenital abnormalities or chronic illnesses are at a high risk of pneumonia. Up to 70% of cases may be caused by viruses, particularly in younger cohorts. Of cases with a bacterial aetiology the commonest organism is streptococcus pneumoniae. Worldwide pneumonia remains the leading cause of death in under 5s; however, this is uncommon in developed countries.

Suspect pneumonia in patients with fever and cough, with increased work of breathing, hypoxia, reduced air entry on auscultation or dullness to percussion. Patients may also demonstrate non-specific symptoms such as lethargy and abdominal pain.

X$_R$ Chest X-ray may show minimal changes, consolidation or widespread bronchopneumonia.

T$_X$ Children with significantly increased work of breathing and/or hypoxia, signs of sepsis (→ *next section*) or those who cannot maintain hydration status will require hospital admission.

Although some pneumonia is caused by viral infections, it is difficult to distinguish these from bacterial causes; therefore, it is recommended that all children with pneumonia are treated with antibiotics (→ *Table 18.4*).

For children well enough for discharge from hospital, oral amoxicillin is recommended as first-line therapy, or a macrolide such as clarithromycin. For those children requiring IV treatment, IV co-amoxiclav is an appropriate choice; however, this may vary depending on local bacterial prevalence and resistance, so local guidance should be followed. Children with cystic fibrosis may present with complicated chest infections, which require specialist advice from the outset.

Pneumonia in older children and adults → p. 220.

OTHER MAJOR ILLNESSES IN CHILDHOOD

Sepsis

Sepsis remains a leading cause of morbidity and mortality in children worldwide. It represents the effect of a dysregulated host systemic inflammatory response to a pathogen (bacterial, fungal or viral). This pro-inflammatory cascade can then lead to vasodilatation, capillary leak, myocardial dysfunction and ultimately multi-organ failure. Unfortunately, the initial presentation of sepsis in children can be very non-specific and deterioration may be rapid and catastrophic.

It may be extremely challenging to differentiate a child with early sepsis from the many other children presenting with a normal physiological response to fever associated with a viral infection. There are currently no screening tools with both good sensitivity and acceptable specificity. Abnormal physiological parameters may act as a trigger to consider sepsis but are not reliable to rule in sepsis in isolation. Blood tests such as FBC and CRP can be normal despite serious infection, particularly where onset is rapid, and they may be falsely reassuring. Height of fever is not generally useful in differentiating serious bacterial infection from viral illness, other than in infants under 3 months (→ *below*). The course of the illness, in addition to observation of the child's demeanour and behaviour by an experienced clinician, may be the most effective method of differentiation.

If there is concern for sepsis, involvement of a senior clinician should be sought and treatment should be initiated promptly – it can later be de-escalated if clinical signs are more reassuring. If a child displays abnormal physiological parameters, but appears 'well' and is happily playing in the waiting room, sepsis is unlikely – in these cases a period of watchful waiting and a review by a senior clinician is a reasonable strategy.

Some groups are particularly vulnerable to sepsis and for these patients a particularly low threshold for initiation of early antibiotic therapy is necessary. These patients include neonates, those with complex neurodisability, and those patients with immunodeficiency. An infant under one month presenting with fever should be assumed to have sepsis until proven otherwise. Under three months of age, a temperature over 38°C should trigger further investigation with blood tests and a urine microscopy at a minimum in almost all cases, along with a review by a pediatrician (exceptions may sometimes be made for post-vaccination fever after review by a senior clinician).

Management

Following recognition of sepsis the following interventions should be initiated:

- Call for senior help (including paediatrics, anaesthesia or PICU depending on centre).
- Monitor and record continuously the heart rate, BP, temperature, respiratory rate, SpO_2, capillary refill time, GCS score, pupillary size/reactions and the spread of any rash.
- Check for and treat hypoglycaemia (→ *p. 346*).
- Oxygen therapy, aiming to maintain oxygen saturations between 94% and 98%. There is increasing recognition that hyperoxia can be detrimental, so reducing supplemental oxygen once safe to do so is encouraged. If oxygen saturations are not recordable due to poor perfusion, assume the need for high-flow oxygen in the first instance.
- Obtain intravenous or intraosseous access and send blood tests including blood cultures, venous or capillary blood gas and lactate, biochemistry including calcium and magnesium, full blood count, glucose and meningococcal PCR. (Low platelets, low WCC, raised urea and creatinine, coagulopathy and a base deficit >–5 mmol/L suggest a poor prognosis.)
- Broad spectrum parenteral antibiotics should be given immediately (do not wait for blood test results) (→ *Table 18.4*).
  - Ceftriaxone is used as a first-line monotherapy in an IV dose of 80 mg/kg (maximum dose = 2 g). It is effective against meningococci, pneumococci and *Haemophilus influenzae*. Cefotaxime (in the same doses) is an alternative and is the first choice in infants aged <3 months with a history of prematurity or jaundice, or if calcium-containing infusions

are also being used. It also has the advantage of being administered as a bolus dose so can be given more rapidly than an infusion of ceftriaxone.
  - The addition of clindamycin is recommended to cover Group A streptococcus which can behave similarly to meningococcal disease
  - To cover listerial infection, IV ampicillin/amoxicillin may be added for neonates and immunosuppressed patients (50 mg/kg four times daily).
  - Consider the addition of aciclovir (10 mg/kg by IV infusion) if there is any suspicion of meningoencephalitis.
- Consider fluid resuscitation with the aim of restoring circulating volume and physiological parameters. Start with an initial bolus of 10 mL/kg repeated as necessary following reassessment up to 40–60 mL/kg. Excess fluid administration can be detrimental with risk of prolonged ventilation, increased ICU length of stay and mortality. Reassess after each bolus, looking for any evidence of increasing respiratory distress or oxygen requirement, crepitations on auscultation or increasing hepatomegaly due to liver congestion. If it has been necessary to give 40–60 mL/kg preparations should be made for intubation and transfer to intensive care.
- Vasopressor/inotropic support is likely to be required if physiological parameters remain significantly abnormal after 40–60 mL/kg fluid. Adrenaline or dopamine infusions, can be given peripherally via IV or IO lines until central access is obtained.
- Correct hypocalcaemia, hypomagnesaemia and hypokalaemia
- Insert urinary catheter and monitor urine output

Meningitis and meningococcal disease

Approximately 25–30% of meningococcal disease cases occur in children under the age of five years. A second peak of disease occurs in late adolescence/young adulthood. Incidence of invasive meningococcal disease has decreased substantially over the past two decades in the UK, largely due to widespread vaccination uptake; however, mortality in confirmed cases remains high at about 10%. Meningococcal group B disease is responsible for >80% of cases, with group C accounting for <10% of infections (since the introduction of the MenC vaccine).

A distinction should be made between meningococcal meningitis and meningococcal sepsis, although the two can co-exist. Meningococcal sepsis consists of overwhelming systemic infection and dysregulated host response and management is as for sepsis (→ *above*). Meningococcal sepsis may present with a non-blanching or purpuric rash, which is well recognised by the public and parents due to extensive publicity. This is not exclusive to meningococcal infection and may not initially be present. However, if a purpuric rash is noted in a pyrexial or unwell child, particularly if the rash begins to spread, or there are other signs of sepsis, immediate treatment must be initiated as for sepsis. Purpura fulminans is indicative of coagulopathy. It is now estimated that approximately 1% of children with fever and a non-blanching rash have meningococcal disease (from 10% to 20% prior to vaccine introduction).

In meningococcal meningitis, photophobia and neck stiffness are relatively unusual features; the most common symptoms are fever, malaise and drowsiness. Headache, vomiting and irritability are also often seen. Raised intracranial pressure (ICP) may lead to confusion, fits, abnormal posturing and florid neurological signs. *Meningitis → below*

Tx see 'Sepsis'

Prehospital treatment

In a patient with suspected meningococcal disease, parenteral antibiotics (benzylpenicillin) should be administered in the community before urgent transfer to hospital only if:

- The patient has a non-blanching rash or
- The patient does not have a rash but there may be significant delays in the patient getting to the hospital

It is no longer recommended that benzylpenicillin be given routinely to patients who do not have a rash before transfer to the hospital.

Prevention of transmission of the meningococcus bacteria

> Meningococcal disease is a notifiable disease in the UK, and local public health teams should be informed of any confirmed case.

The meningococcus is carried in the nasopharynx of many healthy children and adults without causing any disease. Some people, however, may develop invasive disease within a few days of colonisation. Illness occurs in the first few days only after this colonisation and not during established carriage. The incubation period is generally 3–4 days with a range of 2–10 days.

Following contact with meningococcal disease, chemoprophylaxis is recommended for close household contacts (including shared dormitories, those sharing communal kitchens and partners with close contact). The absolute risk of a second case following contact is 1 : 300 within 30 days – this can be reduced by 90% with chemoprophylaxis.

Childminders should be dealt with as part of the family unit, but school contact or other community contact is not generally an indication for prophylaxis.

> Health-care staff require prophylaxis only when they have been exposed to respiratory droplets/secretions of the patient with meningococcal disease during the acute stage of the illness (usually those managing the patient's airway during intubation for example).

Ciprofloxacin is now the antibiotic of choice for close contacts of all ages, including during pregnancy. Rifampicin (or even ceftriaxone) is used when there is a hypersensitivity to ciprofloxacin. *Antibiotic dosages for prophylaxis against meningococci → Box 18.8.* The responsibility for tracing other contacts lies with the department of public health.

> **Box 18.8 Antibiotic dosages for prophylaxis against meningococcal infection**
>
> *Ciprofloxacin by single oral dose*
>   Adults and children aged >12 years = 500 mg
>   Children aged 5–12 years = 250 mg
>   Children aged 1 month to 4 years = 125 mg
>
> *Rifampicin by mouth*
>   Adults and children aged >12 months = 10 mg/kg twice daily × 2 days
>   Children aged <12 months = 5 mg/kg twice daily × 2 days (to a maximum dosage of 600 mg per dose or 1200 mg per day)
>
> *Ceftriaxone by single IM dose*
>   Adults and children aged >12 years = 250 mg
>   Children aged <12 years = 125 mg

Meningitis

Bacterial meningitis occurs all year round although it usually peaks in winter months. Unfortunately, early diagnosis can be difficult and so the possibility of meningitis must always be considered in any patient with an unexplained illness or fever. Symptoms and signs in older children and adults include:

- severe headache
- nausea and vomiting
- fever
- back or joint pains

- drowsiness or confusion
- photophobia
- neck stiffness (often absent!)
- although well known, Kernig's and Brudzinski's signs are not sensitive in the detection of meningeal irritation and their absence is not reassuring.
- raised intracranial pressure (ICP) may lead to confusion, fits, abnormal posturing and florid neurological signs.

Infants may have relatively non-specific signs such as:

- drowsiness and irritability
- poor feeding
- distress on handling
- vomiting or diarrhoea
- high-pitched or moaning cry (often absent)
- tense or bulging fontanelle (often absent)
- apnoeic or cyanotic attacks
- fever
- neck stiffness (often absent)

In meningococcal infection photophobia and neck stiffness are relatively uncommon features; the most common symptoms are fever, malaise and drowsiness.

Management

In patients with suspected meningitis:

- Give oxygen to maintain oxygen saturation at 94–98%.
- Gain IV access. Shock must be treated but in its absence fluids should be given sparingly-excess fluid may contribute to cerebral oedema and increasing ICP
- Obtain routine blood specimens, blood cultures, blood gas, lactate and meningococcal PCR.
- Control fits (→ p. 356).
- Check for and treat hypoglycaemia (→ p. 346).
- Start antibiotics. (→ p. 354).
- The definitive investigation for meningitis is a lumbar puncture. This must not delay the administration of parenteral antibiotics. *Contraindications to lumbar puncture →Box 18.9*
- IV dexamethasone (0.15 mg/kg stat and then four times daily for 4 days) should be used in children >3 months of age, as soon as possible following lumbar puncture that demonstrates:
  - Purulent CSF
  - CSF WCC >1000/μL
  - Raised CSF white cell count and protein >1 g/L
  - Bacteria on gram stain
- This should be as soon as possible after starting antibiotics (ideally within 4 hours). Do not start dexamethasone >12 hours after commencing antibiotic treatment.
- Refer the patient to the paediatric team for further investigation and treatment. Consider the need for a CT scan of the brain to exclude other diagnoses.

> **Box 18.9 Contraindications to lumbar puncture**
>
> - Signs of raised intracranial pressure
>   - Reduced or fluctuating GCS
>   - Relative bradycardia and hypertension
>   - Focal neurological signs
>   - Abnormal posturing
>   - Unequal, dilated or poorly responsive pupils
>   - Papilloedema
>   - Abnormal 'doll's eye' movements
> - After convulsions until stabilised
> - Focal neurological signs
> - Widespread purpuric rash
> - Coagulopathy, platelet count <100 × 10⁹/L, on anticoagulant treatment
> - Shock
> - Respiratory insufficiency (risk of precipitating respiratory failure)
> - Local infection to LP site

Viral meningitis

Many different viruses may cause a meningitis. The clinical picture is very similar to a bacterial infection although the severity of the illness is usually much less. Until the diagnosis is confirmed by lumbar puncture, the treatment is identical to that for bacterial meningitis.

Encephalitis

Coxsackieviruses, other enteroviruses, arboviruses and herpes simplex virus, may all infect the brain. Drowsiness, lethargy and confusion are the most common symptoms, usually with very few hard signs, meaning a low threshold for suspecting the diagnosis is necessary. Herpetic encephalitis in the neonatal period carries a high mortality and risk of neurological sequalae, which can be reduced by prompt treatment with acyclovir. Lumbar puncture may be helpful; a CT scan is usually normal. The treatment is similar to that for suspected bacterial meningitis but with the addition of drugs directed against herpes simplex. Aciclovir 10 mg/kg is given by IV infusion every 8 hours for 10 days (calculated on ideal body weight in obese patients).

Seizures

Around 7% of children have had a seizure by the age of 3 years, but only 0.5% of school-age children have epilepsy. In the neonatal period, birth injury, hypoglycaemia and hypocalcaemia are common causes of convulsions, whereas intracranial infection, encephalopathy and poisoning occur at all ages. Children with neurode-velopmental conditions are also likely to present with seizures.

Febrile convulsions occur in about 3% of children between the ages of 5 months and 5 years. The child may present with prolonged fitting or there may have been a short period of clonic or tonic activity. Sometimes there is a story of an apparently well child suddenly becoming limp and falling to the floor. A history of stiffness, cyanosis, drooling or the eyes rolling upwards is extremely suggestive of a seizure. Pyrexia lowers the seizure threshold and therefore children with a known diagnosis of epilepsy are also more likely to have a fit when pyrexial. It is important to understand that the height of the fever is not believed to be directly related to the development of febrile convulsion, nor does lowering the temperature prevent the convulsion. Seizures may recur during the same illness or future febrile episodes, or this may be an isolated episode. Anti-epileptic medication is not recommended for simple febrile convulsions.

INVESTIGATIONS: The blood glucose should be checked in all cases at the bedside and the SpO_2 monitored. Children with atypical convulsions may need toxicological, infective and metabolic screening together with a CT scan of the brain. An ECG should be obtained in patients presenting with seizures (particularly first and afebrile episodes) as apparent seizure can, occasionally, represent an episode of arrythmia.

Tx
- Support the airway and apply facemask oxygen. Apply monitoring. Check glucose.
- Time the seizure and attempt to obtain IV access.
- If seizure is ongoing at 5 min, buccal midazolam can be given (0.5 mg/kg) if available, without the delays associated with obtaining IV access. Lorazepam 0.1 mg/kg by slow IV injection (or by the intraosseous route) can be given if access is available. IV/IO diazepam emulsion 0.25 mg/kg is an alternative. Rectal diazepam (0.5 mg/kg) is an alternative if buccal midazolam is not available and IV access delayed (→ *Table 18.5*).

Table 18.5 Rectal dose of diazepam

Age (years)	Rectal dose (mg)
>1	5
>3	7.5
>5	10
>12	20
Adult	30

- If seizure is ongoing for a further 5 min following initial dose, a second dose of benzodiazepine can be given at the same dose as above. In most cases, IV/IO access will now be available, in which case the preferred treatment is lorazepam
- After another 5 min of ongoing seizure give levetiracetam 40 mg/kg IV or IO (max 3 g) over 5 min
- Call for help from anaesthetic or critical care teams to prepare for induction of anaesthesia and intubation
- If seizure activity continues 10 min after the levetiracetam infusion has finished, proceed to rapid sequence induction if team is ready
- If there is a delay to RSI, administer 20 mg/kg phenytoin infusion over 20 min (if patient is already taking phenytoin, give 20 mg/kg phenobarbitone)
- Once seizure control has been established, consider the need for CT scan. Most patients with atypical, focal or prolonged seizures should have imaging. A prolonged seizure in a patient with known epilepsy and either an established pattern of similar seizures or a clear trigger, may not require CT.

Discharge and follow up

Children who have had prolonged or recurrent seizures should be admitted. Most other children can be discharged home once recovery is complete and sustained, provided that

- there is a definite diagnosis (known epilepsy or febrile illness in an appropriate age group)
- in febrile convulsions, the focus of infection has been identified and need for treatment assessed
- the parents agree to the discharge
- the home circumstances are satisfactory
- there are adequate arrangements for follow-up.

Some hospitals have a policy of admitting all children with a first febrile convulsion. At a minimum, these patients should be carefully assessed to identify the source of the fever (often a viral illness) and rule out serious bacterial infection. A period of observation is often useful to permit full recovery and reassure parents. Blood tests in this group are low yield and usually not necessary in the absence of other concerns.

Diabetic ketoacidosis in children

Type 1 diabetes is on the increase in the UK, particularly in children aged <5 years. Almost 40% first present in diabetic ketoacidosis (DKA) with 20% having a pH of <7.1. DKA is the most common cause of death in children with diabetes, with one death in every 300 episodes of DKA. Most deaths occur as a result of cerebral oedema (80%), hypokalaemia or aspiration pneumonia. Leading up to presentation there may be a history of increasing polyuria, polydipsia and weight loss. Commonly a concurrent infection precipitates the diabetic crisis. Abdominal pain and vomiting are common symptoms and patients may display a characteristic deep rapid breathing pattern (Kussmaul's breathing). DKA usually results in profound fluid deficit leading to shock in some cases, and the metabolic derangement and electrolyte disturbance may be severe.

Investigations: Any patient presenting with increased thirst, polyuria, weight loss or tiredness and nausea or vomiting, abdominal pain, hyperventilation, dehydration or reduced level of consciousness must have their capillary blood sugar checked at triage. If blood sugar is >11 mmol/L, then blood ketone (beta-hydroxybutyrate) levels should be checked, along with a capillary blood gas if ketones are high.

DKA is defined as

- pH <7.3 or bicarbonate <15 mmol/L
- Blood ketones >3 mmol/L (or ketonuria ++ on test strips if blood ketone not available)
- In most cases, blood glucose will be >11 mmol/L; however, this is not essential for diagnosis, as diabetic patients on insulin may present in DKA with lower blood sugar

Tx *Most hospitals will have established DKA pathways which should be followed carefully according to local guidance.*

- Obtain IV access and send blood samples for FBC, electrolytes and CRP
- Apply oxygen to maintain oxygen saturation at 94–98%
- Ensure an accurate weight has been recorded wherever feasible
- Give 10 mL/kg 0.9% NaCl (or a balanced crystalloid) as an intravenous bolus over 30 min. This should be given more rapidly (15 min) for patients in shock.
- Shocked patients may require further fluid boluses in 10 mL/kg aliquots to restore circulating volume, up to 40 mL/kg. If shock persists at this point consider inotropes.
- Calculate fluid deficit. Clinical assessment is very unreliable and so
  - Assume 5% deficit in patients with pH >7.1
  - Assume 10% deficit in patients with pH <7.1
  - See → Box 18.10
- One hour after starting the fluids for rehydration, start an infusion of soluble insulin at a rate of 0.05–0.1 Unit/kg per hour.

Patients using a subcutaneous insulin pump should have this disconnected whilst on IV insulin.

- Do not give IV bicarbonate to patients with DKA.

 Box 18.10 **Fluids for a child with DKA**

24-hour fluid requirement
= maintenance fluids + half calculated deficit

Fluid deficit in litres = Dehydration (%)
× Body weight in kg

- Assume 5% dehydration in patients with pH >7.1
- Assume 10% dehydration in patients with pH <7.1
- Deficit should be replaced over 48 hours
- For NON shocked patients subtract the initial 10 mL/kg bolus from this calculated deficit
- Do NOT subtract fluid boluses given to SHOCKED patients

Maintenance fluid
- 100 mL/kg/day for the first 10 kg of body weight
- 50 mL/kg/day for the next 10–20 kg
- 20 mL/kg/day for each additional kilogramme above 20 kg

Choice of fluid:
- Use 0.9% saline with 20 mmol KCl in 500 mL (40 mmol KCl in a litre)
- If venous potassium is high on presentation, wait to add potassium to fluids until patient has either passed urine, there is a clear history of passing urine recently or potassium has fallen to normal levels.

- Acute gastric dilatation is common in DKA and so a nasogastric tube may be required, especially if the child is comatose or vomiting.
- Once the blood sugar has fallen to 14 mmol/L, the IV infusion should be changed to 0.9% saline with 5% glucose, with 20 mmol potassium per 500 mL (40 mmol per 1000 mL). Reduce the insulin infusion to 0.05 Units/kg per hour if previously higher. If 0.1 units/kg of insulin is still felt necessary, use 10% glucose with potassium as above.

Recognition and treatment of cerebral oedema →
Box 18.11.

A third of children who develop cerebral oedema in DKA have permanent neurological sequelae.

Box 18.11 Recognition and treatment of cerebral oedema

In DKA, cerebral oedema usually occurs in the first 24 hour after starting rehydration. There are three major diagnostic criteria:

1 A reduced or fluctuating level of consciousness
2 Sustained episodes of bradycardia
3 Incontinence that is inappropriate for the age of the child

and five minor criteria: vomiting, headache, lethargy, hypertension and aged <5 years.
Two major or one major and two minor criteria strongly suggest the diagnosis.
Late signs such as papilloedema, convulsions and coma are associated with an extremely poor prognosis.

Treatment should be started immediately:

- Administer oxygen
- Exclude hypoglycaemia
- Nurse the patient with head elevated
- Give 5 mL/kg 2.7% sodium chloride OR 20% mannitol 2.5–5 mL/kg
- Restrict fluids to 50% of maintenance requirement only and replace the estimated deficit over 72 rather than 48 hours
- Discuss the potential need for intubation with an intensivist.
- Arrange a CT scan of the brain (to exclude other diagnoses)
- Repeat the dose of mannitol after 2 hours if no improvement

COMMON PAEDIATRIC PRESENTATIONS

Herpes simplex stomatitis → *p. 424*. Mumps → *p. 442*.

Fever

High fever is one of the commonest reasons that children present to the emergency department. Parents are often concerned about the height of the fever or concerned that the temperature has not resolved with antipyretic treatments. They should be reassured that fever itself is not dangerous and is in fact a useful part of the immune response to infection. Antipyretic treatment should not be used solely to 'bring the temperature down' but should be targeted towards relieving pain and distress if present – there is no need to wake a comfortably sleeping child to administer paracetamol for example. Outside of early infancy (<3 months), the height of fever is not well correlated with risk for serious bacterial infection.

The clinician must determine firstly whether there are any signs of sepsis or serious bacterial infection (→ *p. 353 and Box 18.12*) and secondly whether a focus for infection can be identified. A child who is a good colour, alert, playing and interacting normally with caregivers has a low likelihood of serious infective illness.

Assessment must include the recording of heart rate, respiratory rate, capillary refill and temperature, Examination must be thorough including an examination of ears and throat and full exposure to assess for any rashes.

Box 18.12 Signs suggestive of serious illness

- Pallor, mottling, blue lips or tongue
- Lack of social response
- 'Appears ill' to a healthcare professional
- Not waking, or not staying awake
- High pitched, weak or continuous cry
- Grunting
- Tachypnoea >60 bpm
- Severe chest recessions/retractions
- Reduced skin turgor
- Bulging fontanelle

Upper respiratory tract infections (URTI) and earache

Young children may have upper respiratory infections as often as 10 times a year. Such infections may precipitate asthma attacks or lead to more serious chest infections. Symptoms of URTI include the following:

- **Cough and/or runny nose**: the most common signs of infection. The barking cough of croup is important to recognise because it may accompany stridor (see above).
- **Sore throat**: this is caused by pharyngitis or enlarged lymph nodes in the neck.
- **Earache**: young children may pull at their ears if they have earache. Otitis media is a frequent accompaniment of URTI in children.
- **Abdominal pain**: this sometimes occurs with an URTI due to mesenteric adenitis. There are usually no localising signs. Specific tenderness may be difficult to

distinguish from appendicitis or urinary tract infection in which case further investigation or referral is needed.

- **Non-specific symptoms**: pyrexia, poor feeding, malaise, crying and vomiting.

Tx Reassurance, fluids and paracetamol are the mainstays of treatment. The former is greatly enhanced if preceded by a thorough examination.

Acute otitis media

A common accompaniment of URTI in children, AOM is painful and may cause significant distress. In most cases of AOM, the cause is viral, and antibiotic treatment is not recommended. The risk of diarrhoea and other antibiotic side effects outweighs any marginal benefit in shortening symptom duration. The exceptions to this are those who are systemically very unwell. Children under the age of 2 with bilateral AOM and those who have otorrhoea are an intermediate group who may be offered delayed antibiotic prescription with advice to use these if symptoms do not improve within a specified time frame. Ear drops with anaesthetic and analgesic (phenazone and lidocaine) may be useful to manage pain and distress. Most AOM will resolve in 3 days with or without treatment.

Tonsillitis

Patients commonly present with sore throat, with or without fever, and lymphadenopathy. Ensure that they are able to maintain hydration orally – if they are struggling due to pain, the use of local anaesthetic spray (benzydamine hydrochloride) is useful to improve comfort. Examine for any evidence of quinsy (→p. 439). The majority of these presentations are viral. The FEVERPAIN score can be used to determine those who may benefit from antibiotics (→ Box 18.13).

Box 18.13 FeverPAIN score

- Fever in past 24 hours
- Absence of cough or coryza
- Symptom onset <3 days
- Purulent tonsils
- Severe tonsillar inflammation

Likelihood of streptococcal infections: 0 points 13–18%, 1 point 14–18%, 2 points 30–35%, 3 points 39–48% 4 or 5 points 62–65%. Consider delayed antibiotics for patients with 2–3 points, and immediate antibiotics for 4–5 points.

Urinary tract infection

Urinary tract infections are a common site of bacterial infection in children. Presenting symptoms and signs are often non-specific, especially in the younger patients, who may be more likely to present with pyrexia, vomiting or vague abdominal pain. *Urinary tract infections in children* → *Chapter 17 p. 335.*

Rashes

The rash in meningococcal disease is classically purpuric but may be macular in the initial stages.

The common exanthemas (rashes) of childhood may be challenging to differentiate. However, their recognition is important for prognosis, detection of severe illness and in some cases public health.

The main types are the following:

- **Purpuric**: a non-blanching red or purple rash is caused by the extravasation of blood. The septicaemia of meningococcal disease is the most serious cause (→ p. 354). It also occurs in IgA vasculitis (Henoch–Schönlein purpura) and platelet deficiency (idiopathic thrombocytopenic purpura, leukaemia or drugs).
- **Urticarial**: blotchy, raised, itchy, red and hot. There is diffuse erythema and sometimes swelling of the face and hands. Areas may look like nettle-stings, which are also caused by histamine release (→ p. 306). Often recognised as an 'allergic' rash, the commonest cause (in the absence of a known trigger) is viral infection. Itchy scratch marks with either little else to see or some urticaria are usually caused by scabies infection (→ p. 427).
- **Vesicular**: small, itchy, fluid-filled vesicles that develop at different rates are typical of chickenpox. Later, they become pustular and, if badly infected, should be treated with flucloxacillin. Vesicles and blisters may also be seen in:
  - herpes simplex (perioral and on the fingers) (→ p. 424)
  - impetigo (→ p. 424)
  - hand, foot and mouth disease: this is a Coxsackie viral infection that starts as painful red dots on the soles, palms and palate before small, clear, blisters develop
  - staphylococcal scalded skin syndrome (Ritter's disease or fourth disease): this occurs mostly in infants. An epidermolytic toxin from a pathogenic strain of *Staphylococcus aureus* causes a widespread but superficial bullous eruption

- insect bites (most commonly found on the legs).
- a single, dark, pus-filled vesicle is often found at the centre of a streptococcal cellulitis.
- **Morbilliform (or measles-like)**: the maculopapular rash of measles is diffuse, irregular and usually bright red. It is accompanied by an URTI, swollen watery eyes (conjunctivitis) and Koplick's spots (white dots on the buccal surface of the cheeks). The old name for this dreaded illness was 'first disease'. *Measles → below*.
- **Pink, red, macular or papular**: scarlet fever is recognised by a diffuse, rough-feeling, red rash with circumoral pallor and a 'strawberry' tongue. These features are preceded by pharyngitis and pyrexia. The old name for scarlet fever was 'second disease' and a milder form of the illness is sometimes called 'scarlatina'. *Scarlet fever → below*.

A large variety of viral infections may cause a diffuse erythematous (and sometimes maculopapular) rash accompanied by pyrexia and upper respiratory symptoms including the following:

Rubella (German measles or third disease): the erythematous rash is accompanied by characteristic postauricular and occipital lymphadenopathy.

Erythema infectiosum (slapped cheek syndrome or fifth disease): an infection with parvovirus B19, which begins with erythema of the cheeks and circumoral pallor. A 'lacy' rash then develops on the extremities, lasting for 7–10 days. This parvovirus can cause fetal loss in the second trimester of pregnancy and also affects the production of red blood cells.

Roseola infantum (exanthem subitum or sixth disease): there are discrete pink macules on the trunk.

There are no 'seventh' and 'eighth' diseases!

Acute (guttate) psoriasis → p. 425.
Erythema nodosum → p. 425.
Lichen planus → p. 426.
Pityriasis rosea → p. 426.

> The diagnosis of Kawasaki's disease should be considered in any child with a febrile illness that persists for longer than 4 or 5 days (→ *p. 362*).

Measles

Although still relatively rare, the incidence of measles is increasing in the UK with a case fatality rate of around 1 in 5000. The patient has 2 and 3 days of severe cough, coryza and conjunctivitis, followed by a red maculopapular rash that starts on the hairline and behind the ears, before it spreads to the face, trunk and extremities.

The temperature is usually >38.3°C, and Koplik's spots may be seen on the buccal mucosa. In some areas of the body, the rash becomes confluent before starting to fade after 3–4 days. Around one in five patients with measles develops one or more complications including:

- pneumonia
- otitis media
- permanent loss of hearing
- diarrhoea (1 in 12).

Rarer complications include subacute sclerosing panencephalitis (SSPE) and death.

INVESTIGATIONS: Rapid diagnosis is required for both clinical and public health action, but clinical diagnosis alone is unreliable. Therefore, one of the following specimens should be taken (discuss with local health protection agencies):

- Urine and/or throat swab (ideally in virus transport medium [VTM] or a dry swab if VTM is unavailable) for PCR testing
- Blood (clotted) for measles IgM testing
- HPA (Health Protection Agency) salivary swab for both PCR and IgM testing.

TX The treatment of uncomplicated measles is symptomatic – oral fluids and ibuprofen or paracetamol. Around 10% of cases require admission to the hospital. The disease is notifiable in the UK and a list should be made of all the people who have been in the ED waiting room at the same time. The incubation period of measles is about 14 days from exposure to the appearance of the rash, and it is infectious from 4 days before to 4 days after the onset of the rash.

> Measles is highly infectious. The virus can remain in the air for up to 2 hours after the patient has left the room. It is important that vulnerable (pregnant or immunocompromised) contacts of measles cases are identified as early as possible because they may require human normal immunoglobulin (HNIg).

Scarlet fever

Scarlet fever is caused by an exotoxin from *Streptococcus pyogenes* and is most common in children aged between 6 and 12 years. The illness starts with a sore throat, fever, cervical lymphadenopathy, headache, myalgia and general malaise. After 12–48 hours a fine, red, rough-textured rash appears on the chest, in the axillae and behind the ears. There is redness of the face with circumoral pallor. The 'sandpaper-like' rash then becomes more generalised but is worse in the skinfolds. It begins to fade after

3 to 4 days and a whitish coating on the tongue and throat peels away to leave a red 'strawberry' tongue. As the patient recovers, desquamation of the skin occurs, initially on the face and axillae, then on the palms, fingers and toes. Scarlet fever is treated with antibiotics (e.g. phenoxymethylpenicillin or clarithromycin). Septic complications such as pneumonia, sinusitis and local abscesses may occur. In rare cases, group A streptococci can also induce immune disorders such as rheumatic fever, glomerulonephritis and erythema nodosum. Scarlet fever is a notifiable disease in the UK (except in Scotland).

Kawasaki's disease

Kawasaki's disease is an acute multisystem inflammatory disease of unknown aetiology. Although uncommon, it is included in this section because of its non-specific features. Eighty per cent of cases occur in children aged <5 years, sometimes in small epidemics. There is an underlying vasculitis. The diagnosis is usually only confirmed if at least five of the following clinical features are present:

- Fever
- Reddening of the oropharyngeal mucosa including the tongue
- Dry, fissured lips
- Conjunctivitis
- Peeling fingers or toes
- Erythema of the hands and feet, which become swollen and indurated (oedema and pain in the extremities may be the predominant symptom)
- A morbilliform, maculopapular or urticarial rash on the trunk and limbs (within 5 days of the onset of the fever)
- Enlarged cervical lymph nodes (in over half of patients)
- Arthralgia
- Thrombocytosis.

During the illness, the coronary arteries can become dilated. This may result in the development of coronary aneurysms and delayed but sudden death.

Tx Patients in whom Kawasaki's disease is suspected should be referred to the paediatric team. The administration of oral aspirin and IV human immunoglobulin can protect the coronary arteries from damage, but only if given within 10 days of the onset of the illness.

Diarrhoea and vomiting

> Children often vomit after minor injuries and during the course of many illnesses.

Table 18.6 Signs of dehydration

% of body weight lost	Signs
<5	Generally well: dry membranes, slight oliguria
5–10	Unwell: apathetic, sunken eyes and fontanelle, reduced skin elasticity, tachypnoea, oliguria
>10	Shocked: tachycardia and vasoconstriction
>15	Moribund

The main dangers of gastroenteritis are dehydration and electrolyte imbalance. Infants are particularly susceptible to dehydration because of their very high turnover of water relative to their size. An infant's normal daily fluid intake of 120–150 mL/kg represents up to 15% of his or her body weight. Clinical signs of dehydration are difficult to interpret and should be considered in combination. *Signs of dehydration may include → Table 18.6.*

> Dehydration may be underestimated in hypernatraemia or in plump children.

In the UK, the most common infectious agents that are isolated from children with enteric infections are rotavirus (56%), *Campylobacter* sp. (28%), *Salmonella* sp. (11%), norovirus (3%), *Shigella* sp. (1%) and verocytotoxin (shiga)-producing *Escherichia coli (E.Coli 0157)* (1%). Bloody diarrhoea occurs in up to 30% of children infected with *Campylobacter jejuni* and in up to 90% of children with *E. coli* 0157 infection. *E. coli* infections should be suspected when there has been a contact with ruminant farm animals (such as cattle, sheep and goats) or environments contaminated with their faeces or when an outbreak of *E. coli* 0157 is present locally. The incubation period for infection is usually 3 to 4 days but may be up to 14 days. *E. coli* 0157 infection leads to haemolytic uraemic syndrome in about 15% of cases (→ p. 271). This may occur up to 14 days after the onset of enteric symptoms. Children with bloody diarrhoea should have blood samples taken for: U&E, FBC, amylase, LFT, CRP and blood gas. Referral to the paediatric team is recommended.

Tx Most children can be managed at home with oral rehydration fluids (although clear liquids do not affect the frequency, amount or duration of loose stools). Vomiting may be reduced by giving fluids frequently and in small amounts. Give an oral fluid challenge to patients with mild–moderate dehydration by asking parents to administer 5–10 mL every 5 min via enteral syringe. Apple juice, diluted to half concentration with water, is likely to be better tolerated and at least as effective as oral rehydration solution.

Use of buccal antiemetics (ondansetron orodispersible) is an option if not tolerating the above, although this may increase diarrhoea in some patients.

Admission to hospital is required for children who are moderately dehydrated if they are unable to tolerate oral fluids. In young children enteral rehydration via NG tube is preferred to intravenous fluid. In severe cases, the plasma electrolytes should be measured; hypoglycaemia may occur.

Haemolytic uraemic syndrome → p. 271.

Intussusception

Although not a common illness, this cause of intestinal obstruction is included in this section because of its often non-specific presentation. Intussusception usually affects children between the ages of 3 months and 3 years and is most common in the first year of life. It occurs when the terminal ileum and the ileocaecal valve invaginate into the caecum and ascending colon. The classic triad of intermittent colicky abdominal pain, vomiting and redcurrant jelly stools is seen in less than 10% of children with intussusception. Lethargy and malaise are the most common signs. There may be a palpable mass in the right hypochondrium.

Investigations: Redcurrant jelly stool is rare, but the faeces usually test positive for blood. Ultrasound scan is the diagnostic study of choice; barium or air enema is a treatment.

Tx All children with suspected intussusception should be referred immediately to a surgeon. Insert a cannula and manage any cardiovascular compromise with a 10 mL/kg fluid bolus repeated as necessary.

NEONATAL PRESENTATIONS

Neonatal Life Support Page → 328

Neonates, prior to receipt of initial vaccinations should, wherever possible, be accommodated in an individual cubicle rather than exposed to the potential of infection in the general waiting room.

The collapsed neonate

Neonates are particularly susceptible to a range of conditions, which may lead to them presenting to the ED in a collapsed state. They are vulnerable to infection and congenital conditions undetected antenatally may become evidence during the first weeks of life.

These are high risk presentations and senior ED and paediatric assistance should be called immediately. Presentations are almost invariably non-specific in nature, and a systematic approach is essential to ensure serious causes are identified and treated promptly.

Follow an ABCDE approach (→ *p. 342*) with particular note of:

- **A:** Neonates have a large occiput meaning neck flexion can compromise airway patency. Use a folded sheet or blanket under the shoulders to allow the head to remain in the neutral position when supine.
- **B:** Very young babies are particularly prone to apnoea as a response to a range of insults. Prepare to provide ventilatory support, by locating and connecting appropriately sized equipment, even if it is not immediately required.
- **C:** Obtaining intravenous access is often easier in neonates than in chubby toddlers. If you have the skills and equipment, consider umbilical vein cannulation. Intraosseous access is often the quickest and easiest method. Ensure the intraosseous needle is sized appropriately – if small-sized needles are unavailable, manual insertion of an 18–20 g lumbar puncture needle is a recognised alternative. Conduct a thorough cardiovascular examination, including pre- and post-ductal saturation, auscultation for murmurs and palpation of femoral pulses. Hepatomegaly may be suggestive of right-sided heart failure or fluid overload.
- **D:** Neonates are prone to both birth and non-accidental head trauma, both of which are likely to present non-specifically. Check the fontanelle and pupils. Assess the infant's tone and assess for abnormal movements.

  Neonatal seizures may be subtle and comprise movements such as lip smacking, eye deviation, limb cycling and asymmetric tone, rather than the tonic-clonic movements more familiar in older children and adults.

  Remember to check the glucose. Low glycogen stores render the neonate particularly susceptible to hypoglycaemia. In the neonatal period (after the first 24 hours of life), a blood glucose of 2.5 mmol/L is considered the lower limit of normal.
- **E:** Examination must be thorough, but it is also essential to ensure that the temperature is maintained. Thermoregulation in neonates is immature and the relatively large body surface area means an infant will become hypothermic rapidly if not appropriately warmed. If possible, management on a resuscitaire is preferable. Look in particular for congenital problems and evidence of trauma. The infant must be examined

top to toe and front to back, including the external genitalia and hernial orifices. Masculinisation of the external genitalia of a female infant may be suggestive of congenital adrenal hyperplasia.

Differential diagnosis and management

Differential diagnosis – *Box 18.14*

- Obtain intravenous or intraosseous access
- Wherever possible obtain venous blood for FBC, U&E, LFT, calcium, glucose and blood cultures
- Obtain venous or capillary blood gas
- In all cases, unless there are clear signs of fluid overload, an initial fluid bolus of 10 mL/kg crystalloid should be administered
- Give antibiotics. Sepsis is by far the most common underlying problem and rapid treatment may be lifesaving. Cefotaxime is an appropriate choice, with amoxicillin to cover for congenitally acquired listeriosis.
- Have a low threshold for giving intravenous acyclovir. Neonatal herpes encephalitis has a devastating prognosis if untreated and often presents without a clear history of herpes virus exposure.
- Duct-dependent cardiac lesions often present in the second week of life as the ductus arteriosus begins to close. Consider intravenous prostacyclin infusion if a duct-dependent lesion is suspected. Prostacyclin infusion can provoke hypotension and apnoea, so intubation prior to commencement of the infusion is often appropriate.

Box 18.14 Differential diagnosis for the collapsed/seriously unwell neonate

- **T** – Trauma (nonaccidental and accidental)
- **H** – Heart disease and hypovolemia
- **E** – Endocrine (e.g. congenital adrenal hyperplasia and thyrotoxicosis)
- **M** – Metabolic (electrolyte imbalance)
- **I** – Inborn errors of metabolism
- **S** – Sepsis (e.g. meningitis, pneumonia, and urinary tract infection)
- **F** – Formula mishaps (e.g. under- or over-dilution)
- **I** – Intestinal catastrophes (e.g. volvulus, intussusception and necrotising enterocolitis)
- **T** – Toxins and poisons
- **S** – Seizures

Common neonatal problems

Poor feeding

Poor feeding is a common presentation of a range of serious conditions. Feeding is amongst the most energy-intensive activities a neonate undertakes and thus breathlessness, sweating, fatigue on feeding are equivalent to exertional symptoms in an older patient. A meticulous examination is essential to identify underlying causes.

For new parents, establishing breast feeding is often very challenging. Breastfeeding rates are far lower than desirable and well-intentioned but misguided advice from healthcare professionals is a contributory factor to this. Refer for expert infant feeding support if the baby is otherwise well rather than offering incomplete or incorrect advice.

Weight loss

A degree of weight loss is expected in the first days of life as feeding is initially established. If this becomes >10% of birth weight, then this is suggestive of dehydration or feeding difficulty and requires referral to a paediatrician for further assessment, and for specialist infant feeding support. Birth weight should have been regained within the first 3 weeks of life.

Crying

Persistent crying of an infant is incredibly distressing and fatiguing for new parents. This is a presentation that must be handled sensitively, with combined enquiry into the condition of both infant and parent. Parents often fear serious undiagnosed pathology, and a thorough examination is essential to both identify serious or treatable causes and reassure the caregivers. A period of observation may be invaluable to observe the behaviour of both the baby and caregivers. Reassurance, discussion of normal infant behaviour and parental expectations and referral for support are important. There is a real, although small, risk of non-accidental injury from exhausted and frustrated care givers in the early weeks of life. http://Purplecrying.info and http://iconcope.org are examples of excellent resources.

Consider:

Corneal abrasion – look for signs of conjunctival injection or discomfort on eye opening.
Hair tourniquet a parent/caregiver's hair can become accidentally wrapped around a digit (or occasionally penis/clitoris) of the infant, compromising distal circulation. If the skin is intact, hair removal cream can be used to dissolve the hair. Alternatively, the hair must be divided with a scalpel to ensure distal circulation is restored.

Infantile dyschezia Infants in the first months of life may appear to be uncomfortably straining at stool and distressed by apparent abdominal discomfort before passage of normal stool. Parents may mistake this for constipation. Dyschezia is due to immature control of the anal sphincter and incoordination with abdominal muscle contraction preceding defaecation. This resolves spontaneously and parents/caregivers can be reassured.

Colic Usually defined as unexplained crying for 3 hours a day, 3 days a week for at least 3 weeks. 'Colic' affects approximately 20% of infants and may be considered part of the wide spectrum of normal infantile behaviour. Over the counter remedies are ineffective, and management consists primarily of parental support and careful explanation.

Post natal depression All contacts with a healthcare professional are an opportunity for empathetic enquiry as to the well-being of the parents or caregivers, with active consideration of the possibility of postnatal depression. If postnatal depression is suspected, follow-up with the mental health team, or GP and midwife/health visiting team, should be arranged.

Vomiting

Gastrooesophageal reflux Many infants (at least 40%) have a degree of reflux, due to immaturity of the gastroesophageal sphincter. This usually starts before 8 weeks of age and may be frequent. In an infant who is gaining weight appropriately and otherwise well, this is best managed with reassurance of the parents or caregivers. Symptoms will resolve in 90% of infants before the age of 1 year.

Bilious vomiting Green bile stained vomitus in an infant is suggestive of an obstructive surgical cause such as malrotation, or duodenal/jejunal atresia. All such patients should be referred for paediatric surgical review.

> Bilious vomiting in an infant is a surgical problem until proven otherwise

Pyloric stenosis Vomiting is often described as forceful/projectile by parents/caregivers, and direct observation of a feed and the vomiting is often useful. Frequent forceful/projectile vomiting in an infant up to 2 months old is suggestive of pyloric stenosis. This is more common in first-born male infants. Only about one in seven cases will have the classic triad of projectile vomiting, visible peristalsis, and a palpable 'olive' mass in the abdomen. A metabolic alkalosis and hypokalaemia are often noted; however, hypokalaemia may take several weeks to develop and its absence should not be considered reassuring. Correct biochemical abnormalities and dehydration prior to surgery.

Safe sleep advice

Rate of SIDS (→ *p. 371*) has reduced by over 80% following the publication of safe sleep guidance in the 1990s. An attendance at the emergency department is an important opportunity to reinforce safe sleeping guidance. Risk is 50% lower if parents share a room with the infant, whereas risk is increased by sleeping on a sofa (x50) or placing the infant prone (x6). Safer sleep advice includes:

- Placing infant on their back with feet to the foot of the bed
- A firm flat mattress with no sleep positioners, bumpers or soft toys
- Avoidance of overheating – no head coverings, room between 16 and 20 degrees.
- Sleeping in the same room as parents for at least the first 6 months
- Avoid exposure to cigarette smoke
- Never sleep with the infant in a car seat, bouncer or on the sofa

Injuries and accidents

Refer to the relevant sections in the appropriate chapters.

Burns → Chapter 10.
Fingertip injuries → p. 134.
Foreign bodies in the ears and nose → pp. 435 and 436.
Impetigo → p. 424.
Minor injuries → Chapter 21.
Poisoning → Chapter 15.
Swallowed foreign bodies → p. 438.
The child who is not moving an arm → p. 119.
The limping child → p. 95.

Poisoning

Detailed information about poisoning → Chapter 15.

Younger children are particularly prone to ingesting substances accidentally or out of curiosity; older children may experiment with drugs or alcohol. Occasionally, inappropriate medication may have been obtained from an adult. Small items such as coins, batteries and magnets are frequently swallowed or placed in orifices. Ingested magnets and button batteries are particularly concerning → *Chapter 15.*

There is usually a history of definite or probable ingestion however less commonly poisoning may be suspected due to non-specific signs such as:

- confusion, agitation and drowsiness
- tachycardia
- dilated pupils
- evidence at the scene (which is of enormous help to hospital staff).

> **Box 18.15 One pill can kill, dangerous ingestions**
>
> - Sulphonylureas
> - Beta-blockers
> - Opiates
> - Tricyclic antidepressants
> - Calcium channel blockers
> - Amfetamines

Due to their small size children are more vulnerable to toxicity from adult therapeutic doses of a medication. In some cases just 'One Pill Can Kill'. → *Box 18.15*

Button battery ingestion → Chapter 15
Magnet ingestion → Chapter 15

Osteochondritis

There are several conditions in which there is an abnormality of bone in an area of growth or at the site where a major tendon is developing its attachment to bone. Children with one of these diseases may present to the ED with pain and reduced movements, often exacerbated by a minor injury. There is often slight swelling around the affected area. These osteochondritides are most commonly seen in the lower limb:

- **Head of the femur**: Perthes' disease (→ *p. 96*)
- **Lower pole of the patella**: Sindig–Laarson disease (→ *p. 102*)
- **Tibial tuberosity**: Osgood–Schlatter disease (→ *p. 102*)
- **Posterior calcaneum**: Sever's disease
- **Navicular bone**: Köhler's disease (→ *p. 109*)
- **Head of a metatarsal bone (usually the second metatarsus)**: Freiberg's disease.

XR The affected area may be deformed or fragmented. It is thought that a deficiency in the blood supply of the growing bone leads to aseptic necrosis.

TX Symptoms usually resolve with time. Rest from sports should be advised and an appointment at the orthopaedic clinic should be given.

Epiphyseal injuries

Injuries to the epiphyses are specific to childhood and adolescence. The epiphyseal plate is a weak area of the bone and so is often damaged. Bilateral or unilateral growth retardation may then occur. The Salter–Harris classification describes five types of epiphyseal injury, of which type II is the most common (→ *Figure 18.2*).

Ankle injuries in children → p. 107.
Elbow injuries in children (and a description of the growing elbow) → p. 119.
Wrist injuries in children → p. 124.

Immunisation in childhood

It is every child's right to be protected against preventable infectious diseases. No child should be denied immunisation without serious thought as to the consequences, both for the individual child and for the community.

> One in 10 children with meningococcal group C infection dies
>
> One in 20 children with *Haemophilus influenzae* B meningitis dies
>
> One in 500 infants with pertussis dies

In ED, good practice in the area of immunisation is essential. No child should be given a single anti-tetanus vaccine. If protection against tetanus is needed, then this should be given together with the other vaccines indicated for that age group (→ *Table 18.7*). Unvaccinated children should be either immunised opportunistically or else referred to the GP and health visitor for follow-up.

Sedation and analgesia for children undergoing procedures in the emergency department

It is inevitable in an ED that distressing and sometimes painful procedures are necessary. Minimising or eliminating pain and distress as far as possible should be a priority. Restraint of young children for painful procedures (sometimes referred to as 'brutacaine'!) is not appropriate and may have long-term impact on the child's relationship and engagement with healthcare staff. Ensure your patient has received appropriate analgesia before opting for sedation.

Distraction and diversional therapies

These are a long-established psychological means of helping with difficult situations. Elaborate coloured pattern and bubble generators are now available as well as traditional diversions such as music and stories. Many departments employ a play specialist who are experts in this specific aspect of care.

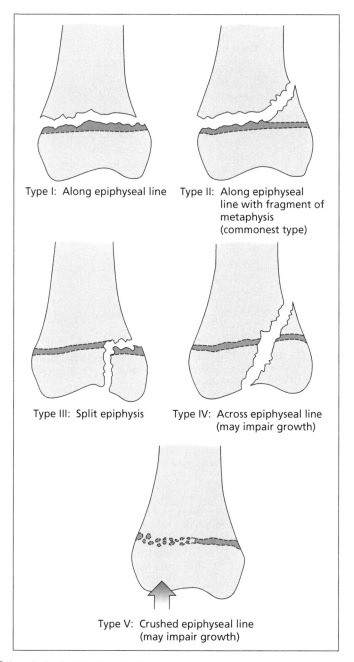

Figure 18.2 The Salter–Harris classification of epiphyseal injuries.

Table 18.7 UK immunisation schedule for children

Age	Target of immunisation	Name of vaccine
2 months	Diphtheria, tetanus, pertussis, polio, *H. influenzae* b and hepatitis B Rotavirus Meningococcus group B	DTaP/IPV/Hib/HBV (6 in 1) Rotarix oral vaccine Bexsero MenB vaccine
3 months	Diphtheria, tetanus, pertussis, polio, *H. influenzae* b and hepatitis B Rotavirus Pneumococcus	DTaP/IPV/Hib/HBV (6 in 1) Rotarix oral vaccine PCV
4 months	Diphtheria, tetanus, pertussis, polio, *H. influenzae* b and hepatitis B Meningococcus group B	DTaP/IPV/Hib/HBV (6 in 1) Bexsero MenB Vaccine
12–13 months	*H. influenzae* b and meningococcus group C Measles, mumps and rubella Pneumococcus Meningococcus type B	Hib/MenC MMR PCV Bexsero Men B vaccine
Age 2 until school year 6 annually	Influenza	Nasal flu vaccine
3 years and 4 months	Diphtheria, tetanus, pertussis and polio Measles, mumps and rubella	DTaP/IPV or dTAP/ IPV MMR
Teenage	Human papilloma virus (main cause of cervical cancer) Tetanus, diphtheria and polio Meningitis ACWY	HPV Td/IPV Meningitis ACWY

Td = tetanus vaccine combined with low-dose diphtheria vaccine. Low-dose (adult) diphtheria vaccine (d) should always be given after the age of 10 years rather than standard full-strength (paediatric) diphtheria vaccine (D). In older patients, use of the D vaccine results in a high number of both localised and generalised reactions.

Rewards such as balloons, badges and bravery certificates can help to soften the trauma of an unpleasant experience. Raisins and sweets – sugar free of course – are also used in some departments.

Breastfeeding

For young infants who are breastfeeding, it may be possible and helpful to feed during an unpleasant procedure (cannulation, immunisation). This is helpful to reduce distress and should be encouraged if feasible and the parent wishes it.

Local anaesthetic creams

Topical local anaesthetic preparations are available. Mixtures such as 'EMLA' (lidocaine 2.5% and prilocaine 2.5% cream) and 'Ametop' (tetracaine 4% gel) are suitable for procedures on intact skin such as venepuncture and splinter removal.

Preparations such as LAT gel (lidocaine, adrenaline and tetracaine) can be applied to wounds requiring suturing and covered by a dressing. After 20 min the blanched areas of skin show the areas which have been anaesthetised.

Local anaesthetic agents

These must be used with care in children as the maximum safe dose is easily exceeded (→ *Box 18.16*).

Box 18.16 Maximum doses of local anaesthetic agents

Bupivacaine	2 mg/kg
Lidocaine	3 mg/kg

Intranasal opiates

Intranasal administration of opiates (usually diamorphine or fentanyl) provides rapid and effective relief of severe pain without need for cannulation. This is an excellent choice for rapid control of pain in patients with burns, fractures and dislocations. Intranasal diamorphine dose is 0.1 mg/kg made up to a volume of 0.2 mL. Initial fentanyl dose is 1.5 mcg/kg and does not require dilution. An atomiser device can be used for administration but is not essential.

Oral morphine suspension

This can be used to alleviate the pain of a procedure where local anaesthesia is not practicable, such as changing a dressing on a large burn. The dose is 0.2–0.4 mg/kg for a child aged >12 months. The elixir must be given at least 60 min before the procedure to give adequate time for it to work.

Oral midazolam suspension

This is an effective sedative for minor or painless procedures in children (e.g. CT scan). The usual dose is 0.5 mg/kg. The onset of sedation occurs within about 20 min and the peak effect may be reached a few minutes later. Recovery is rapid – within <2 hours. The parents of all children who have been sedated should have written aftercare instructions to take home (→ *p. 408*). Some children (around 10%) who have been given midazolam in the above dosage will become hyperexcited. As with all benzodiazepines, the effects of midazolam can be reversed with flumazenil (→ *p. 281*).

> Sedative drugs used in isolation do not provide analgesia.

Parenteral doses of opiate analgesics

These can sometimes be useful in instances where a combination of sedation and analgesia is desirable and oral therapy is not suitable (*Dosages → Box 18.5 on p. 346*).

Gaseous analgesia and sedation

Analgesic gas from a premixed nitrous oxide/oxygen cylinder (e.g. Entonox) should be administered via a demand valve with a low opening pressure. Alternatively, an excellent sedative effect may be obtained with a continuous flow apparatus such as the Quantiflex˙ machine (→ *p. 15*).

Ketamine (→ *Chapter 1 p. 15*)

Ketamine can be used in sedative dose to provide an analgesic and dissociative effect and is a good choice in most children. Avoid in children with neurodevelopmental or behavioural problems, or those with active upper respiratory tract infections. Ketamine sedation must only be undertaken by senior staff with appropriate experience and training.

SAFEGUARDING ISSUES AND NON ACCIDENTAL INJURY

Five main types of child abuse are now recognised:

1 Emotional abuse
2 Neglect
3 Sexual abuse
4 Physical abuse (non-accidental injury or NAI)
5 Exploitation and organised abuse

The above list is in approximate order of prevalence, although the exact ranking is unknown.

Child abuse occurs in every culture and is perpetrated by all socioeconomic groups and genders. Presentation to the ED may be one of few opportunities to identify this and safeguard your patient. A child returned to an abusive environment is at high risk of further injury and potentially death. The emergency physician must be aware of local policies and procedures relevant to child safeguarding.

Certain factors may be associated with inability of parents/caregivers to respond appropriately to the needs of the child and are thus risk factors for neglect or abuse. These include:

- Substance misuse
- Significant mental health problems
- Very young parents
- Unintended pregnancies
- Parents abused as children
- Domestic abuse
- Social stressors – poverty, insecure or inadequate housing, lack of support

The stress of looking after very young children also increases the risk and so:

- a third of NAI occurs under 6 months of age
- a third of NAI occurs between 6 months and 3 years of age
- a third of NAI occurs over 3 years of age.

Diagnosis of non-accidental injury and abuse is a complex problem and experienced advice should be sought early. Parents should be kept informed about the concerns and the process of assessment unless there are concerns this will place the child at further risk. Most parents are understanding the need for investigations to keep children safe, as long as it is explained carefully in a non-accusatory manner.

Physical abuse

Physical abuse can present in a wide variety of ways and is often not immediately obvious. Burns are the most common (15–25% of burns are thought to be abusive in nature), followed by fractures and bruising. There are patterns of physical signs for some types of abuse but the history and the context in which the events occurred are the most important first indicators to alert the clinician. Some features of a history of injury that should raise suspicion of abuse are the following:

- Injury in a non-mobile child (any bruising under the age of 6 months is of particular concern)
- Inappropriate delay in seeking help and advice after a significant injury
- History of previous frequent accidents or multiple attendances to hospital with injury
- The history of the accident is not a likely mechanism for that injury
- A vague, absent or changing account of the mechanism of injury
- Different carers give different explanations for the same injury
- The child gives a different history
- The child is reported to have sustained the injury in a way that is inconsistent with his or her development (e.g. fell over before the child has started walking)
- The adults with the child are either unconcerned or hostile during questioning. Their attention is focused on their own needs throughout.

The following list of signs of child abuse is by no means comprehensive:

- Unexplained head, facial, chest or limb injuries, especially in children who are not able to walk and thus fall (few children walk under the age of 11 months)
- Any bruising in a non-mobile infant
- Symmetrical bruising
- Linear bruising, especially to the buttocks or back
- Bruising around the eye, especially if bilateral
- Bruising around the ears, especially if bilateral
- Other facial bruising including in or around the mouth
- Facial petechiae/subconjunctival haemorrhages
- Tears of the frenulum of the upper lip in non-mobile infants (this is often an accidental injury following a fall in toddlers and young children)

- Grasp marks or fingertip bruising especially to the face, arms or chest
- Unusual cuts and bruises; outline imprints of hands, sticks, cords, shoes, belts and teeth may be present
- Marks to the neck
- Marks to the genitalia
- A tender, red scalp (hair pulling)
- Unusual burns, e.g. those of a glove or stocking distribution or to the perineum or cigarette type
- Injuries of different ages
- Multiple old scars
- Any fractures in children aged <12 months
- Coexisting signs of neglect.

Non-accidental head injury in infants (previously called the 'shaken baby syndrome') → p. 42

All children in whom the diagnosis of non-accidental injury or abuse is suspected should be fully examined from top to toe by an experienced doctor. The investigation and management of a case of possible deliberate harm to a child must be approached in the same systematic and rigorous manner as the investigation and management of any other potentially fatal disease. This is usually undertaken by a trained paediatrician.

XR There are also typical radiological findings of abuse, which are more common in younger children:

- Old unsuspected fractures
- Fractures at different stages of healing (→ *Box 18.17*)
- Rib fractures (posterior rib fractures are particularly specific for abuse)
- Skull fractures in children who cannot walk (especially if multiple, depressed or in areas other than the parietal bones) (→ *p. 43*)
- Spiral fractures of long bones (twisting injuries)
- Injuries to the metaphyses of long bones (twisting injuries); these are very specific for non-accidental trauma
- Periosteal injuries (twisting forces).

Tx

> Look for a specific Child Protection Plan via the local social services portal or by making contact with Children's social care by telephone (→ *p. 403*).

 Box 18.17 Healing of fractures on radiographs

Periosteal new bone formation	10–14 days
Loss of fracture line definition	14–21 days
Soft callus formation	14–21 days
Hard callus visible	>21 days

There will be a local protocol for the management of suspected non-accidental injury and safeguarding concerns. The child should always be discussed with a senior member of the ED or paediatric staff. Most cases should be referred to the paediatric team for further assessment. The duty social worker for child protection must also be notified of the concern as soon as possible. This should be promptly followed up in writing. A full 'child protection medical' may be required following liaison between social care and paediatric staff- local policy should be followed for the completion of this. Children under the age of 2 years may require a 'skeletal survey' (X-ray examination of the entire skeleton) and examination by an ophthalmologist (for retinal haemorrhage).

Legal aspects of child protection, including emergency powers, → p. 403.

Neglect and emotional abuse

Only gross forms of neglect can be recognised in an ED. Some of the characteristics are as follows:

- Short in stature and underweight for age
- Cold, mottled, discoloured extremities
- Poor skin condition (especially in the nappy area)
- Poor nutritional state (wasting, sparse hair, voracious appetite)
- Flat affect
- Lack of energy and failure to play.

Emotional abuse is even more subtle than physical neglect.

Tx As for other forms of abuse, these children should be discussed with local safeguarding teams, children's social services and a senior paediatrician.

Sexual abuse

> Before the age of 16, at least 1 in 10 girls and 1 in 15 boys will have been sexually assaulted. The peak incidence of first assault is at about 8 years of age.

Sexual abuse of children can occur in all socioeconomic, cultural and religious groups and is associated with:

- acute perineal injury
- chronic perineal damage
- genitourinary infection
- sexually precocious behaviour
- sexualised drawings and play

- regressive patterns of behaviour
- eating and sleep disorders
- psychosomatic symptoms
- withdrawal and depression
- self-harm
- promiscuity
- episodes of missing from home

Girls are affected about four times more often than boys. A proportion of patients who present with self-harm as teenagers or adults will later give a history of sexual abuse. Adolescent patients may be victims of grooming and sexual exploitation, which may come to light with careful and empathetic history taking. It is important to recognise that sexual exploitation may be characterised by a negative relationship, with a power differential, in which the adolescent receives something (gifts, alcohol, drugs or affection) in exchange for sexual activity. The young person may consider themselves to be in a relationship with their abuser and not recognise its abusive nature.

HEADDS assessment → Box 18.7
Needs of adolescent patients → p. 347.

Tx All suspected cases should be referred for consideration of the need for child protection as described earlier. Examination of acute injuries should be left to a specialist sexual assault referral centre, unless immediate treatment is required.

Sudden infant death syndrome

This term refers to the unexpected death of an infant under one year of age, which remains unexplained after thorough investigation including post-mortem, assessment of place of death and clinical history taking. One baby in every 1400 live births dies suddenly and unexpectedly for no obvious reason. This sudden infant death syndrome is the most common cause of death in the UK in infants aged >1 month. The diagnosis does not include all sudden infant deaths because some infants die suddenly from well-understood causes. It is recommended that the term SUDI/SUDC (Sudden Unexpected Death in infancy/childhood) is used while investigation is ongoing. SIDS is more common among boys and with premature or low birthweight infants.

- Twins have approximately double the risk of singletons
- Over 80% of cases occur under the age of 6 months
- It is more common in the winter months.
- Most deaths from SIDS seem to occur during sleep.

Safer sleep guidance → p. 365.

Tx Resuscitation attempts should always be initiated whilst information gathering is in progress, unless there is clear rigor mortis. A member of staff should be assigned to support the parents throughout resuscitation attempts. Parents should be allowed to remain with their child continually (if they wish), including during resuscitation and medical procedures with appropriate explanation and support.

If the infant is one of twins, the surviving twin should be admitted to the paediatric ward for monitoring, as risk to the second twin is up to eightfold.

Sudden unexpected death in childhood procedures (SUDIC)

Following an unexpected death in childhood, the following multi-agency procedures must be followed, to enable understanding of the cause and circumstances surrounding the death.

- A thorough examination by a consultant paediatrician and key investigations are essential before the patient is moved to the mortuary. Examination findings may change before post-mortem (especially skin marks and livido). Local procedures should be followed to arrange this. In some areas a designated doctor for child deaths will attend the department promptly for this examination.
- Uniformed police officers often attend the ED after notification from ambulance control. Parents should be reassured that this is a routine part of the SUDIC procedure.
- Children's social care must be notified, to contribute to the investigations as part of the rapid response team.
- In most cases, the named doctor for child deaths and senior investigating police officer will visit the home or place of death to gather additional information surrounding the circumstances of the death.
- An initial multi-agency meeting should take place within 48 hours to identify any immediate risks to other family members, or child protection considerations and to arrange support for the bereaved family.
- Following post-mortem and multi-agency input, the death will be discussed at a Child Death Overview Panel.

The disturbed patient

Antonia Hazlerigg[1,2] and Laura Cottey[2]

[1] Emergency Department, Royal Infirmary of Edinburgh, Edinburgh, UK
[2] Academic Department of Military Emergency Medicine, Royal Centre for Defence Medicine

Psychological disturbance can cause more upset to a patient, and their family and friends than a physical problem. The core principle of managing a patient within the emergency department (ED) is that any patient with a physical or mental health need should have access to ED staff that understand and can address their condition and access to appropriate specialist services regardless of their postcode, GP or time of arrival. The distress experienced by a disturbed patient should never be underestimated and attempts should always be made to try and minimise the detrimental impact that an ED environment can have.

A patient may appear disturbed due to a range of conditions that must be considered in the differential diagnosis, including substance use, head injury or seizures, metabolic conditions and sepsis in addition to mental health disorders (→ *Box 19.1 for common acute presentations of mental disturbance*).

Mental health disorders are common. One in six people in England experiences symptoms of common mental health disorders, like anxiety and depression, in any given week. Worldwide, depression is one of the leading causes of disability, and suicide is the second leading cause of death in 15–29-year-olds. Over the course of a lifetime, 1 in 15 people will attempt suicide.

Rates of dementia are rising, with an estimated million people living with dementia expected by 2025 in the UK.

Drug and alcohol use also remains an important cause of behavioural disturbance. One in 11 adults in the UK report drug use in the previous year, and alcohol excess is the biggest risk factor for death, ill-health and disability amongst 15–49-year-olds.

> **Box 19.1 The presentation of mental health problems to the emergency department**
>
> - Acute psychiatric disturbance (patient with little insight brought to ED by relatives, social workers or the police)
> - Psychological symptoms (patient usually self-referred with depression or anxiety)
> - Exacerbation of symptoms or loss of control in known psychiatric disease (patient usually has good insight and self-refers; may request admission)
> - Personality disorder (patient in a state of crisis, can display behaviours which are considered disruptive, often short-lived but severe in nature)
> - Self-harm
> - Alcohol and drug abuse
> - Acute emotional upset

The task of the ED is to:

- identify those patients who need immediate treatment
- rule out medical conditions as a cause for symptoms and manage them if required
- treat any related injury appropriately
- manage the patient in an appropriate area
- risk assess the patient for suicide and self-harm
- support the patient and accompanying persons
- liaise with the appropriate agencies for further care.

The RCEM Lecture Notes: Emergency Medicine, Fifth Edition. Edited by Catherine Williams and Amy Nickson.
© 2024 John Wiley & Sons Ltd. Published 2024 by John Wiley & Sons Ltd.
Companion website: www.wiley.com/go/LNEM5

INITIAL ASSESSMENT AND MANAGEMENT OF THE DISTURBED OR DISTRESSED PATIENT

A careful systematic approach to the disturbed patient can help to establish the diagnosis and ensure referral to the appropriate services. The ED is a busy and chaotic space and is often not the most suitable environment to assess a disturbed or significantly distressed patient. If possible, conduct the consultation in a quiet area, whilst ensuring personal safety and use a supportive and empathetic approach. For some of these patients, assessment may be most appropriate in a specialist centre or designated area; however, this will be determined by local protocols, always keeping patient-centred care at the heart of decision making.

Ask about

- Presenting complaints as described by the patient and those accompanying them
- The history of the presenting complaint, any triggering or exacerbating factors and accompanying symptoms
- Current drug therapy and other management and support
- Previous psychiatric history: symptoms, duration, diagnoses, admissions and any treatment received
- Coincidental physical illnesses and past medical history
- Family history
- Substance misuse
- Social circumstances and support (e.g. many people with a mental health problem are also affected by debt, homelessness, substance use or contact with the criminal justice system)

Look for

Conduct a mental state examination

Appearance and behaviour:

- Abnormal appearance or behaviour, e.g. appropriately dressed, evidence of neglect, do they appear worried, anxious, fearful, aggressive, eye contact
- Are they alert and orientated? Is there evidence of disorientation, difficulty concentrating or altered conscious level?
- Is there evidence of abnormal movements, e.g. tics, hyperactivity, dystonic movement

Speech:

- What is the rate, form and content of speech? Is the speech logical and coherent? Does it rapidly change topic, e.g. flight of ideas?

Mood:

- Ask about mood, how does he or she feel? What is their view of themselves and their future? Describe the mood from a subjective and objective perspective.

Thoughts:

- Is thought content disordered? Is there evidence of any abnormal beliefs: delusions, misinterpretations and overvalued ideas
- Are hallucinations (visual or auditory) and disorders of perception present?
- Does the patient describe any obsessions and compulsions?

Insight and mental capacity

- What insight does the patient have into their problems?

Concise notes may be augmented by verbatim quotes of the patient's responses to questioning. A brief but comprehensive physical examination is also important to exclude as far as possible 'organic' causes of disturbance (e.g. head injury, hypoglycaemia, infection, drug disturbance, epilepsy, neurological disease, e.g. autoimmune encephalitis and cerebrovascular disease). This must include at a minimum:

- temperature
- heart rate
- examination for any evidence of head injury
- evidence of infection
- blood sugar
- gross neurological signs (walking and talking).

In addition, the following symptoms have been identified as typical of acute behavioural disturbance (ABD) and should be considered a medical emergency and prompt early recognition and interventions ($\rightarrow$ p. 377).

- Tactile hyperthermia (hot to touch)
- Constant or near constant physical activity
- Extreme agitation or aggression.

Management

Therapeutic activity includes the following:

- Verbal calming and de-escalation techniques including review of environmental factors, which should always be attempted prior to any consideration of pharmacological methods. Aim for the least restrictive option which will ensure patient and staff safety.
- Treatment and correction of organic problems (e.g. sepsis, hypoxia and metabolic disturbances)
- Management of associated drug and alcohol ingestion
- **Sedation**: may be required if patient fails to respond to de-escalation techniques. The ED team needs to determine the most appropriate route, bearing in mind the safety of both the patient and team. ($\rightarrow$ Box 19.2)

Box 19.2 Pharmacological sedation/ rapid tranquilisation

There are three groups of drug agents currently used for sedation in the ED:

- Benzodiazepines are mostly commonly used with a number of routes of administration and wide safety profile. Oral lorazepam should be tried initially; intramuscular (IM) use has associated problems of a slow onset and unpredictability. Intravenous (IV) benzodiazepines (lorazepam or midazolam) may also be used but carry with them the challenge and risk of intravenous cannulation of a distressed and agitated patient.
- Ketamine is now the first line parenteral drug as it has a quick onset via IM route at 4 mg/kg. Sympathomimetic side effects, e.g. tachycardia, increased blood pressure should be closely monitored. Emergence phenomenon is a documented side effect and can be managed with benzodiazepines.
- The second line agent is IM droperidol which carries a lower risk of prolonging the QT interval than haloperidol. Avoid in Lewy-Body dementia and Parkinson's disease.
- Promethazine may be a useful option, if available, for a benzodiazepine tolerant patient, or if avoidance of antipsychotics is considered desirable.

All normal precautions for sedation, including full patient monitoring, should be observed regardless of medication choice.

- **Rapid tranquilisation**: This technique is utilised when there is risk to the patient or care staff, which it has not been possible to deescalate in other ways. It is a form of chemical restraint and the aim should be to minimise any physical restraint that may have been utilised and facilitate treatment of patient in their best interests whilst ensuring the safety of staff. Choice and route of agent should be determined by the patient's presentation with consideration of medication previously effective for this patient (if known).
- Discussion of patient options for referral and referral to psychiatry liaison services or other agencies.

Interaction with the disturbed patient

The impression given by staff is very important, and every patient should be treated with respect and kindness, regardless of the situation. It must be recognised that the patient is extremely vulnerable, and both the environment of the ED, and the professionals they come into contact with, have potential to exacerbate a patient's distress. It is therefore important to avoid actions that may be interpreted as threatening and simultaneously to ensure that staff are never put at risk or in a position of vulnerability. Staff must avoid being judgemental and must be sensitive to a patient's affect. They need to be aware of the potential for behaviour which can be difficult to interact with, but must not react to it in a critical manner.

The aim is to support the patient at a time of crisis, manage the immediate medical demands and to identify appropriate agencies that can provide ongoing care. The latter can include the patient's relatives and friends or the patient's own resources. Medication and admission – rarely against the patient's will – may be necessary. Physical restraint may be justified; however this needs to be proportionate to patient presentation. The key principle is to use the least restrictive option, for the minimum necessary duration. Thus, a patient who is distressed and shouting, but not presenting an immediate risk to themselves or others, probably does not warrant physical restraint. If physical restraint is required, it may sometimes require the involvement of security teams or the police.

A patient's distress and associated behaviour can usually be managed with appropriate reassurance, consistent messaging and policies, empathetic interaction and communication. Simple interventions, such as provision of food or drink, can deescalate many situations. Avoid making promises that cannot be kept.

Throughout care in the ED, it is essential to reassure the patient regularly about the intended course of action and to keep the patient up to date with events.

CONFUSION AND PSYCHOTIC BEHAVIOUR

Acute confusional states

Delirium is often subdivided into hyperactive, hypoactive and mixed types. The main features include:

- Disturbance of consciousness
- Change in cognition
- Rapid development over a short period of time (usually hours to days) with a tendency to fluctuate during the course of the day

Delirium is often under-recognised (especially hypoactive and mixed types) and is associated with high rates of mortality and morbidity. Even after treatment of the underlying cause, delirium can persist for up to 6 months. Some patients will never regain full cognitive function.

Patients at risk include the elderly (>65 years), those with underlying dementia, patients with severe illness and those with a hip fracture. There are added patient and system risks with delirium so the aim must always be prevention. Scoring systems can be used in the ED to aid with recognition of delirium, for example the 4-AT (→*Box 19.3*). With suggestion of delirium, a diagnosis should be actively sought and documented, using DSM-V (Diagnostic and Statistical Manual of Mental Disorders) or short CAM (Confusion Assessment Method) scores. Often this will occur beyond the ED after a period of stabilisation and investigation has occurred.

A wide range of underlying conditions may be responsible for confusion and disorientation and so a full history, physical examination and laboratory findings are required to establish the cause.

- Hypoxia may present as a toxic confusional state and a psychosis of rapid onset with disorientation, hallucination and delusions. There will be a clouding of consciousness and impairment of recent memory. These sudden alterations in cerebration are very frightening and sufficient to cause aggression in many patients.
- Hypoglycaemia may cause considerable confusion and aggression.
- Infection, particularly of the central nervous system (CNS), can also cause an acute confusional state. Elderly patients with any infection (e.g. chest or urinary tract) can present in such a way that the underlying medical condition is completely masked.
- Drug intoxication (→ *p. 378 and Chapter 15*).
- Gross metabolic disturbance, including that found with hepatic and renal failure.
- Organic brain lesions, or encephalopathy, may occasionally present in this way.
- Post-ictal states: there may be aggression and agitation in a similar way to hypoglycaemia.
- Constipation is a much-overlooked and easily treatable cause of delirium and a careful history and consideration of a rectal examination are important
- Myocardial infarction (MI) may present with acute confusion in elderly people. There is often a tendency to attribute presentations of delirium to a urinary tract infection in the absence of convincing symptoms. While UTI certainly can contribute to delirium, caution should be exercised to ensure that other potential causes are not overlooked. The PINCHME mnemonic is useful to prompt consideration and treatment of a range of causes → *Box 19.4*

Investigations:

The majority of presenting patients are those who are elderly and those with significant illness. The following investigations should be ordered for the majority of those presenting with suspected delirium.

- Full blood count (FBC), glucose, blood chemistry including calcium, liver function tests (LFTs), thyroid function tests (TFTs) and C-reactive protein (CRP)
- Chest X-ray and ECG

 Box 19.3 4-AT assessment

(1) Alertness	Normal	0
	Mild sleepiness for <10 seconds after waking then normal	0
	Clearly abnormal	4
(2) AMT – Age, date of birth, place, current year	No mistakes	0
	1 mistake	1
	2 or more mistakes/ Untestable	2
(3) Attention – 'Please tell me the months of the year in backwards order'	>7 months correctly	0
	<7 months or refuses to start	1
	Untestable (drowsy, inattention)	2
Acute change or fluctuating course – Evidence of significant change or fluctuation in alertness, cognition or other mental function arising in the last 2 weeks and still evident in the last 24 hours	No	0
	Yes	1

Scoring key: 4 or more – possible delirium/cognitive impairment.
1–3 – possible cognitive impairment.
0 – delirium or significant cognitive impairment unlikely.

Box 19.4 Causes of delirium 'PINCHME'

Pain
Infection
Nutrition
Constipation
Hydration
Medication – consider particularly sedatives and anticholinergic medication
Environment

- Urinalysis is not helpful in the elderly population due to high rates of false positives – this can lead to premature diagnostic closure and harms associated with unnecessary antibiotic therapy (number needed to harm = 3) (N.B. malodorous urine does not correlate well with urinary tract infection).
- Mid-stream urine culture may be appropriate; however, the high rates of asymptomatic bacteriuria must be considered and results correlated carefully with clinical presentation.

Consider the following depending on presentation:

- Serum vitamin B_{12}, folate and ferritin levels
- CT scan of the brain is of low yield in undifferentiated delirium patients, and so is usually not useful in ED in the absence of head injury, anticoagulant treatment or focal neurology.

Tx The key is to identify and treat the underlying cause of delirium-ome diagnoses can be rapidly diagnosed and treated, e.g. hypoglycaemia. In the emergency situation, it is essential to manage the immediate risks that delirium brings.

- Ensure a safe environment and effective communication (including reassurance and orientation); involve family and carers whereever possible.
- Basic observations should be continued and oxygenation and hydration maintained.
- Retention of urine, constipation, pain and discomfort must be avoided and medications should be reviewed.
- If possible, avoid catheterisation and sedation, however this may be required if it is impossible to assess or manage an agitated patient, or the patient presents a risk of harm to self or others. Ensure that adequate analgesia is administered, and splintage is applied.
- **Sedation**: If non-pharmacological means are not sufficient to manage the acute situation, then sedation may be the best option. In practice both benzodiazepines and anti-psychotics may be utilised. Use of small dose of benzodiazepines (often lorazepam or midazolam) can be effective and have a rapid onset of action, but careful observation and monitoring are necessary. A typical antipsychotic can also be utilised (e.g. haloperidol) for acute delirium, but avoid or use with great caution for those with Parkinson's disease or Lewy Body dementia, and those at risk of having a long QT interval. Dosing for all agents should be at the lowest appropriate dose (dose reduction is necessary in the elderly), titrated according to symptoms and should be used in short term only (<7 days). The use of depressant drugs has previously been criticised in hypoxaemia because it may decrease respiratory effort, however occasionally, in situations of extreme agitation, judicious sedation decreases oxygen requirements and makes possible the administration

of high-concentration oxygen by mask – this decision should be made by a senior clinician.

Acute behavioural disturbance (ABD)

ABD (sometimes previously known as agitated delirium) is a medical emergency with a mortality rate around 10%. It has a wide variety of definitions worldwide; however, within the UK, there is consensus that it refers to the patient cohort that exhibits sudden onset of aggressive or violent behaviour with autonomic dysfunction, which is typically associated with acute or chronic drug use, or mental illness. This is an umbrella term rather than a formal diagnosis and may have a variety of underlying causes.

The range of presenting symptoms and signs and range of causes necessitate a broad differential diagnosis, including psychiatric disorder, head injury, sepsis, seizures, hypoglycaemia, hypoxia, serotonin syndrome, neuroleptic malignant syndrome, thyroid storm and deliberate or accidental toxic ingestion/substance misuse.

> High temperatures and heart rate in a patient under physical restraint is a concerning sign which suggests a high risk of adverse outcomes

The ED clinician should suspect and promptly address ABD when a patient arrives being restrained, particularly with high temperatures and heart rate – this is a high-risk presentation which must not be dismissed as merely an 'aggressive' patient.

Hyperthermia is a particularly concerning sign suggestive of significant physiological disruption possibly due to high catecholamine response. ABD has been linked with a number of high-profile deaths in police custody and is often a highly emotive presentation, which can cause significant distress to families, patients and staff.

It is often difficult to complete a full physical examination and perform accurate physiological observations in this situation and combined with potential violence and aggression this leads to significant risk. A rapid run through of the escalation management protocol detailed below should be adopted.

Management: ABD is a medical emergency and requires early recognition, early intervention, proactive treatment and collaboration between all personal involved with care (including police or security as well as medical personnel). Attempts at verbal de-escalation should occur early; however if this fails, then a prompt move to chemical restraint over prolonged physical restraint should be planned.

Physical restraint must be:

- Justifiable
- Reasonable
- Proportionate
- Applied for the minimal time possible

Escalation management protocol for severe agitation:

- Verbal de-escalation
- Physical Restraint – held for as short a time as possible, using recognised techniques only (avoiding prone positioning)
- Chemical Restraint including rapid tranquilisation using oral medication initially where possible (→ *see Box 19.2*)

Once control of the situation has been obtained, a full assessment and targeted investigations addressing the range of possible underlying causes should be undertaken.

Drug-induced psychiatric syndromes

Prescribed drugs

Mental disturbance caused by prescribed drugs is particularly common in elderly people but may occur with CNS-depressant drugs, β blockers, digoxin and cimetidine at all ages. Symptoms include fluctuating clouding of consciousness and restlessness with paranoid delusions and visual hallucinations in severe cases. Although usually a result of overdosage, these reactions may sometimes occur because of intolerance to the normal dose or after withdrawal of the drug. Anti-cholinergic medication burden is cumulative and a significant cause of cognitive impairment in the elderly.

Recreational drugs

Patients may retain full consciousness but experience paranoid delusions and visual hallucinations after ingestion of cocaine, amphetamines, lysergic acid diethylamide (LSD), 'spice', synthetic cannabinoids and psychotropic fungi. Fear and restlessness lead to disruptive and aggressive behaviour. The condition can often be distinguished from schizophrenia by the history and by the extreme nature of the patient's behaviour; however, the possibility of 'dual diagnosis' should be noted.

Treatment of specific poisonings → Chapter 15.

Psychoses

The term psychosis is characterised by a variety of symptoms (for example, hallucinations or delusions) leading to an alteration in the patient's perception, thoughts, mood or behaviour. These symptoms may lead to marked distress and may result in varying degrees of loss of capacity.

Schizophrenia is now no longer thought to be a single condition. The name embraces a heterogeneous group of clinical syndromes in which hallucinations, delusions and thought disorders are present. The intensity of these symptoms is constantly changing, and they may be modified or abolished by drugs. Mood and behaviour are similarly fluctuant.

Patients with both schizophrenia and mania may present acutely to the ED with obvious psychotic behaviour. The distinction between the two conditions can be difficult at times but is not initially important because short-term pharmacological control of symptoms is similar in both conditions.

More commonly, a patient with a known history of schizophrenia comes to the ED with an exacerbation of usually well-controlled symptoms. Loss of therapeutic control may be precipitated by:

- pressure of outside events
- moving area of residence away from long-term support
- omitting depot (long-acting parenteral) therapy
- absence of usual support (friends, relatives or care workers).

Tx Psychotic behaviour may necessitate the administration of neuroleptic drugs (e.g. IV or IM haloperidol 5–10 mg), although oral lorazepam 2 mg and/or oral haloperidol 5 mg may be tried initially. These patients will subsequently require expert care from specialist mental health multidisciplinary teams.

Medical conditions in psychiatric patients

Up to 50% of psychiatric patients have a co-existing medical condition and, in some cases, this may exacerbate psychiatric symptoms. In particular, patients with a diagnosis of schizophrenia have an increased incidence of:

- cardiovascular disease
- endocrine disease
- infection
- nutritional problems.

There is a corresponding increase in mortality from these conditions, and it is essential that medical symptoms in patients with established mental health problems are always be investigated appropriately and not assumed to be due to mental illness. Medical emergencies will always take precedence over psychiatric treatment, although in some circumstances management may need to be undertaken in parallel.

'Ruling out organic causes'

Emergency physicians are often asked to assess patients presenting with ostensibly psychiatric symptoms, to 'rule out' an organic cause for these symptoms. This can be challenging. At a minimum, this should involve a thorough history and appropriately targeted physical examination, which will inform decisions about further investigations. Investigation strategy should be targeted and patient specific rather than 'routine'.

Collateral history is often helpful (this can be friends and family, as well as pre-hospital emergency workers) to risk stratify those that are more likely at risk of a medical condition, and specifically exclude delirium.

In general, older patients presenting with new psychiatric symptoms and those with no prior history of mental health problems will require more extensive assessment and investigation. In these cases, assume an organic cause until this has been ruled out (i.e. these patients will likely require more investigations than those with previous psychiatric illness). Remember that some conditions presenting with apparently psychiatric symptoms (e.g. space occupying lesions in the brain, NMDA receptor antibody encephalitis) may require diagnostic techniques not readily available in the ED.

ALCOHOL-RELATED PROBLEMS

Acute intoxication with alcohol

A potentially intoxicated patient should always be managed carefully with a full clinical examination and relevant investigations to identify other pathology which could either mimic intoxication, e.g. hypoglycaemia, or be coexistent as a result, e.g. head injury. Diagnosis of alcohol intoxication must always be made by exclusion never by neglect – these patients are high risk. Consider other substance ingestion including deliberate overdose of medication.

Observation of the intoxicated patient must be in a safe area of the ED (i.e. where close observation is possible) as alcohol absorption from the gastrointestinal tract will continue for some time after the last ingestion. In comatose patients, blood levels may continue to rise for about 2 hours after presentation. The patient may appear to be becoming quieter and more cooperative, when they are actually becoming more intoxicated.

Respiratory depression and inhalation of vomitus can occur quite suddenly and patients with reduced conscious level need close monitoring and potentially airway protection as the nature of the poison ingested raises rather than lowers the risk of aspiration. Never disregard a patient as 'just drunk'. Nurse intoxicated patients on their side in the 'recovery' position to reduce the risk of aspiration of vomitus.

Signs of intoxication with alcohol and for the treatment of acute alcohol poisoning → p. 294.

Considerations in the intoxicated patient

Injury: People with an alcohol addiction are more prone to injury and very much more susceptible to assault than most people. A full physical examination is essential. Loss of reflex protective mechanisms when drunk contributes to the increased incidence of subdural haematoma as a complication of head injury in those who drink to excess (→ *p. 39*).

Suicide and self-harm: Suicide and self-harm have an increased incidence in people with alcohol addiction and those who drink to excess. Therefore, possible injury and ingestion of other drugs should always be considered.

Alcohol withdrawal states

Alcohol withdrawal is not synonymous with delirium tremens. There are in fact several possible presentations that can follow the cessation of drinking in patients who are physically dependent on alcohol.

Acute withdrawal syndrome

This occurs within 6–12 hours of abstinence and presents as:

- agitation and restlessness (sometimes extreme)
- tremulousness
- sweating
- tachycardia
- anorexia, nausea and retching
- upper abdominal pain (but beware of pancreatitis or ulcer).

Assessment and monitoring Symptom triggered scoring systems are recommended as part of local hospital protocols to assess the severity of symptoms and guide treatment e.g. CIWA-Ar (Clinical Institute Withdrawal Assessment – Alcohol revised) (→ *Figure 19.1*).

Tx Most of the symptoms respond well to benzodiazepines such as diazepam or chlordiazepoxide. High doses may be needed but should be guided by local protocols; the correct dose is apparent by the symptom relief that it affords as assessed by regular review and re-scoring. Upper abdominal symptoms may be helped by antacids. Cautious doses of benzodiazepines should be used in patients with alcoholic liver disease (lorazepam

Clinical Institute Withdrawal Assessment of Alcohol Scale, Revised (CIWA-Ar)

Patient: _____ Date: _____ Time: _____ (24 hour clock, midnight = 00:00)

Pulse or heart rate, taken for one minute: _____ Blood pressure: _____

NAUSEA AND VOMITING -- Ask "Do you feel sick to your stomach? Have you vomited?" Observation.
0 no nausea and no vomiting
1 mild nausea with no vomiting
2
3
4 intermittent nausea with dry heaves
5
6
7 constant nausea, frequent dry heaves and vomiting

TACTILE DISTURBANCES -- Ask "Have you any itching, pins and needles sensations, any burning, any numbness, or do you feel bugs crawling on or under your skin?" Observation.
0 none
1 very mild itching, pins and needles, burning or numbness
2 mild itching, pins and needles, burning or numbness
3 moderate itching, pins and needles, burning or numbness
4 moderately severe hallucinations
5 severe hallucinations
6 extremely severe hallucinations
7 continuous hallucinations

TREMOR -- Arms extended and fingers spread apart. Observation.
0 no tremor
1 not visible, but can be felt fingertip to fingertip
2
3
4 moderate, with patient's arms extended
5
6
7 severe, even with arms not extended

AUDITORY DISTURBANCES -- Ask "Are you more aware of sounds around you? Are they harsh? Do they frighten you? Are you hearing anything that is disturbing to you? Are you hearing things you know are not there?" Observation.
0 not present
1 very mild harshness or ability to frighten
2 mild harshness or ability to frighten
3 moderate harshness or ability to frighten
4 moderately severe hallucinations
5 severe hallucinations
6 extremely severe hallucinations
7 continuous hallucinations

PAROXYSMAL SWEATS -- Observation.
0 no sweat visible
1 barely perceptible sweating, palms moist
2
3
4 beads of sweat obvious on forehead
5
6
7 drenching sweats

VISUAL DISTURBANCES -- Ask "Does the light appear to be too bright? Is its color different? Does it hurt yours eyes? Are you seeing anything that is disturbing to you? Are you seeing things you know are not there?" Observation.
0 not present
1 very mild sensitivity
2 mild sensitivity
3 moderate sensitivity
4 moderately severe hallucinations
5 severe hallucinations
6 extremely severe hallucinations
7 continuous hallucinations

ANXIETY -- Ask "Do you feel nervous?" Observation.
0 no anxiety, at ease
1 mild anxious
2
3
4 moderately anxious, or guarded, so anxiety is inferred
5
6
7 equivalent to acute panic states as seen in severe delirium or acute schizophrenic reactions

HEADACHE, FULLNESS IN HEAD -- Ask "Does your head feel different? Does it feel like there is a band around your head?" Do not rate for dizziness or lightheadedness. Otherwise, rate severity.
0 not present
1 very mild
2 mild
3 moderate
4 moderately severe
5 severe
6 very severe
7 extremely severe

AGITATION -- Observation.
0 normal activity
1 somewhat more than normal activity
2
3
4 moderately fidgety and restless
5
6
7 paces back and forth during most of the interview, or constantly thrashes about

ORIENTATION AND CLOUDING OF SENSORIUM -- Ask "What day is this? Where are you? Who am I?"
0 oriented and can do serial additions
1 cannot do serial additions or is uncertain about date
2 disoriented for date by no more than 2 calendar days
3 disoriented for date by more than 2 calendar days
4 disoriented for place/or person

Total **CIWA-Ar** Score _____
Rater's Initials _____
Maximum Possible Score 67

The CIWA-Ar is not copyrighted and may be reproduced freely. This assessment for monitoring withdrawal symptoms requires approximately 5 minutes to administer. The maximum score is 67 (see instrument). Patients scoring less than 10 do not usually need additional medication for withdrawal.

Sullivan, J.T.; Sykora, K.; Schneiderman, J.; Naranjo, C.A.; and Sellers, E.M. Assessment of alcohol withdrawal: The revised Clinical Institute Withdrawal Assessment for Alcohol scale (**CIWA-Ar**). *British Journal of Addiction* 84:1353–1357, 1989.

Figure 19.1 ECIWA-Ar.

is often used due to shorter half-life) and co-morbidities (COPD, reduced GCS, >70, head injury, pregnancy). The patient may require admission for a reducing dose of oral benzodiazepine. If a patient is discharged from, or chooses to leave hospital following this presentation, it is essential that they understand the risk of sudden cessation of alcohol intake. A planned stepwise reduction with support of local alcohol services is often recommended.

Prophylactic parenteral thiamine and vitamin B and C (e.g. Pabrinex 2–3 pairs 3 times a day for a minimum of 5 days) followed by oral thiamine should be given to harmful and dependent drinkers if at risk of malnourishment or decompensated liver disease.

Typical times of onset of alcohol withdrawal states → Figure 19.2.

Acute alcohol hallucinosis

Around 10% of people withdrawing from alcohol will suffer from auditory and visual hallucinations while fully conscious and situationally aware. The onset is within 12–24 hours of abstinence and resolution occurs within 24–48 hours. The hallucinations are vivid and voices may be described such as those of family or friends, often threatening or degrading in manner. This is a distinct condition, separate from other withdrawal states, which should be discussed with a psychiatrist.

Alcohol withdrawal seizures

Fits tend to be generalised and tonic–clonic in nature. They may be recurrent and require short-term treatment as well as a long-term management strategy. Concurrent head injury must be excluded as a cause.

A short-acting benzodiazepine, e.g. lorazepam can be offered to reduce the likelihood of further seizures alongside review of their drug regimen for alcohol withdrawal. Phenytoin should not be used to treat alcohol withdrawal seizures.

Delirium tremens

This occurs after 24–72 hour of abstinence and is recognised by:

- agitation and restlessness
- tremulousness
- fever and tachycardia
- delirium (acute confusional psychosis with bizarre visual hallucinations often concerning animals or insects)
- fits.

Tx Delirium tremens occurs in 5% of patients undergoing alcohol withdrawal but has a high mortality rate (15–20%) without corrective treatment, so intensive monitoring and observation are mandatory often for up to 72 hours on cessation of drinking. Risk factors include concurrent acute medical illness, heavy daily alcohol use (60+ units), older age and abnormal LFTs. The patient will need adequate sedation (lorazepam can be offered as first-line treatment) and supportive therapy. Parenteral lorazepam or haloperidol can be offered if persistent symptoms.

Alcohol misuse and dependence

Excessive alcohol intake is common throughout the world (*also → p. 294*). Its detection and control are a major global health problem. Patients may present to

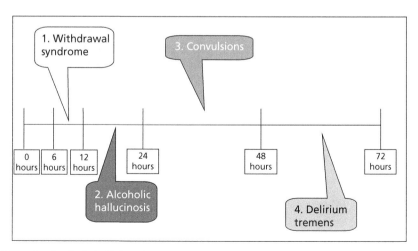

Figure 19.2 Timeline for alcohol withdrawal states.

emergency services with a large variety of medical and traumatic complaints that are related to underlying alcohol misuse and dependency. Alcohol misuse can present in the form of harmful (high-risk) drinking and alcohol dependence → see Box 19.5. Both terms are descriptive and not diagnostic. A diagnosis will be made via the ICD-10 or DSM-IV criteria and will include symptoms being present for over a year. Males are statistically more at risk of alcohol dependence than females, with approximately 4% of the whole population affected.

> The maximum recommended weekly intake of alcohol is 21 units for men and 14 units for women – with at least one or two alcohol-free days. (Definition of a unit → p. 395.)

Recognition of the harm that alcohol can cause has led to national alcohol strategies being instigated. All patients presenting to the ED due to alcohol should have an alcohol history taken and ideally a screening tool should be utilised. Within the ED, the Paddington

Box 19.5 Definitions of alcohol misuse problems

Harmful drinking: pattern of alcohol consumption leads to physiological and physical health problems.
Alcohol dependence: relates to difficulty controlling alcohol intake, a strong desire to drink and related behavioural, cognitive and physiological factor.

Alcohol Test (PAT), Fast Alcohol Use Screening Test (FAST), or AUDIT-C have been found to be useful → see Table 19.1. The screening tools allow stratification for structured brief advice, extended brief intervention and for those with more concerning presentations a referral to specialist alcohol services. It should be noted that local care pathways vary greatly. A slow downward spiral often leads to the loss of driving licence, job and home, and then to residence in a hostel or becoming homeless – interventions are most effective when undertaken early in this pattern.

The following are the main features of alcohol dependency:

- a strong desire or sense of compulsion to drink alcohol
- difficulties in controlling drinking behaviour in terms of its onset, termination or levels of consumption
- a physiological withdrawal state when drinking has stopped or been reduced, as evidenced by the characteristic alcohol withdrawal syndrome (tremor, sweating, anxiety, nausea and vomiting, agitation and insomnia)
- evidence of tolerance,
- progressive neglect of alternative pleasures or interests because of alcohol consumption,

Signs of chronic alcohol misuse include:

- poor nutritional status
- raised γ-glutamyl transpeptidase
- macrocytosis in the absence of folate or vitamin B$_{12}$ deficiency
- multiple rib fractures at various stages of healing on CXR (pulmonary tuberculosis [TB] may also be present)
- atrial fibrillation.

Requests for unplanned detoxification are often made to ED staff. Unfortunately, there are very few acute facilities

Table 19.1 AUDIT C

AUDIT C	0	1	2	3	4	Score
How often do you have a drink containing alcohol	Never	Monthly or less	2–4 times per month	2–3 times per week	4+ times per week	
How many units of alcohol do you drink on a typical day when you are drinking?	1–2	3–4	5–6	7–9	10+	
How often have you had 6 or more units if female, or 8 or more if male, on a single occasion in the last year?	Never	Less than monthly	Monthly	Weekly	Daily or almost daily	
						Total Score

Scoring: A total of 5 or more is a positive screen.
0–4 indicates low risk.
5–7 indicates increasing risk.
8–10 indicates higher risk.
11–12 indicates possible dependence.

available for people requiring acute detoxification. If the patient needs an acute medical admission, then it is important that CIWA-Ar is assessed early in the patient's stay and reviewed later to determine whether inpatient detoxification treatment is required.

If the patient can be discharged from the ED, it is essential that they are advised to avoid sudden reduction in alcohol intake. Information should be provided regarding local alcohol services, which can arrange planned alcohol withdrawal and provide psychological support.

> Treatment of alcohol dependence is more effective if it is started early, before social and physical consequences become well established. Changes in funding for 'alcohol' services in the UK reflect a growing recognition that this help must be accessible by patients presenting to both primary and emergency care facilities.

Complications of chronic alcohol abuse

Many health problems accompany chronic alcohol abuse.

Alcoholic liver disease (Chapter 16)

Patients with alcoholic liver disease can often be picked up incidentally in the ED through abnormal liver function tests or presenting after injury. Screening tests such as Paddington Alcohol Test are useful to identify those with potential alcohol-related problems.

Examination may reveal features of alcoholic liver disease including signs of cirrhosis, jaundice, ascites and non-specific symptoms such as lethargy, abdominal pain and reduced appetite.

Patients should be managed on the basis of clinical presentation as opposed to liver function test abnormality.

Wernicke–Korsakoff syndrome

> In 80% of people with Wernicke–Korsakoff syndrome, the diagnosis is made only at post mortem examination.

The common causation of these two eponymous conditions (failure of cellular metabolism in the brain) has led to the description of one syndrome with two extreme forms:

1 **Korsakoff's syndrome**: the patient develops severe loss of short-term memory which often leads to confabulation. The patient may also be confused or disoriented. This syndrome is often preceded by Wernicke's encephalopathy.

2 **Wernicke's encephalopathy** an acute, reversible condition caused by thiamine deficiency. The classic triad consists of ophthalmoplegia, ataxia and confusion. Peripheral neuropathy is often present and in extreme cases hypothermia, hypotension and coma may also be seen.

The syndrome is often precipitated in alcohol-dependent patients by the stress of an intercurrent illness. It may be very difficult to diagnose, and the classic triad is rarely encountered. Cerebellar degeneration (which is irreversible) may present a very similar clinical picture in intoxicated, alcohol-dependent patients. If in doubt, it is better to treat as Wernicke–Korsakoff syndrome.

Tx Parenteral thiamine and vitamins B and C (e.g. Pabrinex 2–3 pairs 3 times a day for a minimum of 5 days) and oral thiamine commenced after. The patient should be admitted, rehydrated and observed. A CT scan of the brain should usually be performed to rule out alternative causes.

DEPRESSED MOOD AND SELF-HARM

Depression

About one in seven people experiences some of the symptoms of depression in any 1 year and many more will experience an episode of a depressive disorder at some time during their lives. The problem is underdiagnosed and undertreated and so:

- enquire about depressed mood asking
  - During the last month, have you often been bothered by feeling down, depressed or hopeless?
  - During the last month, have you often been bothered by having little interest or pleasure in doing things?
- enquire about suicidal thoughts in anyone who may be depressed.

> Questioning about suicidal intent will not encourage a patient to attempt self-harm.

Severe depression is usually accompanied by disturbance of eating, sleeping and working. Relationships are strained and retardation of all normal activities may be profound. The risk of suicide is paradoxically at its greatest during the early stages of recovery from depression.

Tx If suicidal thoughts are present, if there are profound somatic symptoms or there has been self-harm then a psychosocial assessment should be completed. This is often done by a mental health specialist, and referral made to mental health liaison services. Less severe cases of depression can usually be treated by the GP with referral for talking therapy and/or antidepressant treatment. Supervision of a severely depressed person by a close relative or friend may be required for their safety and mental well-being. Safety planning such as removal of access to means of self-harm may be necessary.

Suicide

Recent statistics indicate that approximately 6000 people take their own lives each year, with three quarters of these being men. Suicide is the leading cause of death for men under the age of 50. The highest rates are in men aged 35–44 years and men aged >85 years. Some professions carry a particularly high risk of suicide: doctors, pharmacists, vets, nurses and farmers. In the UK, the incidence of suicide is increasing in men aged <24 years and in young Asian women.

Most people who die by suicide have informed somebody of their intention before death and therefore such disclosures should always be taken seriously in ED and patients should be referred for appropriate assessment and follow up from mental health services. Enquiring whether an individual has had suicidal thoughts or plans will not increase the risk of completed suicide, but may give the patient the permission needed to disclose the extent of their symptoms. All patients admitted to the ED following attempted suicide or disclosing suicidal intent should be reviewed by a mental health professional before consideration of discharge.

Self-harm

Self-harm accounts for over 200 000 annual ED attendances in the UK and is one of the top five causes of acute medical admission. Patients may harm themselves by either poisoning or physical injury, the latter usually taking the form of cuts to the forearms or neck.

In some cases, it is clear that this episode represented attempted suicide, on some occasions the patient's intent is less certain. Self-harm is also frequently used by patients, as part of a behaviour pattern, to distract from or manage psychological distress, without attendant intention to cause life threatening injury. However, in the 12 months after attending an ED with self-harm, 20% of patients will present again and almost 1% will die by suicide. It is therefore very important to distinguish between the different psychological states that underlie the self-harming behaviour:

- Depression and attempted suicide
- Psychosis and attempted suicide
- Emotional upset and impulsive self-harm
- Sexual or other experimentation and unintentional self-harm.

> Around 40% of patients who poison themselves express a wish to die.

Tx The poisoning or injury must be treated appropriately and sensitively (*Chapter 15*). It is vital that healthcare staff avoid increasing stigma, criticising the patient or using shaming language.

Withholding analgesia or local anaesthetic in wound management and similar punitive behaviours from healthcare professionals are *entirely unacceptable* and counter-productive.

Psychosocial assessment should take place in parallel to the physical treatment rather than waiting for its completion. Guidelines recommend that all patients who have harmed themselves are assessed by a member of a mental health liaison team. This may follow admission for medical treatment or direct referral from the ED. If this is not feasible, then the risk of suicide or further self-harm must be assessed before discharge (→ *Box 19.6*).

 Box 19.6 Assessment of suicide risk

Certain features of the social and medical history coupled with aspects of the presentation suggest serious intention to commit suicide:

High-risk individuals

- Elderly (all self-harm in people >65 should be taken as evidence of suicidal intent)
- Male
- Widowed
- Recently bereaved
- Living alone with little support
- Unemployed

There are special risk factors in women

- Three or more children under the age of 5 years
- Lack of either a close, caring relationship or a job

High-risk backgrounds

- Chronic disabling physical illness
- Previous psychiatric illness or suicide attempt
- Chronic pain
- History of alcohol or other drug abuse
- Family history of mental illness, suicide or alcoholism

Serious circumstances

- Overdose or injury performed in isolated circumstances
- Active precautions taken to avoid detection
- Self-harm timed to reduce likelihood of detection
- Did not confide in a potential helper
- Left a suicide note
- Modified a will or insurance, etc.

Suicidal thoughts

- Wanted, and still wants, to die (asking about this will not increase the risk of a repeat attempt)
- Has had these thoughts and planned suicide for at least 24 hours
- Thought that the method used would succeed in killing him or her
- Is sorry that he or she has recovered
- Has intense feelings of hopelessness and worthlessness

Patients who harm themselves have an increased risk of suicide in the following year.

Deliberate self-harm in young people aged <16 years

Self-harm is common in teenagers with as many as 1 in 10 affected. It is seven times more common in girls than in boys. There may be self-poisoning or various types of physical injury. The most common trigger is an argument with a parent or close friend. As in adults, self-harm in adolescents may reflect a variety of different underlying mental states and patients give many different reasons for hurting themselves. Unfortunately, from a diagnostic perspective, the younger the child, the less likely it is that the severity of the act that they perform reflects the actual seriousness of the urge to harm themselves. In all such cases, consideration needs to be given to the child's mental state, care and protection, and parental involvement. It is the policy of the Royal College of Paediatrics and Child Health, and the Royal College of Psychiatrists that all young people aged <16 years who harm themselves should receive a specialist assessment by an appropriately trained person, usually a child psychiatrist. This may require a temporary admission to a paediatric ward, which in some cases may have additional benefit in providing a 'cooling off' period from stressors at home. Arrangements may depend on the facilities available locally.

> In the UK in 2005, 1 in 10 children had a recognised mental disorder. This prevalence of psychological disease doubles in children whose parents are both unemployed.

SPECIAL SITUATIONS

Compulsory admission and treatment → p. 398 and Box 20.5 on p. 399.

People with learning disabilities

Approximately 3% of the population has a learning disability (defined as an IQ <70). People with all levels of learning disability live in the community, in their family homes and in supported accommodation. Many lead independent lives in their own homes.

They develop similar physical and mental health problems to non-disabled people, although they have a higher prevalence of epilepsy, head injury, and difficulties with hearing and speech. Their presentations may be atypical because of difficulties in communication. This, coupled with apparent tolerance of quite severe symptoms, can make diagnosis challenging. Common presenting problems to the ED include physical injuries, medical illness, self-harm and alcohol misuse. Mental illness may manifest itself as a change in the person's usual pattern of behaviour. These patients should be treated as adults with a normal capacity for making decisions about their health, although simple language may need to be used. Family and carers may sometimes need to be involved but only with the patient's consent.

Personality disorders

Personality disorder can be defined as an enduring condition which interferes with the sufferer's sense of well-being and ability to function in full in ordinary social settings – this may affect an individual in a variety of ways. The aetiology is complex and incompletely understood but probably comprises a complex mixture of psychosocial and neurobiological elements. There is a strong correlation with adverse childhood experiences. Historically, mental health services have provided limited support for patients with this diagnosis, although this shows signs of slowly changing.

From an ED perspective, patients with a personality disorder are relatively more likely to present following risk-taking behaviour, self-harm or in a state of emotional distress. Patients are at a real risk of harm from stigmatisation and potentially judgmental attitudes of staff, or from having all symptoms dismissed a manifestation of personality disorder.

> Brief assessment of a patient presenting with behaviour which appears unreasonable or difficult to manage, tempts the busy healthcare worker to attribute symptoms to long-term personality disorders and to make judgmental decisions. However, patients who have documented mental health conditions can still develop new treatable conditions.

Tx As with any patient, a careful assessment should be made at each attendance. Avoid dismissing new presenting symptoms or attributing all attendances to 'personality disorder.' Similarly, harm may result from over-investigation or over-treatment of patients who attend frequently. The advice of the mental health team or review of the mental health notes can be very useful because many of these patients and their patterns of behaviour are well known to the mental health services. It may not be essential for acute mental health team input on each occasion, although attempts should be made to ensure that community support is available and that appropriate agencies know of the patient's hospital attendance. Good records are essential to help at future presentations.

Anxiety disorders

Anxiety can present in a variety of ways to the ED. This may require an assessment of a presenting physical ailment and appropriate reassurance before attributing symptoms to anxiety. Severe anxiety symptoms can be debilitating and spending some time helping the patient to manage these symptoms with, e.g. breathing and sensory grounding techniques, can be time well spent. Patients usually have some insight into their problems so referral can be made to an appropriate agency, be it mental health liaison, GP or psychologist.

Panic attack

A panic attack is a deeply distressing and unpleasant experience for the patient. There may be a variety of triggers (or none immediately evident), and usually an underlying anxiety state. Symptoms may include palpitations, shaking, dry mouth and nausea. Hyperventilation leads to respiratory alkalosis, leading in turn to reduced ionised calcium levels, which can result in paraesthesia around the mouth and hands, and ultimately carpopedal spasms. This physically evident symptom can reinforce the level of panic and become self-perpetuating. Calm reassurance along with breathing and sensory grounding exercises is the appropriate management strategy.

Depressive states → p. 383

Requests for drugs

Patients sometimes present to an ED with requests for psychotropic drugs such as opiates or benzodiazepines. Generally speaking, it is inappropriate for such prescriptions to be dispensed by doctors who do not have ongoing care of a patient. However, there are no absolutes in medicine and every request should be listened to and dealt with according to the clinical situation – where it is possible to access prior hospital or GP records this may be useful.

> Never feel pressurised into prescribing.

It is helpful to remember that most patients who stop taking heroin do not experience major withdrawal symptoms. 'Cold turkey' is very unusual. According to many ex-users, the discomfort experienced during opiate withdrawal is no worse than a bad dose of flu and is certainly not akin to the life-threatening states caused by the cessation of alcohol intake. However, staying away from recreational drugs in the long term is much more difficult than just stopping for a limited period.

Alcohol withdrawal states → p. 379.

Withdrawal from opioid drugs (narcotic analgesics)

> Why do people take heroin? Most users experience a pleasant, relaxing effect with a sensation of deep inner warmth and complete detachment from all of life's problems.

Patients with physical dependence on opioids commonly present to an ED with psychiatric problems, drug overdose, alcohol intoxication, deep vein thrombosis (DVT) or infections secondary to drug injection. They may require admission to an observation area or ward. Symptoms and signs of withdrawal usually occur

6–12 hours after the last dose of heroin or 18–48 hours after a dose of methadone, as follows:

- Anxiety, restlessness, irritability, insomnia, cravings, dysphoria
- Lacrimation, rhinorrhoea, sneezing, yawning
- Muscle cramps, sweating, piloerection ('gooseflesh')
- Nausea, diarrhoea, vomiting
- Tachycardia, raised BP, dilated pupils.

The state of opioid withdrawal is unpleasant but not dangerous. However, failure to manage it effectively may limit the patient's compliance with other treatments or lead to self-discharge. Symptoms gradually decrease spontaneously over 5–10 days.

Tx The initial level of treatment depends on the clinical features, which can be assessed using the Clinical Opiate Withdrawal Scale (*COWS → Box 19.7*), but it is important

---

 Box 19.7 **COWS score**

Resting pulse rate: (record beats per minute) Measured after the patient is sitting or lying for 1 min.

0 pulse rate 80 or below
1 pulse rate 81–100
  pulse rate 101–120
  pulse rate greater than 120

Sweating: over past half an hour not accounted for by room temperature or patient activity.

0 no report of chills or flushing
1 subjective report of chills or flushing
2 flushed or observable moistness on face
3 beads of sweat on brow or face
4 sweat streaming off face

Restlessness observation during assessment:

0 able to sit still
1 reports difficulty sitting still, but is able to do so
3 frequent shifting or extraneous movements of legs/arms
5 unable to sit still for more than a few seconds

Pupil size:

0 pupil pinned or normal size for room light
1 pupil possibly larger than normal for room light
2 pupils moderately dilated
5 pupils so dilated that only the rim of the iris is visible

Bone or joint aches: If patient was having pain previously, only the additional component attributed to opiates withdrawal is scored.

0 not present
1 mild diffuse discomfort
2 patient reports severe diffuse aching of joints/muscles
4 patients are rubbing joints or muscles and are unable to sit still because of discomfort

Runny nose or tearing: Not accounted for by cold symptoms or allergies.

0 not present
1 nasal stuffiness or unusually moist eyes
2 nose running or tearing
4 nose constantly running or tears streaming down cheeks

GI upset: over last half an hour.

0 no GI symptoms
1 stomach cramps
2 nausea or loose stool
3 vomiting or diarrhoea
5 multiple episodes of diarrhoea or vomiting

Tremor observation of outstretched hands:

0 no tremor
1 tremor can be felt, but not observed
2 slight tremors observable
4 gross tremors or muscle twitching

Yawning observation during assessment:

0 no yawning
1 yawning once or twice during assessment
2 yawning three or more times during assessment
4 yawning several times/minute

Anxiety or irritability:

0 none
1 patient reports increasing irritability or anxiousness
2 patients obviously irritable anxious
4 patients so irritable or anxious that participation in the assessment is difficult

Gooseflesh skin:

0 skin is smooth
3 piloerrection of skin can be felt or hairs standing up on arms
5 prominent piloerrection

Score:

5–12 = mild
13–24 = moderate
25–36 = moderately severe
>36 = severe withdrawal

to reassure the patient that any worsening of symptoms will trigger a review of the therapy. Oral methadone mixture (1 mg/mL) is usually prescribed. Buprenorphine is sometimes given as an alternative and, in an emergency, dihydrocodeine is reasonably effective. Benzodiazepines will also alleviate most of the symptoms of opiate withdrawal. The dose of methadone is 30 mg immediately followed by 10 mg every 4 hours if signs of withdrawal recur (total daily dose up to 60–80 mg). Equivalent doses of methadone are:

Oral methadone 2 mg = injectable methadone 2 mg = injectable diamorphine 1 mg (street heroin is not equivalent to medical diamorphine and so an empirical approach is necessary).

Patients who regularly use drugs should be referred to the community drug team. If already on a registered drug programme, their key worker should be contacted. It is important to consider the welfare of any children who may be in the care of people who use drugs.

Acute poisoning with opioids (narcotics) → p. 291.
Child protection issues → p. 369 and 403.

Withdrawal from other drugs

Patients with a physical addiction to sedatives and tranquillisers may display symptoms similar to alcohol withdrawal; these drugs should not be stopped abruptly. People who regularly use stimulant drugs such as amfetamines or cocaine will not usually suffer from a withdrawal state although they may become quite depressed.

Alcohol withdrawal states → p. 379.

Factitious, fabricated and induced illness (FII)

Factitious illness in patients presenting to the ED is rare.

Patients affected by this behavioural disorder (formerly known as 'Muchausen's syndrome') display a recurrent need to adopt the sick role. Effectively, this means feigning illness through factitious symptoms and signs of physical illness to get attention, analgesia or admission to hospital. The underlying psychology of this behaviour is poorly understood and complex.

The diagnosis should be made by exclusion (and in retrospect if necessary) by an experienced multidisciplinary team. While harm can result from treatment given in good faith to patients with factitious illness,

much more harm may come from incorrectly and prematurely coming to this conclusion.

Factitious illness must be distinguished from:

- Personality disorder, including some self-harm
- Health anxiety
- Functional illness and somatisation disorder
- Exaggeration of symptoms for secondary gain
- Deliberate drug-seeking behaviour due to addiction or criminality
- Undiagnosed physical illness

Features associated with FII may include the following:

- Apparently complex social background, no relatives
- Stranger to the area, 'passing through'
- Numerous previous hospital admissions elsewhere, usually undisclosed
- Classic textbook symptoms and signs, usually of painful conditions (e.g. renal colic)
- Scars from previous surgery
- Negative tests contrasting with positive history (beware of extraneous blood in urine specimens)
- Specific requests for opiate analgesia.

Tx It is not appropriate for this diagnosis to be made in the ED. If a patient presents with this pre-existing diagnosis, senior clinicians should be involved in decision-making about clinical investigation and management.

> It is better to give morphine in good faith to a few patients with fabricated illness than to withhold it inappropriately from one patient with genuine pain. The doctor is not a detective; if there is a suspicion of genuine distress then analgesia should be given.

Fabricated and induced illness in children/perplexing presentations

This is a condition whereby a child, young person (or occasionally an adult) suffers harm through the deliberate action of their parent or caregiver and which is attributed by the adult to an illness or another cause. It is a relatively rare but potentially lethal form of abuse and the usual child protection procedures apply (→ *Chapter 18*). It can lead to physical or emotional harm. The child can be directly harmed, physically and emotionally through the induction of illness and indirectly due to the medical response including investigations and treatments. The diagnosis should be made by an experienced paediatric multidisciplinary team and management includes safeguarding processes (→ *p. 369*).

Functional illness

Patients can present to an ED with symptoms that cannot be explained with an obvious physical cause; however, there is a very real set of symptoms that the patient is experiencing. Differing terminology used within healthcare systems can complicate managing these patients, in both their acute and long-term management. It is important for the Emergency Physician to respond to suspected functional illness compassionately. It is all too easy in a busy department for clinicians to become dismissive or critical; however, this response is potentially harmful. A key factor is to recognise that functional symptoms are distinct from and much more common than 'malingering' or fabricated illness.

Common presentations include seizures, headaches, fatigue, dizziness, blackouts, functional weakness or blindness. Up to 15% of new patients seen in UK neurology clinics are ultimately diagnosed with functional or dissociative illness. Patients can also have a range of contributing conditions including anxiety, depression, chronic pain or significant stress, although these may not be immediately evident.

Certain functional illnesses such as psychogenic seizures and functional neurological disorder (→ *p. 244*) have recognisable characteristics which allow a positive diagnosis to be made. The Emergency Physician may be one of the few professionals to directly witness the seizure, for example and so a clear assessment and description can be invaluable in planning ongoing care.

If the team is confident that this is likely a functional disorder, ED management should include reassurance for the patient, clear explanations to family members and initiating involvement of the multi-disciplinary team. A clear explanation, acknowledging the genuine nature of the symptoms, the common nature of functional illness and the high likelihood of full recovery, is a key part of management.

Good communication within the ED can enhance the long-term care for these patients. Consider giving a range of differential diagnoses, arrange follow-up wherever possible, normalise the experience, give time for recovery and aim for discharge direct from ED whenever possible. Ideally, ongoing care will be delivered by a multidisciplinary team including psychology and neurology input – access to this will vary according to the local health care system.

Psychological support for patients and relatives

There are three main groups of people who may need psychosocial care after traumatic events:

1 Survivors/injured victims.
2 People who have participated in events as rescuers, emergency staff, etc.
3 The families of those who have died or been injured.

Adults, children and people from various ethnic and social groups may all have differing needs. Most people involved will have a normal emotional reaction with features of grief and distress; some may appear dazed and confused by events. The use of standardised individual or group 'debriefing' should be avoided because it is of no proven benefit and may do harm.

Some people will have features of acute stress soon after the traumatic event. Typical early symptoms include fear, anxiety, anger, guilt, sadness, feelings of helplessness and distressing thoughts and dreams. Physical symptoms such as fatigue, muscle aches, tension headaches and dry mouth may also occur. Features may be accentuated by the presence of coexisting conditions such as depression or substance abuse and anxiety, panic or phobic disorders. A few individuals may appear unaffected at first, only to experience problems hours or days later. For most people, symptoms subside without intervention. 'Psychological first aid' consists of the following:

- Information about possible symptoms that may be experienced
- Education for the individual and the family about the reasons for his or her altered attitude, mood and behaviour (including advice to avoid telling the sufferer to 'snap out of it')
- Advice to avoid using alcohol, tobacco or drugs to cope with anxiety
- Practical and social support as required.

The use of antidepressant drugs for adults in this early phase may be helpful if signs of depression are present.

All individuals with ongoing or worsening symptoms should be assessed if:

- symptoms have lasted longer than 1 month
- symptoms are complicated by other mental health problems
- the person has suicidal thoughts
- the person is unable to cope with normal activities
- there is marked hyperarousal.

Post-traumatic stress disorder (PTSD) is usually diagnosed only after a month of persistent symptoms. It is treated with cognitive–behavioural therapy by trained staff and this is associated with good long-term outcomes. Prolonged use of anxiolytic drugs should be avoided, although they may be helpful for adults in the first 2 weeks after a traumatic event to alleviate panic attacks or sleep disturbance. Antidepressant therapy may be required for many months in some patients.

Victim support → p. 393.

Counselling

The constant recollection of distressing thoughts reinforces a negative perception of problems and further lowers mood. Counselling aims to break this cycle.

- Cognitive–behavioural counselling helps a patient to focus on positive rather than negative thoughts.
- Psychodynamic counselling takes a historical view of human mental processes and analyses the effect of past events on present thinking.
- Supportive counselling encourages the patient to focus on current daily problems rather than dwelling on traumatic events.

Bereavement care → p. 171.

Violence and aggression

Violent or aggressive behaviour can be rarely attributed to psychiatric illness on its own and may be provoked by environmental, organisational, situational or attitudinal factors. In the acute hospital setting, over half of all violent incidents occur in the ED; therefore, ED staff need to have knowledge and procedures to manage these incidents, keeping patient centred care at the heart of what we do.

Healthcare staff have a duty of care to their patients, whilst government and organisations also have a duty of care to their staff to ensure that they and their colleagues are not placed at unreasonable risk of injury during the course of their duties. For this reason, the police should be involved early on in any potentially violent situation. Many hospitals now have their own security personnel who can attend at short notice.

Globally, violence against emergency workers is escalating, with resultant law and policies formed to protect the zero-tolerance approach to violence against emergency workers. In the eyes of the law, intoxication with alcohol or drugs is no justification for unreasonable behaviour. The exceptions to this generalisation are functional psychoses and organic confusional states, which are not the direct result of the person's own actions. Thus, before an individual is removed from the ED, these conditions must be excluded.

Risk assessment for violence

Prevention of violence is the most recommended approach to violence in healthcare settings. Front-line staff should have training to enable screening of those that are more likely to escalate to violence during their ED attendance.

Anticipation of violence is a key aspect of violence management. Staff skills should include:

- Assessment of why behaviour is likely to progress to violence (includes personal, mental, physical, environmental, social, behavioural factors)
- Recognition of potential escalating behaviour which may be indicated by:
  - Restlessness and pacing around the floor
  - Increased volume of speech and erratic movements
  - Refusal to communicate
  - Prolonged eye contact
  - Tense and angry facial expressions
  - Delusions or hallucinations with a violent content
  - Verbal threats or gestures.
- Use of methods to diffuse an escalating situation, e.g. verbal de-escalation

Members of staff must recognise that they are responsible for avoiding provocation in potentially violent situations. It is not reasonable to expect a person exhibiting angry behaviour to simply 'calm down'. ED staff must learn to monitor and control their own verbal and non-verbal behaviour such as body posture and eye contact. In addition, they must be able to defuse a difficult situation.

Whether or not there is an underlying medical cause for violence that requires medical treatment, will determine the individual management required. If there is an underlying medical condition, use the escalation framework described earlier in the chapter (*Rapid tranquilisation and ABD → page 377*). If it is determined that there is no underlying cause for this unacceptable behaviour then the police should be involved. Novel solutions are being trialled to reduce this burden on emergency workers, e.g. body worn cameras and permanently based police officers within EDs can act as a deterrence to violence.

Angry relatives

Dissatisfied or frankly aggressive relatives or friends of patients are not uncommon in an ED. There are several frequently met reasons for this:

- Inappropriate reaction to the stress of sudden illness or bereavement

- Guilt and redirection of blame
- Unrealistic expectations of a resource-limited system
- Misunderstanding of the situation (a failure of communication)
- Unexplained delays at any stage
- Understandable reaction to a failure of care.

The departmental staff must reply calmly, politely, clearly and firmly to all expressions of anger. If resolution cannot easily be achieved, then the case must be referred to a senior member of staff. There is a clear procedure to be followed for all formal complaints, which will usually be directed through a central office of the hospital ($\rightarrow$ *p. 406*).

> Do not be frightened of saying that you are sorry. You can express regret that the patient is upset without implying that you are to blame.

20

Medicolegal aspects of emergency medicine

Amy Nickson

Emergency Medicine Consultant, Royal Bolton Hospital, Bolton, UK
Sexual Offences Examiner, Lancashire SAFE Centre, Preston, UK

The advice given in this chapter is drawn from UK medical practice, and the legal framework may vary in other parts of the world.

CLINICAL FORENSIC MEDICINE

Description of injuries

Many descriptions of injury are intended for lay people, the police, or the legal profession. Medical terminology is unlikely to be familiar to them. A pair of erythematous haematomas on the pretibial area thus becomes two red lumps on the shin. Nevertheless, this simplification of terminology must not compromise its accuracy. In both medical records and non-medical documents, the description of a wound must include the following:

1 Site – described in everyday language
2 Side – left or right
3 Shape – circular, V shaped, etc.
4 Size – measured with a ruler
5 Structures that are also involved – such as nerves, tendon, and bone, including radiological findings
6 Sutures – number inserted in the skin.

Drawings or photographs can be very helpful. Some idea of the age of a wound is also desirable, although with older injuries this requires a considerable amount of experience. Opinions as to causation should be expressed only if requested and then only if supported by the doctor's experience.

Types of wounds

According to the Offences Against the Person Act 1861, to wound is to destroy or damage, however superficially, a bodily surface, be it skin or mucous membrane. For the purposes of medicolegal description, there are five main types of wound:

1 **Bruises**: these are also known as contusions or ecchymoses. Blunt force applied to the body surface causes rupturing of small blood vessels and allows blood to escape into the surrounding tissues.
2 **Abrasions**: an abrasion or graze involves only the outer layers of the skin and indicates a point of impact. Direction may also be apparent, as may dirt from the source of trauma.
3 **Lacerations**: whenever blunt force splits the whole thickness of the skin, the wound is called a laceration. Such wounds may be inflicted with sticks or bottles or sustained in falls. The characteristic features are ragged, abraded, contused edges and irregular division of the tissue planes.
4 **Incised wounds**: sharp cutting objects make even wounds with straight, unbruised edges. An incised wound is longer than its depth.
5 **Stab wounds**: a stab wound is different from an incision because its depth is greater than its length. The shape and edges of the wound depend on the object used. A puncture wound is a very small stab wound. The external dimensions of a stab wound are a very poor guide as to the size of the weapon (e.g. knife blade). This is because:

The RCEM Lecture Notes: Emergency Medicine, Fifth Edition. Edited by Catherine Williams and Amy Nickson.
© 2024 John Wiley & Sons Ltd. Published 2024 by John Wiley & Sons Ltd.
Companion website: www.wiley.com/go/LNEM5

- the weapon may be tapered and not introduced to the full extent of its width
- the weapon may not have been used perpendicularly to the skin surface
- the skin contracts after the blade is withdrawn.

Areas of transient redness should also be noted. Erythema may be caused by pressure or a blow. There may be accompanying swelling or tenderness. Such injuries might include the red finger marks on a slapped face or the tender, red scalp that results from hair pulling. Fading occurs within a matter of hours.

Specific mechanisms of injury may give rise to a defined type of wound, such as a burn. Burns are distinct patterns of damage that result from thermal or chemical injury (*for types of burns → Chapter 10 and for child abuse → p. 369*).

> All clothing from a wounded patient should be preserved in a sealed, labelled bag for the attention of the investigating police officers.

Taser injuries → p. 400.

Asphyxia

Attempted suffocation and strangulation may both cause a picture similar to traumatic asphyxia syndrome (→ *p. 80*). Signs of compression of the face or the neck may be present, as may the marks of a violent struggle. Hanging causes death through a mixture of asphyxia, cerebral ischaemia and if associated with a drop, spinal disruption. The asphyxia resulting from a bag over the head, seen in children and sexual asphyxia, usually causes death by hypoxia and subsequent bradycardia.

Drowning → p. 30.

Violent crime

Most of the victims of violent crime who present to an ED are young men. (→ *Box 20.1*). They have often been assaulted in a bar, a club, or in the street, and are often also intoxicated. In contrast, 75% of the attacks on women occur in the home of either the victim, or the assailant.

Injuries to the face, head and hands are the most common, unless weapons are used in the assault. There may be long-term psychological effects including:

- depression
- loss of confidence, fear and anxiety
- irritability, decreased concentration and mood changes

> **Box 20.1 Risk factors for violent crime**
>
> - Male sex
> - Age 16–29 years
> - Low income
> - Single
> - Urban area
> - Alcohol intoxication
>
> Only about half of all violent crimes are reported to the police, with men much less likely to report than women; 50% of victims suffer 80% of all recorded crimes and an unfortunate 4% suffer over half of these.

- lethargy, sleep and appetite disturbances
- headaches, nausea and muscle tension
- behavioural changes (e.g. withdrawal or increased alcohol consumption).
- post-traumatic stress disorder (PTSD) (→ *p. 389*).

Domestic violence

More than 25% of all violent crime reported to the police is domestic violence towards women. It is thought to account for around 1% of all ED attendances. Up to one in four women will be physically assaulted by a partner during her lifetime and around one in 10 will suffer an attack each year. It is estimated that a woman in an abusive relationship will suffer over 30 physical assaults before disclosing the abuse – usually only when asked directly. There are no patterns of presentation with sufficient sensitivity to reliably identify victims of domestic violence, but facial bruising should always alert suspicion. Other associations with abuse are deliberate self-harm and pregnancy.

Abuse may be:

- psychological – shouting, swearing, humiliation or enforced isolation from family and friends
- economic – withholding of money and transport
- sexual
- physical.

Physical injury is the most likely form of domestic violence to present to an ED. The following are possible signs of it:

- Delayed presentation of injuries
- Injuries that are inconsistent with the mechanism described in the history
- Multiple injuries, especially when symmetrically distributed or of differing ages
- Injuries such as bites, burns, scalds or bruises

- Injuries on areas of the body that are normally clothed
- Injuries to the face, neck, breasts, genitals or pregnant abdomen
- Perforated eardrums or detached retinas
- Genital injuries or pelvic pain

> Domestic violence may occur in same-sex relationships and may be perpetrated by women against men. The annual crime survey for England and Wales found a quarter of all domestic abuse crimes in 2018/19 were committed against a male victim.

Tx Injuries should be treated appropriately and enquiries made about the current safety of any children in the family. (The risks of violence to children growing up in an abusive household are substantial. Concerns about the welfare of children should lead to immediate contact with local child protection services → p. 369.) The police can be involved only with the consent of the injured party.

A MARAC (Multi-Agency Risk Assessment Conference) is a way of information sharing between agencies, for the highest risk domestic violence cases. A MARAC referral can be made from the ED if the clinician has serious concerns about the victim's situation.

> Reluctance by victims of domestic violence to involve outside help is common. This may frustrate staff who believe that immediate action is required. However, research has shown that information provided in EDs may be used at a later date when the patient finally feels that the time is right.

Rape and sexual assault

Around 17% of women and 3% of men in the UK state that they have been subjected to non-consensual sexual experiences as adults. About two-thirds of assaults of this type are committed by someone known to the victim. The experience of sexual violence can be life threatening and degrading. Not surprisingly, psychological harm and PTSD are common sequelae. Not all patients who have been sexually assaulted have visible genital (or oral) injuries, although around 50% have other physical injuries. Examination should be left to a forensic medical officer because evidence will need to be collected in a way that does not contaminate it or render it inadmissible. Locard's principle states that 'every contact leaves a trace' – This includes ED staff.

Tx Assess for serious injuries, provide emergency contraception and HIV post exposure prophylaxis if required.

Arrange for transfer of the patient to a sexual assault referral centre. It should be made clear to the patient that referral does not constitute automatic reporting of the offence to the police, but the police should be informed if the patient consents or is a child. Some patients may be wary of police involvement straight away following an assault, but can provide forensic samples that can be used later if they chose to report.

Drug-assisted sexual assault

Alcohol (self-administered or in laced drinks) is by far the most common drug to be associated with sexual assault. However, gamma-hydroxybutyrate (GHB), ketamine, flunitrazepam and zopiclone have all been reported as being used to facilitate sexual assault. Patients drugged and assaulted in this way present a very difficult problem because they will have an impaired memory of events and may just feel that 'something wrong happened'.

Child abuse

Child protection procedures → p. 404.
Types of and signs of child abuse → p. 369.

Abuse of elderly people

Physical abuse of elderly people is surprisingly common; neglect and emotional abuse are even more common. Look of signs of poor nutritional status, unkempt appearance, pressure ulcers, inconsistent injuries and emotional distress.

The Care Act 2014 requires that each NHS trust must make enquiries and act to protect older adults experiencing abuse or neglect. Use local safeguarding processes to alert concerns, or if the risk is immediate or serious it may be appropriate to contact the police, with the patient's consent if they are able to do so.

ALCOHOL AND OTHER DRUGS/ FITNESS TO DRIVE

Misuse of drugs

The Misuse of Drugs Act 1971 prohibits certain activities in relation to 'Controlled Drugs', in particular their manufacture, supply and possession. Controlled drugs are divided into three classes called A, B and C (→ *Box 20.2*) class A being the most harmful. The Misuse of Drugs Regulations 2001 define the classes of people who are authorised to supply and possess controlled drugs and in

Box 20.2 **The Misuse of Drugs Act 1971 and the Misuse of Drugs Regulations 2001**

Controlled drugs are divided into three classes:

- **Class A includes:** cocaine, LSD (lysergic acid diethylamide), diamorphine, morphine, pethidine, methadone, opium, MDMA (3,4-methylenedioxy methamphetamine or ecstasy), methamfetamine, phencyclidine and class B substances when prepared for injection
- **Class B includes:** codeine, standard amfetamines and barbiturates
- **Class C includes:** buprenorphine, cannabis, most benzodiazepines, zolpidem, anabolic steroids and some hormones

The Misuse of Drugs Regulations 2001 five schedules, each with its own specific legal requirements:

- **Schedule 1 includes:** cannabis, LSD and other drugs that are not used medicinally. *Home office licence required to handle.*
- **Schedule 2 includes:** diamorphine, morphine, pethidine, cocaine, ketamine and amfetamines. *Need to be recorded on a controlled drug register.*
- **Schedule 3 includes:** buprenorphine, midazolam, temazepam and gabapentin.
- **Schedule 4 includes:** other benzodiazepines, zolpidem, anabolic steroids and some hormones
- **Schedule 5 includes:** those preparations, such as codeine, that (because of their strength) are exempt from virtually all controlled drug requirements

these regulations, and drugs are divided into five schedules, corresponding to their therapeutic usefulness, 1 being useless (→ *Box 20.2*).

Schedule 2 and 3 prescriptions must be indelible, *signed* by the prescriber, include the *date* on which they were signed and specify the prescriber's *address*. A machine-written prescription is acceptable, but the prescriber's signature must be handwritten. The total volume in millilitres (in both words and figures) of the preparation to be supplied or the number of dosage units (tablets, capsules and ampoules), in both words and figures should be documented.

Requests for drugs in the ED and drug withdrawal → p. 386.

Alcohol and trauma

The direct and indirect effects of Ethyl alcohol coupled with its availability, make it probably the most dangerous substance of abuse in the world. It is so frequently involved in the causation of accidents that no discussion of the work of an ED would be complete without it. In the UK, a tenth of all road accidents that result in injury are a result of the alcohol and almost all other injuries have a significant association with alcohol usage (→ *Figure 20.1*).

Detection and treatment of alcohol abuse → pp. 379–383.
Treatment of alcohol poisoning → p. 294.

Nearly a quarter of all ED attendances are alcohol related. Over a quarter of all male hospital inpatients have a current or previous alcohol problem.

Measurement of alcohol in the human body

Units of alcohol

A unit of alcohol is defined as 10 mL by volume (58 g by weight) of pure alcohol – roughly the alcohol content of a standard measure of 25 mL of many spirits. Half a pint of beer (3% strength) or a glass of wine (125 mL of 8% alcohol) is also roughly equivalent to 1 unit. Within the first hour, a unit of alcohol increases the blood level by approximately 15 mg/dL in an average man.

In a healthy person, about 90% of ingested alcohol is cleared from the blood by the liver. This occurs at a steady rate of about 15 mg/dL per hour.

Requests for specimens for analysis from patients in hospital

The Police Reform Act 2002 provided new powers for taking blood specimens from patients involved in road traffic accidents to test for levels of alcohol or drugs. Under the previous legislation, it was a statutory requirement to obtain consent for blood sampling from the person concerned. Therefore, when a patient lacked capacity to consent (usually because of a depressed level of consciousness), a specimen could not be obtained. This led to people escaping

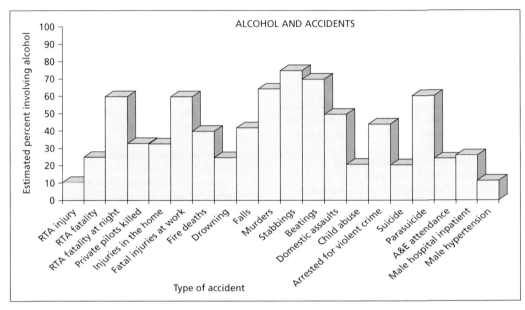

Figure 20.1 The involvement of alcohol in trauma and RTC (road traffic collision).

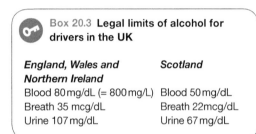

Box 20.3 **Legal limits of alcohol for drivers in the UK**

England, Wales and Northern Ireland	Scotland
Blood 80 mg/dL (= 800 mg/L)	Blood 50 mg/dL
Breath 35 mcg/dL	Breath 22mcg/dL
Urine 107 mg/dL	Urine 67 mg/dL

prosecution for very serious offences, such as causing death by careless driving while under the influence of alcohol.

A police constable may now request that a blood sample be taken from a patient who, for medical reasons, is incapable of giving consent. The sample will be taken by a forensically trained medical professional, in the correct way to ensure a 'chain of evidence'.

As soon as possible, the police will inform the patient that a blood sample has been taken and obtain his or her consent for it to be analysed. As per the Road Traffic Act 1998, failure to supply a sample or give permission for analysis may render the person liable to prosecution. See Box 20.3 for legal limits of alcohol for drivers.

Driving and other drugs

Many drugs may impair the ability of a patient to drive or to operate machinery. Drivers taking minor tranquillisers or tricyclic antidepressants are two to five times more likely to be involved in an accident than untreated control individuals. The early stages of treatment are associated with the highest risk, and the effects of centrally acting drugs are often potentiated by alcohol.

As a result of these risks, patients must always be warned whenever their treatment could alter their ability to drive or perform other activities safely. Discharge advice following sedation → Box 20.11 on p. 409.

Police can stop any road user and ask them to perform a roadside cannabis and cocaine test with a mouth swab.

Frequent users of cannabis are 10 times more likely to be injured or to cause injury to others in motor vehicle accidents than other road users.

Misuse of Drugs Act 1971 and the Misuse of Drugs Regulations 2001 → Box 20.2 on p. 395.

Driving and medical conditions

Medical conditions in drivers contribute to about 1% of the road accidents in the UK that result in injury or death (→ Box 20.4).

There are two sets of medical criteria for fitness to drive: Group one is an ordinary licence and group two is for large lorries and buses. Licence holders have a statutory obligation to notify the licencing authority as soon as they become aware that they have any condition that

> **Box 20.4 Most common causes of collapse at the wheel**
>
> Fits
> Unspecified blackouts
> Hypoglycaemia
> Myocardial infarction
> Strokes

might affect safe driving, unless the condition is not expected to last more than 3 months. Failure to notify is a legal offence.

> The General Medical Council advises that a doctor should notify the licencing authority when a patient is placing him- or herself or others in danger by continuing to drive. This does not constitute a breach of confidentiality.

Safe driving requires good eyesight, judgement, coordination, muscle strength and reaction times. The Road Traffic Act 1988, Section 92, lists prescribed disabilities that bar the sufferer from driving. They are:

A epilepsy
B severe learning disability
C liability to sudden attacks of disabling giddiness or fainting (from any cause)
D disorder of the heart requiring a pacemaker
E inability to meet the eyesight requirements (the number-plate test).

In practice, a person with any of these conditions can drive once he or she has satisfied the licencing authority that he or she does not present any significant risk. The rules for group 2 drivers are more stringent, they require a medical examination every 5 years over the age of 45, and yearly over 65.

For the purposes of the ED, patients should be advised to (temporarily) refrain from driving whenever there is a possibility of a condition being diagnosed that could make driving or other complex tasks dangerous to themselves or others. Such problems may include:

- seizures
- transient loss of consciousness if unknown cause or suspected cardiac cause
- hypoglycaemic episodes where the patient was unaware
- dizziness and vertigo
- head injury
- cardiac dysrhythmias

- myocardial infarction
- CVAs (cerebrovascular accidents) and TIAs (transient ischaemic attacks)
- application of an eye pad in the ED (→ *p. 429*)
- decreased ability to use a limb (e.g. forearm in plaster)
- post-sedation or strong analgesia.

Driving, or other prohibited activities, should only be recommended when:

- the condition has resolved completely
- the diagnosis has been ruled out after specialist investigation
- the condition has been controlled and a symptom-free period has elapsed.

In the UK, the Medical Advisory Branch of the Driver and Vehicle Licencing Authority (DVLA) supplies written and verbal advice for doctors on all aspects of fitness to drive.

LEGAL ISSUES

Consent

In the competent adult, treatment can be given only if the patient gives consent. Any physical contact or treatment without this consent is battery, which does not require harm to have resulted to the patient. Consent may be given verbally, in writing, by gestures or by actions, but not just by the 'absence of resistance'. A signature on a consent form does not by itself prove that consent was valid if the information given to the patient was inadequate. In addition, the following points should be noted:

- Valid consent or refusal is dependent on a patient's ability (capacity) to make decisions, namely to:
  1 understand and retain information
  2 weigh up this information
  3 communicate their decision.
- Capacity to give meaningful consent is governed by the following laws:
  England/Wales: Mental Capacity Act 2005
  Scotland: Adults with Incapacity Act 2000
  Northern Ireland: Mental Capacity Act (NI) 2016.

However, these laws presuppose that all registered medical practitioners are qualified to assess capacity. It also *assumes* that all adults have capacity unless proven otherwise.

> Conscious adults without serious mental dysfunction are always regarded by the law as capable of giving consent.

Children → p. 403.
Patients with mental illness → p. 398.

- Patients may be competent to make some healthcare decisions, even if they are not competent to make others.
- Consent is valid only if the patient understood to what he or she was consenting (i.e. gave informed consent). Doctors must provide information about all material risks and disclose any risk to which a reasonable person in the patient's position would attach significance. This includes any alternatives to the proposed treatment and the risks of having no treatment.
- The patient's right to self-determination takes precedence over the physician's duty to preserve life. A competent adult has the right to refuse any treatment or investigation even if it puts his or her life or health at risk. The patient has no obligation to justify this decision with valid and rational argument. The only exception to this rule is where treatment is for a mental disorder and the patient is detained under the Mental Health Act 1983.

- All practicable steps must be taken to help a patient make a decision.
- A competent pregnant woman may refuse any treatment, even if this would be detrimental to the fetus.
- Consent obtained by deceit or with coercion is invalid.
- Consent may be withdrawn at any time.

Making decisions for incompetent patients

Patients who lack capacity will need decision about their healthcare to be made for them. The following can help in the decision-making process:-

- Advanced decision – allows a competent patient to make decisions about their healthcare for a future date where they might lack capacity. Covers negative decisions, i.e. refusing certain treatments including life-sustaining measures. Cannot dictate or demand which treatment doctors should give. Cannot refuse actions needed to keep a person comfortable, clean and warm
- Lasting power of attorney (welfare power of attorney in Scotland) – donor appointed by the patient to make healthcare decisions on their behalf. Must be registered with the Office of the Public Guardian. Cannot make decisions that are contrary to the patient's best interests.
- Best interests of the patient – decided by healthcare professionals caring for the patient. Only if the decision cannot be postponed to a time where the person may regain capacity. Must be achieved via the *least restrictive* method.

'Best interests' extend wider than just 'medical interests' to include such factors as previous wishes and beliefs and general well-being. People close to the patient may be able to provide valuable information on some of these factors.

To force medical treatment on a patient who is *actively refusing*, it must convincingly be shown to be a medical necessity. The amount of restraint must be *proportional* to the risk the patient is at, e.g. how likely is it that they will come to harm without this restraint, and how serious is that harm? The *least restrictive* method is that which impedes the least on their freedom, liberty and dignity. Giving a patient a sedative tablet or injection is less restrictive than several people holding them down if they are at imminent risk of harm. Providing a patient with a quiet, comfortable place with a cup of tea and an interesting activity is less restrictive than sedating them.

Blood transfusion for Jehovah's witnesses

There are 140 000 Jehovah's Witnesses in the UK and Ireland; their faith does not allow transfusion of blood or its primary components. Administration of blood in the face of a refusal by an informed and rational patient is obviously unlawful. Similarly, if written evidence in the form of a signed and witnessed advance directive exists, this should be acted upon. In the absence of verbal or written instructions from the patient, clinical judgement should take precedence over the opinion of relatives or friends.

Use of tranexamic acid and clotting factors in severe bleeding → p. 26.

The children of Jehovah's Witnesses may be denied blood transfusion by their parents. If the well-being of a child is at risk, a court order (a specific issue order) may be applied to provide legal sanction for an isolated treatment. However, in an emergency, blood should be given to a child as soon as it is needed to save life.

Mental health act

Part I of the Mental Health Act 1983 (England and Wales) and 1984 (Scotland) defines mental disorder as follows:

1 Mental illness
2 Mental impairment (learning disability)
3 Psychopathic disorder
4 Any other disorder or disability of mind.

In Part II, civil detention orders are specified (→ *Box 20.5*). The indication for these orders is that the patient is suffering from a mental disorder of a nature or degree that

Box 20.5 **Orders (sections) of the Mental Health Act (1983 England and Wales) with corresponding provisions for Scotland and Northern Ireland**

Section 2
- Admission for assessment followed by treatment
- Duration up to 28 days
- Application by nearest relative or approved social worker
- Medical recommendation by two doctors (one Section 12 approved)

Section 3
- Admission for treatment
- Duration up to 6 months
- Application by nearest relative or approved social worker
- Medical recommendation by two doctors (one Section 12 approved)

Section 4
- Admission for assessment in cases of emergency
- Duration up to 24 hours
- Application by nearest relative or approved social worker
- Medical recommendation by one doctor (preferably acquainted with patient) who must state that admission under Section 2 will involve undesirable delay

Section 5 (2)
- Detention of patient already in hospital for any form of inpatient treatment
- Duration up to 72 hours
- Invoked by doctor in charge of care or a nominated deputy

Section 5 (4)
- Nurse's holding power applicable to any patient already receiving treatment for a mental disorder

- Duration up to 6 hours while a doctor is found
- Invoked by registered nurses

Section 136
- Police admission order that allows a police officer to remove a person apparently suffering from a mental disorder from a public place to a designated place of safety for assessment by a doctor and a social worker
- Duration up to 24 hours
- Invoked by any police officer

Section 135
- Under this order, and with a magistrate's warrant, a police officer, accompanied by a doctor and a social worker, may enter the residence of a person they believe to be suffering from a mental disorder to take him or her to a place of safety
- Duration up to 24 hours

Corresponding provisions of the relevant legislation in Scotland and Northern Ireland
The following information is given as guidance only:

Mental Health Act 1983 (England and Wales)	Mental Health (Care and Treatment) Act 2003 (Scotland)	Mental Health (Northern Ireland) Order 1986
Section 2	Short term detention certificate	Article 4
Section 3	Compulsory treatment order	Article 12
Section 4	Emergency detention certificate	Article 9
Section 136	Section 297	Article 130

warrants detention of the patient in hospital in the interests of his or her own health or safety or with a view to the protection of others.

In the ED, the sequence of orders would usually be:

- Section 4 (Emergency Admission Order) or
- Section 136 (Police Admission Order), changed as soon as possible to:
- Section 2 (Assessment Order), converted later in hospital to:
- Section 3 (Treatment Order).

Patients detained under a police admission order (Section 136 of the Mental Health Act 1983)

Police officers may bring patients to an ED under Section 136 of the MHA (Mental Health Act 1983) if it is felt there are concurrent physical health needs. This police admission order can be invoked by any police officer and has a maximum duration of 24 hours (→ *Box 20.5*). This was reduced from 72 hours by the Policing and Crime Act 2017.

The stated purpose of the order is to allow police officers to remove a person who is apparently suffering from a mental disorder from any place other than a private dwelling to a safe area where the person can be assessed by an approved mental health professional.

The police should stay with the patient until the time when either they are discharged or detained under a different section of the MHA. The Police have a right to search the patient for harmful items, and the patient has a right to legal advice should they request it.

Patients cannot receive treatment against their will under section 136 if they have capacity, but can be treated as per the Mental Capacity Act above if they lack capacity. Patients with acute mental health disorders *do not* automatically lack capacity.

The violent and uncontrollable patient

Occasionally, a patient who is obviously dangerously disturbed and violent may be brought in by the police or paramedics. The most common causes are:

- drug intoxication (usually amfetamines or other stimulant drugs)
- hypoglycaemia
- post-ictal confusion
- head injury
- acute psychiatric illness.

There is a duty to protect hospital staff, police and other patients in the ED. Sedation is often necessary to allow the removal of force and assessment of the patient. The quickest and safest way of achieving this is with an intramuscular injection of ketamine or droperidol. The usual rules regarding the administration of sedating drugs must be applied (→ p. 15). Whilst the intravascular route may be faster acting, it is very difficult to safely secure venous access in a very agitated patient. A benzodiazepine in increasing aliquots is a useful adjunct. Once the patient is calmer, monitoring equipment can be applied and a more detailed assessment can be performed in relative safety.

The absconding patient

Patients with mental health presentations can often be vulnerable and high risk of absconding from hospital. The emergency department should ensure that patients at risk of absconding have mental health triage performed as soon as possible, which should include

- An assessment of their capacity (as per MCA 2005) and any signs of serious mental illness
- A description of their physical appearance
- Consideration of whether regular visual observations are needed (e.g. every 15 min)

A patient who is threatening to leave should have early input from a senior clinician to assess the patient whilst trying to de-escalate. ED personnel do not have powers to detain under the MHA 1983. Options are limited to requesting a Section 4 or 2 assessment or police assistance who can use an s136 in the ED. Reasonable and proportionate force can be used for patients who pose an immediate risk to themselves or others (under common-law doctrine of necessity).

If a patient has left without assessment, then the information known about the patient should be used to assess their risk of harm. Attempt to locate them in the immediate area, use CCTV if available and ring the patient and their next of kin. If these measures fail, the senior clinician should decide whether there is a real risk to the patient's life that requires the police to be called to search for them. Other options include contacting the patient's GP or community mental health team to review as an outpatient.

The patient in police custody

The fact that a patient is in police custody does not affect the duty of care that a doctor has towards him or her. Nor should reasonable constraints on his or her freedom prevent an adequate examination. The police do not have an automatic right to the information shared between doctor and patient and can be asked to wait outside if it is felt safe to do so.

Handcuffs may cause a circumferential reddening of the wrists. Occasionally, abrasions and even anaesthesia in the distribution of the superficial radial nerve may be found.

The decision of 'fitness to be detained' is one for a forensic medical professional to make, as is the similar examination for 'fitness to be interviewed'. A patient discharged to police custody should be one ordinarily fit to be discharged home with a relative. Close monitoring such as vital signs or head injury observations is not provided.

Taser injuries

'Tasers' are hand-held electrical devices that can be used to incapacitate. They belong to a group of so-called 'non-lethal' weapons, designed as an alternative to firearms in critical situations. The taser fires two barbed probes into its target, which are attached to the 'gun' by a pair of thin wires. A high-voltage current is then immediately discharged down these wires, causing painful and overwhelming muscle contractions in the victim. Although such weapons are in fairly common use, they are not entirely without risk, particularly when used against vulnerable individuals with pre-existing medical conditions, suffering from drug intoxication, psychiatric illness or extreme agitation. When fired at the torso, there is the potential for inducing cardiac dysrhythmias and cardiac arrest. The most common medical complications are probably secondary injuries from the sudden fall to the ground induced by the shock. If presenting to the emergency department after having been tasered the patient should be asked about any cardiac symptoms, particularly chest pain and an ECG performed if appropriate. The barbs can usually be removed by firm and rapid perpendicular traction whilst bracing the skin to prevent tenting. Other considerations include an Obstetric/foetal well-being check for pregnant patients and a pacemaker check for those with a permanent pacemaker.

Concealed drugs

Police may bring an arrested patient to hospital due to their suspicions of internal drug trafficking, of which there are three main types:

- **Body packers**: swallow large quantities of well wrapped, but high purity drugs, to attempt to cross borders. A leaking or ruptured package can be rapidly fatal.
- **Body stuffers**: ingest a smaller quantity of drugs, usually in a flimsy package such as cling film, often taken in haste to avoid detection.
- **Body pushers**: conceal drugs in small plastic containers in the rectum or vagina.

Clinicians are not permitted to perform intimate examinations or investigations on patients in police custody without their consent. The first-line investigation is a low-dose CT scan (LDCT), to assess the location and approximate number of packages. The report may be used as evidence to remand a detainee under s152 of the Criminal Justice Act 1998 (up to 192 hours) to retrieve the remaining drug packages.

Patients should be treated based on the toxidrome they present with if symptomatic and be observed for at least 8 hours if asymptomatic. Body packers with symptoms and a positive LDCT will need urgent surgical removal of remaining packages. Any passed or removed packages must be handed directly to Police.

Release of information to the police

Most information requested by the police relates to injuries sustained by victims of assaults. It is provided on a standard form with the patient's written consent (*'Statements by professional witnesses'* → p. 403). However, police officers sometimes request information about

Table 20.1 Personal and sensitive information

Personal information	Sensitive information
Names or initials	Sexuality
Date of birth	Ethnicity
Gender	Physical or mental health conditions
Address or postcode	Religious or similar beliefs
Occupation	Political opinions or memberships
Identity number (e.g. NHS or National Insurance number)	Offences committed or court proceedings

Under the Data Protection Act 2018 and the NHS Caldicott guidance, there is a duty to keep personal and sensitive information on patients (and staff) confidential and secure.

patients who are suspects rather than victims (e.g. 'Did a young man attend with a hand injury last night?'). Most circumstances require the disclosure of personal rather than sensitive or clinical information (→ *Table 20.1*). Clinical information should almost never be divulged without the informed written consent of the patient. The laws that control the release of information to the police in England and Wales and the situations in which they apply are described below.

> Police should be informed whenever a victim of an injury by a gun, knife or other dangerous weapon arrives at a hospital. This does not include accidental or self-harm wounds from a knife. This is to allow police officers to consider the risk of further harm to the patient, hospital staff or other members of the public. At this stage of initial contact, personal information should not normally be disclosed.

Legal duty to disclose, even without consent

Terrorism: under the provisions of the Terrorism Act 2000, there is a statutory duty to immediately inform the police if any information is gained either personally or professionally about suspected terrorist activity.

Motor vehicle offences: Section 172 of the Road Traffic Act 1988 makes it a statutory duty to provide the police, on request, with the names and addresses of drivers who are allegedly guilty of offences under this act. Clinical information should not be given.

Court orders: where the courts have made an order, the required information must be disclosed unless the decision is challenged at a higher court.

Legal power to disclose, but must consider implications of gaining consent

Public interest disclosures: the Police and Criminal Evidence (PACE) Act 1984 describes offences that are considered serious (see *Box 20.6*) and can be used as suitable guidelines for the release of non-clinical information, without patient consent. The public interest served by disclosing must outweigh the public interest in protecting the confidentiality of the individual. Seek senior clinical and legal advice if considering this.

Child protection: under Section 47 of the Children Act 1989, a local authority must make all necessary enquiries to safeguard or promote a child's welfare. In such a situation, information should be released without the consent of either parent or child (and without an obligation to inform them) unless 'to do so would be unreasonable in the circumstances of the case'. If you suspect that a child is being abused, then you have a legal power to disclose information to social services (under 'vital interest' conditions of the Data Protection Act) or to the police (under PACE Act).

> **Box 20.6 Serious arrestable offences (Police and Criminal Evidence act, PACE, Section 116)**
>
> An arrestable offence is 'serious' if its commission (or threatened commission) has led to or is intended or likely to lead to the consequences listed below:
>
> - Serious harm to the security of the state or to public order
> - Serious interference with the administration of justice or with the investigation of an offence
> - The death of any person (including by dangerous driving)
> - Serious injury to any person, which includes any disease or any impairment of a person's physical or mental state
> - Substantial financial gain to any person
> - Serious financial loss to any person. Loss is defined as 'serious' for the purposes of this section if, having regard to all the circumstances, it is serious for the person who suffers it

Female Genital Mutilation (FGM) (Serious Crime Act 2015): It is illegal in UK law to excise, infibulate or otherwise mutilate the whole or any part of the labia majora or clitoris of another person.

If FGM is discovered or disclosed during a patient's journey, then it is mandatory that this is recorded by the healthcare professional in the patient's notes. Women over the age of 18 who have undergone FGM do not need to be referred to social services or the police. They should be supported and offered relevant follow-up, should they want it.

Other females within their immediate or extended family (especially those under the age of 18) should be identified and consideration given to their risk of FGM and need for protection. Any child (less than 18 years of age) who presents with symptoms of FGM, who discloses the fact, or you suspect that they are at risk of FGM, then it is your responsibility to report this to the police and implement relevant safeguarding procedures as with any child abuse case. This information must be shared with the GP and health visitor as part of safeguarding actions.

Data Protection Act 2018 Exemptions: the police may also seek personal information under an exemption of the Data Protection Act 2018. Schedule 2 Exemptions allow information to be provided by an organisation about an individual without consent. This is used when the police believe that the seeking of consent would prejudice their enquiries regarding either the prevention or detection of crime or the apprehension or prosecution of offenders. The hospital can then assess the merits of the request and decide whether to apply the exemption.

The freedom of information act

The Freedom of Information Act 2000 gives everyone in the UK greater rights of access to the information held by public authorities such as NHS trusts. Requests can be made by anyone (e.g. members of the public, the media and pressure groups) to access information such as reports, policies, guidelines, correspondence, emails and minutes of meetings. The Act applies to all public bodies and specifies that the request must be met within 20 working days.

Statements by professional witnesses

Clinicians who work in ED will often receive requests from the police for written statements about patients whom they have seen. These police statements should be carefully and legibly written using the case notes and should follow the format as shown in → *Box 20.7* and use the correct description of injuries (→ *p. 392*).

Box 20.7 Statement by a professional witness

This is the statement of Dr. [Name]. My qualifications are [Qualifications] and my GMC registration number is [Number]. I am employed as a [Grade of doctor] in the Emergency Department of [Name of hospital]. On [Date of incident] I was on duty when I examined [Name of Patient, Date of Birth, Do Not Give Address (1)] who attended the hospital (or was brought to the hospital by ambulance) at [Time of registration using 24-hours clock].

[Name of patient] alleged [Brief history and details of the incident as reported to doctor (2)].

On examination, there were [Clinical findings in layman's terms (3)].

These injuries were treated with [Details of treatment (4)].

He or she was referred to [Details of any referral or follow-up]. He or she was discharged from the hospital at [Time of departure using 24-hours clock].

The relevant medical records can be produced to the court if required, labelled exhibit [Your initials with a number].

Notes on the above

(1) **No address**: to protect the victim from possible intimidation when the statement is made available to the defence.
(2) **Details of incident**: the history is part of the complete medical examination and so is more than hearsay evidence. A brief description such as 'said that he was hit on the head with a baseball bat' will suffice. Do not be tempted to expand this or other sections in relation to either causation or outcome. This statement is the evidence of a professional witness not the opinion of an expert witness.
(3) *Clinical findings* → *p. 392.*
(4) **Treatment**: including number of stitches, etc.

The witness statement form must be signed and dated in the space provided at the top of the form and after the last handwritten word on the statement.

Going to court

ED clinicians may even have to go to court to give evidence as a professional witness. This is different from appearing as an expert witness. The professional witness must give an accurate account of his or her findings and actions but is not expected to be the ultimate authority on the subject. He or she should be:

- punctual, appropriately dressed and courteous
- well informed and willing to answer all questions without evasion
- in possession of copies of the relevant notes (however, these notes can be consulted in court only with the permission of the bench)
- honest about the limitations of his or her own knowledge of the subject
- able to describe the work of his or her profession in a way that everyone can understand.

Cases are tried in either Magistrate's or Crown Courts in England or Sheriff's or High Courts in Scotland depending on the nature of the alleged crime.

RESPONSIBILITIES TO CHILDREN

Consent and confidentiality for children

In UK law, a person's 18th birthday draws the line between childhood and adulthood (Children Act 1989.) Once children reach the age of 16 they are presumed by law to have capacity to consent to treatment (Mental Capacity Act 2005) However, unlike adults, their refusal of treatment can, in some circumstances be overridden by someone with parental responsibility or a court. We have an overriding duty to act in the best interests of a child in circumstances where refusal would likely lead to death, severe permanent injury or irreversible mental or physical harm.

Children under 16 may be competent to consent to or refuse treatment depending on whether they have sufficient maturity to understand the decision at hand. This so-called 'Gillick competence' comes from a case where a mother challenged the Department of Health guidance which enabled doctors to provide contraceptive advice and treatment to girls under 16 without their parents knowing (Gillick v West Norfolk 1985). The judges ruled that children under 16 can consent if they have sufficient understanding and intelligence to fully understand what is involved in a proposed treatment, including its purpose, nature, likely effects and risks, chances of success and the availability of other options.

This type of decision is called common law, i.e. it is not written in statute, but if the same question comes up again in any lower court, the previous decision of the higher court must be followed. Lord Fraser was one of the judges in this case, and he set out guidelines for doctors prescribing contraceptives for children under the age of 16 who refuse to inform their parents (Fraser guidelines).

If a child lacks competence, then consent should come from a parent or person with parental responsibility.

- Only one parent is required to give consent
- If a parent refuses to give consent and the treatment is felt to be in the best interests of the child, the courts can override the parents' decision
- In an emergency, where delays will cause harm to the child, treatment can proceed without consent

Blood transfusion in the children of Jehovah's Witnesses →
p. 398.

Children have the same right to confidentiality as adults, however there are some caveats to this.

- Confidentiality must be broken if a child is at risk of harm or abuse. The doctor should consider informing the patient that information will be shared.
- A parent can request to see the medical records for their child (subject access request), but if the child saw a doctor on their own and requested their parents not know, then these notes need not be disclosed (provided the child was competent for this decision).

Child protection procedures

The Children and Social Work Act 2017 replaced local safeguarding children boards (LSCBs) with multi-agency safeguarding arrangements, which fully came into force in September 2019. They require the Local Authority, Clinical Commissioning Group (CCG) and Police involvement.

This is known as the Safeguarding Board in Northern Ireland and the Child Protection Committee (CPC) in Scotland.

Anyone who has concerns about a child's welfare should make a referral to Local Authority children's social care and should do so immediately if there is a concern that the child is suffering significant harm or is likely to do so. This triggers statutory actions under the Children's Act 1989.

Section 47 enquiries

The child's social worker leads an initial multiagency enquiry to be completed within 45 days. This will often include a medical assessment, usually by a Paediatric Consultant and can include X-ray skeletal surveys. Following section 47 enquiries, an initial child protection conference will be held to analyse the information and form a child protection plan.

The emergency protection order

The Emergency Protection Order (EPO) is obtained by a judge at family court to remove the child into care. It may be made for a maximum of 8 days and extended for up to

a further 7 days. Any person may apply for this order but applications are usually made by employees of either a social services department or the NSPCC (National Society for the Prevention of Cruelty to Children). The local authority take on limited parental responsibility of the child during this time, but foster parents do not.

In Scotland, the equivalent is the Child Protection Order (CPO).

The police protection order

The Police Protection Order (PPO) gives a police officer the power to take a child 'into police protection' for up to 72 hours if he or she believes that the child is at immediate risk. Police may bring the child to the ED if it is felt they need urgent medical treatment. This order can also be used to prevent the removal of a child from the ED – at much shorter notice than the EPO.

DEATH

Reporting of death and the role of the coroner

The coroner must be informed if death is associated with any of the following:

- poisoning by any toxic substance or medicinal product, e.g. bleeding in a patient on anticoagulants
- violence, trauma or injury
- self-harm or suspected suicide
- neglect, including self-neglect
- any treatment or procedure, e.g. during surgery
- an injury or disease attributable to any employment held by the person
- any other unnatural cause, e.g. accidents or environmental exposure
- the cause of death is unknown
- while in custody or subject to detention under the mental health act
- the identity of the deceased is not known

> If in doubt, discuss the patient with the coroner or his/her deputy.

A coroner will hold an inquest if there is reasonable cause to suspect that the deceased has died:

- a sudden death of which the cause is unknown
- a violent or otherwise unnatural death
- in prison or in such a place or in such circumstances as to require an inquest under any other Act.

Doctors involved in the care of the patient may be asked to give evidence at inquests to assist the coroner in answering three questions:

- Who was the deceased?
- Where and when did they die?
- How did they come about their death?

Inquests are held in coroner's court, which will usually be attended by members of the deceased's family who can also ask questions to witnesses. It is an inquisitorial process not an adversarial one, i.e. nobody is 'on trial', but if the verdict is unlawful killing or neglect there will be a police investigation and possibly criminal charges.

Coroners may produce a 'report to prevent future deaths' or a 'Regulation 28 Report', following an inquest if they feel that an organisation needs to take action following a death. The organisation has 56 days to provide a response.

Medical Examiners are doctors who are specially trained to liaise with bereaved families and scrutinise the medical notes of deceased patients. This process is to ensure the quality of the death certification process, allow the bereaved to raise any concerns and ensure proper scrutiny of all deaths outside of the coronial process (The Coroners and Justice Act 2009.)

In Scotland, there is no coroner. Instead, fatal accident enquiries (FAIs) are conducted by a special unit of the Crown Office and Procurator Fiscal Service (COPFS). FAIs are conducted before a Sheriff following investigation by the Procurator Fiscal who presents the evidence.

Mandatory FAIs:

- Work related
- Death in custody
- Child detained in secure accommodation
- Discretionary FAIs (instructed by Lord Advocate):
- Sudden, suspicious or unexplained
- Serious public concern

Clinical diagnosis of death

For most purposes, death is signalled by the irreversible failure of respiration, circulation and innervation. Diagnosis of death in an apparently lifeless patient should thus depend on the following:

- Absence of respiratory movements or breath sounds
- Absence of central pulses or heart sounds
- Absence of the protective reflexes of the eye (e.g. the corneal reflex)
- Absence of the pupillary response to light.

The Academy of Medical Royal College's Code of Practice for the diagnosis and confirmation of death recommends that the patient should be observed by the person responsible for confirming death for a minimum

of 5 min to establish that irreversible cardiorespiratory arrest has occurred.

A state of near-death simulated by hypothermia, cold-water drowning or sedative poisoning must be excluded. Rigour mortis is usually fully established 12 hours after death, lasts about 12 hours and then wears off over the next 12 hours.

Diagnosis of death using neurological criteria

Sometimes a patient may be brought to an ED with a functioning circulation but no other apparent signs of life. The criteria necessary for the diagnosis of death using Neurological criteria were updated by the Academy of Medical Royal Colleges in 2008.

Essential preconditions to testing

Before a diagnosis of brainstem death can be considered all the following must coexist:

1 The patient is completely unresponsive.
2 The patient is maintained on a ventilator because spontaneous respiration had previously become inadequate or had ceased.
3 There is no doubt that the patient's condition is caused by irremediable, structural brain damage.

Necessary exclusions

Before proceeding to testing, the following must be ruled out:

1 Coma secondary to drugs, hypothermia or metabolic disorder
2 Respiratory failure and unresponsiveness secondary to neuromuscular blocking agents. Spinal reflexes should still be present.

Testing for absent brainstem function

Seizures and abnormal posturing (decorticate or decerebrate) imply that there is a passage of nervous impulses through the brainstem, which therefore has live neurons in it.

The brainstem findings used to confirm death in the UK code are as follows:

- No pupillary response to light
- No corneal reflex
- No vestibulo-ocular reflexes
- No motor responses within the distribution of the cranial nerves in response to adequate stimulation of any somatic area

- No gag reflex and no cough reflex response to bronchial stimulation by a suction catheter passed down the trachea
- Apnoea over a 5 min period during which the patient is oxygenated by diffusion and the $paCO_2$ rises by greater than 0.5 kPa; failure of the respiratory centre is the ultimate sign of loss of brainstem function.

Tests should be carried out by an experienced clinician, in the presence of another doctor. Retesting is performed after an interval of 2 to 3 hours for the purposes of ensuring that:

- there is no observer error
- there is no change in signs.

These tests are usually performed on an Intensive Care Unit (ICU), after withdrawal of sedating and neuromuscular blocking drugs.

Organ and tissue donation

The law regarding organ donation has changed recently in the UK from an 'opt in' to an 'opt out' system. The understanding now is that all adults agree to become organ donors when they die, unless they have made it known that they do not wish to donate.

Excluding donations from a living donor, there are two main types of organ donation described by the World Health Organisation:

1 **Donation after brain death (DBD)**: follows death certified using neurological criteria
2 **Donation after cardiac death (DCD)**: follows; death certified using cardiorespiratory criteria

Patients initially assessed in EDs in whom DBD is a possibility should be admitted wherever possible to an ICU in order that their clinical and broader interests (including the potential for donation) can be fully assessed. Specialist nurses in organ donation (SN-ODs) are vital to liaise with NHS Blood and Transplant and counsel families on the process. There are some absolute contraindications to organ donation (→ Box 20.8).

 Box 20.8 Patients who are not suitable for organ donation

Patients with the following conditions should not be referred as potential donors:

- Variant Creutzfeldt–Jakob disease (CJD)
- HIV disease (but not HIV infection)
- Ebola virus disease
- Active cancer with spread outside affected organ

The law requires that treatment be given only if it is in the patient's best interests. However, if an individual expressed a wish to be an organ donor, treatments that facilitate that wish and do not cause the person harm or distress are regarded as in their best interests.

OTHER ED ISSUES

Complaints

Any public organisation must have a well-structured system for dealing with complaints. Problems that are dealt with in a rapid, efficient, and courteous manner will often resolve satisfactorily.

The most common areas of complaint to a department of emergency medicine are:

- waiting times
- attitude of staff
- communication and information given
- aspects of clinical care.

Local resolution

Face-to-face – discussion of the problem usually follows a direct approach to a member of the clinical or clerical staff at the time of treatment. It can often be resolved by listening carefully to the issues and responding sensitively:

- Ensure the patient has given consent for you to discuss their care, if the complainant is a relative.
- Do not be confrontational or defensive.
- Express sympathy and say you are sorry. You can empathise with a patient's distress without admitting liability or error (e.g. 'I am sorry that you are unhappy with your treatment').
- Ask questions and obtain the full facts about concerns.
- Do not attempt to justify; explain if appropriate.
- Agree a course of action and ensure that it is carried out quickly and efficiently.
- Provide information about the NHS complaints system if the complainant wishes to take the matter further.
- Document the content and conclusion of the discussion in the patient's case notes.

A complaint can be a useful piece of feedback for an ED and can prompt important change and quality improvement so do not be afraid to thank a patient for their feedback.

Written complaints – should be made within 12 months of the problem revealing itself and are forwarded to the hospital complaints manager who then gathers information from the relevant clinical staff. The chief executive subsequently replies in writing within 6 months and a meeting with the patient or the relatives may be convened.

Each NHS trust has a Patient Advice and Liaison Service (PALS) to listen to concerns independently of the treating medical team and can refer to the Independent Complaints Advocacy Service.

Investigation by the health service commissioner

The next level of the system is a complaint to the Parliamentary and Health Service Ombudsman. The Ombudsman is independent of the NHS and acts as a final arbiter of both complaints and complaints procedures.

Chaperones

The use of a chaperone is recommended for any intimate examination of a patient. You should use another medical professional, not a family member of the patient. If the patient refuses to have a chaperone present but you feel that one is necessary, you should explain why to the patient and if they still refuse, offer to try and find another clinician who is willing to perform the examination without a chaperone. Ultimately, the patient's clinical needs take precedence, and this should be recorded carefully in the notes.

Notifiable diseases (and other notification duties of registered medical practitioners)

In the UK, registered medical practitioners attending a patient are required to notify the proper officer of the local authority in which the patient resides when they have 'reasonable grounds for suspecting' that the patient:

- has a notifiable disease as listed in the Notification Regulations (→ *Box 20.9*)
- has an infection not included in the Notification Regulations which, in the view of the doctor, could present significant harm to human health (e.g. emerging or new infections)
- is contaminated (such as with chemicals or radiation) in a manner that, in the view of the doctor, could present significant harm to human health

---

 Box 20.9 **Notifiable diseases in the UK**

[Schedule 1 of the Health Protection (Notification) Regulations 2010 with additions for Scotland and Northern Ireland]

Acute encephalitis (not Scotland)
Acute bacterial meningitis***
Acute poliomyelitis***
Acute infectious hepatitis*** (not Scotland)
Anthrax***
Botulism***
Brucellosis***
Chickenpox (Northern Ireland only)
Cholera***
COVID-19
Diphtheria***
Enteric fever (typhoid or paratyphoid fever)***
Food poisoning*** (not Scotland)
Gastroenteritis in children aged <2 years (Northern Ireland only)
Haemolytic uraemic syndrome (HUS)***
Haemophilus influenzae type b (Scotland only)
Infectious bloody diarrhoea*** (not Scotland unless *Escherichia coli* O157)
Invasive group A streptococcal disease***

Legionnaires' disease*** (not Scotland)
Leprosy (not Scotland or Northern Ireland)
Malaria (not Scotland)
Measles***
Meningococcal septicaemia***
Mumps
Necrotising fasciitis (Scotland only)
Plague***
Rabies
Rubella
Severe acute respiratory syndrome (SARS)***
Scarlet fever (not Scotland)
Smallpox***
Tetanus***
Tuberculosis
Tularemia (Scotland only)
Typhus
Viral haemorrhagic fever (VHF)***
West Nile Fever (Scotland only)
Whooping cough***
Yellow fever
***URGENT = notify immediately by telephone and then send paper/electronic version within 3 days.

Doctors should not wait for laboratory confirmation or results of other investigations to notify a suspected case. This ensures the prompt transfer of information so that health protection interventions and control measures can be initiated as soon as possible. Notification requires the completion of the appropriate form but urgent cases should be notified by telephone as well (within 24 hours of any suspicions at the latest). In Scotland, written notification should be undertaken electronically via the Scottish Care Information (SCI) Gateway.

Notifiable diseases in the UK → Box 20.9.

Fit notes

Most patients discharged from the ED will need only a few days away from work. Self-certification is allowed for 7 days absence before a note from a doctor is required. If a patient will be unable to work for more than 7 days, it may be appropriate to issue a Med 3 certificate for this period (see *Box 20.10*).

Patients who have received sedative or opioid drugs in the ED

Many patients receive drugs likely to cause sedation as part of their treatment in the ED. For both practical and medicolegal reasons, these patients need to be given verbal and written warnings about the possible residual effects of these drugs. → *Box 20.11* summarises suggested information for the patient to take home.

Box 20.10 Form Med 3

 Closed statements – has return to work date

The note is for less than 2 weeks from the day of examination. It should indicate the earliest day on which the patient is likely to be fit for work.

Open statements – no return to work date

If a doctor is unable to issue a closed statement as above, then an open statement may be issued by entering a period during which the absence from work is likely to continue. This period may not be for more than 6 months from the date of issue unless the patient has been certified as unfit to work for the previous 6 months. When a patient who has been given an open statement recovers, he or she must be given a closed statement as above to terminate the spell of incapacity and allow a return to work:

Safe discharge

To send a patient home you must be sure of the following:

- The symptoms can be adequately controlled in the environment in which the patient lives.
- Any further investigation or treatment that the patient may need can be arranged
- The patient has access to further help, and carers, should it be necessary.
- You have communicated your plan for present and future management to both the patient and any others necessary for this care (e.g. relatives, GP, health visitor, district nurse, social worker).

Generic discharge information, made bespoke appropriately, should be given; this should include:

- Advice about pain relief and prescriptions given by the ED
- Advice about fitness to work and fitness to drive
- Further appointments and follow-up arrangements
- Injury or illnesses specific information (often on a separate leaflet)
- Advice about symptoms or signs that should prompt further assessment
- Contact information for both the ED and patient advice and liaison service

Box 20.11 **Instructions about the care of a patient who has received sedative medicines in the ED**

Your relative/child/friend has received sedative medicines or injections in the ED. These drugs may cause:

- drowsiness
- unsteadiness and loss of balance
- poor coordination and clumsiness

Some of these effects may last for up to 24 hours. As a result of this, a person who has received sedatives should:

- be accompanied home
- be escorted when going upstairs
- take care when using the toilet or bathroom

They must NOT:

- be left alone in the house until fully recovered (e.g. overnight)

- drive or go cycling
- go out walking alone
- use machinery or go into situations where poor balance or coordination could be dangerous
- drink alcohol
- sign any legally binding documents

However, they can:

- eat and drink light meals
- take painkillers and regular medicines

If you have any worries or problems with this patient, then telephone the ED helpline.

21

Small wounds and localised infections

Emergency Medicine Consultant, Royal Bolton Hospital, Bolton, UK
Health Education North West, Manchester, UK

SMALL WOUNDS

Small does not mean trivial. The wound may be:

- the only visible manifestation of a significant deep injury
- simple yet serious if not treated promptly or properly
- capable of leaving a considerable amount of disfigurement or loss of function
- of no consequence in the doctor's eyes but worrying to the patient.

> Inadequately treated small wounds cause much distress for patients, a lot of worry for doctors and a considerable amount of work for lawyers.

Assessment of wounds

Careful assessment of wounds is essential to ensure underlying injury is not overlooked and high-risk features are managed appropriately. Consider:

- **Mechanism of injury**:
  What forces were involved? Could there be an underlying fracture? Wounds cause by a sharp object (e.g. knife, glass) are more likely to involve damage to underlying structures. Wounds caused by broken glass should always have X-rays obtained to rule out retained foreign body
- **Site of injury**:
  Consider the underlying structures. In an injury to the trunk, perineum or neck, cross-sectional imaging and formal exploration may be required to rule out serious injury. For wounds near a joint consider joint position at time of injury and whether joint penetration may have occurred. Consider underlying neurovascular structures.
- **Time of injury**: wounds more than 6 hours old are more likely to become infected
- **Place of injury**: field or garden injuries carry a greater risk of contamination with tetanus and gas-forming organisms.
- **Interpersonal violence and safety concerns**: Was this injury inflicted by another person? Does the patient feel safe at home or have somewhere safe to return to? Consider domestic violence and seek advice if concerned. Wounds believed to be inflicted by knife or gunshot must be reported to the police in the UK → *p. 401*.

> A butcher's knife may be contaminated with many organisms from animal carcasses. When boning a carcass and holding the knife with both hands, it is possible to receive a deep, penetrating and highly contaminated wound.

The RCEM Lecture Notes: Emergency Medicine, Fifth Edition. Edited by Catherine Williams and Amy Nickson.
© 2024 John Wiley & Sons Ltd. Published 2024 by John Wiley & Sons Ltd.
Companion website: www.wiley.com/go/LNEM5

Also ask about

- Allergies to drugs including antibiotics
- Previous injuries: in paediatric patients, this may relate to concerns about safeguarding (→ p. 369)
- Past medical history – immunosuppression or diabetes increase risk of infection which may influence management
- Current medication – some drugs may affect local treatment (e.g. anticoagulants)
- Is the patient vaccinated against tetanus? → p. 415.

Look for

- **Site and size of the wound**: it is a good idea to measure the wound if possible. Consider the direction of the force that inflicted the injury, and the position of joints at the time – this will help identify potential underlying structures which may be at risk of damage.
- **Wound depth**: superficial wounds are those not fully penetrating the skin (e.g. some abrasions). Deeper wounds will require exploration under local anaesthesia. Truncal wounds and those over high-risk areas like the neck should not be explored in ED.
- **Character of the wound**: use of these specific terms can carry medicolegal implications, and so in cases of uncertainty it may be best to avoid using these descriptors.
  - An abrasion (graze) is due to a blunt injury applying friction and is usually superficial.
  - An incised wound is caused by a sharp object (e.g. knife) and have sharp, straight edges.
  - A 'stab' wound is deeper than it is wide.
  - Lacerations are tears to the skin caused by blunt injury. The edges are usually irregular and may be bruised.
- **Injury to deep structures**:
  - **Tendon injury**: Tendon function must be isolated and individually examined. Complete division of a tendon will be evident from loss of function; however, a tendon may be partially divided and retain function initially. Wounds must therefore be explored under local anaesthesia and tendons visualised. It is important to move the tendon through its full range of movement under direct vision to rule out a partial division.
  - **Nerve injury**: Any altered sensation distal to a wound should be assumed to be a nerve injury until proven otherwise. Sensory loss does not need to be complete to be significant as some function is often retained in the early phase even with nerve transection. Examine sensory and motor components of each nerve individually.
  - **Vascular injury and bleeding**: Examine distal pulses and perfusion. Control active bleeding with direct pressure for 5–15 min. If bleeding persists, consider using a 'glove tourniquet' in the short term to achieve a bloodless field and enable adequate wound assessment. Topical tranexamic acid or lignocaine with adrenaline can be used to achieve haemostasis. Bleeding is exacerbated by anticoagulants, partial (rather than complete) tears of vessels and continued interference with wounds. If there is a potential for significant bleeding, intravenous (IV) access should be established and appropriate equipment and monitoring available prior to attempts at exploration. Scalp wounds in particular can lead to profuse and persistent bleeding, which may result in haemorrhagic shock.
  - **Wound contamination**: Assess the degree of wound contamination and the nature of any contaminating material. Do not send microbiology swabs from fresh wounds – these will just demonstrate skin commensals and are unhelpful. Swab older wounds with evidence of infection.

Pain may be extreme with some small injuries. Less painful and more serious injuries may have been inflicted in the same incident and can easily be missed. Local anaesthetic may be needed before further investigation occurs; sensory loss must be recorded first.

Anaesthesia for wounds

All wounds must be explored and cleaned before the closure is contemplated. This usually requires anaesthesia, as does the subsequent closure. A general anaesthetic may be required when the areas involved are multiple or large, or belong to children or anxious adults (→ Boxes 21.1 and 21.2).

Cleaning and exploration of wounds

Wounds must be thoroughly cleaned to reduce the risk of infection. In particular, the removal of any contaminating substances (e.g. soil, gravel) is essential. In most cases, clean tap water is appropriate for wound cleaning, and the patient can undertake initial wound cleaning themselves. Pressure irrigation using a bag of saline may be helpful for more stubborn dirt. Local anaesthesia will be required for deeper and more heavily contaminated wounds, which may require scrubbing with a nailbrush or toothbrush to ensure adequate decontamination. Do not use hydrogen peroxide which risks damaging healthy tissue. Chlorhexadine is preferred over povidone-iodine solution if antiseptic is

Box 21.1 Local infiltration

Maximum doses of local anaesthetics → p. 368.

Treatment of severe local anaesthetic toxicity → Box 21.3.

- In most cases, lidocaine without adrenaline is appropriate. Lidocaine with adrenaline may be useful where there is active bleeding. Bupivicaine is an option if longer periods of anaesthesia are likely to be required.
  - 2% lidocaine is suitable for nerve blocks; in a digital ring block, this reduces the volume required and hence the risk of vascular compression
  - 1% lidocaine is appropriate for general use
  - 0.5% lidocaine should be used when large areas of tissue are involved and more than 10 mL anaesthetic are required
- Infiltration of local anaesthetic is painful. Consider buffering the local anaesthetic (10 mL lidocaine with 1 mL 8.4% bicarbonate) and warming to room temperature to reduce pain of injection.
- Clean the wound edge with an antiseptic solution. If local anaesthetic is injected before the antiseptic has dried, then the patient will be given a painful subcutaneous injection of both
- It may be necessary to trim hair for at least 2 cm around the wound, before injecting local anaesthetic. The aim is to expose the wound fully and to prevent hair from interfering with the sutures. Scissors are usually adequate. A razor is sometimes necessary. Never shave the eyebrows
- Using a short 23 G needle, inject a small amount of lidocaine under the wound edge, either through the wound edge if the wound is fresh and socially clean or through the skin if the wound is grossly contaminated or contused (safer but more painful)
- Once this small area is anaesthetised inject through it to raise a weal a little further on. Wait and then repeat. In this way, the patient feels only the first injection

Box 21.2 Ring block

This is effective for procedures involving distal wounds of the finger. There is a risk of damage to, or spasm of, the digital arteries, and it must not be used if there is a history of upper limb circulatory problems.

- Use plain lidocaine (2% for an adult). The risks of causing digital ischaemia with injected adrenaline are greatly overstated and evidence

has not shown significant adverse events from the use of adrenaline in digital wound repair; however, it is rarely required. Clean the base of the finger with an antiseptic solution
- Insert a 23 G needle into the dorsolateral border of the base of the finger. The tip of the needle should end up near the bone on the palmar side of the finger. Aspirate and if blood is seen withdraw the needle and start again
- Inject 1 mL, and then another 1–2 mL as you withdraw the needle, to block both palmar and dorsal digital nerves. Repeat on the opposite side of the finger
- An alternative approach is a single volar injection of approximately 3 mL lidocaine at the midpoint of the digital palmar crease.
- Wait for at least 5 minutes for full anaesthesia of the finger
- If digital artery spasm occurs, stop the procedure. Massage the base of the finger where the anaesthetic has been injected and instruct the patient to move the finger vigorously. These manoeuvres should dissipate the fluid and release the spasm

Box 21.3 The treatment of severe local anaesthetic (LA) agent toxicity

Signs of severe LA toxicity include sudden loss of consciousness, convulsions, cardiovascular collapse, cardiac conduction disturbances, tachydysrhythmias, asystole and ventricular fibrillation (VF).

- Institute cardiopulmonary resuscitation (CPR) if required
- Attend to the ABCs
- Control convulsions with standard drugs
- Control cardiac dysrhythmias with standard therapy
- Treat cardiac arrest with lipid emulsion, continuing CPR throughout for up to an hour. (This is a relatively new approach. Intralipid 20% has been shown to reverse LA-induced cardiac arrest in animal models and in some human case reports. It has also been used successfully in life-threatening LA toxicity without cardiac arrest.) An intravenous bolus of 20% Intralipid 1.5 mL/kg is given over 1 min followed by an infusion of 0.25 mL/kg per min. The bolus injection can be repeated twice at 5-min intervals if an adequate circulation has not been restored and the rate of the infusion can be doubled. Monitor patients for signs of pancreatitis after use of Intralipid.

used, although there is little evidence that this reduces infection rates significantly compared to the use of saline. Dirt left in a wound may cause infection or be taken up by inflammatory cells to produce a permanent tattoo effect.

Exploration of a wound is essential to identify:

- the depth and extent of damage
- structures exposed or damaged
- foreign bodies.

An appreciation of the direction and force of the injuring agent will facilitate exploration.

Resection of tissue

- Use a scalpel to remove dead tissue and trim the edges of old wounds.
- Be very cautious in the scalp, foot and hand. Do not trim wound edges in these areas as skin is at a premium here – have a low threshold for seeking expert advice. Significant, deep or complex wounds to the face should almost always be referred for specialist management due to the profound psychological impact of scarring in this area.

Radiographs for foreign bodies

If there is a suspicion of a foreign body, soft tissue X-ray should be undertaken in most cases. Metallic, glass and stone foreign bodies are usually detectable. It can be difficult to differentiate foreign bodies on the skin surface (e.g. glass fragments) with embedded foreign bodies, so cleaning the wound and a fresh dressing is important prior to X-ray. Radio-opaque skin markers can be useful to identify areas of concern. The radiograph request must indicate that a foreign body is being sought so that the radiographer can adjust the exposure accordingly. Ultrasound can be useful to identify radiolucent foreign bodies (e.g. wood).

Foreign bodies act as a nidus for infection and can cause ongoing pain and irritation, so should always be removed from an open wound wherever possible. Small fragments, obvious on a radiograph, can sometimes be very difficult to find and remove when embedded in soft tissue. Occasionally, less damage is done by leaving them *in situ*. This decision must be made after consultation with a senior colleague.

Patients sometimes re-present to the ED with ongoing symptoms and concern about possible embedded foreign body. Ultrasound or radiographs can be used to confirm the presence and localise the foreign body – removal in this circumstance is usually best carried out in theatre by specialist teams.

All wounds involving glass must have radiographs to exclude retained fragments.

Closure of wounds

- **Primary**: For most recent wounds, primary closure is the appropriate option. If the wound is contaminated, this should occur after thorough cleaning. There is no absolute time period from injury that precludes primary wound closure.
- **Delayed primary**: Traditional teaching recommended delayed primary closure after 3–5 days, for crush injuries, or for wounds that have presented 'late' (>6 hours) to the emergency department. Delayed closure aims to reduce wound infection; however, there is very little evidence available to support decision-making in this regard. Factors affecting decision-making will include location of wound and cosmetic impact, risk of infection (high in large wounds, lower limb wounds and diabetes), patient preference and availability of follow-up options.
- **Secondary (i.e. by natural processes)**: When surgical closure is impossible or inappropriate (e.g. infected wounds), granulation and epithelialisation are encouraged.

Tissue glue

Useful for superficial and low tension wounds, and with the additional advantage of being quick and painless. Do not use in wounds over joints or near the eyes. Oppose the wound edges before applying glue to the wound and hold for 30–60 seconds while the glue hardens. Patients should be advised to keep the area dry for the first 5 days.

Tissue glue is applied to the carefully opposed external skin surfaces and not into the open wound.

Adhesive strips

Useful for superficial wounds. Not recommended in moist areas (e.g. axillae) or in wounds under tension. Closure with adhesive strips is particularly useful for wounds with thin and fragile skin such as pretibial lacerations, where sutures would cut through the skin. Use of tincture of bezoin can help adhesion.

Hair apposition technique

An effective technique in scalp laceration is to use the patient's hair as effectively an embedded suture. Twist approximately five hairs together on one wound edge, and do the same on the other side. These two 'bunches' can then be twisted together and secured with glue. This technique compares favourably with suturing in trials.

Sutures

For most wounds, non-absorbable sutures should be used. 4/0 sutures are appropriate for limb wounds, 3/0 for scalp and trunk wounds and finer sutures (5/0 or 6/0) for hands or facial wounds. Absorbable sutures should be used to close subcutaneous spaces if required.

- Handle wound edges with toothed forceps
- Use the instrument tie technique
- Plan sutures strategically – do not just start at one end. For irregular wounds, oppose the wound edges along the length of the wound prior to starting and place sutures to secure key points initially.
- Use interrupted sutures – not continuous or subcuticular because these cause increased risk of infection tracking along the suture.
- Do not close a wound under significant tension

Suturing skills cannot be learned from a book.

Skin loss: When closing defects in the skin, excessive tension should be avoided at all costs. If there is extensive skin loss or any loss on the face or hand, seek advice. Small skin defects elsewhere may be closed by undermining. This is achieved using a scalpel about 3 mm below the skin in the horizontal plane. A tissue plane may then be opened up using blunt scissors.

Aftercare of wounds

Dressings may not be required (e.g. on the face) or may be of simple non-adherent type. Splintage should be minimal but may be necessary if a wound is over the extensor aspect of a joint.

Removal time for sutures varies with the site: 3–4 days on the face, up to 10 days in lower limbs or over joints, but usually about 7 days for most other parts of the body. Earlier replacement with adhesive strips may

avoid permanent puncture-mark scars. Sutures may be removed by community nursing teams or according to local agreement.

Resuturing wounds

Patients returning with wounds that have broken down should have a senior opinion. Such wounds must be cleaned and dressed until ready for re-suture. If there is evidence of local infection oral antibiotics will be required. Facial wounds need a specialised opinion and wounds in children may need reclosure under general anaesthetic. The possibility of a retained foreign body should always be considered.

Reimplantation of body parts

Successful reimplantation of amputated body parts is possible using microsurgical techniques. Clean injuries without contamination or contusion have the best chances of success. Suitable structures for reimplantation include:

- the whole or part of a finger (with amputations proximal to the distal interphalangeal joint only)
- the penis
- ears
- large pieces of scalp
- hands, feet and more extensive parts of a limb.

Patients with these injuries should be discussed as soon as possible with the nearest plastic surgery unit. The amputated part should be wrapped in saline-soaked gauze and then put in a plastic bag in a container full of crushed ice. The body tissue must not come into direct contact with the ice as tissue necrosis may occur.

Prevention of wound infection

This is achieved in most cases by:

- cleaning the wound
- excising necrotic tissue
- closing the wound as appropriate
- dressing the wound carefully
- using antibiotics when indicated (→ *Box 21.4*)
- anticipating the presence of spore-forming organisms (→ *p. 415*).

Patient concordance in aftercare is very important, so a clear explanation is essential.

Most wounds do not require prophylactic antibiotics, and the mainstay of reducing infection is thorough cleaning prior to wound closure. Penetrating

> **Box 21.4 Indications for antibiotics in wound care**
>
> Antibiotics are indicated for wounds that:
>
> - are already showing signs of infection when seen
> - are more than 12 hours old and in need of primary closure
> - have a definite history of contamination with problem organisms (e.g. human and cat bites)
> - are possibly contaminated with deep areas that are not amenable to cleaning (e.g. some puncture wounds)
> - have exposed or damaged deep structures (e.g. bone in compound fractures, tendon or nerve)

and deep puncture injuries that cannot be cleaned as easily may benefit from prophylactic antibiotics, as may crush injuries to fingertips with distal phalanx fractures. The most common wound contaminants are bacteria from the skin, so flucloxacillin or clarithromycin is adequate cover. In bites or highly contaminated wounds, a wider spectrum of organisms is involved and so co-amoxiclav or clarithromycin should be prescribed.

Spore-forming organisms are more likely to contaminate wounds incurred on sports fields or in gardens and injuries of the lower limb. They will flourish in areas of hypoxia, e.g. deep, penetrating and contused wounds. Primary prevention involves scrubbing all wounds under effective anaesthesia and surgically removing all necrotic tissue. All foreign material must be removed.

Gas gangrene can be prevented if wounds are managed as outlined above. Long-acting penicillins are no substitute for adequate wound toilet.

Prevention of tetanus

Diagnosis and treatment of tetanus → p. 245.
Routine UK immunisation schedule for children → Table 18.7 on p. 368.
Summary of tetanus prophylaxis → Table 21.1.

There are still occasional cases of tetanus reported in the UK, although prophylaxis against tetanus is cheap and safe. Infection is caused by contamination of a wound with the spores of the bacillus *Clostridium tetani*, which may be present in soil or manure. Days or even weeks after infection, local multiplication of

Table 21.1 Tetanus prophylaxis

Patient immunisation status	Tetanus prone wound	High-risk tetanus prone wound	Clean wound
Those aged 11 years and over, who have received an adequate priming course[a] of tetanus vaccine with the last dose within 10 years	Nothing required	Nothing required	Nothing required
Children aged 5–10 years who have received priming course and preschool booster			
Children under 5 years who have received an adequate priming course			
Received adequate priming course of tetanus vaccine but last dose more than 10 years ago	Immediate reinforcing dose of vaccine	Immediate reinforcing dose of vaccine HTIg at a different site	Nothing required
Children aged 5–10 years who have received an adequate priming course but no preschool booster			
Not received adequate priming course of tetanus vaccine	Immediate reinforcing dose of vaccine	Immediate reinforcing dose of vaccine	Immediate reinforcing dose of vaccine
This group includes uncertain vaccination status and those born before routine vaccination rollout in 1961	HTIg at a different site	HTIg at a different site	

HTIg, human tetanus immunoglobulin.
[a] Adequate priming course = at least 3 doses of tetanus vaccine.

the organism occurs with release of its neurotoxin (→ *p. 245*). Until recently, most cases of tetanus in the UK were in people aged >65 years who had not been previously immunised, more recently there have been sporadic outbreaks amongst people who inject drugs. Even the most trivial of wounds can introduce tetanus into the body, but some wounds carry a particularly high risk. *For factors that identify tetanus-prone wounds* → *Box 21.5*.

In the UK vaccination programme, tetanus is always given as a combined immunisation with either just diptheria and inactivated polio or also including pertussis or additionally with haemophilus influenza type B and hepatitis B. Combined vaccines should also be used when boosters against tetanus are required in the ED to provide comprehensive protection.

Tetanus toxoid vaccine confers active immunity. It stimulates the production of antibodies, which may take several weeks to reach a peak. Therefore, in some cases, patients with high-risk wounds (→ *Box 21.5*) may also require passive immunisation with human tetanus immunoglobulin (HTIg). The two injections should be given into separate areas. Patients with impaired immunity may not respond to active immunisation and may therefore also need HTIg.

Box 21.5 **Tetanus-prone wounds**

Wounds that are considered tetanus-prone include:

- puncture-type injuries acquired in a contaminated environment, e.g. gardening or farming injuries
- wounds containing foreign bodies
- wounds or burns with systemic sepsis
- certain animal bites and scratches including deep puncture wounds or where the wound has occurred in an agricultural setting (domestic animal bites should not contain tetanus spores)

Particularly high risk tetanus prone wounds are those that also:

- have heavy contamination with material likely to contain tetanus spores, e.g. soil, manure
- wounds or burns that show extensive devitalised tissue
- wounds or burns that require surgical intervention that is delayed for more than 6 hours

---

Active immunisation against tetanus was introduced into some areas of the UK as part of the primary immunisation of infants from the mid-1950s and was adopted nationally from 1961. It was provided by the British armed forces (mostly to men!) from 1938 onwards. Knowledge of these dates and the age of the patient will help to determine the likelihood of previous immunisation.

Patients with doubtful or unknown immune status to tetanus require a full primary course of vaccine (three doses at 1-month intervals) which the patient should be advised to arrange via their GP.

Human tetanus immunoglobulin

Human tetanus immunoglobulin (HTIg) gives rapid passive immunity. It is a preparation of human antibodies, which is not associated with significant side effects or allergy, unlike the previously used horse serum. The dose is 250 IU by deep IM injection. This may be increased to 500 IU if more than 24 hours have elapsed or if there is a risk of heavy contamination or after large burns.

Tetanus and diphtheria immunisation for children

The administration of an unscheduled tetanus and diphtheria immunisation to a child may cause great difficulty with the correct timing of other immunisations. For this reason, concurrent administration of the other recommended immunisations for that age group or referral to the child's health visitor is usually the better practice.

Routine UK immunisation schedule for children → *Table 18.7 on p. 368.*

Wound botulism

This related clostridial infection has recently reemerged in the UK.

Diagnosis and treatment of wound botulism → *p. 246.*
Treatment of clostridial and other necrotising soft-tissue infections → *p. 274.*

SPECIFIC TYPES OF WOUNDS

Abdominal wounds → *p. 82.*
Burns → *p. 141.*
Chest wounds → *p. 75.*

Facial wounds → p. 64.
Forensic aspects of wounds → p. 393.
Neck wounds → p. 63.
Scalp wounds → p. 39.
Serious hand injuries → p. 132.
Wrist wounds → p. 123.

Abrasions

Motorcyclists and children may present with dirty abrasions.

Tx The basic care is as for any wound. However, the ingrained dirt must be removed to prevent infection and to avoid the development of a permanent 'tattoo'. Scrubbing with a swab or a small brush may be necessary. Analgesia for this purpose can be obtained by:

- application of local anaesthetic gel
- infiltration of local anaesthetic
- general anaesthesia.

Crush wounds

Where there is an element of crush or bursting in the mechanism of injury there is widespread damage to tissues. Extracellular fluid accumulates and the tissues continue to swell for 24–48 hours.

Tx The wound should be cleaned, explored and then dressed.

> If crush wounds are closed immediately, interstitial pressure will rise, resulting in tissue necrosis and infection.

The patient must be reviewed on the following day. Severe crush injuries require admission for elevation and observation. Decompression may sometimes be needed, especially if the crush has damaged deep tissues without tearing the skin or if there is a deep, closed compartment.

Compartment syndrome → p. 112.

Degloving injuries

When skin is traumatically removed from limbs in this way, it is tempting to simply replace and suture it. However, the injured skin is always contused and often dead. The risks of necrosis and sloughing are very great. A patient with a degloving injury must be referred for inpatient surgical management.

Roller injuries

These have features of both degloving and crush injuries. The injury may seem trivial at first but widespread tissue necrosis can occur. Admission, elevation and careful observation are essential. Vascular compromise is suggested by:

- failure to blanch on pressure
- failure of capillary refill
- paraesthesia.

Flap wounds

Flaps are caused by initial contact at the apex of the wound and then a tearing of the skin towards the base. Contusion of the skin flap is inevitable. Narrow, distally based flaps have a poor blood supply.

Tx If the flap has a wide base or is thick with obviously viable tissues, it may be sutured in the normal way. If not, consider defatting the flap and replacing it as a skin graft with a pressure dressing. The skin of children is very elastic and a V-shaped cut may appear to have lost tissue or have a narrow base as a result of contraction. The skin flap should be stretched back to its normal position without undue tension before viability and skin loss are assessed.

Stab wounds

Stab wounds are defined as wounds that are deeper than they are long. As such they have an invisible deep part. The risk of severe damage relates to the anatomical site of the injury, but particular areas of concern are

- the chest – back or front (→ pp. 63, 75, 80)
- the neck (→ p. 63)
- the abdomen (→ p. 82)
- near joints
- near large limb vessels.

> The presence of distal pulses does not exclude vascular damage. Swelling is always worrying.

XR The vast majority of patients with stab wounds to the trunk will require trauma CT imaging. If X-ray of a limb is taken following a stab wound, air in a joint space should alert the clinician to synovial penetration.

Tx Stab wounds must be assessed by an experienced doctor. The majority of stab wounds should be admitted under specialist teams for formal exploration and closure. Uncomplicated injuries are best treated by cleaning and simple dressing; immediate closure tends to trap any haematoma that forms. All patients with this type of injury should be either admitted for observation or reviewed on the following day.

Legal aspects of stab wounds → Chapter 20.

Gunshot wounds

Gunshot wounds have a twofold potential for damage:

1 Direct injury to structures along the track
2 Damage to neighbouring structures from dissipated kinetic energy. This depends on the type of weapon involved. High-velocity weapons fire bullets that transfer a large amount of energy to the surrounding tissues. Damage is greatest to solid organs in closed spaces. Bone splinters may cause secondary damage. Vascular injury can be overt and extensive or confined to the endothelium (with intact pulses); delayed thrombosis may result.

XR As for stab wounds above.
Tx All patients with gunshot wounds require:

- resuscitation (*Major trauma → Chapter 2*)
- admission and observation
- trauma CT imaging if the wound involves trunk, head or neck.

Most need surgical exploration of the bullet track to remove necrotic tissue and clothing fragments.

Legal aspects of gunshot wounds → Chapter 20.

Animal bites in the British Isles

Bite wounds account for up to 2% of all attendances at an ED. Dog bites are the most common mammalian bites and bites from humans and other primates are usually the worst.

Tx Bite wounds are typically a combination of puncture wounds, laceration and in some cases considerable crush injury and contusion. They are at risk of infection and the key to avoiding this is extremely thorough wound cleaning, including consideration of and removal of any foreign material (e.g. teeth). In large or deep bite wounds, or those in special areas (face, genitalia, hands), this is probably best done by specialist teams under general anaesthesia. Classical dogma dictated avoidance of primary closure of dog bites; however, more recent evidence indicates that they can be safely sutured at presentation. This is especially important in cosmetically sensitive areas. There is no benefit to delayed closure and 'loose closure' should be avoided.

Most dog bites do not need antibiotics at first presentation unless there is considerable tissue damage, a high risk area is involved (hands, feet, face and genitals), or the patient is particularly vulnerable to infection (e.g. immunocompromise, diabetes). Patients with cat bites, human bites or deep puncture wounds should be given a short course of co-amoxiclav (or doxycycline and metronidazole if allergic to penicillins) to protect against anaerobic infections. All patients must be covered against tetanus infection (→ *p. 415*). Cat bites carry a small risk of a painful, fulminating cellulitis due to deep inoculation with *Pasteurella multicida.*

Human bites may carry a risk of hepatitis B transmission. *For prophylaxis against blood-borne viruses → p. 422.*

'Fight bites'→ Chapter 9 p. 133.
Envenoming (especially adder bites) → p. 299.
Rabies → p. 265.

Insect and spider bites in the British Isles

The horsefly (*Haematopota pluvialis*) is also known as the cleg fly and has a very painful bite for a small creature. The female flies use their sharp mandibles to rip a triangular hole in the skin of humans and other mammals and then suck up the blood that oozes out of the wound. These insects easily spread bacteria from host to host and so a bite of this type may often become cellulitic → *p. 423.* **The Blandford fly** (*Simulium posticatum)* is a species of black fly. It is small and dark and is usually found near water, mostly in the south of England. Unlike other biting flies, Blandford flies will crawl through clothing and often bite in the middle of the day rather than the evening. The females use their jagged mouths to bite through skin and then feed on blood, just before mating. Allergic reactions can occur and, if the bites are contaminated with bacteria, then local infection is possible.
The false black widow spider (*Steatoda nobilis*) is the most venomous of the 12 biting spiders found in the British Isles. It arrived in Britain 200 years ago and is closely related to the true black widow spider. It is mostly found in the south of England and only the female spiders bite. Enough poison is delivered by a single envenoming to cause severe pain and inflammation. Victims describe a burning sensation that spreads out from the bite and also flu-like symptoms lasting for up to 3 days. This is thought to be a mild form of neurotoxic araneism (spider poisoning). Antihistamines provide some relief of symptoms.

Stings in the British Isles

Wasp and bee stings: the stings from almost all arthropods of the *Hymenoptera* cause local pain, redness and swelling but rarely result in severe problems. Exceptions are anaphylactic reactions and intraoral swellings, both of which need appropriate treatment (→ *pp. 166 and 306*). (It is said that up to 0.5% of the population is hypersensitive to either bee or wasp venom.) Unlike wasps, bees leave their stings imbedded in the skin, and these should be removed with splinter forceps. The acid bee venom may then be neutralised by the application of bicarbonate, while vinegar may help to soothe the caustic wasp sting. The inflammation from all stings can be treated with local applications of calamine lotion, antihistamine cream or hydrocortisone 1% cream.

Caterpillar stings: the brown tail moth (*Euproctis chrysorrhoea*) is common throughout central and southern Europe, including the south of England, and is found in all types of habitat. The hairs of its caterpillars may cause an extremely painful rash if touched. (This ordinary-looking caterpillar is brownish grey with red spots along its back and is not particularly hairy.) Hydrocortisone cream may ease the pain. The oak processionary moth (*Thaumetopoea processionea*) has a similar distribution to the brown tail moth but the toxin on its insignificant-looking brown caterpillars is irritant to the skin, eyes and bronchi of humans and animals. These moths are considered to be a significant human health problem when populations reach outbreak proportions, such as those in The Netherlands and Belgium in recent years.

Weever fish stings: the lesser weever fish (*Trachinus vipera*) is found in shallow sandy water around the shores of the British Isles; the greater weever fish (*Trachinus draco*) is caught by anglers in deeper water. The dorsal and gill cover spines of both fish may give a very painful sting. The venom can be denatured by immersing the injured part in very hot (but not >45°C) water.

Jellyfish stings: the Portuguese man-of-war jellyfish (*Physalia physalis*) has friable and venomous tentacles, as do several other jellyfish found in British waters. Adherent tentacles should be removed with forceps and then a strong solution of sodium bicarbonate applied to the injured area. The stings from other British species of jellyfish, e.g. the lion's mane jellyfish (*Cyanea capillata*), are also treated with alkaline solutions unlike tropical species (such as the box jellyfish [*Chironex fleckeri*] of Australasia) for which vinegar is an essential first-aid remedy.

Bites and stings from exotic creatures

Exotic pets may inflict exotic bites and stings on their keepers. In addition, world travellers may encounter poisonous insects, spiders, snakes, fish, corals, hydroids, anemones, jellyfish and octopi. Bat bites carry a risk of rabies (including in the UK) → *p. 265*.

T͟x͟ All such wounds must be cleaned thoroughly and then dressed. Tetanus prophylaxis must be ensured. It may occasionally be necessary to give antivenom, and it is important that each ED knows where the nearest supply is kept (the *British National Formulary* contains up-to-date telephone numbers of regional depots). In the UK, 24-hour help and advice can be obtained from the following centres:

1 The Liverpool School of Tropical Medicine
2 The Hospital for Tropical Diseases in London.

In the case of travellers, expert local advice is essential for both diagnosis and treatment.

Envenoming (especially adder bites) → p. 299.
Non-venomous injuries from the spines of sea urchins and other marine creatures → p. 421.
Rabies → p. 265.

Cutaneous myiasis

Myiasis is rare in the UK. Travellers (and military personnel) from tropical regions may present with large red boils which may have a central aperture through which a living creature is visible. The human bot fly (*Dermatobia hominis*) is found in Latin America, and the tumbu fly (*Cordylobia anthropophaga*) is resident in Africa, Arabia and southern Europe. Tumbu maggots may be partially asphyxiated by the application of petroleum jelly and then squeezed out of their home. Bot fly larvae are more resistant but will usually crawl out of the central punctum of the burrow if 2% lidocaine is injected around and into the swelling (the lidocaine seems to reduce the maggots' ability to grip the sides of their burrows → *Figure 21.1*). No other treatment is required unless there is significant surrounding infection.

Pretibial lacerations

Pretibial lacerations are common in elderly patients and often follow comparatively minor trauma. The area has a poor blood supply and little deep tissue to support the skin. Despite this, most pretibial wounds heal well, albeit slowly. More problems can be anticipated with:

- distally based flaps
- very contused flaps
- very elderly patients
- patients with very thin skin or those on steroids.

T͟x͟ Most pretibial lacerations should not be sutured – the stitches tear the thin skin. Adhesive strips are ideal but must not be applied until the wound has been adequately

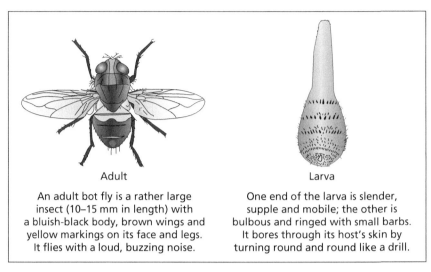

Adult	Larva
An adult bot fly is a rather large insect (10–15 mm in length) with a bluish-black body, brown wings and yellow markings on its face and legs. It flies with a loud, buzzing noise.	One end of the larva is slender, supple and mobile; the other is bulbous and ringed with small barbs. It bores through its host's skin by turning round and round like a drill.

Figure 21.1 The human bot fly and its larva.

cleaned, usually under local anaesthesia. Tension should be avoided when laying back the skin. Blood clots must be removed and the flap laid closely on to a clean bed. A secure non-adherent pressure dressing can then be applied.

The patient should be encouraged to continue ankle movements but to elevate the foot when at rest. Initial follow-up should be arranged for a couple of days post-injury and then as appropriate. Admission for bed rest may be required for frail patients with extensive wounds. In extreme cases, plastic surgical advice may be needed.

Pretibial haematomas

After injury, patients may present with a large tender, pretibial haematoma. This carries the risk of skin necrosis due to vascular compromise of the overlying skin.

Tx A large haematoma should be evacuated via an incision. Needle aspiration is unlikely to succeed. The mode of anaesthesia for the procedure depends on the patient and the size of the haematoma. Local infiltration, regional block, or Entonox will be suitable in many patients; however, some may require general anaesthesia. A yankauer suction catheter can be used to evacuate the haematoma via the laceration or a small incision, before application of adhesive strips and a pressure dressing.

Puncture wounds of the feet

Puncture wounds of the feet are common and often caused by nails, needles and glass. There is usually a tender but unremarkable wound on the sole.

XR Radiographs are indicated for any suspicion of foreign body and with all glass wounds. A retained fragment is common with wounds from a needle and with glass but not when a nail is involved. A skin marker, applied to the skin at the site of entry, will greatly help with localisation on a radiograph.

> Retained foreign bodies can be very difficult to locate, even if they appear superficial on a radiograph.

Tx The wound must be cleaned, an antiseptic dressing applied and anti-tetanus prophylaxis given if indicated. The patient should be instructed to return if there are any signs of infection.

Foreign bodies must be removed in a suitable environment – usually an operating theatre – by an experienced doctor working in good conditions (fine instruments, a bloodless field and adequate anaesthesia).
    Patients returning with obvious infection must be seen by a senior member staff. In antibiotics, further consideration of the possibility of foreign bodies and follow-up are indicated. Infections in puncture wounds can be very difficult to treat. Exploration of the track and IV antibiotics may be required in some cases.

> *Pseudomonas* sp. likes to live in the damp environment of training shoes and similar footwear.

Nails through hands or feet

It is quite common for a patient to present with a nail protruding from a finger or a foot. The patient should be asked if the nail is from a nail gun. The nail fired from this tool has two copper barbs on it, which impede withdrawal. Sensation must be assessed before local anaesthesia is administered and then movements assessed after the nail is removed.

Xʀ Initial radiographs can be helpful if there is difficulty removing the nail. Otherwise, they should be obtained after removal to look for bony damage.

Tx The nail should be removed under local anaesthesia and the wound protected with an antiseptic dressing. If there is bony damage, antibiotic cover is indicated (flucloxacillin or clarithromycin).

Foreign bodies in the feet or hands

The removal of a foreign body from the palm of the hand or the sole of the foot can be particularly difficult despite often appearing straightforward. It may require:

- a bloodless field and hence a tourniquet
- good anaesthesia, usually general
- skill and experience
- adequate equipment – a metal detector may be helpful.

Management should be discussed with a senior colleague; inpatient care may be required. Some foreign bodies can be removed in the ED. These will be:

- superficial
- easily palpable
- recently implanted
- discussed with a senior member of staff.

Other foreign bodies

Other foreign bodies (e.g. airgun pellets) need localisation and then a similar consideration given to the mode of removal.

Sea urchin spines

Patients may present with sea urchin spines embedded in their hands or feet, usually acquired while swimming in the Mediterranean Sea. The dark-brown spines are very friable and so are difficult to remove intact – they may result in local irritation, infection and granuloma formation. Softening the skin with either acetone or salicylic acid 2% ointment, applied overnight, may facilitate the process. Analgesia can be achieved with local anaesthetic cream before attempting to remove the larger pieces with a hypodermic needle. Smaller pieces may be scrubbed out with a toothbrush. Fortunately, with appropriate dressings and analgesia, the injury settles down very quickly.

Other spine-bearing marine creatures including stingrays, scorpion fish, stonefish, weever fish, catfish and crown-of-thorns starfish may inflict painful puncture wounds on the unwary. The pain is usually very marked in the case of venomous species. Expert local advice is essential for both diagnosis and treatment.

Envenoming → p. 299.
Stings from weever fish spines → p. 419.

Fish hooks

Fish hooks can be removed under local anaesthesia (ring block or infiltration of lidocaine). The barbed end of the hook should be pushed forwards through the anaesthetised skin and the hook cut in two with K-wire cutters. It can then be withdrawn easily.

Splinters under the nail

Splinters under the nail should be removed under ring block. Attempts may be made with splinter forceps initially, but it is often necessary to trim back or remove the nail. Thorns can cause serious infections including tetanus and must be removed.

Subungual collections

Subungual haematomas can be drained by trephining (→ p. 139). This procedure does not introduce infection and thus antibiotics are not required for an associated fracture. Collections of pus under the nail may require removal of the nail under a ring block.

Hair tourniquets around the digits

An infant is sometimes found to have a tight ring of hairs (usually an adult's long thick hairs) wrapped around the base of a finger or toe (this can be the reason for a crying or otherwise distressed child). The hair tourniquet has often eroded deeply into the skin, but distal ischaemia is rare. The constricting band of hair must be removed. Hair removal cream is effective for this purpose where skin is not broken, otherwise divide the hair carefully with a stitch cutter, ensuring that no residual hair rings remain buried in the circumferential wound.

Injection injuries to the digits

EpiPen adrenaline injection injuries → p. 133.
High-pressure hose injection injuries → p. 133.
Oil-based veterinary vaccine injection injuries → p. 133.

Blood and body fluid exposure incidents ('needlestick injuries')

Post-exposure prophylaxis after sexual exposure or needlestick injury (to blood-borne viruses) (PEP) → p. 332.

Both hospital staff and members of the public may present after a needlestick injury or other body fluid exposure incident. Hepatitis B, hepatitis C and HIV are the major blood-borne viruses (BBVs), but several other pathogens may also be transmitted by this route. Exposure incidents include the following:

- Piercing of the skin by any contaminated sharp objects
- Splashes into the eyes with body fluids
- Contamination of broken skin by body fluids
- Significant human bites
- Sexual contact.
- Ingestion by the mouth of body fluids.

An assessment of risk must be made. → p. 332. The UK prevalence of hepatitis C amongst people who inject (or have previously injected) drugs has fallen over recent years and is currently estimated at around 17%. The prevalence of HIV in the same population is much lower at between 0.5% and 1.2%.

Tx Skin exposures should be washed with soap and water. HIV cannot be transmitted through intact skin. Small wounds and punctures may be cleaned with an antiseptic such as alcohol hand hygiene solution which is viricidal to HIV and hepatitis B and C. Eyes or mucosal splashes should be copiously irrigated with water. Wounds must be cleaned and dressed and prophylaxis against tetanus ensured. The general risks from BBVs and the risk from this particular incident should be discussed with the patient.

The patient's GP and/or occupational health department must be notified of the type and date of the injury, the action taken and any further action or follow-up required.

Hepatitis B immunisation → Box 17.4 on p. 332

LOCALISED INFECTIONS AND INFLAMMATIONS

Hot red joints

Patients may present to an ED with a single acutely inflamed joint. This may be caused by:

- septic arthritis including gonococcal arthritis
- crystal arthropathy (e.g. gout or pseudogout → p. 423)
- a bursitis in the area of the joint (→ pp. 102 and 114)
- a connective tissue disorder (rarely).

Septic arthritis

Risk factors for septic arthritis include

- Prosthetic joint
- Underlying joint disease (i.e. rheumatoid arthritis, osteoarthritis)
- Age >80 years
- Immunosuppression
- People who inject drugs
- Local soft tissue infection or ulceration
- Other systemic infections (haematogenous spread)
- Recent joint surgery or previous corticosteroid joint injection

The most common joints to become infected is the knee, but any joint can be affected. The joint is held in position of maximum joint volume (e.g. knee in extension, hip flexed and externally rotated), and all movements are typically restricted by intense pain. Up to 20% of cases are polyarticular – do not rule out the diagnosis if more than one joint is affected. Many patients (about 40%) will be apyrexial.

XR Loss of joint space may be seen in septic arthritis; however, X-rays are often normal.

Tx If there is doubt, then the patient should be assumed to have a septic arthritis until proved otherwise. Diagnostic joint aspiration should be undertaken, with synovial fluid culture and microscopy, to confirm or refute the diagnosis. Hip aspiration will usually require ultrasound-guided joint aspiration. Do not aspirate a prosthetic joint – refer patients promptly to the orthopaedic team for assessment.

Intravenous antibiotics should be commenced after joint aspiration, and blood tests are taken (unless this causes unreasonable delay). Refer to the orthopaedic team for admission and management.

Acute gout

The first metatarsophalangeal joint is the most common site for acute gout although the knee may sometimes be primarily affected. The patient presents with severe local pain and a red, swollen joint. There is extreme tenderness such that even the weight of the bedclothes can be unbearable. A pyrexia may accompany the inflammation. Other causes of a painful joint must be excluded. A serum urate is of no utility in the acute phase, having neither the sensitivity nor specificity to confirm or refute the diagnosis. Serum urate often falls during an acute attack and a normal urate level cannot rule out the diagnosis.

Tx A wool and crepe bandage may be useful to protect the joint, together with non-weight-bearing crutches. The inflamed area should be rested and elevated. A makeshift 'cage' to protect a painful foot at night can be made by cutting a hole out of a large cardboard box. Initial analgesia and anti-inflammatory activity are provided by nonsteroidal anti-inflammatory drugs (NSAIDs). In severe cases, an additional short course of oral steroids (prednisolone 30–40 mg a day) gives fast and effective relief.

The patient should be referred back to the GP with a view to exclusion of precipitating causes and consideration of preventative therapy with allopurinol (after 4–6 weeks). Allopurinol should not be commenced during an acute attack but should be continued if already on treatment.

Osteomyelitis

This diagnosis should always be considered when there is spontaneous or unresolving bony pain. In adults, osteomyelitis most commonly affects the vertebrae, whereas in children long bones are more commonly infected. In ED patients, the distal phalanges of the hands and the feet are common sites of osteomyelitis due to the incidence of local trauma. Infection may occur by either local contiguous or haematogenous spread. There may be a history of a minor injury or local infection, but then pain, swelling and redness persist beyond the expected time of resolution. There may be an associated septic arthritis. Following haematogenous spread, symptoms may be insidious – consider osteomyelitis in patients with back pain accompanied with systemic symptoms. The inflammatory process can be relatively acute or more chronic. The major risk factor for developing osteomyelitis is an immunosuppressive state (such as diabetes mellitus, chronic steroid use or alcohol excess), and the most commonly isolated pathogen is *Staphylococcus aureus.*

> Bone tumours may masquerade as bone or joint infection.

XR Plain radiographs are usually the initial mode of imaging if osteomyelitis is suspected; however, early in the infective process radiographs are often normal. After 10–14 days, radiographs show absorption of the underlying bone, giving a characteristic moth-eaten appearance. However, almost 50% of the bone structure must be destroyed before there is detectable radiological lucency. Elevation of the overlying periosteum may also be seen. The neighbouring joint space may be lost if infection has spread to the joint.

Tx Patients with suspected osteomyelitis must be referred to the orthopaedic department. Treatment consists of IV antibiotics and surgical debridement.

Cellulitis

Infection of the skin may arise around a wound or without any obvious port of entry. The patient is usually tired and anorexic with a raised temperature; slight nausea is common. The skin is red, swollen and hot, but the degree of pain is variable. A cause should be sought but is usually not found.

Tx Symptomatic treatment and antibiotics should be prescribed. The infection may be streptococcal or staphylococcal, and initial treatment is usually with flucloxacillin. Clarithromycin can be given to patients who are allergic to penicillins. Admission for observation and IV therapy may be required for extensive or progressing infections, or for those with significant systemic upset. Less severe cases can be treated with oral antibiotics at home but should be reviewed within 24–48 hours. The limits of the infection should be marked on the skin with a pen so that changes are obvious at review. Patients should be advised to rest and elevate the affected area.

> Lower limb cellulitis is almost invariably unilateral. Patients with bilateral erythematous skin changes to the legs are rarely suffering from cellulitis. Consider acute lipodematosclerosis, lymphoedema, chronic venous eczema and vasculitis.

Athlete's foot: is a fungal infection, which gives rise to an itchy whitish area between the toes. It may be the cause of an ascending cellulitis and should always be excluded whenever there is cellulitic infection of the lower leg. Athlete's foot is treated with a topical antifungal cream such as clotrimazole.

Erysipelas

Erysipelas is a type of skin infection that is caused by group A β-haemolytic streptococci (*Streptococcus pyogenes*). It was formerly known as St Anthony's fire. It differs from cellulitis in several ways:

- The affected skin is fiery-red, swollen, hot, tender and indurated.
- The affected area has raised edges and a sharply demarcated border. Vesicles, bullae and petechiae may occasionally occur.
- There is regional lymphadenopathy and, sometimes, lymphangitis.
- Fever and systemic upset are common (rigors, headaches, nausea and muscle pains). These symptoms may be prodromal.
- It involves the dermis rather than deeper subcutaneous tissues.
- It is caused by streptococci rather than by staphylococci.

Erysipelas targets the face (20%) and the legs (70%), usually in older adults. Immunodeficiency or general ill health predisposes an individual to the condition. Erysipelas is treated with phenoxymethylpenicillin, clarithromycin or clindamycin. The infection recurs in around 25% of patients.

Impetigo

A localised staphylococcal infection of the skin may cause an area of weeping inflammation with a yellow crust. This is impetigo and is a highly infectious condition. It is most commonly seen in children, usually in the peri-oral region but may spread to other parts of the patient or to relatives and medical staff.

Tx All patients should be advised of measures to contain the spread by:

- frequent and appropriate hand washing
- avoidance of contact with the infected area
- using own towel and cutlery, etc.

An anti-staphylococcal cream should be prescribed (e.g. mupirocin or fusidic acid). Severe cases or those with systemic upset will need oral flucloxacillin.

Herpes simplex infections

Herpes simplex may cause painful yellow blisters with surrounding inflammation on the fingers or face. There is often accompanying malaise, pyrexia and enlargement of related lymph nodes. Herpetic whitlow of the finger may be mistaken for paronychia but should not be incised to avoid the spread of infection. → *Paronychia p. 426.* Antiviral treatment may be useful for patients presenting within 48–72 hours of development of lesions.

Primary herpetic gingivostomatitis in children may be highly painful and distressing. Symptoms such as painful swallowing may necessitate admission. Treatment with aciclovir is recommended within 72 hours of symptom onset. Use of benzydamine muscosal spray provides symptomatic relief.

Large abscesses

A great variety of large abscesses is inevitably seen in patients presenting to an ED. Among the most common types are found in the following areas:

- Axillary – often loculated and may be recurrent
- Breast → *p. 335*
- Perianal → *p. 324*
- Pilonidal → *p. 324*
- Gluteal → *p. 324*
- Labial → *p. 335.*

These painful and distressing conditions should be treated under general anaesthesia in the privacy of an operating theatre. Recurrent abscesses of the groin, perineum and axilla may be a result of hidradenitis suppurativa – a condition of unknown aetiology that leads to blockage and infection of apocrine sweat glands. There may be local fistulae and skin tags. The problem is treated by excision of all the surrounding hair-bearing skin and its related apocrine glands.

Boils (furuncles)

A boil is an abscess arising from a hair follicle. The problem may be multiple or recurrent.

Tx Small abscesses in appropriate sites in adults may be drained in the ED under local anaesthesia. Others need inpatient care.

Most abscesses should be drained with an incision along the lines of cleavage of the skin. In the limbs, a longitudinal incision is more appropriate to avoid damage to nerves, vessels and tendons. Achieving adequate local anaesthesia may be difficult. Local anaesthesia can be injected into the roof of the abscess and in a ring around the collection. Take care not to exceed the maximum local anaesthetic dose as a surprising amount of lidocaine may be needed to achieve adequate anaesthesia for this procedure. The cavity can then be opened with a longitudinal incision and pus evacuated, followed by irrigation with a syringe of saline. Packing is no longer considered essential for small and superficial abscesses. A dressing should be applied over the whole area.

The patient will require oral analgesics to take home. The wound should be reviewed on the following day and the dressing changed.

Infected sebaceous cysts

Sebaceous cysts may become infected and painful. The resulting tender, red lump may be distinguished from a boil by:

- the history of a pre-existing swelling
- the site (cysts are common in certain areas such as the back and the neck)
- the presence of a central punctum (only sometimes visible)
- the contents of the swelling (white, cheesy material).

Tx In the early stages of infection, the inflamed cyst may respond to antibiotics. However, incision and drainage are often necessary and management is then identical to that detailed above for a boil. Sometimes an infected sebaceous cyst will disappear after discharging its contents but often the wall will need surgical removal at a later date.

Panton-Valentine-Leucocidin associated staphylococcal infection

Panton-valentine-leucocidin (PVL) is a toxin that destroys white blood cells and is associated with increased virulence of staphylococcal infections. Clusters may occur in close contact settings, e.g. military barracks, gyms and prisons. Consider the diagnosis in patients with recurrent soft tissue infections, necrotising soft tissue infections, or where a cluster of infections occurs in a close contact setting. PVL staphylococcal infection can cause invasive infections, in particular a haemorrhagic pneumonia with high mortality.

Initial management is as for other skin and soft tissue infections. Testing for PVL staphylococcus requires a specific assay, and so it is essential to inform the laboratory of the concern when sending microbiological samples.

Kerion

A kerion is a large fluctuant abscess to the scalp as a result of an immune response to a dermatophyte fungal infection (tinea capitis). It may cause hair loss in the overlying area. Kerion should be treated with oral antifungal agents for 6–8 weeks (e.g. terbinafine, itraconazole).

Skin lesions acquired from animals (zoonoses)

Orf begins as painless vesicles, which progress to red nodules with sunken centres containing pus. The lesions then gradually discolour, crust and heal. No specific treatment is required. The causative virus is acquired from sheep and goats.

Cutaneous anthrax starts as a small vesicle, which becomes purulent. A painless skin lesion then develops at the site with a black eschar and a considerable amount of surrounding oedema and induration. Anthrax can be an occupational disease of people who work with large herbivorous mammals or their hide products but has also been spread by terrorist action. If inhaled, the spores of *Bacillus anthracis* cause a haemorrhagic pneumonia and septicaemia. Anthrax is a notifiable disease.

Systemic anthrax → p. 269.

> Anthrax should be considered as a possibility in IV drug users with severe soft-tissue infections or other sepsis including meningitis.

Tularaemia presents as pyrexia and indurated skin ulcers with lymphadenopathy. It is transmitted to humans by close contact with rabbits. Tularaemia is not endemic in the UK, but occurs in Scandinavia, eastern Europe and the USA. If inhaled, *Francisella tularensis* may cause plague-like pneumonia.

Monkeypox → *p. 268.*

Other skin lesions

Patients with an enormous variety of other skin lesions may present to an ED over the years. Their detailed description is beyond the scope of this book. However, the following lesions cause confusion more often than most:

- **Erythema nodosum:** the characteristic fiery-red, infiltrated lesions of erythema nodosum are seen on the knees, shins and forearms. They are very tender with an ill-defined border. Bruising may occur. Erythema nodosum is sometimes mistaken for an allergic reaction; larger patches may look like cellulitis. The condition is a reactive vasculitis to systemic diseases, infections and drugs. A recent streptococcal illness is by far the most common precipitant.
- **Acute guttate psoriasis:** this is most common in children and adolescents. A shower of small, round, erythematous papules appears 1–3 weeks after an

infection (usually streptococcal in nature). It is thought that streptococcal superantigens may resemble an antigen on keratinocytes. Crops of papules appear over about 2 weeks and soon develop characteristic psoriatic scaling. The lesions are most prominent on the trunk but may also affect the scalp, face and limbs. The rash settles slowly over several weeks and is often mistaken for a reaction to antibiotics.

- **Pityriasis rosea:** this self-limiting benign illness occurs in clusters in spring and autumn and is most common in women aged 15–40 years. A primary plaque (the 'herald' patch) first appears, usually under the costal margin. It is oval shaped, 1–2 cm in diameter and salmon coloured with a dark-red periphery. The two areas are separated by a fine, scaly ring. This primary lesion is sometimes accompanied by vague prodromal symptoms and is followed after 3–21 days by a distinctive rash that appears in crops following the lines of cleavage of the skin. The secondary lesions are smaller than the herald patch but similar in appearance. They are distributed symmetrically on the truck, neck and proximal limbs and last for between 2 and 6 weeks. There is a variable amount of pruritis. Despite the clustering of contacts, no causative agent has ever been identified. No treatment is required other than reassurance.
- **Lichen planus:** this dermatosis of uncertain aetiology is encountered far more frequently in MRCP examinations than in reality. Shiny pink papules appear on the wrists, shins and lumbosacral area, often with involvement of the mucous membranes. Itching is a variable feature. The rash can look non-specific with an atypical distribution and so often gives rise to confusion. Treatment is aimed at controlling the itching with steroid creams and calamine lotion.
- **Juvenile spring eruption and polymorphic light eruption** is a fairly common rash caused by a delayed hypersensitivity response to UV light. The rash is polymorphous and typically appears a few hours after UV exposure. Juvenile spring eruption is a localised reaction of a similar aetiology typically affecting the exposed helices of the ears. Small itchy erythematous papules may blister and crust before healing. Treatment involves avoidance of sun exposure and topical corticosteroids.

Common rashes of childhood → p. 360.

Paronychial infections

Infections around the nailfolds of the fingers are a common cause of presentation to an ED. Following initial inflammation, a pus-filled collection gathers in the potential space under the nailfold (→ *Figure 21.2*). As this enlarges, it becomes evident.

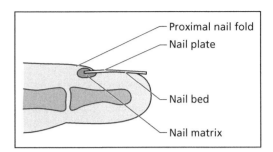

Figure 21.2 Anatomy of the eponychium.

Tx Antibiotics are ineffective once an abscess has formed. Soaking the digit, with gentle blunt retraction of the nailfold often results in the abscess discharging. If drainage is required, the aim is to lift the eponychium/nailfold by blunt dissection and avoid incision. A blunt needle or splinter forceps should be inserted under the nailfold longitudinally to release the pus → *Figure 21.3*. For larger collections, consider inserting a wick (small piece of gauze) to facilitate ongoing drainage. Ring block may be used but is usually not required.

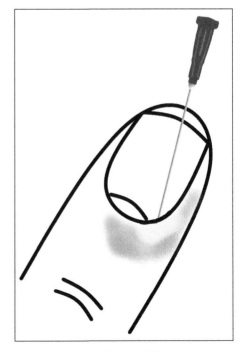

Figure 21.3 Drainage of paronychia.

Felon

A subcutaneous abscess of the finger pulp is often caused by minor trauma such as splinters or fingerprick glucose monitoring. Tight fibrous septae from the periosteum of the distal phalanx to the epidermis prevent the expansion of the tissue space and so the infected finger pulp becomes tense and very painful. Erythema and swelling do not extend proximal to the distal interphalangeal joint – proximal extension suggests flexor tendon sheath infection. Early felon may be treated with oral antibiotics, however, most will require incision and drainage, usually by a hand surgeon.

Ingrowing toenails

This paronychial infection of the big toe commonly presents to an ED. The area alongside the distal toenail is red and tender. There may be a yellow exudate and, in chronic cases, tissue granulation.

Tx Local policy varies according to the availability of chiropody services. A chiropodist will usually perform a wedge resection of the side of the nail and give advice on foot care. Recurrent cases should have the germinal matrix of the nail destroyed with phenol.

In the absence of a chiropodist, severe infection may be treated by removal of the entire nail under ring block. The patient then requires an antiseptic dressing, crutches and analgesia. They must be told to rest and elevate the foot. The dressing should be changed on the following day.

Frostbite

Cold injury is most likely to affect peripheral exposed parts such as fingers and toes and is not only seen in extreme climates. The frostbitten area is initially pale and extremely painful but, if exposure continues, the pain subsides. On re-warming, there is erythema, oedema and blistering and eventually a line of demarcation will appear at the junction with the undamaged tissue.

Tx Analgesia should be given (together with IV fluids if more than fingers or toes are involved). Rapid rewarming of acute cases is achieved by total immersion of the affected part in warm water. The degree of permanent damage cannot be assessed when first seen and so admission for observation may be indicated.

Trench foot

This is a similar condition where tissue damage and maceration result from prolonged contact with cold, wet, muddy footwear. Treatment follows the same principles.

Wanderer's foot

No discussion of foot problems in a textbook of emergency medicine would be complete without a mention of this condition. The patient presents with macerated soles of the feet that are causing pain while walking. The shoes and socks are usually in poor condition and extremely smelly. There may be a history of homelessness and prolonged walking.

Tx The feet should be washed and then soaked in antiseptic. Blisters should be deroofed and dressed, and any obvious infection treated. Crutches may be needed. Definitive treatment necessitates a place to stay so as to rest and bathe. New footwear may be required.

Homelessness → p. 12.

Scabies

Infestation by the scabies mite causes intense itching, which is worse at night. Other close contacts may be affected.

At first, the mites affect only the areas where they burrow – between the fingers, wrists, genitalia, buttocks, axillae, waistline and the soles of the feet in children. Small linear tracks of papules may be the only evidence. Later, a sensitivity reaction to the mite causes a widespread papular eruption.

Tx Malathion 0.5% aqueous lotion is applied to all areas of the body including the head and the face. It is left to dry naturally and then washed off after 24 hours. Only one application is necessary provided that all areas are covered (e.g. the web spaces and under the fingernails). This will eradicate scabies in around 75% of cases. For those with persistent symptoms, a second application after 1 week is recommended. Permethrin 5% cream is a more expensive – and possibly more effective – alternative. It is applied to the whole body, washed off after 8–12 hours and then reapplied after a week. The whole family and any close contacts must be treated, whether or not they have a rash; the GP should be asked to coordinate this. An oral sedative antihistamine may be required at night to control the itching.

22

Ophthalmic, ENT and facial conditions

Amy Nickson

Emergency Medicine Consultant, Royal Bolton Hospital, Bolton, UK
Sexual Offences Examiner, Lancashire SAFE Centre, Preston, UK

THE EYES

Assessment of the eye

- Obtain an accurate history.
- Ask about vision and test the visual acuity (→ *Box 22.1*).
- Examine the eye with a light source looking for redness, discharge and other gross abnormalities. Look also for asymmetry and irregularity of the pupils.
- Note the pupillary response to direct light and test the afferent pupillary response. When the damaged eye is illuminated, absence of pupil constriction in the opposite eye indicates an interruption of the visual pathway.
- Assess ocular movements, visual fields and eyelid movements.
- Check for exophthalmos (proptosis) and enophthalmos

In the presence of blepharospasm (inability to open the eyes), further examination may require the application of local anaesthetic eyedrops, e.g. tetracaine (amethocaine) 1% or oxybuprocaine 0.4%.

- Evert the eyelids to allow examination of the fornices.
- Instil orange-coloured fluorescein drops to highlight any corneal damage – the injured epithelium appears bright green under cobalt blue light
- Examine the eye systematically from front to back using a slit lamp and an ophthalmoscope. This may sometimes necessitate the administration of a short-acting mydriatic (a drug that dilates the pupil) such as tropicamide.

The anterior chamber may contain blood, which collects inferiorly in the erect patient to produce a fluid level called a hyphaema (→ *Figure 22.1*). A white exudate containing inflammatory cells in the anterior chamber is called a hypopyon.

Damage to the lens or pupillary muscle will result in irregularities in the shape of the iris and disorganised or absent constriction to light. A laceration through the cornea will allow aqueous humour, muscle and even part of the lens to herniate anteriorly. Vitreous humour may be opacified by bleeding and the fundus thereby totally obscured.

> Whenever local anaesthetic has been applied to the conjunctival sac in the ED, it is advisable to pad the eye for protection for a few hours.

Additional information can be obtained by asking the patient to look at the chart through a pinhole. This improves vision in patients with a refractive or corneal abnormality but worsens vision in those with macular problems.

Corneal abrasions

Corneal abrasions may result from a scratch or other injury to the eye. Sometimes they follow prolonged rubbing of an irritated eye:

- The eye is red, injected (enlarged conjunctival blood vessels), painful and watering.

The RCEM Lecture Notes: Emergency Medicine, Fifth Edition. Edited by Catherine Williams and Amy Nickson.
© 2024 John Wiley & Sons Ltd. Published 2024 by John Wiley & Sons Ltd.
Companion website: www.wiley.com/go/LNEM5

Box 22.1 **How to test visual acuity**

Test each eye separately with patient wearing normal spectacles.

Acuity equation = Distance from eye to print in metres / Number adjacent to smallest line of print readable on chart

- Snellen letter chart is 6 m in front of patient (or equivalent distance using a mirror)
- Largest print on top line is usually 60
- Smallest print on bottom line is usually 5
- A patient with normal acuity can read down to line 6 and has '6/6' vision
- With excellent acuity this may be '6/5' vision
- A patient who cannot read the top line has vision 'worse than 6/60'
- If the test is repeated at 3 m and the top line can now be read, vision is '3/60'
- If the patient is unable to read letters from any distance, then assess if fingers can be counted or if light can be perceived.

Box 22.2 **Padding an eye**

- A single pad will not keep an eye closed
- To apply a double pad, fold one pad in half and place it over the closed eyelids. Place a second, flat pad over the first and secure it in place with three pieces of tape
- The patient must be advised not to drive. Monocular vision impairs judgement of speed and distance.
- If both eyes require pads, leave this until the patient is at home
- All patients require spare pads and tape to take away

- Antibiotic ointment (e.g. chloramphenicol 1%) three times a day for 3 days if there is a possibility of infection; however, the risk after minor trauma is low.
- Consider a drug with Gram-negative cover in contact lens wearers (e.g. levofloxacin or gentamicin)
- Consider a firm eye pad for 2 hours if topical local anaesthetic is used (→ *Box 22.2*)
- Instructions not to wear contact lenses until treatment is complete
- Instructions to return if there is not a marked improvement within 24–48 hours.

Most abrasions heal spontaneously within 2 days. Remember to check tetanus immunisation status.

Nonsteroidal anti-inflammatory drug (NSAID) drops or ointment are very effective at relieving pain but concerns regarding the complications of long-term use suggest that only short term use with follow-up should be adopted.

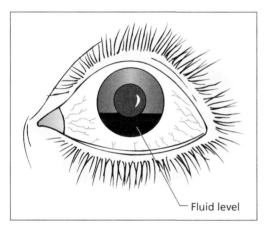

Fluid level

Figure 22.1 Hyphaema – blood in the anterior chamber of the eye.

- There is often pronounced blepharospasm.
- There may be a sensation of a foreign body.
- The abrasion should be visible on fluorescein examination.

Tx A foreign body must be excluded, especially a subtarsal one (→ *below*). The patient then requires the following:

- Ocular lubricants for symptomatic relief (available over the counter).

Subtarsal foreign body

Foreign material may lodge in the conjunctival sac. There is an anatomical trap under the upper eyelid.

- The eye is red, injected and watering.
- There is pain and blepharospasm.
- There is a marked foreign body sensation.
- There is increased discomfort on blinking (but small children may keep their eyes tightly shut for relief).
- Linear scratches to the superior cornea are extremely suggestive of a subtarsal foreign body.

Tx Evert the eyelid and remove any foreign material with a moistened cotton bud. Dramatic relief of the pain provides a good indication of foreign body removal, if the procedure can be tolerated without topical anaesthesia.

Superficial foreign bodies imbedded in the eye

Fragments may fly into the eye while working (e.g. grinding) or may be blown in by the wind:

- The patient complains of a red, painful, watering eye.
- There is marked blepharospasm.
- The eye is injected and vision may be slightly blurred.

Always consider the possibility of deeper damage with higher velocity injuries (→ *below*).

Tx Superficial fragments may be removed from the anaesthetised cornea using a cotton bud or a hypodermic needle. The resulting corneal injury should then be treated in the same way as a corneal abrasion.
Rust rings: metallic, ferrous foreign bodies produce rust rings if left in the cornea for more than a few hours. If the rust is not removed completely, the patient should be reviewed at the eye clinic after 48 hours when the softened area of damage will easily 'shell out'.

Photokeratitis

Also known as 'arc' eye, this condition occurs in a welder, skier or ultraviolet sunbather with inadequate eye protection. The condition is caused by corneal absorption of ultraviolet light. Problems usually start several hours after exposure:

- Both eyes may be affected.
- The eyes are painful, weeping and red.
- There is usually blepharospasm and a sensation of a foreign body.
- Fluorescein may reveal multiple tiny 'punctate' corneal erosions.

Tx Symptoms can be relieved by the instillation of local anaesthetic. The patient is then given topical antibiotics and advised to use cold compresses and wear sunglasses. The condition should settle within 48 hours.

Chemical splashes

Chemicals may cause inflammation of the conjunctiva or even a corneal burn. Patients present with a painful, watery, red eye. Alkalis cause more serious damage due to liquefactive necrosis.

Tx Apply a topical anaesthetic and irrigate the eye with copious amounts of saline. This is best achieved using 500-mL bags through a standard giving set or by using a purpose-built irrigator (such as a Morgan lens) until pH is 7–8 (1–2 L is often required). Fluorescein drops will help reveal the extent of the damage. Topical antibiotic and lubrication should then be prescribed. The patient should be seen by ophthalmology within 24 hours.

Haziness of the cornea and limbal ischaemia (pallor of part of the darker outer ring of the iris) convey a worse prognosis and should be referred immediately.

Management of specific chemical injuries:

Cement powder: cement reacts with moisture in the eye to form highly alkaline calcium hydroxide. Before irrigation (as above) quickly brush off any remaining dry dust whilst wearing face protection. Use a moist cotton bud to remove particles from the fornices.

'Tear gas': a group of several agents used by law enforcement, which cause irritation of eyes, skin and respiratory tract. Blow cool dry air on the patient's face to vaporise the gas and then irrigate as above. Permanent harm is very rare.

Hydrofluoric acid: HF burns are more serious than other acids due to the release of fluoride ions (→ *p. 148*). Hexafluorine is thought to be the most effective decontamination solution for ocular HF burns.

'Super Glue': If eyelids are accidentally glued together with cyanoacrylate glue, wash gently with warm water and apply a patch, the eye will open again in 1–4 days.

Penetrating injuries to the eye

Deep, foreign bodies are difficult to identify, produce greater morbidity and yet, initially, may not be as painful as superficial lesions. A good history is essential. There is a high risk of intraocular damage in patients with eye pain who have worked with:

- a hammer and chisel
- glass
- machinery that emits high-speed fragments
- high-pressure water jets.

The presence of hyphaema or prolapse of intraocular contents indicates severe injury, as does distortion of the pupil. Positive Seidel's test (a stream of fluid leaking from a wound on fluorescein exam) is specific for penetrating injury. Retained ferrous fragments can cause blindness as they are neurotoxic.

> The degree of pain that follows ocular trauma is not a reliable indicator of the severity of the injury.

XR Fluorescein-aided corneal examination is followed by radiology of the eye. Lateral views with the eye looking up and down (so that the opacity appears to move) are particularly helpful in distinguishing intraocular and extraocular foreign bodies. Accurate localisation sometimes requires CT.

Tx Immediate specialist referral is essential, but acuity should be assessed first and an eye patch applied. Do not apply any pressure on the eyeball and advise the patient to avoid coughing and straining. Check tetanus status.

Blunt trauma to the eye

Damage to the globe of the eye most commonly results from assaults and sports injuries, e.g. squash balls that are small enough to enter the eye socket. Pressure on the eyeball or coughing and straining by the patient must be avoided.

Hyphaema: blood in the anterior chamber is caused by rupture of internal blood vessels (→ *Figure 22.1*). The patient is at risk of acute (secondary) glaucoma and requires tonometry to check intra-ocular pressure (IOP). A hyphaema may occasionally be accompanied by iridodialysis – rupture of the insertion of the iris.

Traumatic mydriasis: fixed dilatation of the pupil is a relatively common observation after blunt injury. The pupil may be distorted. Mydriasis is sometimes permanent. Traumatic miosis (constriction of the pupil) may also occur.

Dislocation of the lens: this is uncommon, although trauma is the most common cause. Cataract may also occur.

Iridodialysis: Avulsion of the iris root can lead to a D shaped pupil.

Posterior segment injuries: suspected where there is a sudden reduction in visual acuity. Injuries include vitreous haemorrhage and retinal damage such as tears, haemorrhage and detachment. Choroidal rupture and even globe rupture are occasionally seen.

Retrobulbar haemorrhage: An ophthalmological emergency requiring urgent treatment. Following trauma, the features include eye pain, proptosis and progressive visual loss. It can be diagnosed on CT scan, but treatment should not be delayed if there is decreased visual acuity. Lateral canthotomy (an incision to lateral canthal ligament to relieve the high intra-ocular pressure) followed by immediate referral to an ophthalmologist (→ *Figure 22.2*).

Tx The presence of any of the above conditions is an indication for an urgent ophthalmic opinion.

Lateral canthotomy: for most Emergency clinicians this will be a procedure that one will never need to perform, but which should be learned and practiced on a model in case it is ever required. (→ *Figure 22.2*)

1 Ensure the patient is as comfortable as possible. Identify the lateral canthus and clean. Inject 1–2 mL of 1% lidocaine in and around lateral canthus.

2 Crush the lateral canthus with forceps for 1–2 min to reduce bleeding during the procedure. Cut the crushed tissue with scissors.

3 Pull the lower lid away from the globe with forceps. 'Strum' the tissue below the lateral canthus with scissors to identify the inferior crus of the ligament. Cut the ligament with the scissors pointing inferiorly.

4 If vision remains poor, cut the superior crus of the ligament in a similar fashion. Ensure Ophthalmology are on their way to provide definitive treatment.

'Blow-out' fractures of the floor of the orbit → p. 71–72.

Subconjunctival haemorrhage

Post-traumatic subconjunctival haemorrhage is common and usually trivial. Fluorescein may be used to reveal any conjunctival lacerations. Failure to visualise the posterior border of the haemorrhage may suggest orbital or retro-orbital trauma.

Spontaneous subconjunctival haemorrhage may follow coughing or straining or in the presence of hypertension. It is alarming to the patient but is usually of no consequence.

Tx No specific treatment is required but the patient should be warned that the discolouration may take several weeks to resolve.

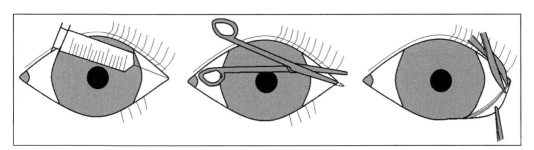

Figure 22.2 Performing a lateral canthotomy.

> **Box 22.3 Assessment of the acute red eye: key observations to help in diagnosis**
>
> - Is the problem bilateral?
> - Is there any associated visual loss?
> - Is there a sensation of a foreign body?
> - Is the eye uncomfortable and irritated or is it painful?
> - Are the eyelids puffy or the conjunctiva oedematous?
> - Is there any photophobia?
> - Is the pupil irregular, dilated or unreactive?

Assessment of the red eye

Determining the cause of the acutely red or painful eye requires careful history taking and examination. Key observations are shown in → *Box 22.3*.

Infective conjunctivitis

This may be caused by several different agents:

- It is often bilateral.
- The eye is red, injected and uncomfortable with a gritty feeling.

Bacteria cause the classic, sticky eye, which is worse on waking.
Viral conjunctivitis results in itchy, watery eyes. There may be a concurrent upper respiratory tract infection (URTI). Injected follicular swelling in the lower fornix and a preauricular lymph node are characteristic findings.
Adenovirus causes a more painful conjunctivitis, sometimes with visual blurring due to keratitis. The condition is slow to resolve and very infectious.

Tx As it may be difficult to differentiate between the types of infectious conjunctivitis, it is usual practice to treat them all with a topical antibiotic (e.g. chloramphenicol ointment) and advise bathing the eye with warm, wet cotton wool.

> Ocular conditions that have not significantly improved after 24 hours of treatment, merit a specialist opinion.

Allergic conjunctivitis

This is caused by exposure to eyedrops, plants or other allergens and is associated with atopy. Chloramphenicol, neomycin and atropine are the most common drug offenders:

- It is the most common cause of a puffy, red eye.
- There is lid swelling with a cobblestone appearance under the lid and conjunctival oedema (chemosis).
- Itching is the predominant symptom.

Tx Remove the offending substance. Eyedrops containing an antihistamine or mast cell stabiliser (e.g. olopatadine 0.1% or sodium cromoglicate 2%) or an oral antihistamine may be helpful.

Episcleritis

Idiopathic inflammation of the layer between the conjunctiva and sclera which is self limiting.

- It is uncomfortable with a stinging feeling.
- A discrete area of conjunctiva is injected and swollen.

Tx Outpatient ophthalmological referral is required. NSAIDs can be helpful.

Scleritis

Presents similarly to episcleritis but with more intense, 'boring' eye pain.

- Sclera is oedematous with a slight violet hue.
- Pain may be worse on moving the eyes and may wake the patient at night.

Tx Ophthalmological referral is required, the usual treatment is with NSAIDs and corticosteroids. The patient will then need investigation for autoimmune connective tissue diseases which are related to this condition.

Pre-septal and orbital cellulitis

Pre-septal cellulitis involves structures anterior to the orbital septum, and orbital cellulitis affects structures posteriorly. It is more common in young children and arises from a bacterial infection of an adjacent sinus or eyelid.

- The eyelids are puffy and red.
- Swelling may be painless at first but within hours there is pain, fever and distress.
- Proptosis, painful eye movements and reduced vision suggest orbital cellulitis although it can be difficult to differentiate in early infection.

Tx Admission and treatment with intravenous (IV) antibiotics is required. CT scan can be useful to assess the extent of infection. Referral is to an ENT (ear, nose and throat) surgeon, ophthalmologist or paediatrician, as suggested by the most likely origin of the infection and local policy.

Complications: orbital cellulitis can lead to several other serious conditions, including cavernous sinus thrombosis, meningitis and abscess.

Corneal ulcers (keratitis)

Dendritic ulcers: these are caused by herpes simplex infection of the cornea:

- The eye is red and the patient is photophobic.
- There is a branching 'dendritic' ulcer that stains with fluorescein.

Referral and therapy with ganciclovir 0.15% is required. Immunocompromised patients warrant same day referral due to the risk of retinitis.

Bacterial corneal ulcers: these may be related to minor corneal trauma or chronic ocular surface disease.

- The eye is red and painful, there may be discharge.
- There is a corneal opacity which stains which fluorescein.

Refer to eye clinic for culture of corneal scrapings before antibiotics are started. Contact lens-related infections tend to be due to Gr-species such as *Pseudomonas* or occasionally an amoebic infection called Acanthamoeba which is extremely painful and difficult to treat.

Marginal keratitis: is characterised by small, white patches within the cornea, close to the limbus, which do not stain well with fluorescein. These are sterile inflammatory infiltrates.

Uveitis (iritis)

Inflammation of the anterior intraocular structures which is usually autoimmune or idiopathic. It is often recurrent and in young adults may be associated with ankylosing spondylitis. There is:

- a red and painful eye with circumcorneal injection.
- tenderness of the eye.
- photophobia.
- adhesions between the pupillary margin and the lens (synechiae), which may cause irregular shaped pupil.
- a haze over the cornea, especially the lower half or even hypopyon.

Tx Urgent referral to an ophthalmologist is required. Local anaesthetic does not relieve symptoms; a cycloplegic

(e.g. cyclopentolate) may be prescribed once angle closure has been ruled out as well as a topical steroid.

Glaucoma

Acute angle-closure glaucoma is a disease of the over-40s and especially elderly people. It is associated with severe long-sightedness (hypermetropia). Impaired outflow of aqueous humour from the anterior chamber of the eye causes raised intraocular pressure (IOP). Drugs with anticholinergic effects can cause secondary angle-closure. Clinical features include the following:

- A red, painful eye, which is injected and tender and feels hard on palpation through the lid.
- Visual loss, with the appearance of haloes around lights.
- A semi-dilated, ovoid pupil, which does not react to direct or consensual light stimuli.
- Corneal haze caused by oedema.
- Malaise, headache and vomiting (can be the presenting complaint).

Tx Immediate ophthalmic referral is essential. Discuss initial treatment, that may include:

- Parenteral analgesics and antiemetics
- Pilocarpine 2–4% eye drops
- Acetazolamide 500 mg orally or by slow IV injection

The eyelids

Injuries → p. 72.

Blepharitis

Inflammation of the eyelids should be treated with a topical antibiotic ointment and advice on bathing the eyelids. Refractory cases will benefit from a non-urgent referral to ophthalmology clinic.

Lumps on the eyelids

Small cystic swellings of the eyelid glands are common (hordeolum/styes or chalazia). They may become inflamed. Advise the patient on warm compresses and lid massage and prescribe a topical antibiotic ointment. Refractory cases will benefit from a non-urgent referral to ophthalmology clinic.

Sudden loss of vision

Retinal detachment

- Visual loss often described as 'like a curtain'
- Sensation of flashing lights

- Detached retina appears dark through an ophthalmoscope
- Associated with hypermetropia and trauma to the eye
- **Tx** – surgery or gas bubble injection, refer within 24 hours.

Retinal venous occlusion

- Sudden, unilateral visual loss of varying degrees
- Congested, haemorrhagic 'snowstorm' retina
- May involve a tributary of the retinal vein and hence one quadrant of the retina
- Increasing incidence with age, hx of diabetes and hypercoagulable states
- **Tx** – prevention of macula oedema using steroids, biological agents and laser therapy.
- Refer within 24 hours.

Retinal arterial occlusion

- Acute, unilateral visual loss
- Pale, ischaemic retina with a 'cherry-red spot' at the macula and a swollen optic disc
- Similar risk factors to stroke → *p. 240*
- May be associated with temporal arteritis (check erythrocyte sedimentation rate [ESR]) → *p. 239*
- Patients with an accessory cilioretinal artery can retain central area of the visual field
- Visual acuity at presentation often predicts final acuity, so aim is to dislodge any clots within 90 min
- **Tx** – Try gentle pulsing pressure over the closed eye, vasodilation with nitroglycerin or intra-ocular pressure-lowering drugs such as acetazolamide. There may be some benefit from intra-articular thrombolysis.
- Urgent input needed from ophthalmology and stroke teams

Amaurosis fugax

- A resolved episode of retinal artery occlusion is called amaurosis fugax and should be treated like transient ischaemic attack (TIA) → *p. 242*

Vitreous haemorrhage

- Associated with diabetes, trauma, sickle cell disease and sub-arachnoid haemorrhage
- Bleeding into the posterior eye causes obscured, blurred vision with floaters
- Absent red reflex/retina cannot be visualised
- Blood clears gradually, but refer patient to eye clinic for IOP monitoring

Optic neuritis

- Can develop suddenly or over days, with foggy or blurred vision, where colours look washed out.
- Can be worse when the patient is warmer (Uhthoff's phenomenon)
- Causes include viral infections, autoimmune conditions but most commonly, demyelination, e.g. multiple sclerosis.

Others

Cortical blindness: this condition follows a head injury and may persist for several hours.
Acute maculopathy: fluid leakage, bleeding, infection or inflammation can occur with or without chronic macular disease. Needs urgent ophthalmology referral.
Migraine: can present with scintillating scotoma and field defects → *p. 239*.
Psychological and functional disorders: bilateral blindness can be a feature of functional neurological disorder or conversion disorder.

THE EARS

Barotrauma → p. 246.
Haemotympanum and bleeding from the ear canal → p. 45.
Injuries to the pinna → p. 71.
URTI in children → p. 359.

Otitis media

- Gradual onset of pain with a red bulging drum on otoscopy
- Acute suppurative otitis media also has discharge and tympanic membrane rupture
- Consider oral antibiotics only in patients with otorrhoea and children under 2 with bilateral infection
- Admit patients with signs of sepsis, meningitis or facial nerve palsy

Mastoiditis – spreading infection from the middle ear can form an abscess in the mastoid air spaces of the temporal bone. Patients are usually unwell with fever, the pinna is pushed forwards and there is boggy oedema over the mastoid. Diagnosis often includes a CT scan, and the patient will need admission under ENT.

Otitis externa

- Known as 'swimmer's ear', usual pathogens are *Pseudomonas* spp. or *Staphylococcus* spp.
- The ear canal is swollen and red with creamy exudate
- **Tx** ear drops containing an antibiotic and steroid. Advise patient to keep the ear dry
- Refer patients with signs of pinna cellulitis or perichondritis, acutely stenosed canals or facial nerve palsy

Necrotising otitis externa – a condition causing osteo-myelitis of the temporal bone, more common in patients with diabetes and immunocompromise. It is character-ised by severe, deep pain and requires admission and CT scan.

Rupture of the tympanum

- **Infection**: otitis media, mostly in children → *above*
- **Direct trauma**: something poking into the auditory canal, e.g. cotton bud
- **Indirect trauma**: usually a slap to the pinna that sends a pressure wave down the auditory canal; this may occur in domestic violence → *p. 393*
- **Barotrauma**: diving or air travel in susceptible indi-viduals → *p. 246*
- **Blast injury**: a primary injury from blast overpressure (shock) waves → *p. 30*
- **Lightning strike or high-voltage electric shock**: often bilateral rupture → *p. 150*
- **Fracture of the base of the skull**: more commonly a haemotympanum occurs → *p. 45*.

Tx Management of the underlying cause is essential. Some degree of hearing loss is inevitable after damage to the eardrum and ENT follow-up is usually advisable. Advise patients to keep the ear dry and to use a cotton ball rolled in petroleum jelly placed gently in the canal whilst bathing.

Problems with earrings

The missing components of an earring stud can become embedded in an inflamed earlobe, especially in the days following ear piercing.

Tx The ear should be anaesthetised using an auricular block (→ *Box 22.4 and Figure 22.3*). The foreign body can then be easily and painlessly removed using splinter forceps. The area should be treated with a local antiseptic.

Foreign bodies in the ear

Patients may present acutely with a missing foreign body or chronically with a discharging ear. In an adult, the lost object is usually the tip of a cotton bud; in a child, more variety can be expected!

Tx Loops can be used, as can Hartmann's 'crocodile' forceps and wax hooks. The method used depends on personal experience and patient compliance. If removal is unsuccessful, referral should be arranged to the next ENT clinic. A slight delay before removal is not important but inexpert manipulation, with inadequate instruments, a poor light and a struggling child can cause injuries to the tympanic membrane.

Insects can crawl or fly into the auditory canal where their movements cause great distress. Before removal, they can be killed by pouring olive oil into the canal or paralysed by instilling 2% lidocaine.

> Cold liquids instilled into a patient's ear canal can cause nystagmus and vertigo, so remember to warm them slightly beforehand.

 Box 22.4 Auricular ring block

This technique provides anaesthesia to the entire ear

- Disinfect skin at the base and superior aspect of ear
- Insert needle into the skin just inferior to the attachment of the earlobe to the head
- Advance needle just anterior to the tragus, aspirate while advancing (note the proximity of the temporal artery)
- Inject 2–3 mL of local anaesthetic while slowly withdrawing needle
- Redirect the needle posteriorly, behind the pinna, aspirating whist you advance the needle
- Inject 2–3 mL of local anaesthetic whilst withdrawing needle

- Remove needle and reinsert just superior to the attachment of the helix to the scalp superiorly
- Advance needle to just anterior to the tragus, aspirating whilst you while advance the needle
- Inject 2–3 mL of local anaesthetic whilst withdrawing the needle towards to the original puncture site
- Redirect and advance the needle, posterior to the pinna in an inferoposterior direction
- Inject 2–3 mL of local anaesthetic whilst withdrawing the needle
- Allow at least 5 min to elapse for the block to take effect before commencing the procedure

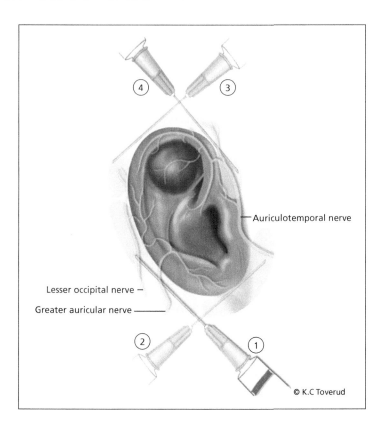

Figure 22.3 Auricular ring block.
© K.C. Toverud.

Sudden hearing loss

Sudden hearing loss is commonly caused by the movement of accumulated wax in the ear canal. This causes an obstructive type of deafness. Wax can be removed by syringing, a procedure usually performed at the local health centre. There are also drops available over the counter to loosen the wax (e.g. Exterol).

Sudden sensorineural hearing loss is an indication for urgent ENT/audiology referral. Patients are often prescribed steroids, e.g. 60 mg prednisolone reducing over 10 days for idiopathic cases. Consider secondary causes such as ototoxic drugs, Cogan's syndrome (hearing loss associated with acute keratitis), Meniere's disease, Lyme disease and stroke.

THE NOSE

Nasal foreign bodies

Usually a paediatric presentation, they can be removed in the ED but often they are deep and surrounded by crusty exudate, having been in place for some days. There may be a purulent discharge.

> Unilateral nasal discharge in a small child is usually caused by a retained foreign body, even if this history is denied.

Tx Try occluding the unblocked nostril with gentle alar pressure and getting the parent to blow a quick blast of air into the child's mouth with their lips encircling (like mouth to mouth breaths). An alternative is to suck the object out with a Yankauer sucker with the side holes taped up. If these measures fail, early specialist referral is recommended. Inexpert probing with forceps or artery clips may push the object further back and cause airway obstruction.

Epistaxis

Epistaxis is common and often mismanaged. Arterial bleeding can originate from Little's area (Kiesselbach's plexus) on the anterior wall of the nasal septum and occasionally from a posterior branch of the sphenopalatine artery which can cause severe bleeding and often appears to be bilateral. In children, nasal bleeding usually comes from the retrocolumellar vein and follows infection or trauma (with a finger).

> Pressure to stop a nosebleed should be applied by firmly squeezing the soft part of the nose between the fingers. The most common reasons for failure are misplaced compression over the nasal bones and lack of constant pressure.

Tx

- Attempt to arrest haemorrhage with alar pressure. A swimmer's nose clip can be used for this purpose. Keep the patient upright and encourage them to spit out any blood.
- Consider the need for cross-match, full blood count (FBC) and clotting studies. Resuscitate if necessary.
- After 20 min of continuous alar pressure, gently suction clots and examine the area.
- Consider cauterisation with silver nitrate for a small visible anterior bleed.
- Use of topical tranexamic acid and vasoconstrictors is not supported by robust evidence.
- Treat continued anterior bleeding with a wet nasal tampon or a pack (→ *Figure 22.4*). A hydrocolloid gel balloon tampon (e.g. the 'Rapid Rhino®') is ideal. It is comfortable for the patient and excellent at achieving haemostasis by both platelet aggregation and direct tamponade.
- Bleeding from a more posterior site can be controlled by the careful insertion and inflation of a balloon catheter. However, long (7 cm) hydrocolloid gel balloon tampons are now available that are both effective and comfortable for the patient.

- If bleeding continues, consider inserting bilateral packs and reversing any anticoagulation the patient is taking. Contact ENT as patient may need to go to theatre.
- Antiseptic cream (e.g. Naseptin) should be prescribed to prevent recurrent bleeding, especially in children.

THE MOUTH AND THE THROAT

Management of choking → p. 205.
Other airway obstruction, including foreign bodies → p. 213.

Small foreign bodies stuck in the throat

Patients commonly complain of a foreign body stuck in the throat, often after eating fish. Ask about the ability to swallow solids, fluids and saliva; this is usually unaffected.

Examination requires a good light and a cooperative patient. Remove dentures and examine for completeness. Examine in the mouth; the area around the fauces is a common site to find a fish bone. Foreign bodies often lodge in the piriform fossae and are usually radiolucent. A mucosal tear may produce identical symptoms to an impacted foreign body.

XR A lateral radiograph of the soft tissues of the neck will occasionally show a radio-opaque object such as a chicken bone but should not be relied on to rule out a foreign body.

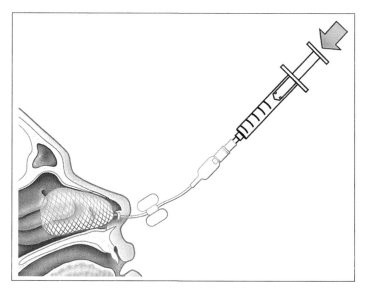

Figure 22.4 Anterior nasal packing.

Tx Any obvious foreign body should be removed; a topical anaesthetic spray may help. Patients with a foreign-body sensation where no cause is found should be discussed with an ENT surgeon; they can usually be reviewed in the next clinic (except where the item is thought to be caustic such as a button battery).

Oesophageal food bolus impaction

A patient may have sudden onset of dysphagia during a meal – often after an attempt to swallow a lump of meat. The blockage is usually reported to be in the 'upper chest'. In the most severe cases, the obstruction extends to fluids, and a drink of water causes regurgitation within a few seconds. Patients with oesophageal conditions such as oesophagitis and stricture are particularly prone to this problem and patients are sometimes found to have a new diagnosis of oesophageal cancer following this presentation.

Tx Some cases resolve spontaneously but there is little hard evidence for the use of many anecdotal treatments, such as effervescent drinks, glucagon and buscopan. Most patients should be referred for surgical assessment and oesophagoscopy.

Swallowed foreign bodies

This is generally a problem of children and some patients with psychiatric conditions. Rounded objects such as coins are the most frequently swallowed. There may be initial coughing but thereafter the patient is usually symptomless. It can be difficult to determine whether the object was inhaled or swallowed, particularly in the case of a lost tooth during facial trauma. Examination should include the fauces, upper airways and lung fields.

The narrowest sites for obstruction are at the cricopharyngeal sphincter, the upper third of the oesophagus at the level of the aortic arch and the cardia. Objects that pass into the stomach will usually traverse the entire gastrointestinal tract within 2–6 days but may not uncommonly take 2–4 weeks. The exceptions are:

- Irregularly shaped articles such as open safety pins – which may impact, especially on the pylorus.
- Multiple magnets – which may attract one another through bowel wall.
- Long, straight objects >5 cm – which may not be able to negotiate the duodenal loop.

> Most foreign bodies that cause a problem are lodged in, or have damaged, the oesophagus.

XR Radio-opaque objects can be localised using radiographs of the chest, abdomen and neck (in that order). For a small child this takes only one film. Thin aluminium objects (e.g. can ring-pulls) and some dental prostheses are not radio-opaque.

> Any patient with persistant oesophageal symptoms should undergo endoscopic evaluation.

Tx
Airway → p. 205.
Pharynx or oesophagus: refer to an ENT surgeon/gastroenterology endoscopist for removal.
Stomach or bowel: usually pass uneventfully, although this may take several weeks. Patients should return if abdominal symptoms develop.
Sharp objects: require observation and either removal or tracking with frequent radiographs.
Glass: Glass may be seen on a radiograph; it is usually harmless.

Ingestion of 'button' batteries

→ see also Chapter 15

Small 'button cell' batteries are sometimes swallowed by children. They may stick and damage the bowel electrically or disintegrate and release toxic contents. There are different types of button battery, mercury batteries being the most dangerous.

Button batteries cause mucosal injury when they become lodged in the gastrointestinal tract, most often the oesophagus. The severity of damage is related to the length of time that the battery is lodged, and injury may occur as early as 2 hours after ingestion.

Late symptoms include:

- fever
- abdominal pain
- vomiting
- blood in the stools.

XR Obtain radiographs of the chest, neck and abdomen until the exact position of the battery is established. Remember to image the entire GI tract as more than one battery may have been ingested. A battery can be recognised by the double ring shadow.

Children with button cells in the stomach need daily abdominal films to show transit and to detect disintegration. Batteries in the bowel should be tracked every 3 or 4 days.

Tx
Foreign bodies in the airway → p. 1, 205.

Box 22.5 Indications for referral for removal of button batteries

- Any button cell in the airway
- Any button cell in the oesophagus
- Any button cell remaining in the stomach for more than 48 hours
- Any button cell static in the gut for a prolonged period
- Any button cell where the ingestion is accompanied by signs of peritonitis
- Mercury cell in the stomach for more than 24 hours
- Mercury cell that appears (on radiograph) to be disintegrating in the stomach (it is advisable to measure mercury concentrations in the blood and urine when leakage is thought to have occurred)

Chemical burns in the mouth suggest that the battery was leaking before ingestion.

- Treat suspected button battery ingestion as an emergency.
- A 10 mL spoonful of honey every 10 min may help to reduce battery corrosion.
- Button batteries in the stomach usually pass from the bowel without problems but all children who have swallowed button batteries should be followed up after 24 hours with a repeat radiograph.

Button batteries that are localised above the stomach or are not passing through the gut satisfactorily or are leaking may require removal. *Indications for referral for the removal of button batteries → Box 22.5.* Endoscopic or magnetic removal is often possible.

All children who have swallowed button-cell batteries must be admitted or followed up in clinic.

Sore throat

Pharyngitis, laryngitis and tonsillitis are common and usually result from a viral infection.

Tx Symptomatic relief with paracetamol and ibuprofen is usually sufficient. Medicated lozenges may also help, as may a single dose of steroid, e.g. oral dexamethasone. Most patients get better without antibiotics and there are rarely any complications from withholding antibiotics. FeverPAIN or CENTOR scores can help distinguish the patients who may benefit from antibiotics. →*Box 18.13 Page 360*

Amoxicillin has been reported to cause a florid rash in patients with glandular fever, hence phenoxymethylpenicillin is often recommended for suspected streptococcal throat infections. Recent studies suggest the incidence of this rash is much lower than previously suggested.

Infectious mononucleosis, cytomegalovirus infection and toxoplasmosis may cause a prolonged sore throat with systemic symptoms.

Quinsy

Peritonsillar abscess presents as a large, unilateral swelling in an unwell patient with a history of tonsillitis. The oedematous uvula is displaced to the opposite side. Dysphagia, halitosis and trismus are inevitable. The throat pain is often unilateral and accompanied by earache and tender cervical nodes. Treatment is with antibiotics as above and referral for needle drainage.

Diphtheria

Diphtheria is caused by infection with the bacterium *Corynebacterium diphtheriae* or *Corynebacterium ulcerans*, which is droplet spread with an incubation period of 1–5 days. Since 1940, widespread vaccination has made this a rare condition, and in 2018 there were just 11 reported cases in the UK. The first symptom of diphtheria is usually a mild pharyngitis causing pain with swallowing. The following are other typical features:

- Low-grade fever (<38.5°C)
- Headache, nausea and vomiting
- Inflammation of the larynx and nasal passages
- Pharyngeal exudate forming a thick greyish 'pseudomembrane'
- Swollen lymph nodes ('bull-neck' appearance)
- Pallor and tachycardia.

Complications include:

- respiratory obstruction
- pneumonia
- otitis media and sinusitis
- myocarditis, peripheral neuritis and nephritis
- shock and organ failure.

Tx Patients with suspected diphtheria should be admitted and discussed with a specialist in infectious diseases. Impending respiratory obstruction may require intubation or even tracheostomy. Diphtheria is treated with benzylpenicillin and antitoxin in severe cases. It is a notifiable disease →*p. 407.*

Epiglottitis

Haemophilus influenzae B, β-haemolytic streptococci or even staphylococci may be responsible. It should be suspected when the 'three Ds' of drooling, dysphagia and distress occur, especially where there is hoarseness or stridor.

Tx

- Reassure the patient and work calmly. Do not examine the throat.
- Summon skilled anaesthetic and ENT help immediately.
- Position the patient for maximum comfort.
- Administer high-flow oxygen.
- Consider using nebulised adrenaline (5 mg) by mask until help arrives.

IV cefotaxime or ceftriaxone is used to treat *H. influenzae* epiglottitis. Non-infectious causes of epiglottitis include caustic ingestions, thermal injury and occasionally as a manifestation of graft versus host disease.

Stridor in children → p. 348.

Deep neck space infections

Retropharyngeal abscess

This condition most commonly affects young children, typically aged 2–4 years but can affect any age group. Infection of the upper respiratory tract leads to a pyogenic adenitis of the retropharyngeal lymph nodes. The resulting abscess is limited to one side of the midline by a median raphe → *Figure 22.5.* The child is obviously unwell and can have:

- a high pyrexia
- a sore throat with dysphagia and odynophagia
- hoarseness, noisy breathing or stridor
- restricted neck movements (a differential diagnosis of torticollis)
- a smooth unilateral swelling of the posterior pharyngeal wall may sometimes be seen.

XR A lateral soft-tissue view of the neck may show marked soft-tissue expansion in the retropharyngeal space which, in severe cases, can push the trachea

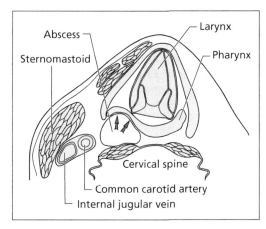

Figure 22.5 Retropharyngeal abscess.

forwards. (The pre-vertebral soft tissue, anterior to C1–4, should normally be no wider than half of the adjacent vertebral bodies.) A CT scan may be performed to provide more information about the swelling.

Tx ENT referral is required for IV antibiotics and, possibly, surgical drainage. Sepsis and mediastinitis may occur.

Submandibular space infections

Lower molar infection can lead to a dangerous infection of the floor of the mouth (Ludwig's angina). It is a rapidly spreading cellulitis that can lead to airway compromise. There is symmetrical 'woody' submandibular swelling. The mouth is often held partially open with a protruding or lifted tongue. *S. viridans* is the most common responsible organism. Diabetes is a risk factor.

Tx Surgical drainage may be required in addition to IV antibiotics. Conditions compromising the airway should be treated in the same way as epiglottitis → *p. 439.*

Swollen salivary glands

Salivary glands may swell because of obstruction, tumour or infection. Obstruction by a stone may cause increased symptoms when the production of saliva is increased (i.e. eating). Mumps must be remembered as a common parotid infection → *p. 442.* Bacterial parotitis may occur in debilitated patients.

Other throat and neck symptoms

Several conditions can be associated with unusual symptoms in the throat. In particular:

Dystonia: bizarre intermittent problems with speech and swallowing may be the only signs of an acute dystonic reaction → *p. 307.*
Tetanus: tetanus ('lock-jaw') may start with jaw stiffness and trismus → *p. 245.*
Pneumomediastinum: the most common symptoms caused by air in the mediastinum are neck pain and dysphagia → *p. 203.*

Bleeding after tonsillectomy

Patients (usually children) may be brought to an ED with post-tonsillectomy bleeding. This may occur a few hours after the procedure or, if secondary to infection, after a few days. Bleeding may occasionally be severe enough to threaten the airway or lead to haemorrhagic shock.

Tx The ENT surgeon should be informed of ALL post tonsillectomy bleeds, urgently if still bleeding. Gentle suctioning may help to clear the airway. Obtain IV access and resuscitate with blood products. IV tranexamic acid may be of some benefit. Most patients will not tolerate pressure on the bleeding area whilst fully awake, so anaesthetic assistance may be required.

Acquired haemophilia and anticoagulation problems → pp. 271, 272.

Dental emergencies

Dentoalveolar abscess

A dentoalveolar abscess is an acute lesion characterised by localisation of pus in the structures that surround the teeth. Odontogenic infections are polymicrobial, with an average of five different causative bacteria. The dominant isolates include genera such as *Bacteroides*, *Fusobacterium*, *Peptococcus* and *Peptostreptococcus* and *S. viridans*.

The lower third molar is the most frequent culprit, followed by other lower posterior teeth. There is localised pain, tenderness and swelling, extending towards the buccal side of the gum and into the gingival–buccal reflection. Severe facial swelling, pyrexia, trismus and dysphagia may also occur.

Tx Definitive treatment should be provided by a dentist. Antibiotics are not advised for otherwise healthy people who do not have signs of sepsis or spreading infection. Good analgesia is important, but remember to enquire about analgesia already taken, as dental pain is a common reason for patients to take a therapeutic excess of paracetamol.

Bleeding after dental extraction

This can occur in the first day or two following an extraction, normally if the clot dislodges or the patient is anticoagulated.

Tx Apply damp gauze or gauze soaked in tranexamic acid or adrenaline with lignocaine. If unsuccessful, try haemostatic agents such as hemocollagen or surgicel or local infiltration of adrenaline with lignocaine.

Acute necrotising ulcerative gingivitis

Also known as Trench mouth or Vincent's angina, it is characterised by a febrile illness with pseudo-membranous inflammation of the gingiva secondary to bacterial infection. There is often a malodourous smell present. It is thought to be due to overgrowth of anaerobic bacterium such as bacteroides, fusobacterium and spirochetes. It is usually only seen in immunodeficiency states.

Tx chlorhexidine mouth washes, a 3 day course of metronidazole or amoxicillin and encourage improved oral hygiene. Patients should be advised that they need urgent assessment by a dentist.

Dental injuries → p. 70.
Numbering system used to describe teeth → p. 70 (Box 5.2).

THE FACE

Facial pain

Sinusitis

This can occur in any of the four groups of sinuses. There may be facial pain and tenderness in the affected area together with headache, purulent nasal discharge and pyrexia. Only consider antibiotics (phenoxymethylpenicillin 1st line) when the symptoms have been longer than 10 days or the patient is systemically unwell.

Shingles

Herpes zoster infection may cause acute unilateral facial pain. Oral aciclovir therapy is recommended for non-truncal shingles within first 72 hours (remembering to adjust the dose in renal failure). Hutchinson's sign, where there is rash on the tip of the nose, can signal shingles of the ophthalmic division of the trigeminal nerve. This may result in damage to the cornea and thus requires ophthalmic review.

Trigeminal neuralgia

TN is a sudden, unilateral, stabbing, pain in the distribution of one or more branches of the trigeminal nerve. Pain occurs in paroxysms lasting from a few seconds to a few minutes, sometimes up to a 100 times a day. Treatment is with carbamazepine or sodium valproate → *p. 227.*

Facial palsy

Bell's palsy is an idiopathic condition causing a unilateral lower motor neuron paralysis of the face. It develops over 72 hours accompanied by mastoid discomfort, hyperacusis and taste disturbance. It must be differentiated from a stroke affecting the face. The classic sign used for this purpose is the failure to wrinkle the forehead on the affected side in Bell's palsy. In an upper motor neuron lesion this movement is likely to be unaffected because the upper part of the face has bilateral cortical representation.

Look in the ears of patients with facial palsy. A herpetic infection of the meatus and tympanic membrane may be identified (Ramsay Hunt syndrome). Earache, vertigo, deafness, loss of taste and vesicles in the fauces or soft palate may occur.

Tx Bell's palsy resolves spontaneously over a few weeks in 90% of patients. Steroid treatment can be started if within the first 72 hours (e.g. 50 mg daily for 10 days.) patients who have difficulty in closing one eye also need a supply of eye pads to protect the cornea at night and lubricating eye drops.

Patients with facial palsy accompanied by a discharging ear, a cholesteatoma or vesicles should be referred to an ENT specialist.

Mumps

Infection with the mumps paramyxovirus has a long incubation period (16–25 days.) Mumps parotitis causes pyrexia, malaise and progressive tender facial swelling around the angle of the jaw. In 80% of cases, both parotid glands are affected. The illness usually resolves spontaneously within 7–10 days. Complications include meningoencephalitis, pancreatitis and inflammation of almost any other glandular tissue. Orchitis is seen in about a third of postpubertal males with mumps. It is usually unilateral and may lead to testicular atrophy. Mumps is a notifiable disease →*p. 388.*

Complications of aesthetic procedures

Dermal fillers are used in aesthetic medicine to shape and fill the contours of the face and lips. Most fillers contain either hyaluronic acid or collagen and have effects lasting 6 months to 2 years before being biodegraded. Some silicone fillers are non-biodegradable and last forever.

The most important complication to be aware of is vascular compromise caused by accidental injection into an artery. This will present as a pale or dusky area of skin with pain, that will become an area of skin necrosis is not treated promptly. It can be difficult to differentiate from bruising in the early stages but must not be missed. Most aesthetic practitioners carry hyaluronidase to immediately inject and dissolve the filler if this occurs, but the patient may present to the ED with these symptoms. Nitroglycerin paste can be applied and warm compresses until hyaluronidase can be acquired. Follow-up is with plastic surgeons.

Other potential complications include allergic reaction and anaphylaxis and soft tissue infection.

23

Global health

A.D. Redmond

Humanitarian and Conflict Response Institute, University of Manchester, Manchester, UK

A widely accepted definition of global health has been provided by Kaplan and colleagues writing in the Lancet. They described global health as:

> '... .an area for study, research, and practice that places a priority on improving health and achieving equity in health for all people worldwide. Global health emphasises transnational health issues, determinants, and solutions; involves many disciplines within and beyond the health sciences and promotes interdisciplinary collaboration: and is a synthesis of population-based prevention with individual-level clinical care'.

Emergency medicine is a critical component of any healthcare system and has a fundamental role to play in underpinning global health. This is reflected in the WHO Global Health Strategy and its inclusion in its three pillars of

- universal health coverage,
- health emergencies,
- better health and wellbeing.

Importantly, all three pillars working together are required to support the satisfactory and equitable provision of healthcare globally; and each is intimately linked with and dependent upon the others. Furthermore, global health is not solely dependent upon a country's healthcare and health systems. It is dependent upon the provision and equitable distribution of wider resources, including for example wealth and education, and ultimately therefore the product of political and economic policies. These may be the direct effect of a nation's own policies or the indirect effect of another. There are consequently major inequalities in the provision of, and access to, healthcare across the world.

GLOBAL HEALTH AND EMERGENCY MEDICINE

These inequalities are reflected in emergency medicine, and there are parts of the world where basic *essential emergency healthcare* is either not available for lack of facilities, inaccessible for lack of transport, or unaffordable to those who cannot pay. This will only be fully addressed when there is *Universal Health Coverage*, defined by WHO as:

> 'ensuring that all people have access to needed health services (including prevention, promotion, treatment, rehabilitation and palliation) of sufficient quality to be effective while also ensuring that the use of these services does not expose the user to financial hardship.'

This is why *universal health coverage* has become a major goal for health reform in many countries, one of the pillars of its global health strategy, and a priority for WHO.

> 'No one should die for the lack of access to emergency care, an essential part of **universal health coverage**. We have simple, affordable and proven interventions that save lives.'
>
> Dr Tedros Adhanom Ghebreyesus, WHO Director-General

The Global Burden of Disease (GBD) study reveals that the overall health of the world's population, as measured by age-standardised DALY rates, is improving ($\rightarrow$ *Figure 23.1*), global life expectancy at birth has increased overall from 67·2 years in 2000 to 73·5 years in 2019, and the chances

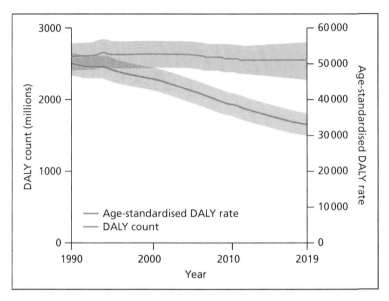

Figure 23.1 Global DALYSs and age-standardised DALY rates.

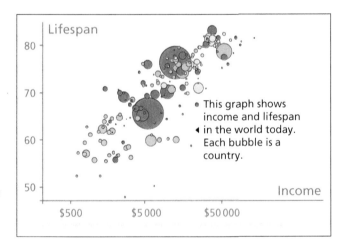

Figure 23.2 Income and lifespan. Each bubble is a country, and its size reflects its population. Taken from Gapminder | Unveiling the beauty of statistics for a fact based world view.

of living not only a longer but a healthy life have similarly increased for the majority of countries.

However, ischaemic heart disease, diabetes, stroke, chronic kidney disease and lung cancer continue to contribute significantly to poor health, with HIV/AIDS still taking a considerable toll on the world's health, but where available, antiretroviral treatment is reducing its impact. There have been significant reductions too in the burden of disease borne by children, driven largely by reductions in major infectious diseases, particularly lower respiratory tract infections, diarrhoeal diseases and meningitis; each of which declined by more than

60% between 1990 and 2019, although they can still place a significant burden on communities.

Sadly, such improvements are not shared equally; the poor and the old carry a greater burden of disease than the young and the wealthy and have the least capacity to address its consequences. (see Figure 23.2).

Such inequalities extend into the management of health emergencies, which in any setting are rarely entirely unheralded, and within an adequate healthcare system can often be avoided, mitigated, or treated. Many 'emergencies' also mark the end point of years of prolonged poor health. An acute myocardial infarction for example may present as an emergency, but it would have been predicted and therefore potentially prevented by adequate recognition and treatment of underlying conditions such as diabetes and hypertension. Those living without access to an adequate healthcare system are therefore more prone to develop conditions that may ultimately present as an emergency, and when they present, do so to a facility inadequately staffed or equipped for its proper management. This is most pronounced in low-/middle-income countries.

WHO has established a number of initiatives through its Violence and Injury Prevention programme that look to support emergency medicine and trauma care in low-/middle-income countries. The WHO **Emergency Care System Framework** (→ *Figure 23.3*) defines a set of key essential functions within an emergency care system that are required to guide its structure and development. It is aimed at a government level and details what must be in place in order to deliver essential emergency healthcare.

To assist a government in benchmarking its current system, there is an accompanying WHO **Emergency Care System Assessment tool** that facilitates the identification of gaps in the existing Emergency Care System Framework and therefore the priorities for system development.

To support the development of pre-hospital and emergency department care, WHO, working with relevant specialists, has developed the WHO **Basic Emergency Care course,** an open-access training course for frontline healthcare providers who work with limited resources. It promotes a systematic approach to the initial assessment and management of patients in those circumstances where early intervention saves lives. The package includes a Participant Workbook and a set of slides to accompany each module. It works alongside and integrates the guidance from WHO Emergency Triage, Assessment and Treatment (ETAT) for children with the Integrated Management of Adult/Adolescent Illness (IMAI).

An important component of any emergency care system is the management of severe injury. Overall, injury accounts for 11% of the total Global Burden of Disease and 10% of all deaths; almost a third more than those from malaria, tuberculosis and HIV/AIDS combined. In turn, these injuries contribute to a trend towards disability taking an increasing share of the overall burden of disease.

The WHO **Global Alliance for the Care of the Injured (GACI)** is a network of governmental, intergovernmental, and non-government organisations that collaborate for the improvement of the care of the injured from the pre-hospital setting through their hospital care to recovery and rehabilitation. The management of severe injuries is a particularly significant part of emergency healthcare in low-/middle-income countries. It is a sad fact that those from poorer economic backgrounds bear over two-thirds of the world's trauma burden, with far higher rates of death from injury, and with more non-fatal injuries, than in higher-income countries. The problem is compounded by those with life-threatening, but survivable injuries in these settings being 6 times more likely to die (36% mortality) than in a high-income setting (6% mortality). Even within affluent countries, those with low socio-economic status and those living in less affluent areas are also more vulnerable to injury, and still tend to die to a greater extent from those injuries. Road traffic crashes, acts of deliberate self-harm, and interpersonal violence, disproportionately affect adolescents and young adults, contributing significantly to the years of potential and productive lives lost to a society.

The WHO **Trauma Care Checklist** (→ *Figure 23.4*) is designed for use in emergency departments and emphasises the key life-saving elements in the successful reception and treatment of the injured patient. It details a systematic approach through a tick box progression to ensure that all essential life-saving interventions are performed in a timely fashion and no quickly reversible life-threatening conditions are missed.

Emergency medical humanitarian assistance

Although Global Health and Emergency Medical Humanitarian Assistance are often viewed alongside each other, they are not necessarily synonymous; although responding to major health emergencies and humanitarian crises is an important contribution that global emergency medicine makes to overall global health.

'Humanitarianism' is often used to simply describe the act of doing something perceived to be inherently good, relieving suffering, or helping those in dire need. It is though more than this and draws on a set of values that date back to, amongst others, Henri Dunant and his foundation of the International Committee of the Red Cross (ICRC) in the mid-nineteenth century. The ICRC led to the Geneva conventions and ultimately to the formulation of the modern humanitarian principles and international humanitarian law, with which all humanitarian organisations must comply.

The humanitarian principles

- **Humanity**: Human suffering must be addressed wherever it is found. The purpose of humanitarian action is to protect life and health and ensure respect for human beings.
- **Neutrality**: Humanitarian actors must not take sides in hostilities or engage in controversies of a political, racial, religious, or ideological nature.

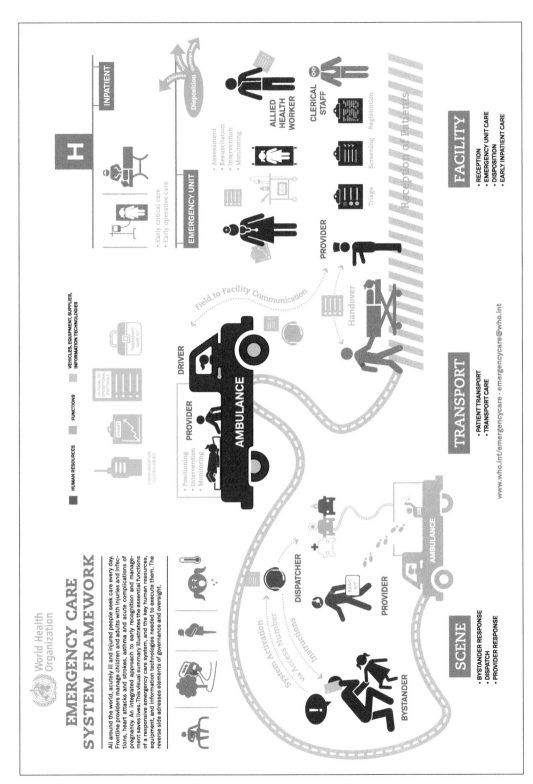

Figure 23.3 Emergency Care system framework.

Trauma Care Checklist

Immediately after primary and secondary surveys:

IS FURTHER AIRWAY INTERVENTION NEEDED? May be needed if: • GCS 8 or below • Hypoxaemia or hypercarbia • Face, neck, chest or any severe trauma	☐ YES, DONE ☐ NO
IS THERE A _TENSION_ PNEUMO-HAEMOTHORAX?	☐ YES, CHEST DRAIN PLACED ☐ NO
IS THE PULSE OXIMETER PLACED AND FUNCTIONING?	☐ YES ☐ NOT AVAILABLE
LARGE-BORE IV PLACED AND FLUIDS STARTED?	☐ YES ☐ NOT INDICATED ☐ NOT AVAILABLE
FULL SURVEY FOR (AND CONTROL OF) EXTERNAL BLEEDING, INCLUDING:	☐ SCALP ☐ PERINEUM ☐ BACK
ASSESSED FOR PELVIC FRACTURE BY:	☐ EXAM ☐ X-RAY ☐ CT
ASSESSED FOR INTERNAL BLEEDING BY:	☐ EXAM ☐ ULTRASOUND ☐ CT ☐ DIAGNOSTIC PERITONEAL LAVAGE
IS SPINAL IMMOBILIZATION NEEDED?	☐ YES, DONE ☐ NOT INDICATED
NEUROVASCULAR STATUS OF ALL 4 LIMBS CHECKED?	☐ YES
IS THE PATIENT HYPOTHERMIC?	☐ YES, WARMING ☐ NO
DOES THE PATIENT NEED (IF NO CONTRAINDICATION):	☐ URINARY CATHETER ☐ NASOGASTRIC TUBE ☐ CHEST DRAIN ☐ NONE INDICATED

Before team leaves patient:

HAS THE PATIENT BEEN GIVEN:	☐ TETANUS VACCINE ☐ ANALGESICS ☐ ANTIBIOTICS ☐ NONE INDICATED
HAVE ALL TESTS AND IMAGING BEEN REVIEWED?	☐ YES ☐ NO, FOLLOW-UP PLAN IN PLACE
WHICH SERIAL EXAMINATIONS ARE NEEDED?	☐ NEUROLOGICAL ☐ ABDOMINAL ☐ VASCULAR ☐ NONE
PLAN OF CARE DISCUSSED WITH:	☐ PATIENT/FAMILY ☐ RECEIVING UNIT ☐ PRIMARY TEAM ☐ OTHER SPECIALISTS
RELEVANT TRAUMA CHART OR FORM COMPLETED?	☐ YES ☐ NOT AVAILABLE

WWW.WHO.INT/EMERGENCYCARE

Figure 23.4 Trauma Care checklist.

- **Impartiality**: Humanitarian action must be carried out on the basis of need alone, giving priority to the most urgent cases of distress and making no distinctions on the basis of nationality, race, gender, religion, class, or political opinions.
- **Independence**: Humanitarian action must be autonomous from the political, economic, military or other objectives that any actor may hold with regard to areas where humanitarian action is being implemented.

There is often an outpouring of offers of assistance when major crises dominate the news cycle, and those working in emergency medicine for example may feel compelled to respond. However, the arrival of uninvited medical teams or even medical individuals into a country in the middle of responding to a major disaster can add an additional logistical problem rather than relieve those with which they are already trying to cope. There is a paradox here in those countries most in need of outside help may equally have less than robust systems for controlling who crosses their borders. It is incumbent upon the responders themselves therefore to ensure their actions comply at all times with the four prima facie principles of good medical practice. Medical teams must respect the **autonomy** of the patient and so be accountable to them through registration with/authorisation by the host government. They should be fully trained and experienced in working in humanitarian emergencies and practise only within their recognised competencies to ensure **beneficence** and **non-maleficence** for their patients. They will also need comprehensive insurance including medical indemnity insurance, as they do at home. The victims of disasters and/or patients in low-/middle-income countries deserve **justice** and access to reparation no less than do patients in high-income countries. Authorisation to practice can be expedited by the host government for those who they wish to invite in, and therefore joining a well-established humanitarian organisation is the most straightforward way of offering your services. Such organisations will also ensure that you are appropriately insured and not a burden on the host country by enabling you to be self-sufficient and not look to draw already limited resources from the stricken country. In general, only go if you are asked, and when in country do what is asked of you by the local health authorities, are good guiding principles. Responding to complex emergencies/civil wars and conflicts is not always so straightforward and can raise very difficult questions about who might be the legitimate authority for granting authorisation to practice. Again, working with established and recognised humanitarian organisations such as UK-MED, ICRC, or MSF will give you the benefit of their long experience of navigating such troubled waters. You may wish also to consider working with the UN/WHO.

As in all aspects of emergency medicine, appropriate training should be completed before independent practice. The consensus view is that those preparing to deploy should have first completed their specialist training and then completed additional 'adaption' training for the humanitarian environment. Finally, it is important to have trained with colleagues and become familiar with the working environment and equipment, particularly if working in a tented field hospital. Organisations will have their own, or refer you to another organisation's, pre-deployment 'simulated' deployments where teamworking and interpersonal skills are tested and developed. An essential component of this pre-deployment training is security training. Immediately before deployment, there may be a short training session on any special features/requirements such as detailed PPE donning and doffing training for deployment to an outbreak. → *Figure 23.5 Training for deployment*

There have been substantial improvements in the coordination and implementation of humanitarian aid in recent years. Major developments include:

The Humanitarian Charter. This was drafted initially in 1997 when a number of humanitarian agencies, including the Red Cross/Red Crescent movements, looked to make the delivery of humanitarian assistance more accountable to its recipients. Within the charter was the recognition of the rights and duties laid down in international law and the fundamental principles of the right to life with dignity, the right to receive humanitarian assistance, and the right to protection and security. At the same time, they identified a set of humanitarian standards to be applied in all humanitarian responses – the Sphere Standards. These are grouped into four sections – (1) water supply, sanitation and hygiene promotion (WASH); (2) food security and nutrition; (3) shelter and settlement; and (4) health.

The United Nations Office for the Coordination of Humanitarian Affairs (OCHA) developed two important initiatives following the earthquake in Armenia in 1988. The huge outpouring of international assistance had highlighted the need for better coordination of international offers of assistance and improvements in its quality assurance and standardisation.

- A **United Nations Disaster Assessment and Coordination team (UNDAC)** was established by drawing on a range of international experts from across a broad range of specialties who could be mobilised at very short notice to deploy to the affected country, and working with the relevant authorities, carry out a rapid needs assessment and disseminate its findings. This would facilitate a more targeted aid response, and with the establishment of an On-Site Operations Coordination Centre (OSOCC), the team could also help to coordinate the incoming humanitarian aid.

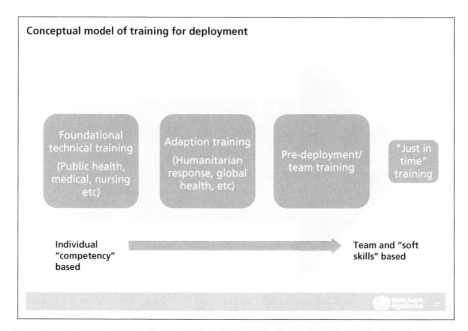

Figure 23.5 Training for Deployment. Camacho, N. A., Hughes, A., Burkle, F. M., Ingrassia, P. L., Ragazzoni, L., Redmond, A., Norton, I., & von Schreeb, J. (2016). Education and training of emergency medical teams: Recommendations for a global operational learning framework. *PLOS Currents Disasters*. Oct 21. Edition 1.

- The **International Search and Rescue Advisory Group (INSARAG)** was established to quality-assure the capabilities of search and rescue teams responding to large-scale disasters. Recognising that verifying the quality and relevance of offers of assistance in the immediate aftermath of a large-scale disaster would be extremely difficult, and likely to divert precious time and resources from the disaster itself, the international search and rescue community, working with the UN, established an advisory group to agree in advance of a disaster a set of general criteria and capabilities from which a classification system could be formulated (e.g. light, medium, and heavy, depending on the type of equipment carried). Search and rescue teams could initially classify themselves against these criteria when offering assistance in order to assist the affected government in choosing which teams to invite, and where to deploy them in country. INSARAG also established a training programme and a system of verification whereby the classification and capability of teams could be independently verified. In this way, affected countries could be assured of the quality and capability of search and rescue teams offering their assistance.

The **Global Health Cluster** was established in 2005 by the UN Interagency Standing Committee as part of a broader 'Cluster System' established to strengthen the humani-

tarian coordination system by building partnerships across UN agencies, Non-Government Organisations and International Organisations (→ *Figure 23.6*). The lead agency for health is WHO, and its secretariat is based at WHO in Geneva. The Cluster approach:

'ensures that international responses to humanitarian emergencies are predictable and accountable and have clear leadership by making clearer the division of labour between organizations, and their roles and responsibilities in different areas. It aims to make the international humanitarian community better organized and more accountable and professional, so that it can be a better partner for affected people, host Governments, local authorities, local civil society and resourcing partners'.

The Global Health Cluster supports Health Clusters/Sectors in the affected countries, building the capacity of their Health Cluster staff and gathering and disseminating relevant and reliable information to guide the response. In particular, they look to identify and address gaps in technical knowledge to ensure the health response follows global best practices and standards.

Just as the response to the earthquake in Armenia in 1998 gave rise to a series of UN initiatives, so concerns about the emergency medical response to the earthquake in Haiti in 2010 gave rise to the WHO **Emergency**

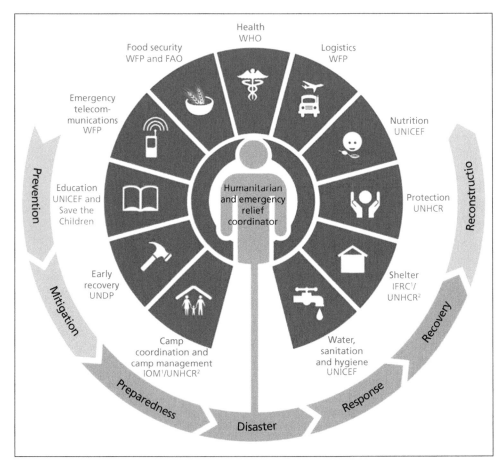

Figure 23.6 The cluster system and UN lead agency.

Medical Teams (EMT) Initiative. This led to the establishment of a set of minimum standards and, similar to what was achieved by INSARAG for search and rescue teams, a classification system for medical teams responding to humanitarian emergencies (→ *Figure 23.7*).

Within the initiative is the capacity to establish a **WHO Coordination Cell (WHOCC)** within the Ministry of Health (MoH) of the affected country to coordinate international medical assistance. Requests for and offers of assistance, including the types by classification of teams needed, are posted on a **Virtual On-Site Operations Coordination Centre (VOSOCC)** and matched by the WHOCC/MoH. On arrival in country, teams can be more efficiently dispatched to where they can be of most benefit.

It is critical that any help that is offered relieves rather than adds to the burden of the affected country. To that end the EMT initiative expects teams to have been fully trained, fully equipped, self-sufficient in food water and medications for at least 2 weeks, and have the experience

and supply chains in place to replenish their stocks without draining the resources of the affected country. Teams can look to be verified by WHO as meeting the standards for their declared classification through a verification process that concludes with a team inspection. WHO verification allows affected countries to make more informed choices about outside medical assistance (→ *Figure 23.8*).

Sudden onset disasters

A disaster is defined by the UN as 'a serious disruption of the functioning of a community or a society involving widespread human, material, economic, or environmental losses and impacts, which exceeds the ability of the affected community or society to cope using its own resources.' Sudden onset disasters by their very nature mean there will be insufficient time for the complete evacuation of the at-risk population. Whilst the frequency

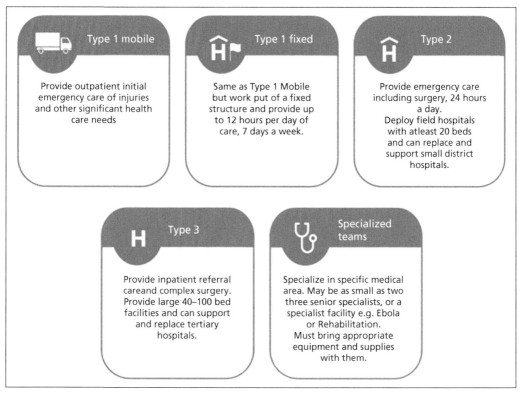

Figure 23.7 WHO classification of emergency medical teams.

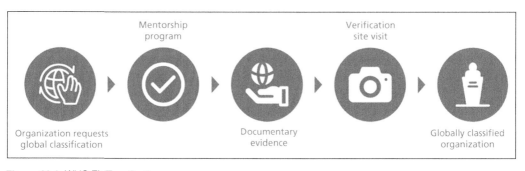

Figure 23.8 WHO EMT verification process.

and impact of disasters upon communities are increasing, paradoxically the deaths from these disasters are going down (Figure 23.9). On the one hand, this reflects improved responses, but it also means that more people are living with the consequences of disasters. These and other phenomena, including war, climate change, migration and rapid urbanisation, can lead to concentrations of people, usually poor people, in some of the most vulnerable areas; although worldwide the death toll has gone down, it is now concentrated in the poorest people living in the poorest communities.

When considering the response to sudden onset disasters, it is worth bearing in mind that as with all emergencies, there are recognised patterns that determine the type of medical response required, as illustrated in → Figures 23.10 and 23.11.

It is important to note that in an earthquake there may be two or three severely injured survivors for every death,

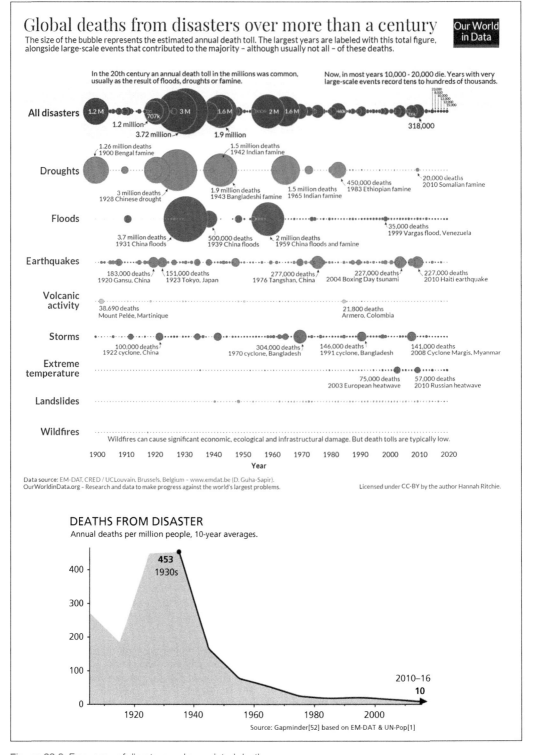

Global deaths from disasters over more than a century

The size of the bubble represents the estimated annual death toll. The largest years are labeled with this total figure, alongside large-scale events that contributed to the majority – although usually not all – of these deaths.

Our World in Data

In the 20th century an annual death toll in the millions was common, usually as the result of floods, droughts or famine.

Now, in most years 10,000 - 20,000 die. Years with very large-scale events record tens to hundreds of thousands.

All disasters 1.2 M 707k 3 M 1.6 M 2 M 1.6 M 460k 230k
1.2 million
3.72 million
1.9 million
318,000

Droughts
1.26 million deaths
1900 Bengal famine
1.5 million deaths
1942 Indian famine
3 million deaths
1928 Chinese drought
1.9 million deaths
1943 Bangladeshi famine
1.5 million deaths
1965 Indian famine
450,000 deaths
1983 Ethiopian famine
20,000 deaths
2010 Somalian famine

Floods
3.7 million deaths
1931 China floods
500,000 deaths
1939 China floods
2 million deaths
1959 China floods and famine
35,000 deaths
1999 Vargas flood, Venezuela

Earthquakes
183,000 deaths
1920 Gansu, China
151,000 deaths
1923 Tokyo, Japan
277,000 deaths
1976 Tangshan, China
227,000 deaths
2004 Boxing Day tsunami
227,000 deaths
2010 Haiti earthquake

Volcanic activity
38,690 deaths
Mount Pelée, Martinique
21,800 deaths
Armero, Colombia

Storms
100,000 deaths
1922 cyclone, China
304,000 deaths
1970 cyclone, Bangladesh
146,000 deaths
1991 cyclone, Bangladesh
141,000 deaths
2008 Cyclone Margis, Myanmar

Extreme temperature
75,000 deaths
2003 European heatwave
57,000 deaths
2010 Russian heatwave

Landslides

Wildfires
Wildfires can cause significant economic, ecological and infrastructural damage. But death tolls are typically low.

1900 1910 1920 1930 1940 1950 1960 1970 1980 1990 2000 2010 2020
Year

Data source: EM-DAT, CRED / UCLouvain, Brussels, Belgium – www.emdat.be (D. Guha-Sapir).
OurWorldinData.org – Research and data to make progress against the world's largest problems.

Licensed under CC-BY by the author Hannah Ritchie.

DEATHS FROM DISASTER
Annual deaths per million people, 10-year averages.

453
1930s

400

300

200

100

0

2010–16
10

1920   1940   1960   1980   2000

Source: Gapminder[52] based on EM-DAT & UN-Pop[1]

Figure 23.9 Frequency of disasters and associated deaths.

Effect	Earthquakes	High winds (without flooding)	Tidal waves/flash floods	Slow-onset floods	Landslides	Volcanoes/ Lahars
Deaths[a]	Many	Few	Many	Few	Many	Many
Severe injuries requiring extensive treatment	Many	Moderate	Few	Few	Few	Few
Increased risk of communicable diseases	Potential risk following all major disasters (Probability rising with overcrowding and deteriorating sanitation)					
Damage to health facilities	Severe (structure and equipment)	Severe	Severe but localized	Severe (equipment only)	Severe but localized	Severe (structure and equipment)
Damage to water systems	Severe	Light	Severe	Light	Severe but localized	Severe
Food shortage	Rare (may occur due to economic and logistic factors)		Common	Common	Rare	Rare
Major population movements	Rare (may occur in heavily damaged urban areas)		Common (generally limited)			

[a]Potential lethal impact in absence of preventive measures.

Figure 23.10 Short-term effects of major disasters. Source: Taken from 'Natural disasters; protecting the public's health' PAHO 2000.

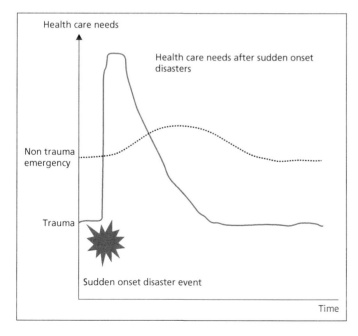

Figure 23.11 Healthcare needs after sudden onset disasters. Source: Taken from "A guidance document for medical teams responding to health emergencies in armed conflicts and other insecure environments." WHO 2021.

whereas after a tsunami there may be only one injured survivor for every nine deaths. When planning a response, it is clear that the surgical requirements in the aftermath of an earthquake are far greater than after a tsunami.

Equally important is an understanding of how the case-load changes over time. The majority of injured patients will require treatment in the hours and days that follow the onset of the disaster, which is often before international medical teams, even the most efficient, can arrive. Any immediately life-saving intervention will likely have been carried out by those present at the time or within no more than a few hours travelling time of the disaster. International teams, however quickly mobilised, will be unlikely to arrive in time to salvage those with severe chest or abdominal injuries, but may have a role to play in the management of non-immediately life-threatening injuries and certainly in assisting with reconstructive surgery. However, coincidental emergencies continue to present to what is now a very stressed health system, and international medical assistance can also be important in supporting and maintaining the delivery of *essential emergency healthcare*. Maternal and child health in particular will always need support, and WHO expects all medical teams that respond to have the capability for dealing with maternal and child health including delivery.

Almost by definition, disasters occur when the capacity of the healthcare system to respond is overwhelmed. Whilst we often use the term 'natural disasters', it is worth considering whether this phrase is always appropriate. There are obviously natural phenomena, earthquakes for example, but the disaster that follows too often represents a failure to prepare, and this like so much in global health is linked to socio-economic status. For example, buildings can be made earthquake resilient, but this costs money, and so the poor are disproportionately more vulnerable to the effects of natural phenomena. Just as we have largely removed the use of the word *accident* in medical practice, accepting there are no true accidents as they can usually be prevented, so we might wish to reconsider the use of the word *natural* when applied to disasters.

Just as good health is not entirely dependent on good healthcare alone but also requires political social and economic support; so effective emergency medical humanitarian assistance is equally dependent on a range of other inputs, most importantly the adequate supply of fresh drinking water, adequate sanitation, and food; shelter, and security.

EMTs must work in support of the national effort and not duplicate existing systems. By working through the UN/WHO channels, they will ensure that they fit into the national health system and can refer patients appropriately. Almost from the start of the deployment, the team must be planning its exit strategy so patients can be appropriately and safely referred back into the system that will continue to manage their care once the EMT has returned home.

EMTs working in disasters are required to make a medical record for each patient that complies with the national MoH requirements and obtain informed consent from patients, in their own language, for all procedures. Each patient should be given a discharge summary in their own language, and teams must liaise with national and UN authorities if they need assistance with translation.

Trauma and surgical care

It is important that the type of trauma care given has been appropriately adapted to the facilities in which the team is working and the constraints of the referral chain imposed by the wider impacts of the disaster. Resuscitation will be limited to life-saving initial care at the incident site, through to advanced trauma life support, depending on the type of EMT facility. A type I outpatient team, for example, will provide triage and assessment of injuries with basic stabilisation of fractures and wound cleaning and immediate discharge, or onward referral of patients who require general anaesthesia to a type II or type III facility. In general, in disasters, any procedure that can be carried out under local or regional anaesthesia should be, with general anaesthesia preserved for those cases where there is no alternative. Type II and type III facilities will deliver in-patient trauma care with wound debridement, closed fracture management with splintage and external fixation, and damage control surgery. Internal fixation is not recommended in these circumstances, as the risk of post-operative infection is too high. It is important that the medical team ensures appropriate follow-up for patients is established, e.g. the removal of external fixation.

There are established protocols for wound care in these environments, such as those developed by the ICRC. The key principles involve effective wound toilet, debridement, and delayed primary closure; the wounds inevitably involve an element of crush and contamination. In a type II/III facility, surgical capacity must extend to the construction of basic flaps and skin graft procedures to cover wound defects following debridement.

Careful consideration must be given to the role of amputation. The disability imposed by the loss of a limb for someone already living in impoverished circumstances is considerable. Even if supplied with a prosthesis by the initial team, the chances of the patient getting it replaced can be small. There can also be a social stigma associated with amputees in some cultures. EMTs should therefore try and preserve limb/limb-length as much as possible, and so are required to have an appropriately trained surgeon in their team when responding to emergencies where amputation is likely to be required. Guillotine amputations are no longer an acceptable surgical procedure and should be avoided. Decision-making in these circumstances can be facilitated by reference to the Mangled Extremity Scoring System and consensus guidelines.

Reconstructive surgery is an important feature of the surgical response after earthquakes in particular, and can be incorporated within the EMT itself or by the deployment of a specialist reconstructive surgical team to augment another EMT or a local health facility.

There are specialist burns management teams that deploy to disasters involving large numbers of burned patients. The management of individual burns must though be within the competencies of all EMTs.

Whether in a tent or in a more substantial facility, all EMTs carrying out surgery have to meet the minimum standards for instrument sterilisation as laid down in the WHO EMT *Blue Book*, with thorough cleansing of instruments followed by steam sterilisation or autoclave between every case.

Pharmacy and medicines management are core elements of an EMT and ensure appropriate and safe prescribing. The WHO model list of essential medicines is a good guide to generic medicine supplies for EMTs, but additional specialist medications will be required, for example when responding to outbreaks. If pharmaceuticals and/or equipment are to be donated when the team leave the country, then this must be done with the knowledge and consent of the local MoH and be at least 1 year from expiry/or meet the requirements of the national MoH.

Advances in technology mean that even in a field hospital, adequate imaging can be facilitated. At the very least, a portable ultrasound should be part of the equipment, but many teams also take portable X-ray facilities. Similarly point-of-care testing has greatly improved the laboratory support available to EMTs responding to a sudden onset disaster.

The surgical skills required are broad. They are often not present in a single individual or encapsulated in a single/subspecialty-orientated training programme, so additional training to broaden surgical expertise is recommended. One such course is the Surgical Training for the Austere Environment at the Royal College of Surgeons of England. Some teams may be able to accommodate the breadth of surgical expertise required by incorporating a number of individual specialists into the team. However this is achieved, teams will be expected to treat surgical cases in both adults and children, as well as surgical emergencies unrelated to the sudden onset disaster. Obstetric emergencies in particular require that each team has the capability to carry out a Caesarean Section safely, and if required, to support the local health service by relieving some of the burden of routine surgery and in particular non-disaster-related surgical emergencies.

Rehabilitation

Including rehabilitation expertise in the EMT ensures the rapid and safe discharge of patients thereby increasing capacity for new admissions. Rehabilitation itself can also deploy as a specialised facility to 'bolt on' to another team or embed within a MoH facility.

Outbreak response

The need for EMTs to respond to surgical health emergencies such as earthquakes is currently outweighed by the increasing demand for medical support to disease outbreaks. The WHO global surveillance system continuously monitors threats to public health and when necessary will activate the **Global Outbreak Alert and Response Network (GOARN)**. The EMT initiative is an important component of the global response, with teams increasingly responding to disease outbreaks including COVID-19, diphtheria, measles and ebola in recent years. As well as providing additional healthcare professionals to strengthen the response network, EMTs also provide technical support and training when requested. Teams are required to have been trained in safe working practices in the presence of dangerous pathogens and have in place robust protocols for the safe donning and doffing of PPE.

Conflicts

Delivering medical aid in a conflict adds another layer of complexity, not least because of the danger. It can also raise ethical issues, particularly when trying to adhere to the humanitarian principles. Aid agencies may consider one party to the conflict as being in much greater need than another, or even the innocent victims of an unprovoked violent campaign, but they must maintain their neutrality, impartiality and independence. There is international humanitarian law to guide all parties, but when this is ignored, the already considerable difficulties faced by humanitarian agencies can only be compounded. Nevertheless, 'humanitarian' agencies must continue to position themselves in the 'humanitarian space' (defined by the UN as the operational environment that allows humanitarian actors to provide assistance and services according to humanitarian principles and in line with international humanitarian law) and not align themselves with one party or another, perceived or otherwise; as perceptions can become distorted, either accidentally or deliberately. Agencies must be vigilant and continually reflect upon their work.

Unlike a sudden onset disaster where a single event precipitates an influx of casualties, medical teams working in conflicts must be prepared for repeated surges of patients, as hostilities wax and wane. The level of care that can be offered to patients is dependent very much on the maintenance of supply lines and evacuation routes. These are inevitably disrupted at times, or sometimes continuously, during conflicts. If a patient cannot be safely evacuated up a referral chain to definitive care, then teams must consider carefully how far they continue with resuscitation and interventions in an individual patient, knowing that the definitive care they need is not available in their forward station, and evacuation blocked by the conflict. As in so much in emergency humanitarian assistance, the level of care to an individual and its impact on resources, must be balanced against the broader standard of care that might be maintained if those same resources were distributed to a group or population.

There are obviously considerable risks inherent in responding to armed conflicts that cannot be removed but may be mitigated by detailed pre-deployment planning and preparation. Ill-prepared or ill-advised interventions bring significant risks to those who deploy, but also to their patients, and threaten the confidence of the affected population in humanitarian relief. It is imperative that those who deploy understand the detailed background to the conflict and the position within it of those who they are working alongside. Managing healthcare in such an environment requires a great deal of experience if interventions are not to be misconstrued or misrepresented, and a difficult situation made worse. There are guiding principles. Just as in medical practice everywhere, adherence to the four principles of ethical medical care (respect for autonomy, beneficence, non-maleficence and justice) must still be maintained along with technical standards and quality assurance. Importantly, there is international humanitarian law and the humanitarian principles. When these are breached, particularly with regard to impartiality, neutrality and independence, then the very concept of a *humanitarian space* can be brought into question.

The key features of international humanitarian law demand that combatants must

- not target people who are no longer engaged in the fighting;
- allow for impartial humanitarian assistance to be given to the civilian population and all wounded and sick in general, including those who have taken direct participation in hostilities ('hors de combat');
- not target those who are providing medical or humanitarian assistance;

- ensure that *all* wounded and sick receive medical care and the civilian population receive humanitarian assistance.

WHO has prepared a guidance document for medical teams responding to health emergencies in armed conflicts and other insecure environments (the "Red Book") to accompany the classification and standards for deployment to sudden-onset disasters (the "Blue Book).

Essential emergency healthcare

As indicated above, in both conflicts and sudden-onset disasters, coincidental emergencies continue to present, as represented by the dotted line on the graphs in *Figure 23.12*. Whatever the nature of the emergency to which they have been asked to respond, unless they are a specialist team embedding in another facility, EMTs must be prepared at all times to deliver and maintain *essential emergency healthcare*. In a crisis, patients will present to the nearest medical facility regardless of what those working in that facility consider their purpose to be; a patient in need will not discriminate. In essence, this means that teams must have protocols in place to manage three types of presentation:

- the direct consequences of the incident (e.g. trauma),
- coincidental emergencies that present during the crisis (e.g. acute myocardial infarction, complications of labour/pregnancy),
- chronic, non-urgent conditions that present to an emergency medical facility when this is likely to be the only source of medical support. Replenishing medication for chronic conditions (e.g. diabetes, hypertension and asthma) is a common presentation and teams should have a supply of such medications for outpatient use.

Dealing with the dead

When responding to disasters, including conflicts, it is almost inevitable that at some point there will be a large number of unburied dead. This is very distressing, the smell is overwhelming, and their presence provokes the fear of epidemics in the survivors. This fear is not unreasonable but is unfounded and not supported by the evidence. At its worst, this fear leads to precipitous burial and mass graves, with all the terrible long-term consequences for families in establishing whether their loved ones have died, and if so, where their bodies might lie. However, in a sudden-onset disaster (rather than a disease outbreak), the unburied dead pose little or no threat to the living. If there is to be a spontaneous disease outbreak, it will be

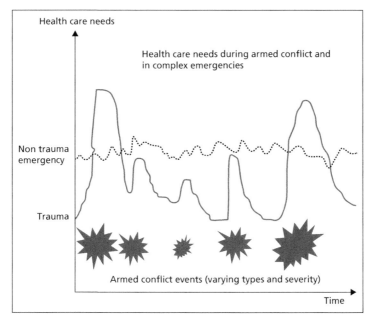

Figure 23.12 Healthcare needs during armed conflict. Source: Taken from "A guidance document for medical teams responding to health emergencies in armed conflicts and other insecure environments." WHO 2021.

from the mass movement of the living into inadequate living conditions with its consequent poor water quality, sanitation, and hygiene (WASH), leading to increased cases of diarrhoeal disease. Of course, if death is from an infectious disease that lives on after death, then there is a risk, but in practice this is essentially limited to the viral haemorrhagic fevers and cholera. It is to be noted that cholera is not an inevitable consequence of a sudden-onset disaster. Inadequate WASH can facilitate its transmission but when and where it is already endemic. For example, the cholera epidemic that followed the earthquake in Haiti, where it was not endemic, came some months afterwards, and is now recognised as having been brought into the country by international workers.

Index

Note: Page numbers followed by "*f*" refer to figures; "*t*" refer to tables and "*b*" refer to boxes

ABCDE assessment 1, 48–9
abciximab 195
abdomen
  examination 28, 29, 311*b*
    in pregnancy 326
  injuries 81–6
    hip symptoms 94
    imaging 84–5
    in pregnancy 32, 85–6
    spinal injuries 50
  pain 84, 310–23
    assessment and
      management 310
    central and lower
      abdomen 316–23
    children 365
    collapse 310, 311*b*
    genitourinary tract 323–4
    non-specific 322
    non-surgical causes 323
    oesophagus and upper
      abdomen 312–16
    perineal problems 324–5
    radiography 263, 316, 317, 319
  abdominal aortic aneurysm,
    leaking 317–18
abducens palsy 47
abductor pollicis brevis 123
abrasions 392, 411
abrin 304
Abrus precatorious 304
abscesses 424
accidents 19*b*, 454
  see also road traffic accidents
ACE inhibitors 195, 275
acetaminophen *see* paracetamol
acetazolamide 247, 263, 433, 434
N-acetylcysteine (NAC) 284–5,
  285*b*, 293
  adverse reactions 284
Achenbach's syndrome 131
Achilles tendonitis
  (tendonosis) 104
Achilles tendon rupture 104, 105
aciclovir 204, 354, 356, 441
acid burns 148–9

acquired immune deficiency
  syndrome (AIDS) 221, 337*b*
acromioclavicular joint
  disruption 114
activated charcoal for
  poisoning 280
  antidepressants 288
  aspirin 287
  beta blockers 287
  calcium channel blockers 288
  carbamazepine 290
  ibuprofen 287
  mefenamic acid 287
  mushroom poisoning 293
  paracetamol 282
  phenothiazines 291
  phenytoin 290
  salbutamol 287
  SSRIs 289
  theophylline 289
acute behavioural disturbance
  (ABD) 377–8
acute coronary syndromes
  (ACS) 185
  biochemical markers 191
  chest pain decision tools 194*b*
  diagnosis 185–6
  ECG 185, 186
  investigations 186
  without ST elevation 193–5
acute dystonic reactions 307–8
acute porphyrias 263, 263*b*
acute radiation syndrome (ARS)
  154–6, 155*b*
acute respiratory distress syndrome
  (ARDS) 80, 212
acute tubular necrosis 258*b*
acute vestibular syndrome 242–3
acute withdrawal syndrome 379–81
adder bites 299–300
Addison's disease 257, 259
adenosine 177, 179, 181
adenovirus 432
adhesive tapes 69
adrenal crisis 257
adrenaline

airway swelling, reducing 2
  anaphylaxis 306, 307*b*
  asthma 215
  bradycardia 175
  cardiac arrest 163, 166, 170
  cautions in hypothermia 249
  children
    bradycardia 175
    bronchiolitis 350
    croup 349
    meningococcal disease 354–5
    stridor 348
  dental extraction, bleeding
    after 441
  epiglottitis 440
  EpiPen injection injuries to
    hand 133
  hypothermia 169
  partial upper airway
    obstruction 209
adrenocortical suppression 10*b*
Adults with Incapacity Act
  (2000) 397
advance directives 398
advanced life support (ALS) 158
  adults 160*f*
  choking 205
  defibrillation 158
  drugs 158*b*
  trauma (ATLS) 20
    chain of care 21–2
    definitive care 29–30
    primary survey and resuscita-
      tion 20, 22–7
    secondary survey 21, 27–8
    training 20*b*
aerocele 45
aerosols 302
age factors *see* children; elderly
  people
age-standardised DALY rates 443,
  444*f*
aggression 294, 377
  head injuries 35
  hypoglycaemia 254
  relatives 390

The RCEM Lecture Notes: Emergency Medicine, Fifth Edition. Edited by Catherine Williams and Amy Nickson.
© 2024 John Wiley & Sons Ltd. Published 2024 by John Wiley & Sons Ltd.
Companion website: www.wiley.com/go/LNEM5

agonal rhythm 175
AIDS 221
airway 1–3
  allergic reactions 306
  artificial *see* artificial airway
  burns 142
  cardiac arrest 157, 158
  children 342
  collapsed patient 233
    cardiac arrest 161
    facial fractures 64
    head injuries 37, 38*b*
  obstruction 1–3
  surgical 2, 205
  trauma patients 22–3
alcohol and intoxication 379–83,
    394–7
  aggressive patients 294, 377
  blood samples 395–6
  brachial plexus injuries 117
  burns 143
  epigastric pain and
    tenderness 313
  forearm and wrist wounds 123
  head injuries 39, 40, 41*b*, 42, 44,
    46, 47
  hypoglycaemia confused with
    intoxication 254
  hypomagnesaemia and
    magnesium therapy 261
  legal limits for drivers 396*b*
  Mallory–Weiss syndrome 312
  pancreatitis 316
  peripheral neuropathies 244
  poisoning 278–80, 294–6
  variceal haemorrhage 314
  withdrawal 323, 388
alkaline burns 148
allergic conjunctivitis 432
allergic reactions 306–7
allopurinol 423
alteplase 192*b*, 229, 231, 241
altitude-related illness 247
altitude sickness 247
Amanita phalloides 293
amaurosis fugax 434
amethocaine 428
Ametop 368
amfetamines
  poisoning 294
  withdrawal 388
aminophylline 166, 215–7, 352
amiodarone
  cardiac arrest 163, 166
  CPR drugs 163
  first-degree heart block 173
  refractory VF/shock-resistant
    VF 161

shockable rhythm drugs 161
  torsade de pointes 181
  ventricular tachycardia 181
amitriptyline 204
ammonia poisoning 302, 303
ammonium nitrate poisoning 303
amnesia 36*b*, 40, 238
amniotic fluid embolism 167
amoxicillin 218, 221, 353, 364,
    439*b*, 441
amphetamines 292
ampicillin 354
AMPLE mnemonic, history
    taking 10
anaesthesia
  facial wounds 68
  hypoxic patient 3
  stridor in children 348
  see also local anaesthesia; general
    anaesthesia
anal fissure 325
analgesia 11
  abrasions 417
  acromioclavicular joint
    disruption 114
  acute coronary syndromes
    without ST elevation 193
  aortic aneurysm, leaking
    abdominal 317–18
  biliary disease 315–16
  bowel obstruction 320
  burns 141, 145, 146, 149
  children 346, 366
  clavicular fractures 113
  collapse 234
  distal radius fracture 127
  disturbed patients 377, 384
  elbow dislocation 120, 121
  frostbite 427
  head injuries 39
  humeral fractures 117, 118
  influenza 225
  limb problems 88
  migraine 239
  oesophageal pain and bleeding
    after vomiting 312–13
  pancreatitis 316
  paraphimosis 339
  peritonitis 317
  pleurisy 204
  pneumomediastinum 203
  porphyrias, acute 263
  pulmonary embolism 231
  radial fractures 124
  rib fractures 78
  rotator cuff injury 115
  scapular fractures 117
  and sedation 13, 14

shoulder dislocation 116, 116*b*
sickle cell disease 270
STEMI 190
temporal arteritis 239
tension headache 240
trauma patients 27, 30*b*
ulnar fractures 124
ureteric colic 323–4
vaginal bleeding in
    pregnancy 330
anaphylaxis 166, 299, 306, 307*b*
angina
  mesenteric 318
  stable (angina pectoris) 196–7
  unstable 185, 193, 197
angio-oedemas 274–6, 307
anion gap 235*b*, 279, 295–7
ankle problems 104–6, 105*f*, 106*b*
antacids 312, 313
antepartum haemorrhage 326–7
anterior cord syndrome 53
anthrax 269, 425*b*
antibiotics
  biliary disease 316
  bronchiectasis 218
  children 350, 350*t*
  chronic obstructive pulmonary
    disease 218
  hand injuries 133, 134, 140
  infective endocarditis 253
  limb problems 89
  oesophageal pain and bleeding
    after vomiting 313
  olecranon bursitis 123
  pancreatitis 316
  peritonitis 317
  pleurisy 204
  pneumonia 220, 221, 223, 353
  rocky mountain spotted fever 268
  sepsis and septic shock 251
  surgical emphysema 76
  trauma patients 28*b*
  urinary tract infection 335
  variceal haemorrhage 314
anticoagulation 180*b* 272, 273
anticonvulsants 346
antidepressants, poisoning 288
antidotes 281
antiemetics 14
antifreeze 295
antivenom 281, 299–300, 419
aortic aneurysms 5, 61*b* 317
aortic dissection 184, 197–9, 197*f*,
    198*t*
aortic flow 25*b*
APACHE (Acute Physiology and
    Chronic Health Evaluation),
    score 33

Apgar score 328*b*
apnoea, brain impact 47
appendicitis 319
'arc eye' 430
armed conflict 457*f*
arterial embolism 110
artesunate 265
artificial airway
    complete upper airway
        obstruction 209
    consciousness, depressed level
        of 2
    physical obstruction, bypassing 2
    trauma patients 22*b*
asphyxia 31, 80, 208, 393
aspiration pneumonia 32, 223
aspirin
    acute coronary syndromes
        without ST elevation 193
    contraindications 193
    Dressler's syndrome 201
    Kawasaki's disease 362
    migraine 239
    pericarditis 201
    poisoning 285–7
    STEMI 190
    stroke 241
    temporal arteritis 239
    transient ischaemic attack 242
asthma 213–8, 213*b*
    adults 213
    cardiac 219
    cardiac arrest 166
    children 216, 351–3
    investigations 214
    pre-discharge checklist 216*b*
    pregnancy 216
asystole 161, 170, 173
atelectasis 226
athlete's foot 423
atlantoaxial rotary subluxation 59
atrial fibrillation (AF) 177
    anticoagulation patients 180*b*
    fast 175*b*, 179, 181
    management 179–80
    stroke 180*t*, 241
    transient ischaemic attack 242
atrial flutter 177
atrial tachycardia 177
atrioventricular nodal re-entry
        circuits 176, 176*b*
atrioventricular nodal re-entry
        tachycardia (AVNRT) 176
atrioventricular re-entry tachycardia
        (AVRT) 176
atropine
    bradycardia 175, 195
    conjunctivitis 432

and ketamine 15
    poisoning 280
        beta blockers 287
        calcium channel blockers 288
        organophosphorus 304
    sinus bradycardia 195
    spinal cord injuries 54
autonomy 448
automated external defibrillator
        (AED) 158
avascular necrosis of the
        lunate 130
AV fistulas problems 130–1
avian influenza 225
AVPU scoring system 8
    head injuries 35
    sedation 14*b*
    trauma patients 27

Bacillus anthracis 269, 425
Bacillus cereus 266
back
    examination 28
    injuries 58–63
    pain 60–2, 60*b*, 61*b*
bacterial meningitis 355, 356
bacterial tracheitis 349–50
bad news, breaking 171
Baker's cyst rupture 102
balanitis 339
barotrauma from diving 246
Bartholin's gland abscess 335
Barton's fracture 127
basic life support (BLS) 158, 159*f*
Beck's triad 80
bee stings 419
Bell's palsy 442
beneficence 448
Bennett's fracture 139
benzatropine 307
benzodiazepines 14, 281, 290–3,
        291*t*, 307, 309
benzydamine 70
benzylpenicillin 246, 355, 440
bereaved relatives
    cardiac arrest 171
    trauma fatalities 32
bereavement nurses 172
berries, poisonous 298
beta blockers
    poisoning 287
    psychiatric syndromes 378
Bezold-Jarisch reflex 5
bicarbonate therapy
    cardiac arrest 163–4
    hyperkalaemia 260
    metabolic acidosis 264*b*
    poisoning 289

see also sodium bicarbonate
biceps, rupture of the long head
        of 115
bifascicular block 182–3
bilevel positive airway pressure
        (BPAP) 212
biliary colic 315
biliary disease 315–16
bird flu 225
bites 418
    adder 299–300
    cat 418
    dog 418
    to ear 71
    exotic creatures 419
    to face 69
    human 133, 136*b*, 418
    insect 418
    spider 418
bitumen burns 149–50
blackwater fever 265
bladder rupture 87
bladder stones 324
Blandford fly bites 418
blast injuries 30
bleach, poisoning 298
bleeding *see* blood loss
blepharitis 433
blepharospasm 428–30
blindness
    acute 434
    cortical 47, 434
    prevention in arteritis 239*b*
blink reflex 47
blood-borne viruses (BBVs) 422
blood components, transfusion
        of 270*b*
blood gas analysis
    asthma 214
    carbon monoxide poisoning
        300–1, 300*t*
    chronic obstructive pulmonary
        disease 217
    head injuries 35
    immediate 10
    organ perfusion 25*b*
    respiratory distress 218
blood loss
    antepartum 326–7
    AV fistulas 131
    cardiac arrest 167
    after dental extraction 441
    epistaxis 436–7
    intra-abdominal 318
    limbs 91
    management 5, 6*f*, 25–7
    postcoital 332
    from scalp 39

after tonsillectomy 441
trauma patients 24-7, 25*t*
blood pressure
cardiac arrest 170
children 343
circulation problems 5
orthostatic syncope 236
see also hypertension;
hypotension
blood transfusion 5
Jehovah's Witnesses 398
trauma patients 25-6
blow-out fracture of the orbit 71-2
blunt injury 80
body fluid exposure incidents 422
Boerhaave's syndrome 312
Böhler's angle, loss of 107, 108*f*
boils 424-5
Bornholm's disease 204
Borrelia burgdorferi 268
botulism 245, 246, 416
boutonnière deformity 138
boxer's fracture 136
box jellyfish 419
brachial plexus injuries 117
bradyarrhythmias 172
bradycardia 172, 173
children 175
poisoning 281, 287, 303, 304
sinus 195
spinal cord injuries 54
breast conditions 335
breathing 3
abnormal rate 3
allergic reactions 306
children 343*b*, 353
collapsed patient 233
head injuries 37
Kussmaul's respiration 263
oxygen therapy 3
paradoxical respiration 3, 53, 79
trauma patients 24
ventilatory support 3
breathlessness (dyspnoea) 3,
209-10, 224, 226
Briefings/debriefings 17
broad complex tachycardias 180
bromocriptine 308
bronchiectasis, acute
exacerbations 218-19
bronchiolitis 350-1
bronchitis, chronic 217
bronchodilators 351
bronchoscopy 213
bronchospasm 287, 304, 306
bronchus 79
Brown-Séquard syndrome 53
brown tail moth 419

brucellosis 269
bruises 392
B-type natriuretic peptide
(BNP) 219
bubonic plague 269
buccal mucosa, injuries 70
Budd-Chiari syndrome 314
budesonide 303, 349
bullous pemphigoid 273
bundle-branch block (BBB)
182, 182*t*
bunions 422
bupivacaine 94*b*, 95*b*
buprenorphine 388
Burkholderia mallei 269
Burkholderia pseudomallei 269
burns 141-56
forensic medicine 393
large 141-6
Lund-Browder chart 142, 144*f*
rule of nines 142, 143*f*
small 146-7
specialist services 146*t*
'button' batteries, ingested 298,
438-9, 439*b*

caesarean section 32
calamine lotion 419
calcaneal fracture 107
calcium channel blockers,
poisoning 287-8
calcium therapy 149, 163, 259-61
calcium chloride and calcium
gluconate, comparative
strength 261*b*
calf muscle strain/tear 104
Campylobacter jejuni 362
Canadian C-Spine rule 54-5, 55*f*
candidiasis 334
cannabinoid hyperemesis
syndrome 322-3
cannabis 293, 396*b*
capacity (to give consent) 397
capillary refill time 4
carbamazepine 177, 280, 290
carbon monoxide poisoning 142,
300-1, 300*t*
carboxyhaemoglobin (COHb) 300,
301*b*
cardiac arrest 157
advanced life support and
defibrillation 158
asystole 161, 170
basic life support 158, 159*f*
bereaved 171-2
cardiopulmonary
resuscitation 158
chain of survival 157

children 157, 163, 169-70, 342
drugs 163-4
electrocution 150
end tidal CO_2 162
extracorporeal CPR 164
fibrinolytics 164
fluids 164
gastric decompression 168
high-quality chest
compressions 161
hypothermia 169*b*, 248*b*
interventions and considerations,
CPR 161
magnesium 163
mechanical chest compression
devices 162
non-shockable rhythms 161
post-resuscitation care 170-1
potentially reversible
causes 162-3
pulmonary embolism 229
pulseless electrical activity 161
recognition 157-8
refractory VF/shock-resistant
VF 161
reversible causes 162-3
shockable rhythms 158, 161
sodium bicarbonate 163-4
special circumstances 165-9
ultrasound 164-5
unsuccessful resuscitation 171,
175
ventricular fibrillation 158, 168
cardiac asthma 219
cardiac contusion and
concussion 80
cardiac dysrhythmias 157, 172
agonal rhythm 175
atrial fibrillation, fast 179, 181
atrial flutter 177
atrial tachycardias 177
bifascicular block 182-3
bradycardia 172, 173, 175, 195
broad complex tachycardias 180
bundle branch block 182
heart block 172-3, 173*f*
intraventricular abnormalities of
conduction 183
irregular broad complex
tachycardia 181
junctional tachycardias 175
long Q-T syndromes 181-2
narrow complex tachycardia 175
pacemakers 173, 182, 182*t*
poisoning 281, 294
principles 172
regular broad complex
tachycardia 180, 181

cardiac dysrhythmias (*cont'd*)
    regular narrow complex
        tachycardia 177
    supraventricular
        tachycardia 176–7
    tachyarrhythmias 175
    tachycardia 178*f*
    torsade de pointes 181
    ventricular tachycardia 180–1
cardiac function 4
cardiac index 4
cardiac markers 186, 191, 192*f*, 193
cardiac output 4, 5
cardiac pacing 183
cardiac pain 323
cardiac tamponade 163, 168, 253
    head injuries 80
    trauma patients 24, 27
cardiogenic shock 250–2
cardiopulmonary resuscitation *see*
        resuscitation
cardiorespiratory arrest 4
cardiovascular parameters 343
cardiovascular problems
    cardiac tamponade 253
    endocarditis 252–3
    myocarditis 252
    palpitations 254
    shock 250–2
cardioversion 172, 177, 180, 181
carers *see* relatives and friends
carpal bones 127, 127*f*
carpal dislocation 128
carpal fractures 127
carpal tunnel syndrome 129
castor oil seeds 304
cataracts 150
cat bites 418
caterpillar stings 419
catheter problems 335
cauda equina syndrome 62–3
cauliflower ear 71
cefalexin (cephalexin) 336
cefotaxime
    bacterial tracheitis 350
    children 354, 364
    epiglottitis 440
ceftriaxone 354
cellulitis 423
    orbital 432–3
    pre-septal 432–3
central cord injury 64*b*
central cord syndrome 53, 53*b*
central pulse 4
    children 4, 343
    and fluid replacement 5
central venous cannulation 168, 170
central venous pressure 5

cephalohaematoma 44
cerebral contusions 47
cerebral malaria 238, 265
cerebral oedema
    after asphyxia 208
    children
        abuse 43
        diabetic ketoacidosis 357
        fits 346
    diabetic ketoacidosis 256, 357
    high-altitude 247
    hypothermia 248
    mannitol 38
    recognition and treatment 359*b*
cerebral pontine myelinolysis 262
cerebrospinal fluid (CSF)
    Guillain–Barré syndrome 245
    leakage 65
cerebrovascular events 240–2
    driving after 242
    transient ischaemic attacks 242
    vertebrobasilar 242*b*
cervical intervertebral disc
        prolapse 59
cervical nerve root pain 59
cervical spine
    clearance 54–8
    dislocation 53
    head injuries 34, 37, 37*b*, 38*b*
    imaging, children 55
    injuries 34, 54–5, 64–5
    lateral view 56–7, 56*f*
    protection
        airway intervention 2*b* 2–3
        head injuries 36*b*
        trauma patients 23
    radiography 29, 56
    trauma patients 23, 29
    see also neck
cervical spondylosis 59
cervical vertebral disc, traumatic
        herniation 53
Chagas' disease 252
chalazia/chalazion 433
charcoal *see* activated charcoal for
        poisoning
Charcot's triad 316
checklists usage, ED 17
chemicals
    burns 148, 439*b*
    contamination 151–2
    poisoning 301–2
chemotherapy 273
chest compression 158, 161–4,
        168–70
chest drains 24, 75, 76, 76*f*
chest examination 28
chest injuries 73–87

assessment and
        management 73–4
    chest wall and lungs 75–81
    radiography 74
    trauma patients 20, 24, 27
    ventilatory support 3
chest pain 184–204
    angina pectoris 196–7
    assessment and
        management 184
    dissecting aneurysm of the
        thoracic aorta 197–9
    intra-abdominal causes 204
    myocardial infarction and the
        acute coronary
        syndromes 185–97
    oesophagitis 204
    pericarditis 199
    pleurisy 204
    pneumomediastinum 196, 203
    pneumothorax 196, 201
    pulmonary embolism 184
    risk stratification 186
    shingles 204
    tracheitis 204
chest X-ray (CXR) 74*b*
    abdominal injuries 81–2
    anthrax 269
    asthma 214, 352
    blast injuries 30
    bronchiectasis 218
    chest pain 184, 186, 195,
        196, 203
    collapse in elderly people 236
    endocarditis 253
    great vessel injuries 80–1
    haemoptysis 232
    immediate 12
    interstitial lung disease 219
    lower airways 213
    myocarditis 252
    oesophageal food bolus
        impaction 438
    pancreatitis 316
    pleurisy 203
    pneumomediastinum 203
    pneumonia 221, 223
    pneumothorax 201
    pulmonary embolism 229
    renal failure 258
    respiratory distress 210, 231
    rib fractures 76–9
    stab wounds 417–18
    sternal fractures 79
    thoracic aortic dissection 198
    trauma patients 29, 30
    tuberculosis 225
chickenpox 204*b*

Chikungunya fever 267
child abuse 369–70, 394
 burns 146*b*
 head injuries 44*b*
 poisoning 305
 police, release of information
  to the 401
 see also safeguarding and non
  accidental injury
Child Protection Committee 404
Child Protection Conference 404
Child Protection Order 404
Child Protection Plan/
  Register 370*b*, 404
children 341–2
 abuse *see* child abuse
 analgesia 346
 assessment and
  management 342–8
 bacterial meningitis 355
 blood loss 5, 6*f*
 bradycardia 172, 175
 burns 142, 144–6
  abuse 146*b*
  Lund–Browder chart 142, 144*f*
 cardiac arrest 157
  advanced life support and
   defibrillation 158, 160*f*
  basic life support 158, 159*f*
  pulseless electrical activity 161
  ventricular fibrillation 158
 collapse 233
 communication with 347
 confidentiality 403–4
 congenital abnormalities 353
 consent 403–4
 cricothyroidotomy 22, 23*b*
 dentoalveolar abscess 441
 diabetic ketoacidosis 255, 357–8
 diarrhoea 362
 drowning 30–1
 dystonic reactions, acute 307
 earache 359
 elbow 113, 118
 encephalitis 356
 epiphyseal injuries 366
 epistaxis 436–7
 facial injuries 64, 68, 71
 facial palsy 442
 fits 9, 346
 flap wounds 417
 fluid replacement 5
 forearm fractures 124
 foreign bodies
  in ear 435
  eye 430
  in lower airways 213
  in nose 436

 swallowed 438
 throat 437–8
gastroenteritis 321
guttate psoriasis, acute 425–6
haemolytic uraemic
  syndrome 272
haemophilia 94
hand injuries 134, 137
head injuries 37*b*, 38*b*, 42–4
 cervical spine imaging 37, 38*b*
 non-accidental injury 42–3
 skull radiology 44, 44*b*
 transfers 40
hip problems 94, 96
hypoglycaemia 256
hypothermia 249
immunisation 347, 416
impetigo 424
intussusception 363
of Jehovah's Witnesses, blood
  transfusion 398, 404
Kawasaki's disease 361*b* 362
knee problems 102*b*
limp 95–6, 96*b*
malaria 265
measles 361
meningococcal disease 238,
  354–5
orbital cellulitis 432
osteochondritis 366
poisoning 365–6
 abuse 305
 activated charcoal 280
 adder bites 299
 beta blockers 287
 carbon monoxide 300
 cyanide 303
 emesis 298
 gastric lavage 280
 iron 295
 opioids 291
 organophosphorus 304
 paracetamol 282–4
poliomyelitis 266
protection 402
rashes 360–1
respiratory distress/
  problems 348–53
 asthma 213, 351–3
 bronchiolitis 350–1
 choking 205–8, 206*f*, 207*f*
 foreign bodies in lower
  airways 213
 investigations 210
 pneumonia 220, 353
 pulmonary embolism 227–31
 stridor and partial upper airway
  obstruction 208–9, 348–50

 wheezing in pre-school
  age 351
 retropharyngeal abscess 440
 safeguarding and non accidental
  injury 369–70
 scarlet fever 361–2
 sedation 13–14, 13*t*, 366–9
 self-harm 379, 383
 shoulder and upper arm
  problems 113
 size 341–2
 splenic injuries 84
 sudden infant death
  syndrome 371–2
 tibial fractures 103
 tonsillectomy, bleeding
  after 441
 torticollis 59
 trauma 22, 23*b*, 30, 31
 urinary tract infection 335*b*,
  335–6, 360
 viral meningitis 356
 vomiting 362–3
 see also infants
Children Act (1989) 402, 403
Children's Coma Scale 42, 345*b*
chin-lift manoeuvre 2
Chironex fleckeri 419
chloramphenicol 147, 429, 432
chlordiazepoxide 379
chlorine poisoning 302
chloroquine 265
chlorphenamine 307
chlorpromazine 263, 291, 308
choking 1*b*, 205–8, 206*f*, 207*f*
cholangitis 316
cholecystitis 204, 315, 316
cholera 267
cholinesterase inhibitor
  poisoning 304
chronic obstructive pulmonary
  disease (COPD)
 acute exacerbations 216–18
 oxygen therapy 3
 and pneumonia, distinguishing
  between 221
cimetidine 378
ciprofloxacin
 anthrax 269
 biliary disease 316
 Legionnaires' disease 223
 meningococcal disease 355
 pneumonia 222
 prostatitis 336
 typhoid fever 267
 variceal haemorrhage 314
circulation 4
 allergic reactions 306

circulation (*cont'd*)
  children 344
  collapsed patient 233–4
  head injuries 38
  poisoning 293
  trauma patients 24–7
circumferential burns 148
cirrhosis 314*b*
citalopram 182*b*
Civil Contingencies Act (2004) 12
civil detention orders 398
civility 18
civil wars and conflicts. *see* complex
    emergencies
clarithromycin
  cellulitis 423
  erysipelas 424
  nails through hands or puncture
      wounds 421
  pneumonia 221, 223, 353
  scarlet fever 362
  torsade de pointes 181
clay shoveller's shoulder 58
cleaning materials, poisoning 298
cleg fly bites 418
clergyman's knee 102
climbers 247
clindamycin 269, 274, 424
clinical forensic medicine *see*
    forensic medicine
clopidogrel 46, 190, 193, 196
closed loop communication 17
Clostridium botulinum 246
Clostridium perfringens 245, 274
Clostridium tetani 245, 415
clotrimazole 423
cluster headache 237, 240
Cluster System 449, 450*f*
coagulopathy 26
  of trauma 26*b*
co-amoxiclav
  bites 69, 418
  phlebitis 111
  pneumonia 221–3
  urinary tract infection 335
cocaine
  cardiac arrest 177
  chest pain 196
  poisoning 292
  psychiatric syndromes 378
  rhabdomyolysis and
      myoglobinuria 262
  withdrawal 388
coccyx, injury to the 63
codeine 291, 292
colic 365
collapse 233–46
  abdominal pain 310, 311*b*

acute vestibular syndrome 242–3
altitude-related illness 247
assessment and
    management 233–5
botulism 246
brainstem stroke 240
cerebrovascular events 240–2,
    250–4
children 235
cluster headache 240
convulsions (seizures) 243–4
decompression sickness 246–7
dermatological conditions 273–6
driving after 242
elderly people 235–6
Guillain–Barre syndrome (acute
    polyneuritis) 245
haematological conditions 270–3
headache 237–8, 237*b*
head injury 238
hyperpyrexia and
    hyperthermia 249–50
hypothermia 247–9, 249*b*
intracranial infection 238
labyrinthitis 243
of the lung 226
metabolic and endocrine
    disorders 254–64
migraine 239
neurological problems 236–46
non-epileptic attack disorder 244
peripheral neuropathies 244–5
poisoning 235
subarachnoid haemorrhage 238
syncope 236
temporal arteritis 239
tension headache 240
tetanus 245–6
transient global amnesia 242
transient ischaemic attacks
    242, 242*b*
transient loss of
    consciousness 236–7
venous thromboembolism
    prevention 258
ventriculoperitoneal shunts 240
at the wheel 397*b*
zoonoses and diseases 264–70
collateral ligament injury (of the
    knee) 98*b* 99
Colles' fracture 117, 126–7, 126*f*,
    126*b*–7*b*
coma
  brainstem stroke 240
  after cardiac arrest 165, 166
  collapse 234*b*
  hyperosmolar (non-ketotic)
      diabetic 256–7

hypoglycaemia 10*b*
  myxedema 257
  poisoning 287–96, 299, 300, 303
community-acquired
    pneumonia 221
compartment syndrome 89, 90, 112
complaints 406
complex emergencies 448
complex regional pain
    syndrome 130
computed tomographic pulmonary
    angiography (CTPA) 228,
    229, 230
computed tomography (CT)
  abdomen 84
  back pain 61
  bowel obstruction 320
  calcaneal fracture 107
  encephalitis 356
  facial injuries 65, 67, 72
  great vessel injuries 81
  headache 238
  head injuries 36, 37, 36*b*–8*b*, 41,
      41*b*, 43*b*, 45–7
    abducens palsy 47
    aerocele 45
    apnoea, brain impact 47
    cerebral contusions 47
    children 43*b*
    cortical blindness 47
    extradural haematoma 45
    skull fractures 43*b*, 44, 45
    subarachnoid
        haemorrhage 47, 238
    subdural haematoma 46
  hip 91
  hyponatraemia 262
  meningitis 355–6
  pelvis 86
  pneumothorax 201
  retropharyngeal abscess 440
  shoulder and upper arm 113
  sickle cell disease 271
  spinal trauma 49*b*
  subarachnoid haemorrhage 47,
      238
  transient ischaemic attack 242
  trauma patients 29
  ureteric colic 324
  Wernicke–Korsakoff
      syndrome 383
concussion 47
conestat alfa 276
confidentiality 402–4
confusional states 3, 375–7, 390
congenital abnormalities 353
conjunctival oedema, acute 432
conjunctivitis 432

consciousness
assessment in children 345
AVPU see AVPU scoring system
depressed level of 238, 255
airway 1–3
alcohol 39b
children 42
disability 5, 8
extradural haematoma 45
head injuries 34–6, 41, 45
hypoglycaemia 10b
poisoning 277, 291
trauma patients 23
loss of 34
transient 236
consent 397–8, 401–4
contact lens abrasions 433
contamination 151–6
continuous positive airway pressure
(CPAP) 211, 219, 220, 224, 303
contraceptive pills
emergency 332
venous thrombosis 110
controlled drugs 394, 395b
convulsions 243–4
alcohol withdrawal 379
antidepressant poisoning 288
see also fits and seizures
COPD see chronic obstructive
pulmonary disease
copper sulphate solution 149
Cordylobia anthropophaga 419
core/periphery temperature
gradient 25b
corneal abrasions 428–9
corneal erosion, recurrent 430
corneal ulcers 433
coronary artery bypass graft (CABG)
surgery 196
coronary heart disease (CHD) 185
coroners 405
cor pulmonale 217
cortical blindness 47, 434
cortical necrosis, acute 258
corticosteroids
adrenocortical suppression 10b
chronic obstructive pulmonary
disease 217
erythroderma 274
Guillain–Barré syndrome 245
Corynebacterium diphtheriae 439–40
co-trimoxazole 223
cough
bronchiectasis 218
chronic obstructive pulmonary
disease 217
pneumonia 220
rib fractures 76, 79

counselling 390
court orders 402
CPAP (continuous positive airway
pressure) 211, 219, 220,
224, 303
crack cocaine 292
cricothyroidotomy
complete upper airway
obstruction 205
facial injuries 64
needle 22b, 23b
partial upper airway
obstruction 209
site for 23f
surgical 22b
trauma patients 22, 23b
Crohn's disease 320
croup 349
cruciate ligament injury 99
crush–flexion injury 134f, 135f
crush wounds 417
crutches 91, 99–101, 103, 104, 106,
109, 110
crying infants 364
cryoprecipitate 270b
crystal arthropathy 100, 122, 123
CT see computed tomography
CURB-65 criteria, pneumonia
220, 221
Cushing's response 36, 38
cutaneous myiasis 419
CXR see chest X-ray
Cyanea capillata 419
cyanide poisoning 303
cyanosis 2b
cyclical vomiting syndrome 322
cyclizine 155
cyclopentolate 433
cyproheptadine 309
cystitis 324
cytomegalovirus (CMV)-negative
blood 26b, 32

damage control resuscitation 85
dantrolene 281, 308
Data Protection Act (1988) 402
D-dimer test
deep vein thrombosis 111
mesenteric vascular disease 319
pulmonary embolism 198, 224, 228
deadly nightshade 298
death 456–7
accidental 19, 42–3
alcohol-related 19, 383
aortic aneurysm, leaking
abdominal 317
asthma 213
botulism 246

cardiac arrest 157, 171, 172
cerebrovascular disease 240
children
abuse 44b
diabetic ketoacidosis 357
measles 361
sudden infant death
syndrome 371
cholangitis 316
clinical diagnosis 405
coronary heart disease 185
coroner 405
Covid-19 223
delirium tremens 381
diabetic ketoacidosis 255, 357
diphtheria 439–40
domestic violence 393–4
ectopic pregnancy 331
electrocution 150
gastrointestinal
haemorrhage 313b
generalised pustular psoriasis,
acute 273
glanders 269
Guillain–Barré syndrome 245
haemolytic uraemic
syndrome 272
head injuries 34b 42
hip fractures 92b
hypothermia 248b
influenza 224
irradiation 154
malaria 265
measles 361
mediastinitis 312
melioidosis 269
myocardial infarction 185
organ and tissue donation 406
pneumonia 220, 353
poisoning 282, 288, 293, 294, 296,
304
psychiatric patients, medical
conditions in 378
rabies 266
reporting 404–5
sudden infant death
syndrome 371
tetanus 245
trauma 19, 32–3
variceal haemorrhage 314
death cap mushrooms 293
decision-making 455
decompression sickness 246
deep hand space infections 140
deep vein thrombosis (DVT)
lower limb 110–111, 111t
pulmonary embolism 227, 229
upper limb 130

defibrillation 158, 161, 249
definitive care 12
  burns 145–6
  trauma patients 29–30
degenerative disease of the hip 94
degloving injuries 417
dehydration, children 344, 362
deliberate self-harm 385
delirium 375–9, 375b, 381
delirium tremens 381
demeclocycline 262
dementia 373, 376
dengue fever 267
dental extraction, bleeding
      after 441
dental injuries 70f, 70b
dentoalveolar abscess 441
depression 383–4
de Quervain's tenosynovitis 129
Dermatobia hominis 419
dermatological emergencies 273–4
dermatomes 50, 51f, 91
desferrioxamine 295
dexamethasone 224, 247, 356
dextrose 35, 346, 352
diabetes 444
  abdominal pain 323
  burns 143
  children 357
  cholecystitis, acute 315
  coronary heart disease 185
  endocarditis 252
  hyperosmolar (non-ketotic)
      diabetic coma 256, 257
  macular disease 434
  poisoning 288
  vitreous haemorrhage 434
diabetic ketoacidosis (DKA) 3,
      255–6
  children 357–8
dialysis-associated steal
      syndrome 130–1
diamorphine 190, 193, 369, 388
diaphragmatic irritation 323
diaphragmatic rupture 81
diarrhoea
  children 344, 362–3
  gastroenteritis 321
  travellers 266–7
disaster
  accident 454
  definition of 450
  frequency, deaths 452f
  healthcare needs 453f
  life-saving intervention 454
  natural 454
  short-term effects 453f
diazepam

alcohol withdrawal states 379
  convulsions 244
  dystonic reactions, acute 291
  fitting children 357
  head injuries 35, 39
  hyperthermia 281
  poisoning 307, 308
  rectal dose 357t
  sedation 14
diclofenac 324
dicobalt edetate 281, 304
diffuse axonal injury (DAI) 34, 47
digital nerve injuries 135
digoxin 163, 173, 177, 288, 378
dihydrocodeine 388
diltiazem 287
dimercaprol 305
dimercaptosuccinic acid
      (DMSA) 305
diphtheria 416, 439–40
dipyridamole 177
disability 5, 8
  children 345
  collapse 234
  trauma patients 19, 27
discharge criteria
  asthma 216
    children 353, 357
  epilepsy 244
  head injuries 42, 42b
  paracetamol poisoning 282
  sedation 15, 408
discitis 62
dishwasher products,
      poisoning 298
dissecting aneurysm of the thoracic
      aorta 197–9
distal interphalangeal (DIP)
      joint 134
distal phalangeal fractures 140
disturbed patient 374
  alcohol-related problems 379–83
  angry relatives 390
  anxiety disorders 386
  assessment and
      management 374–5
  confusion and psychotic
      behaviour 375–9
  counselling 390
  depressed
      mood and self-harm 383–5
  drugs
      requests for 386
      withdrawal from 386–8
  factitious, fabricated and induced
      illness (FII) 388–9
  interaction with 375
  learning disabilities 385

panic attack 386
  personality disorders 385–6
  post-traumatic stress
      disorder 390
  psychological support 389–90
  risk assessment, violence 390
  violence and aggression 390
diversional therapies 366–8
diverticular disease 319
dobutamine 231, 252b, 281, 287, 288
dog bites 418
domestic violence 393–4, 394b
do not attempt cardiopulmonary
      resuscitation decisions
      (DNACPR) 16–17
dopamine 354
dorsal penile nerve block 339b, 339f
doxapram 218
doxycycline 218, 221, 223, 268,
      269, 418
dressings 414
  burns 147
  skin grafts 417
Dressler's syndrome 201
driving
  after collapse/sudden illness
      cerebrovascular accident/
      transient ischaemic
      attack 242
      labyrinthitis 231
  and drugs 396
  and medical conditions 396–7
drooling, in partial upper airway
      obstruction 2
drowning 30–1, 168–9
drug-assisted sexual assault 394
drug-induced psychiatric
      syndromes 378
drug abuse
  anthrax 269, 425b
  botulism 246
  driving 396
  endocarditis 252
  forensic medicine 392
  gas gangrene 274
  head injuries 40
  hyperthermia 249
  hyponatraemia 261
  intra-arterial injection 110
  ischaemia of the hand 130
  necrotising soft tissue
      infections 274
  peripheral neuropathies 244
  poisoning 279, 282, 289, 291, 292
  psychiatric syndromes 379
  requests for drugs 386
  rhabdomyolysis and
      myoglobinuria 262

tetanus 245
venous disease 112
withdrawal 386–8
drunkenness *see* alcohol and
    intoxication
dyspepsia 313
dyspnoea 4, 208, 211, 213, 219
dystonic reactions, acute 307–8

earache 359–60, 442*b*
ear problems 71, 434–6
    burns 153
earring problems 434–6
Ebola fever 266
ECG *see* electrocardiography
echocardiography
    endocarditis 253
    pericarditis 199
    pulmonary embolism 230
    pulse and blood pressure 5
echo in life support (ELS) 164
eclampsia 167, 327–8
ecstasy (MDMA)
    hyperthermia 249
    hyponatraemia 261
    poisoning 292
    rhabdomyolysis and
        myoglobinuria 262
ectopic pregnancy 331–2, 331*f*
elbow 118, 119*b*, 119*f*
elderly people
    abuse 394
    accidental deaths 19
    bullous pemphigoid 273
    burns 145
    central cord syndrome 53, 53*b*
    chest pain 186, 204
    choking 205
    cholangitis 316
    cholecystitis, acute 315
    collapse 235–6
    confusional states 375–6
    diabetic ketoacidosis 255
    drug-induced psychiatric
        syndromes 378
    facial injuries 64*b*, 66
    forearm problems 122
    giant cell arteritis 239
    glaucoma 433
    haemolytic uraemic
        syndrome 272
    haemophilia, acquired 271
    head injuries 36, 37, 46
    hip problems 94
    hypercalcaemia 260
    hyponatraemia 261
    hypothermia 248
    hypovolaemia 24

immediate investigations 12
influenza 224
knee problems 98
liberty, deprivation of 398
malaria 265
mesenteric vascular disease 318
oxygen saturation 3
pelvic fractures 86
peritonitis 317
pneumonia 220
pretibial lacerations 419–20
pulmonary embolism 227
sedation 14
sepsis and septic shock 251
shoulder and upper arm
        problems 115
spinal cord injuries 53
stroke 241
syncope 236
temporomandibular joint
        dislocation 66
tetanus 245, 415–16
urinary tract infection 335*b*
electrical burns 143, 147, 148
electrocardiography (ECG)
    acute coronary syndromes 185,
        186
        without ST elevation 193
    antidepressant poisoning 288
    aortic aneurysms, leaking
        abdominal 317
    atrial flutter 177
    atrial tachycardias 177
    atrioventricular nodal re-entry
        tachycardia 176
    atrioventricular re-entry
        tachycardia 176
    bundle-branch blocks 182*t*
    cardiac arrest 165, 170
    cardiac dysrhythmias 172
    cardiogenic shock 252
    chest pain 184, 186
    electrocution 150
    endocarditis 253
    haemoptysis 232
    heart and great vessel injuries 79
    hyperkalaemia 259
    hypokalaemia 260
    hypothermia 248
    immediate 10, 12
    long Q-T syndromes 181
    myocardial infarction 186,
        189, 190*b*
    palpitations 254
    pericarditis 199
    pulmonary embolism 229, 229*b*
    reperfusion therapy 187–90
    respiratory distress 231

STEMI 187, 188
supraventricular tachycardia 176
torsades de pointes 181*f*
ventricular tachycardia 180
electrocution 150–1
electromechanical dissociation
    (EMD) *see* pulseless
    electrical activity
elevated lactate
    (LLACTATESS) 234*b*–5*b*
emergencies 444
Emergency Care course 445
Emergency Care System Assessment
    tool 445
Emergency Care System
    Framework 445, 446*f*
emergency contraception 332
Emergency Medical Teams
    (EMT) 449–50, 451*f*
emergency medicine 443
    humanitarian assistance 445
    income and lifespan 444*f*
    low-/middle-income
        countries 445
emergency procedures, general
    ABCDE assessment 1
    airway 1–3
    breathing 3
    circulation 4
    disability 5, 8
    environment and exposure 8–9
    fits 9
    glucose 9–10
    history 10
    immediate next steps 10
    management 11–12
    point of care ultrasound 10–11
    pulse and blood pressure 5
    sedation and general
        anaesthesia 13–18
Emergency Protection Order
    (EPO) 404
Emergency Triage, Assessment and
    Treatment (ETAT) 445
emesis 298
Emla cream 368
emotional abuse of children 371
emphysema 217
encephalitis 238, 268, 269, 356
endocarditis 252–3, 253*b*
end-of-life care 15–16
endoscopy, variceal
    haemorrhage 314
endotracheal intubation 2
    burns 142
    children and infants 343
    upper airway obstruction 209
end tidal CO_2 162

enoxaparin 193, 230*b*
Entamoeba histolytica 266
Entonox 15, 369
envenoming 299
environment 8–9
    children 345
    collapsed patients 234
epicondylitis 122
epididymis pain 324
epididymo-orchitis 336
epiglottitis 209, 440
    children 349
epilepsy 244
    abdominal pain 323
    burns 143
    children 357
EpiPen injection injuries 133
epiphyseal injuries in children 366
episcleritis 432
epistaxis 436–7
eptifibatide 195
ergometrine 327
erysipelas 424
erythema infectiosum 361
erythema nodosum 425
erythromycin 181
Escherichia coli
    cholangitis 316
    neutropenic sepsis 273
    O157 267
        bloody diarrhoea in children
            362
        haemolytic uraemic syndrome
            272
    prostatitis 336
    urinary tract infection 335
escitalopram 182*b*
esmolol 161
essential emergency healthcare
    443, 456
ethambutol 226
ethyl alcohol 294
ethylene glycol poisoning 295–297,
    297*f*
euglycaemic diabetic ketoacidosis
    255
Euproctis chrysorrhoea 419
examination
    immediate 11
    trauma patients 27–8
exanthem subitum 361
explosions 30
exposure 8–9
    children 345
    collapse 234
    trauma patients 27
extracorporeal CPR (ECPR) 164
extradural haematoma 45, 45*b*, 46

eyelid problems 72, 416
eye problems 65, 69, 71–2, 428–34
    burns 147

face
    injuries 64–72
        burns 147
        fractures 64–8
        wounds 68–9
    pain 441–2
    palsy 442
    sensory loss 65, 66*b*
    surgical emphysema 65, 66*b*
factitious and induced illness 388–9
fainting 236
falls
    biomechanics 21*b* 34
    calcaneal fractures 107
    clavicle fracture 113
    deaths from 19
    facial injuries 64
    great vessel injuries 81
    head injuries 34, 45
    hip injuries 94
    humeral neck fracture 117
    multiple injuries 19
    pelvic injuries 86
    radial head/neck fractures 121
    sprained wrist 128
    supracondylar fractures 120
false black widow spider 418
family *see* relatives and friends
fascia iliaca block 94*b*
feet
    bones 108*f*
    calcaneal fractures 107
    foot drop 244
    forefoot fractures 109–10
    foreign bodies 421
    hair tourniquets 421
    nails through 421
    pain 109
    puncture wounds 420
    talar fractures 107
    tarsometatarsal fractures/
        dislocations 109
    toe fractures 110
femoral artery occlusion 110
femoral fractures 91–3, 93*b* 95
femoral hernia 92, 93*b* 94
femoral nerve block 95*b*
femoral stretch test 94
femoral vein 112
fentanyl 14, 369
fetocardiotocography (FCTG) 86
fibrinolytics 164
fibular fractures 100, 103
fifth disease 361

filgrastim 273
finger injuries 136–9
first-degree heart (AV) block 172–3
first disease 361
fish, scombroid (toxic effects) 299
fish hooks 421
fits and seizures
    anoxic 236, 243
    after cardiac arrest 165, 166
    children 346, 356–7
    collapse 234
    head injuries 35, 39
    see also convulsions
fixed second-degree heart block
        173
flail segment 79
flap wounds 417
flecainide 181
flexor tendon injuries 135*b*
flexor tendon sheath infection 140
flucloxacillin
    bacterial tracheitis 350
    cellulitis 423
    endocarditis 253
    impetigo 424
    limb problems 89
    nails through hands or feet 421
    rashes 360
    spinal epidural abscess 62
fluid replacement 5
    burns 145*b*
    children 345
    electrocution 151
    see also intravenous (IV) fluids
flumazenil 14, 281, 291, 369
flunitrazepam 394
fluorescein 430, 431, 433
fomepizole 296
fondaparinux 193
food poisoning 267, 300
foot *see* feet
foot drop 244
forearm problems 123–30
forefoot fractures 109–10
foreign bodies
    in airway 1–2, 1*b*
        upper airway 205
    in ear 435
    in eye 430
    in hands and feet 421
    inhaled 342*b*
    in limbs 89
    in lower airway 213
    in nose 436
    radiography 413
    in rectum 324
    subtarsal 429–30
    swallowed 438

in throat 437–8
in vagina 334
forensic medicine
  asphyxia 393
  child abuse 394
  description of injuries 392
  domestic violence 393–4
  elder abuse 394
  rape and sexual assault 394
  types of wounds 392–3
  violent crime 393
fosphenytoin sodium 244
Fournier's gangrene of the scrotum 274
frail injured patients (FRIPs) 31
Francisella tularensis 425
Freedom of Information Act (2000) 402
fresh frozen plasma (FFP), transfusion 270*b*
frostbite 427
frozen shoulder 117–18
functional illness 389
furosemide 220, 260, 262
furuncles 424–5
fusidic acid 424

gag reflex 2*b*
Galleazzi fracture of radius 124*f*
gallstones 315–16
gamma-hydroxybutyrate (GHB)
  poisoning 293
  sexual assault 394
garden substances, poisonous 298
gases, noxious 303
gas gangrene 245, 274, 415
gastric carcinoma 313
gastric decontamination 280–1
gastric dilatation 84
gastric lavage 280, 293
gastric ulcer 313
gastritis 313
gastroenteritis 321–2
  children 362
  intestinal obstruction misdiagnosed as 320*b*
gastrointestinal haemorrhage 313–14
GCS *see* Glasgow Coma Scale
general anaesthesia
  drugs 14–15
  facial injuries 68
  facilities for the administration of 13–14
  head injuries 134
  rib fractures 78
  skin grafts 417
  small wounds 418, 424

see also sedation
generalised pustular psoriasis, acute 273
genitourinary problems 323–4, 335–40
gentamicin 253, 316, 429
German measles (rubella) 361
giant cell arteritis 239
giant hogweed 149
Gillick ruling 403
gingival injuries 70
glanders 269
glandular fever 439*b*
Glasgow Coma Scale (GCS) 34–5, 35*t*
  children 345
  head injuries 34–6, 35*b*–8*b*, 39–41, 41*b*
  sedation 14*b*
  trauma patients 27
glaucoma 433
Global Alliance for the Care of the Injured (GACI) 445
Global Burden of Disease (GBD) 443
global health
  conflicts 455–456
  definition of 443
  outbreak response 455
Global Health Cluster 449
Global Health Strategy
  pillars 443
Global Outbreak Alert and Response Network (GOARN) 455
glucagon 10, 255, 281, 287, 346
glucose 9–10
  acute coronary syndromes without ST elevation 195
  cardiac arrest 165
  children 346
  collapse 234
  diabetic ketoacidosis 255
  hypoglycaemia 10*b*, 254
  trauma patients 27
  see also hyperglycaemia; hypoglycaemia
glyceryl trinitrate (GTN) 184–5
  acute coronary syndromes without ST elevation 195
  angina pectoris 196
  oesophagitis 204
  pulmonary oedema 220*b*
  STEMI 190
glycol poisoning 296
glycoprotein IIb/IIIa inhibitors 193, 195
golfer's elbow 122
gonorrhoea 100

gout, acute 423
great vessel injuries 80–1
Greenstick fractures 125
GTN *see* glyceryl trinitrate
Guillain–Barré syndrome (acute polyneuritis) 245
Guillotine amputations 455
gunshot wounds 30, 76, 418
gurgling sounds, partial upper airway obstruction 2
guttate psoriasis, acute 425–6
gynaecological problems 323, 326–40

haemarthrosis of the knee 99, 100
haematocrit 5, 24–6
Haematopota pluvialis 418
haematuria in the absence of signs of infection 336
haemopericardium 80
haemophilia 26–7, 94
  acquired 271, 313
Haemophilus influenzae
  bacterial tracheitis 349
  chronic obstructive pulmonary disease 218
  type b (Hib)
    epiglottitis 440
haemoptysis 218, 225, 227, 232
haemorrhage *see* blood loss
haemorrhagic fevers 266
haemorrhoids 325
haemothorax 75–6
haemotympanum 45
hair tourniquets around the digits 421
hallucinosis, acute alcohol 381
haloperidol 377, 378, 381
Hamman's sign 203
hands 132
  burns 147–8
  finger injuries 136–9
  foreign bodies in the 421
  hair tourniquets 421
  immediate assessment and management 132–3
  infections 140
  ischaemia 130
  median and ulnar nerve supply to muscles involved in movements of the 123*b*
  metacarpal fractures 136
  nails through 421
  thumb injuries 139–40
  wounds 133–5
Hartmann's solution 5, 259
head
  examination 28

head (*cont'd*)
  injuries 34
    advice to discharged
      patients 42
    ambulant patients 40–4
    biomechanics 34
    in children 42–4
    collapse 234*b*
    complications 41, 47
    consciousness, depressed
      level of 34–5
    electrocution 151
    non-accidental 42–3
    observation following 41
    radiology 44
    specific injuries 44–7
headache 237–8, 237*b*
health emergencies 443
Health Protection (Notification)
    Regulations (2010) 407*b*
health reform 443
hearing loss 435, 436
heart blocks
  complete 173, 173*f*
heart failure 252, 257
heart injuries 80
heart sounds, absent/quiet 4
heart transplant patients 177
heat exhaustion/heat stroke 250
heavy metal poisoning 305–6
Heimlich's manoeuvre 205
Helicobacter pylori 313
Heliox 209, 215
heparin
  acute coronary syndromes
     without ST elevation 193
  atrial fibrillation 180
  diabetic ketoacidosis 256
  low platelets 271
  pulmonary embolism 227
  STEMI 192*b*
  venous thrombosis
hepatic encephalopathy 257–8
hepatitis 315
  B 332*b*, 416, 422
  C 422
Heracleum mantegazzianum 149
heroin
  anthrax 269
  withdrawal 386
herpes simplex infections 424
herpes zoster 323
hidradenitis suppurativa 424
high-pressure hose injection
    injuries 133
HiNTS exam 243*b*
hip 91–7
  extra-articular problems 94

history taking
  children 346
  collapse 234
  hand injuries 132
  head injuries 36*b*, 40, 44
  immediate 10, 11
  trauma patients 27
HIV 238, 252, 337–8
  blood and body fluid exposure
    needlestick injuries 422
    sexual exposure 338
hoarseness, partial upper airway
    obstruction 2
homelessness 12
Horner's syndrome 117
hospital-acquired pneumonia 222
hot tar burns 149–50
household substances,
    poisoning 298
housemaid's knee 102
human bot fly 419, 420*f*
human factors, ED 17–18
human immunodeficiency virus
    see HIV
humanitarian principles
  adaption 448
  autonomy 448
  beneficence 448
  humanitarian charter 448
  humanity 445
  impartiality 448
  independence 448
  justice 448
  maleficence 448
  neutrality 445
humanitarian space 455–456
humanitarianism 445
humanity 445
human tetanus
    immunoglobulin 416
hydrocortisone
  adrenal crisis 257
  adrenocortical suppression 10*b*
  allergic reactions 299
  asthma 215
    children 352
  chronic obstructive pulmonary
    disease 218
  sepsis and septic shock 251
  stings 419
  sunburn 143
  thyrotoxicosis 257
hydrofluoric acid burns 148–9
hydrogen sulphide poisoning 303
hydroxocobalamin 303, 304
Hymenoptera 419
hyperbaric therapy 247
hypercalcaemia 260

hyperemesis gravidarum 330
hyperglycaemia 27, 38
hyperglycaemic hyperosmolar
    syndrome 256–7
hyperkalaemia 258, 259, 259*b*, 262
hyperlipidaemia 185
hyperosmolar (non-ketotic) diabetic
    coma 256, 257
hyperpyrexia 249–50
hypertension 445
  coronary heart disease 185
  malignant 254
hypertensive encephalopathy 254
hyperthermia 249–50
hyperventilation 37, 214, 231
hyphaema 428, 429*f*
hypocalcaemia 26, 148, 149, 260–1
hypoglycaemia 10*b*, 254–5
  children 32, 345*b*, 346, 356, 363
  consciousness, depressed level
    of 8*b*, 9–10
  disturbed patients 374, 376
  head injuries 35
  trauma patients 27, 32
hypokalaemia 162, 165, 214, 260
hypomagnesaemia 261
hyponatraemia 261–2
hyposplenism 221
hypotension
  antidepressant poisoning 288
  head injuries 38
  spinal cord injuries 54
hypothermia 247–9
  burns in children 144
  cardiac arrest 162, 169
  caused by rapid blood
    transfusion 26
  trauma patients 26*b*, 27*b*
    children 32
hypothyroidism 257
hypovolaemia
  abdominal trauma in
    pregnancy 82
  autonomic response 5
  cardiac arrest 162, 168
  fluid replacement 5
  heart rate, slow 4
  limb problems 88*b*
  oxygen therapy 3
  spinal cord injuries 54
  trauma patients 24
    pregnancy 32
hypovolaemic shock 250
hypoxia
  anaesthesia, emergency
    induction of 3
  carbon monoxide poisoning 300
  cardiac arrest 162, 168

disturbed patients 376
drowning 30
heart rate, slow 4
oxygen therapy 3
pulmonary oedema 219
trauma patients 24
pregnancy 32
ventilatory support 3

iatrogenic priapism 340
ibuprofen
children 346b
poisoning 287
icatibant 276
iloprost 133
immediate assessment and
management 11b
airway 1–3
analgesia 10
breathing 3
circulation 4
disability 5, 8
environment and exposure 8–9
fits 9
glucose 9–10
history 10, 11
investigations 10, 12
point of care ultrasound 10–11
pulse and blood pressure 5
immunisations
children 347, 366
diphtheria 416, 439–40
tetanus 416
immunocompromised patients
blood transfusion 26b
irradiation 142
measles 361b
neutropenic sepsis 273
osteomyelitis 423
impartiality 448
impetigo 424
incised wounds 392
independence 448
indigestion symptoms 186
inequalities 443, 444
infants
abuse 44b
bronchiolitis 350
cardiac arrest 167
central pulse < 60 beats/min 4
choking 205
colic, three months, 365
crying 365
drowning 30
fluid replacement 5
hair tourniquets around the
digits 421
head injuries 40, 42

hypoglycaemia 27
supraventricular tachycardia 177,
179
trauma 22
infections, localised 422–7
infective endocarditis 252
inflammations, localised 422–7
inflammatory bowel disease 319–20
influenza 224–5
immunisation 245
infraorbital fracture 66
infraorbital nerve 65
ingrowing toenails 427
inhalation injury 141–2, 145b
Injury Severity Score (ISS) 33
inquests 404–5
insects
bites 418
in ear 435
insulin
acute coronary syndromes
without ST elevation 195
diabetic ketoacidosis 255
hyperkalaemia 259
hyperosmolar diabetic coma 256
hypoglycaemia 254
poisoning 288
Integrated Management of Adult/
Adolescent Illness (IMAI) 445
interferon-γ-release assay (IGRA) 225
intermediate phalangeal fractures
138
intermittent positive-pressure
ventilation (IPPV)
chronic obstructive pulmonary
disease 218
haemothorax 76
heart injuries 80
pneumothorax 76
pulmonary oedema 220
International Committee of the Red
Cross (ICRC) 445
international humanitarian law 456
International Liaison Committee on
Resuscitation (ILCOR) 157
International Search and Rescue
Advisory Group
(INSARAG) 449
interphalangeal joint,
dislocation 140
interstitial lung disease 219
intestinal obstruction 320
intra-abdominal bleeding 318
intra-arterial injection 110
intracranial haematoma 37, 37t, 41,
41b, 42, 44b
intracranial infection 238
intracranial pressure (ICP), increased

Cushing's response 36, 38
extradural haematoma 45
head injuries 36–9, 45
intubation in non-paralysed
patient 24b
meningococcal disease 355
Intralipid 412b
intraosseous cannulation 344b
intrauterine contraceptive devices
(IUCDs) 332
intravenous (IV) crystalloids 25
intravenous (IV) fluids
burns 145, 145b
cardiac arrest 169
contraindications 25
diabetic ketoacidosis 255
hyperemesis gravidarum 330
hypothermia 248
rhabdomyolysis and
myoglobinuria 262
sepsis and septic shock 251
spinal cord injuries 54
trauma patients 25
warmed 8, 25
intravenous urography (IVU) 324
intraventricular abnormalities of
conduction 183
intubation
endotracheal see endotracheal
intubation
head injury patients 37, 38b
trauma patients 24
intussusception 363
investigations
immediate 10
trauma patients 28–9
ionising radiation, types of 152b
IPPV see intermittent positivepres-
sure ventilation
ipratropium 215, 217
iritis 433
iron poisoning 295, 295t
irradiation 151–6
irritable hip 96
ischaemic colitis 318
isoniazid 226
isoprenaline 177, 281, 287
itraconazole 181

jaw-thrust manoeuvre 2, 48
Jehovah's Witnesses 398
jellyfish stings 419
Jequirity bean 304
jugular venous pulse (JVP), raised 4
junctional tachycardias 175

Kanavel's signs 140
Kawasaki's disease 361, 362

keratitis, marginal 433
ketamine
    children, sedation with 369
    poisoning 293
    sedation 15
    sexual assault 394
ketoconazole 181
Klebsiella spp. 273 335
    K. pneumoniae 223
Klein's line 97
knee problems 98–102
Köhler's disease 109
Korsakoff's syndrome 383
Kussmaul's respiration 255
Kussmaul's sign 80

labetalol 253, 254
labial abscess 335
laburnum seeds 298
labyrinthitis 243
lacerations 392
    pretibial 419-20
large bowel obstruction 320
laryngitis 439
laryngoscopy 205, 209
larynx
    injuries 79
Lassa fever 266
lateral epicondylar fractures 121
lead poisoning 305–6, 323
leaking abdominal aortic
        aneurysm 310b, 317–18
learning disabilities, people
        with 385, 398
Le Fort fractures 67, 67b, 67f
left bundle-branch block
        (LBBB) 170, 182, 189
    treatment 190
left ventricular aneurysm 195
left ventricular failure (LVF) 219
legal issues *see* medicolegal issues
Legionnaires' disease 221, 223
lenograstim 273
leptospirosis 315
levonorgestrel 332
liberty, deprivation of 398
lichen planus 426
lidocaine
    boils 424
    cardiac arrest 161, 163
    chest drain insertion 77b
    children 360
    cutaneous myiasis 419
    ear problems 435
    EpiPen injection injuries to
        hand 133
    fish hook injuries 421
    paraphimosis 339

pneumothorax 203
    torsade de pointes 181
    ventricular tachycardia 181
life-threatening electrolyte
        disorders 165–6
lightning injury 150–1, 151b
limbs
    bleeding 89
    compartment syndrome 89
    crutches 91
    examination, trauma patients 28
    fractures 88–9
    general approach to
        problems 88–91
    immediate assessment and
        management 88–9
    local injection of steroids 91
    occlusion 89
    pain 89
    physiotherapy 90
    plaster casts 89–90
    radiographs 89
    sports injuries 91
    vascular problems 89
    wounds 89
    see also lower limb; upper limb
limping child 95–6
lion's mane jellyfish 419
Lisfranc's fracture 105, 106, 109
lithium poisoning 290
liver damage/disease
    ethylene glycol poisoning 296
    paracetamol poisoning 282–4
local anaesthesia
    chest drain insertion 77b
    children 369
    eye problems 428b
    facial injuries 68, 69
    hand injuries 132–4
    limb problems 89
    pneumothorax 203
    sea urchin spines 421
    toxicity 412b
localised infectious and
        inflammations 422–7
Local Safeguarding Children Board
        (LSCB) 404
log roll 49b
long Q-T syndromes 181–2, 182b
loose bodies in elbow 122
lorazepam
    convulsions and fits 244, 357
    disturbed patients 377–9, 381
    head injuries 35, 39
lower airways and lungs 209
    acute breathlessness 209–10
    acute respiratory distress
        syndrome 212

asthma in adults 213–16
bronchiectasis, acute
        exacerbations 218–19
chronic obstructive pulmonary
        disease, acute
        exacerbations 216–18
collapse of lung (atelectasis) 226
cough 232
foreign bodies 213
haemoptysis 232
hyperventilation syndrome 231
influenza 224–5
interstitial lung disease 219
investigations in respiratory
        distress 210
Legionnaires' disease 223
pleural effusion 226–7, 227b
pneumonia 220–3
pulmonary embolism 227–31,
        229b, 230b
pulmonary hypertension 231
pulmonary oedema 219–20,
        219b, 220f
pulse oximetry 210–11
Q fever 223
respiratory arrest 209
respiratory failure 211–12
severe acute respiratory
        syndrome (SARS) 223–4
tuberculosis 225–6, 225f
vaping 232
lower leg 102–4
lower limb
    ankle 104–6
    foot 106–10
    hip 91–6
    knee 98–102
    lower leg 102–4
    thigh 91–6
    vascular conditions 110–12
low-molecular-weight heparin
        (LMWH)
    acute coronary syndromes
        without ST elevation 193,
        195
    diabetic ketoacidosis 256
    hyperosmolar diabetic coma 257
    pulmonary embolism 230, 231
    venous thrombosis 111
Ludwig's angina 440
lumbar disc lesions 94
lumbar puncture 238, 356
    contraindications 356b
lumbar spine 60, 61b, 94
lumbosacral spine injury 56
lunate, avascular necrosis of
        the 130
Lund–Browder chart 142, 144f

lungs *see* lower airways and lungs
Lyme disease 173, 252, 268–9
lymphogranuloma venereum
  (LGV) 325
lysergic acid diethylamide
  (LSD) 293, 378

macular disease of the eye 434
'magic mushrooms' 294
magnesium therapy 182, 261
  asthma 216
  cardiac arrest 161, 163, 165–7
  eclampsia 328
  torsade de pointes 181
  ventricular dysrhythmias 181,
    182*b*
magnetic resonance imaging (MRI)
  Achilles tendonitis 104
  Achilles tendon rupture 104
  ankle 106
  back pain 59, 62
  contraindications 37
  diffuse axonal injury 47
  hip 93, 94
  knee 99
  spine 58
  subarachnoid haemorrhage 238
  wrist 128
magnet ingestion 298–9
Maisonneuve's fracture 100, 107
major incidents 12
malar fractures 66–7
malaria 265
malathion 427
maleficence 448
mallet finger 138–9
Mallory–Weiss syndrome 312
mandibular fractures 65–6, 66*b*
mannitol 38, 262
Marburg fever 266
march fracture 110
marginal keratitis 433
marijuana 293
mast cell tryptase 307
MDMA *see* ecstasy
measles 361
mechanical chest compression 162
mechanical ventilation
  head injury patients 37, 38*b*
  trauma patients 24
medial epicondylar fractures 121
median nerve 128, 129, 133
mediastinitis 312
medicolegal issues 392
  alcohol and other drugs/fitness to
    drive 394–7
  blood transfusion for Jehovah's
    Witnesses 398

chaperones 407
children, responsibilities to 403–4
clinical forensic medicine 392–4
common law, treatment
  under 403
complaints 406–7
consent 397–8
death 404–6
Freedom of Information Act 402
incompetent patients 398
legal issues 397–403
mental health act 398–400
notifiable diseases 407–8, 407*b*
police, release of information to
  the 401–2
police custody 400–1
professional witnesses 402–3
sedative/opioid drugs 408
witness statements 403
mefenamic acid 287
melioidosis 269
Mendelson's syndrome (aspiration
  pneumonia) 32
meningitis 238, 355–6
  bacterial 355
  children 356
  meningococcal 356
  viral 356
meningococcal disease 238
  children 354–5
  travel 238
meniscal injuries of the knee 99
Mental Capacity Act (2005) 397, 403
mental disturbance *see* disturbed
  patient
Mental Health Act (1983), 398–400,
  399*b*
mental state
  examination 374
  organ perfusion 25*b*
  poisoning 305
  see also consciousness
mephedrone poisoning 294
meralgia paraesthetica 94
mercury poisoning 305
mesenteric angina 318
mesenteric infarction 318
mesenteric vascular disease 318–19
mesenteric venous thrombosis 319
metabolic acidosis 248, 259, 263–4
  poisoning 277, 279
    aspirin 285
    calcium channel blockers 287
    ethylene glycol 296
    methanol 295, 296
    theophylline 289
    tricyclic antidepressants 288–9
metabolic alkalosis 264, 264*b*

metabolic disorders 234, 254–64
  acute porphyrias 263, 263*b*
  Addison's disease 257
  adrenal crisis 257
  diabetic ketoacidosis 255, 255*b*,
    256*b*
  hepatic encephalopathy 257–8
  hypercalcaemia 260
  hyperglycaemic hyperosmolar
    syndrome 256–7
  hyperkalaemia 259, 259*b*
  hyperpyrexia 249–50
  hyperthermia 249–50
  hypocalcaemia and tetany 260–1
  hypoglycaemia 254–5
  hypokalaemia 260, 260*b*
  hypomagnesaemia and magne-
    sium therapy 261
  hyponatraemia 261–2
  hypothermia 247–9
  inherited metabolic diseases 263
  metabolic acidosis 263–4
  metabolic alkalosis 264, 264*b*
  myxoedema coma 257
  potassium redistribution 259–60
  renal failure 258–9
  rhabdomyolysis and
    myoglobinuria 262
  thyrotoxicosis 257
metacarpal fractures 136
metacarpophalangeal (MCP) joint
  dislocation 136–7, 140
  ligament injuries 137
  thumb 139–40
metatarsal fractures 109–10
metatarsalgia 109
metformin 288
methadone
  long Q–T syndromes 182*b*
  respiratory rate, slow 3
  withdrawal 388
methaemoglobinaemia 292, 302–3
methanol poisoning 295–7, 297*f*
methionine 285
methotrexate 332
methylprednisolone 239
methylthioninium chloride
  (methylene blue) 302
meticillin-resistant *Staphylococcus
  aureus* (MRSA) 253, 273
metoclopramide 193, 190, 239, 330
metronidazole
  bites 418
  botulism 246
  dentoalveolar abscess 441
  gas gangrene 274
  peritonitis 317
  tetanus 246

midazolam
  convulsions and fits
    children 357
  disturbed patients 377
  elixir 369
  sedation 14
mid-cycle pain 334
migraine 237, 239, 242, 243, 323, 434
milk
  gastroenteritis 322
  poisoning 298
missing prostate sign 86
Misuse of Drugs Act (1971) 394, 395*b*
Misuse of Drugs (Notification of and Supply to Addicts) (Northern Ireland) Regulations (1973) 394–5
Misuse of Drugs Regulations (2001) 395*b*
Misuse of Drugs (Supply to Addicts) Regulations (1997) 394
mitral regurgitation 196
Mobitz type, 1 heart block 173
Mobitz type, 2 heart block 173
Monteggia fracture of ulna 124*f*
mortality *see* death
mountain sickness, acute (AMS) 247
mouth problems 437–41
  burns around the mouth 147
  injuries inside the mouth 65, 69–71
MPH (Microporous Polysaccharide Hemospheres) 27
MRI *see* magnetic resonance imaging
MRSA 253, 273
multiple injuries
  Advanced Trauma Life Support 20
  chain of care 21–2
  epidemiology 19–20
  prehospital care 21, 21*b*
  preparation for patient reception 20
  primary survey and resuscitation 20, 22–7
  secondary survey 21, 27–8
  spinal cord injuries masking 50
  see also trauma, major
multiple sclerosis (MS) 244–5
mumps 442
mupirocin 424
musculoskeletal chest pain 204
mushroom poisoning 293–4
mustard gas poisoning 301

myalgia, viral 204
myasthenia gravis 245
Mycobacterium tuberculosis 225
mydriasis, traumatic 431
myelitis, acute (transverse) 244
myocardial infarction (MI) 184, 444–5
  back pain 61*b*
  biochemical markers 191
  complications 195–6
  diagnosis 185–6
  electrocardiography 187–90, 188*b*, 190*b*
  heart block 173
  non-ST elevation myocardial infarction (NSTEMI) 193
  oesophageal pain 312
  post-infarction pericarditis 200
  pulmonary oedema 219
  pulseless electric activity 161
  subendocardial infarction 193, 194*b*
  treatment 195–6
  see also ST-segment elevation myocardial infarction
myocardial ischaemia 319, 323
myocardial pain 312*b*
myocarditis 252
myoglobinuria 262
myxoedema 257

nails through hands or feet 421
naloxone 14, 35, 292
narcosis 34
narrow complex tachycardia 175
nasal problems 436–7
  burns 142
  fractures 67–8
nasotracheal intubation 22*b*
National Institute for Health and Clinical Excellence (NICE) 90
National Society for the Prevention of Cruelty to Children (NSPCC) 404
natural disasters 454
navicular bone, prominent 109
neck
  examination 28
  injuries 58–64
  pain 59
  see also cervical spine
necrotising fasciitis 274
necrotising soft tissue infections 274
needle cricothyroidotomy 22*b*, 23*b*, 205
needlestick injuries 422
needle thoracocentesis 77*b*

neglect of children 371
neomycin 432
nephrotic syndrome 259
neurogenic shock 54
neuroleptic malignant syndrome 291, 308
neurological assessment 36
neurological problems
  acute vestibular syndrome (vertigo) 242–3
  botulism 246
  brainstem stroke 240
  cerebrovascular events 240–2
  convulsions (seizures) 243–4
  Guillain–Barré syndrome (acute polyneuritis) 245
  headache 237–8, 237*b*, 240
  head injuries 238
  intracranial infection 238
  migraine 239
  non-epileptic attack disorder 244
  peripheral neuropathies 244–5
  subarachnoid haemorrhage 238
  temporal arteritis 239
  tetanus 245–6
  transient global amnesia 242
  transient ischaemic attack 242
  transient loss of consciousness 236–7
  ventriculoperitoneal shunts 240
neurosurgical consultation guidelines 39–40
neutrality 445
neutropenic sepsis 273
NICE 90
nifedipine 247, 288
nimodipine 47, 238
nitrates 184, 190, 195, 220
nitrofurantoin 335, 336
nitrous oxide
  analgesia 15
  ankle dislocation 107
  sedation 15
non-accidental head injury (NAHI) 42–3
non-invasive ventilation (NIV) 212, 212*b*, 215, 218
non-shockable rhythms 161
non-ST elevation myocardial infarction (NSTEMI) 193
non-steroidal anti-inflammatory drugs (NSAIDs)
  Achilles tendonitis 104
  back pain 58
  degenerative disease of elbow joint 122
  epicondylitis 122
  eye problems 429*b*

frozen shoulder 118
migraine 239
olecranon bursitis 123
pericarditis 200
peripatellar bursitis 102
peritendonitis crepitans 129
phlebitis 111
plantar fasciitis 109
pleurisy 204
poisoning 287
supraspinatus tendinitis/
    subacromial bursitis 115
tension headache 240
ureteric colic 324
whiplash injury 58
noradrenaline 288
Noro (Norwalk) virus 266, 322
nose see nasal problems
notifiable diseases 407–8, 407*b*
NSAIDs see non-steroidal anti-
    inflammatory drugs
NSPCC 404

oak processionary moth 419
obesity
    coronary heart disease 185
obstetric problems see pregnancy
occlusion, vascular (of the limbs) 89
octreotide 314
oculogyric crises 245, 307, 308
oesophageal food bolus
        impaction 438
oesophageal injuries 81
oesophageal pain 312
oesophageal spasm 312*b*
oesophagitis 204, 312
Offences Against the Person Act
        (1861) 392
Office for the Coordination of
        Humanitarian Affairs
        (OCHA) 448
oil-based veterinary vaccine
        injection injuries 133
older people see elderly people
olecranon bursitis 122–3
olecranon fractures 121
Ombudsman (for health) 407
omeprazole 32, 312, 313
ondansetron 155
On-Site Operations Coordination
        Centre (OSOCC) 448
opiates/opioids
    children 346*b*
    head injuries 39
    limb problems 89
    poisoning 291–2
    sedation and analgesia 14–15
    withdrawal 386–8

opiate toxicity 35
oral contraceptives
    poisoning 295
    venous thrombosis, risks of 110
oral rehydration solution 322*b*
orbit, blow-out fracture of the 71–2
orbital cellulitis 432–3
orf 425
organ donation 406, 406*b*
organophosphorus poisoning 304
organ perfusion 25*b*
orotracheal intubation 22*b*
orthopantomograms (OPTs/
        OPGs) 66
orthostatic syncope 236
oseltamivir 225
Osgood–Schlatter disease 102
osmolar gap 234, 235*b*, 279, 297
osmotic demyelination syndrome 262
osteoarthrosis
    carpometacarpal joint 130
    elbow 122
    hip fractures 92
    knee problems 100
    tibial condyle fractures 100
    whiplash injury 58
    wrist 130
osteochondritis 366
osteochondritis dissecans 100, 101*f*
osteomyelitis 423
osteoporosis
    back pain 60, 61
    calcaneal fracture 107
    collapsed vertebra 323
    distal radius fracture 126
    hip fractures 91, 92*b*
    tibial condyle fractures 100
otitis externa 434–5
otitis media 359, 360, 434
ovarian cysts 323, 334
ovarian hyperstimulation
        syndrome 334
oxybuprocaine 428
oxygen saturation 3
oxygen therapy 3
    acute coronary syndromes
        without ST elevation 193
    asthma 217
    breathlessness, acute 209
    bronchiectasis 218
    carbon monoxide poisoning 301
    cardiac arrest 168
    children 343
    chronic obstructive pulmonary
        disease 217
    cyanide poisoning 303
    partial upper airway
        obstruction 209

pulmonary embolism 231
respiratory failure 211
STEMI 190
traumatic asphyxia syndrome 80
oxytocin 327

Pabrinex 381, 383
pacemakers
    codes 182*t*
    identification 172, 182
Paddington Alcohol Test 382, 383
paediatrics see children
pain
    assessment 10*b*
    head injuries 39
    relief of 11, 13*b*
        see also analgesia
    trauma patients 24
pallor
    breathing problems 3
    cardiac dysrhythmias 172
    chest pain 185*b*, 186
    circulation problems 4
palpitations 254
pancreatitis 197, 204, 316
PaO$_2$
    asthma 214
    burns 142*b*
    chronic obstructive pulmonary
        disease 218*b*
    estimation of expected 211
    respiratory failure 211
paracetamol (acetaminophen)
    hyperpyrexia 249
    migraine 239
    poisoning 258, 282–5, 283*f*
    sore throat 439
    tension headache 240
paralysis 50
    late onset after spinal injury 54
paralytic ileus 320
paraphimosis 339
paronychial infections 426
paroxysmal hemicrania 240
Participant Workbook 445
Pasteurella multicida 418
patella 98*b*-9*b*
    bipartite 101*f*
    dislocation 101
    injuries 101
patellar apprehension test 101
patellofemoral
        osteochondritis 101–2
peak expiratory flow rate (PEFR)
    asthma 214, 215
    children 351, 352*f*
    predicted (adults) 214
pelvic binder 26*f*

pelvic inflammatory disease (PID)
323, 333–4, 333b
pelvis
avulsion fractures 94–5
injuries 25, 29, 86–7
trauma radiograph 29
pemphigoid, bullous 273
penetrating injury 80
penicillamine 305
penile discharge 337
pepper spray 302
peptic ulceration 193, 204, 313
percutaneous coronary intervention
(PCI, percutaneous
transluminal coronary
angioplasty) 190–1, 199
perianal abscess 324
perianal irritation 325
pericardiocentesis 253
pericarditis 199
constrictive 314
perineal problems 87, 324–5
burns 148
peripatellar bursitis 102
peripheral neuropathies 244–5
peritendonitis crepitans 129
peritonitis 316–17
permethrin 427
personality disorders 385–6
Perthes' disease 96–97, 97f
pethidine 263
pharyngitis 439
phenobarbital 280, 284
phenol 148, 152
phenothiazines 291
phentolamine 133
phenylephrine 340
phenytoin 244, 289, 290, 357, 381
phlebitis 111
phlegmasia cerulea dolens 90
phosgene poisoning 303
phosphorus burns 149
Physalia physalis 419
physiotherapy
Achilles tendonitis 104
bronchiectasis 218
calf muscle strain/tear 104
degenerative disease, hip 94
epicondylitis 122
frozen shoulder 118
knee problems 99
limb injuries 90
patella dislocation 101
patellofemoral
osteochondritis 101
peritendonitis crepitans 129
plantar fasciitis 109
rotator cuff injury 115

shoulder dislocation 116
supraspinatus tendinitis/
subacromial bursitis 115
thoracic outlet obstruction 118
pilocarpine 433
pilonidal abscess 324
piperacillin 222, 273, 314, 316,
317, 319
pituitary damage 43b
pityriasis rosea 426
plague 269
plantar fasciitis 109
plants, poisoning 298
Plasmodium falciparum 265
Plasmodium malariae 265
Plasmodium ovale 265
Plasmodium vivax 265
plaster casts 89–90
ankle problems 107
foot problems 110
lower leg 89
thumb injuries 139
wrist fractures 125
platelet concentrates,
transfusion 270b
platelets, low 271
pleurisy 203–4, 323
Pneumocystis jiroveci
pneumonia 223
pneumomediastinum 203, 441
pneumonia 220–3
abdominal pain 323
aspiration 32, 223
atypical pathogens 223
children 353
community-acquired 221
hospital-acquired 222
increased risk of infection 221
Legionnaires' disease 223
Pneumocystis jiroveci 223
pneumonic plague 269
pneumothorax 75–6, 75b, 201–3
aspiration technique 203b
asthma 213b
oxygen therapy 3
spontaneous 201
tension 24, 75, 75b, 77b, 201
traumatic 24, 75
ventilatory support 3b
point of care ultrasound
(POCUS) 5, 10–11
poisoning
atypical reactions to drugs and
other substances 306–9
biochemical abnormalities
279–80, 279b–80b
cardiac arrest 166
children 365–6, 384

abuse 305
chronic 289, 305
considerations 305–6
forensic aspects 306
general principles 277–82
heavy metal 305–6
information services 282
mental state and psychiatric
assessment 305
self-harm 384
with common medicines 282–91
with harmful agents released into
environment 301–5
with recreational and illegal
drugs 291–4
with substances found at home
and at work 295–301
police
custody, patients in 400–1
release of information to
the 401–2
requests for blood samples 396
Police and Criminal Evidence
(PACE) Act (1984) 402
Police Protection Order (PPO) 404
Police Reform Act (2002) 395
poliomyelitis 266
polonium-210, 153b 154
polytrauma see multiple injuries
popliteal artery, damage to 98
porphyria 263, 323
portal hypertension 314
Portuguese man-of-war
jellyfish 419
positive end-expiratory pressure
(PEEP) 303
posterior cord syndrome 53
posterior segment injuries
(eye) 431
post-exposure prophylaxis after
sexual exposure (PEPSE) 338
postpartum haemorrhage 327
post-resuscitation care 170–1
post-traumatic amnesia (PTA) 40
post-traumatic stress disorder
(PTSD) 390, 393
potassium permanganate 153
pralidoxime 304
prasugrel 190
precipitant delivery 326, 327b
prednisolone
asthma 215, 216
children 353
chronic obstructive pulmonary
disease 218
croup 349
facial palsy 436
gout, acute 423

sciatica 62
temporal arteritis 239
pre-eclampsia 328
pregnancy 328–30
   asthma 216
   blood transfusion 25–6
   carbon monoxide poisoning
      301
   carpal tunnel syndrome 129
   cardiac arrest 166–7
   consent issues 397–8
   diabetic ketoacidosis 256
   ectopic 331–2
   hyperemesis gravidarum 330
   malaria 265
   maternal health 347
   pulmonary embolism 230
   Q fever 223
   trauma in 32, 85
   vaginal bleeding 330
   vasovagal syncope 236
prehospital care
   ketamine 15
   trauma patients 21
preparation for reception of trauma
      victims 20
pressure sores 93
pretibial haematomas 420
pretibial lacerations 419–20
pretibial pain 103–4
priapism, iatrogenic 340
prilocaine 127b, 368
procainamide 181
prochlorperazine 239, 243, 263
procurator fiscal 405
procyclidine 291, 308
prolapse of an intervertebral disc
      (PID) 62
propofol 14
propranolol 287
prostatitis 336
Proteus spp. 335 336
prothrombin complex concentrate
      (PCC), 271, 272b
proximal interphalangeal (PIP) joint
      injuries 137–8
proximal phalangeal fractures 137,
      137f 140
pruritis ani 325
Pseudomonas spp. 420b
   P. aeruginosa 273
psoriasis 273, 274
   acute guttate 425–6
psychiatric assessment, in
      poisoning 305
psychiatric patients, medical
      conditions in 378–9
psychoactive substances 294

psychological disturbance *see*
      disturbed patient
psychoses 378
pubic rami fractures 93
pulled elbow 119–20
pulmonary embolism (PE) 90, 167,
      184, 197, 227–31
pulmonary oedema 219–20, 219b
   high-altitude 247
   neurogenic 38
   traumatic asphyxia syndrome 80
pulse 5
pulseless electrical activity (PEA) 4,
      161
pulse oximetry
   airway obstruction 2
   asthma in children 215, 348, 350
   breathing problems 3
   carbon monoxide
      poisoning 301b
   chronic obstructive pulmonary
      disease 217
   oxygen therapy 3
   respiratory distress 210
   sedation, patient selection for 14
   upper airway obstruction 208
pulsus paradoxus 80
puncture wounds of the feet 420
purpura fulminans 355
purpuric rash 354
pustular psoriasis, acute
      generalised 273
pyelitis 324
pyelonephritis 328, 335, 336
pyrazinamide 226

Q fever 223
quadriceps injuries 101
Quantiflex machine 15
quinidine 181
quinine 265
quinsy 439

rabies 265–6, 266b
radial fractures 127
radial styloid fracture 127
radiation sickness 154, 154b, 155
radioactive substances 152–3
radioactivity/radiation
      measurement 153b
radiography
   ankle 106, 106b, 107
   chest 74, 74f
   elbow 118–19, 119b
      in children 113
   face 64–5
   femoral shaft fractures 95
   foot 107, 109, 110

forearm and wrist 123
foreign bodies
   in lower airways 213
   swallowed 438
haemothorax 75
hand 133–5, 137–9
hip 91–4
immediate 12
knee 99b, 99, 100b
limb problems 89
lower leg 103, 103b
mesenteric vascular disease 319
nails through hands or feet 421
oesophageal food bolus
      impaction 438
oesophageal injuries 81
osteomyelitis 423
pelvic injuries 86
pneumothorax 75
pulmonary embolism 227–31
pulmonary oedema 219–20,
      219b, 220f
septic arthritis 422
shoulder and upper arm 113
spine 54–8
   back pain 60–1
   whiplash injury 58
stab wounds 417
sternal fracture 79
surgical emphysema 76
tension pneumothorax 77b
trauma patients 27–9
tuberculosis 225–6
upper airway obstruction 208
ureteric colic 323
radius, fractures 121
Ramsay Hunt syndrome 442b
ranitidine 32
rape and sexual assault 394
   post-exposure prophylaxis 332–3
rashes
   children 360–1
rattling sounds, partial upper airway
      obstruction 2
reconstructive surgery 455
recovery position
   airway protection 2
   sedated patients 14
rectal bleeding 324–5
rectal examination 311b
rectum, foreign bodies in the 324
red cell concentrates,
      transfusion 270b
red eye 432
referred pain at shoulder 118
refractory VF/shock-resistant
      VF 161
refusal of treatment 403

rehabilitation 455
reimplantation of body parts 414
relatives and friends
  angry 390–1
  bereaved see bereaved relatives
  cardiac arrest patients 171
  communication 11
  consent 397–8
  distressed 374
  head injury patients 37*t*,
    38*b* 42–4
  trauma patients 27*b*
renal calculi 323, 324*b*
renal colic 204, 310*b*, 323–4
renal failure 236, 253, 254, 256–9,
  262, 263, 265, 268
renal injuries 84
Renshaw cells 245
reperfusion therapy
  ECG 187
  STEMI 190–1
rescue breaths 169
respiration see breathing
respiratory arrest 209
respiratory depression 281, 293, 303
respiratory distress 205
  lower airways and lungs 209–32
  upper airways 205–9
respiratory failure 53–4, 206, 217
resuscitation
  cardiac arrest 157, 164–7
    post-resuscitation care 170–1
    unsuccessful resuscitation 171
  children and infants 371–2
  contamination 153
  fluid replacement 5
  head injuries 35*b*, 39*b*
  hypothermia 249
  irradiation 155
  newborn 328*b*
  sedation/general anaesthesia,
    facilities for the administra-
    tion of 14
  trauma patients 20–1, 27
Resuscitation Council (UK) 157,
  177
resuscitative hysterotomy 167*b*
resuscitative thoracotomy 27
reticular activating system (RAS) 8
retinal arterial occlusion 434
retinal detachment 433–4
retinal venous occlusion 434
retrobulbar haemorrhage 67
retrograde amnesia 40
retroperitoneal injuries 84
retropharyngeal abscess 440
Revised Trauma Score (RTS) 33
re-warming in hypothermia 249*b*

rhabdomyolysis 261–2
rheumatoid arthritis 55
rib fractures 76–9
Richter's hernia 320
ricin 304
Rickettsia prowazeki 268
Rickettsia rickettsi 268
rifampicin 226, 253, 269, 284, 355
right bundle-branch block
  (RBBB) 182
right ventricular myocardial
  infarction 195, 188*b*
ring block, 412*b* 421, 426
risk management 17
road traffic accidents 19*b*
  biomechanics 21*b*, 34
  blood specimens 395
  drugs 396
  great vessel injuries 81
  head injuries 34, 42
  medical conditions 396–7
  police, release of information to
    the 401–2
  whiplash injuries 58
Road Traffic Act (1988) 396, 397,
  401
rocky mountain spotted fever 268
roller injuries 417
roseola infantum 361
rotator cuff injury 115
rubella 361
rule of nines 142, 143*f*, 150
rust rings in the cornea 430

safeguarding and non accidental
  injury 369–70
safety netting 17
SAG-M blood 26
St John's wort 284
salbutamol
  allergic reactions 306
  asthma 215, 216
  children 351, 352
  burns 141, 142
  chronic obstructive pulmonary
    disease 217
  hyperkalaemia 259
  poisoning 287
saline
  alcohol poisoning 279
  diabetic ketoacidosis 255
    children 351
  hyponatraemia 262
  metabolic acidosis 263
  metabolic alkalosis 264*b*
  variceal haemorrhage 314
salivary glands, swollen 440
Salmonella spp. 266

S. paratyphi 266, 267
S. typhi 267
Salter–Harris classification of
  epiphyseal injuries 366,
  367*f*
Salter Harris III fracture 107
sandfly fever 267
SaO_2
  acute breathlessness 209
  asthma 214, 215
    children 350, 351
  breathing problems 3
  burns 141
  chronic obstructive pulmonary
    disease 218
  pulse oximetry 210–11
scabies 427
scalds 142, 146, 146*b*
scaphoid bone fracture 127, 128*f*
scarlatina 361
scarlet fever 361–2
schizophrenia 378
sciatica 62
scintigraphy (technetium bone
  scanning) 128
SCIWORA (spinal cord injury
  without radiological
  abnormalities) 31
scombroid fish, toxic effects of 299
scrotal pain 324
sea urchin spines 421
sebaceous cysts, infected 425
second-degree heart (AV) block 173
second disease 361
sedation 13–16
  assessment of level of 14
  children 366–9
  contraindications 15
  discharge criteria 15
  disturbed patients 374
  drugs 14–15
  grades classification 13*t*
seeds, poisonous 298
see-saw respiration, partial upper
  airway obstruction 2
seizures see fits and seizures
selective serotonin reuptake
  inhibitors (SSRIs) 289
self-determination, right to 398
self-harm 379, 384
Sengstaken–Blakemore tube 314
sensory dermatomes 51*f*
sepsis 273
septicaemia 258*b*, 268, 269, 360
septic arthritis 96, 100, 422
septic shock 250–1
serotonin syndrome 289, 308–9
serum lactate 25*b*

severe acute respiratory syndrome (SARS) 223
sexual abuse of children 371
sexual assault and rape 394
  post-exposure prophylaxis 332–3
sexually transmitted infections 336–7
Sgarbossa criteria 189, 190*b*
shaken baby syndrome 43
shared mental model 17–18
Shiga toxin-producing *E. coli* (STEC) 272
shingles 204, 441
shin splints 103
shock 250
  cardiogenic 250–2
  distributive 250
  hypovolaemic 250
  index 25*b*
  neurogenic 54
  obstructive 250
  septic 250–1
  signs of 25*b*
  spinal 53
shockable rhythms 158, 161
shoulder problems 113–18
sickle cell disease 270–1
Simulium posticatum 418
Sindig-Laarson disease 102
sinus bradycardia 195
sinusitis 441
sixth disease 361
skier's thumb 139
skin
  coolness 4
  grafts 417
    burns 147
  hypothermia 248
  lesions 425
  loss 414
skull
  fractures 39, 43–5
    child abuse 44*b*
  radiography 37, 41, 43, 44*b*
slapped cheek syndrome 361
slings 113–15, 114*b* 117, 121, 122, 125
slipped upper femoral epiphysis 97, 97*f*
small bowel obstruction 320, 320*b*
smallpox 268
small wounds 410–16
  abrasions 417
  aftercare 414
  anaesthesia 411
  assessment 410–11
  botulism 416
  cleaning and exploration 411–13
  closure 413–14

crush wounds 417
degloving injuries 417
flap wounds 417
infection prevention 414–15
radiographs for foreign bodies 413
reimplantation of body parts 414
resuturing 414
roller injuries 417
tetanus prevention 415–16
tissue resection 413
Smith's fracture 127
smoking 185, 232
Snellen chart 429*b*
snoring 2
social problems 12
sodium bicarbonate
  cardiac arrest 163–4
  hyperkalaemia 260
  hyponatraemia 262
  jellyfish stings 419
  poisoning
    aspirin 285–6
    ethylene glycol 296
    iron 295
    methanol 296–7
    tricyclic antidepressants 288–9
  rhabdomyolysis and myoglobinuria 262
sodium calcium edetate 305
solvent abuse 294
somatostatin 314
sotalol 181, 297
spider bites 418
Spikes model, breaking bad news 16*f*
spinal concussion 53
spinal cord
  anatomy 48
  clearance 54–8
  epidural abscess 61–2
  imaging 55
  infections 62
  injuries 50–9
    children 50
    cord syndromes 50, 53
    electrocution 150
    hip symptoms 94
    initial management 48–50
    localisation 50
    neck and back injury 58–63
    see also cervical spine; thoracolumbar spine
spinal cord injury without radiographic abnormality (SCIWORA) 58
spinal immobilization 49
spinal shock 53

splenic injuries 84
splintage 89
  avascular necrosis of the lunate 130
  carpal tunnel syndrome 129
  de Quervain's tenosynovitis 129
  disturbed patients 377
  elbow dislocation 121
  femoral shaft fracture 95*b*
  humeral shaft fracture 118
  lower leg 103*b*
  mallet finger 139
  partial avulsion of fingertip 134
  peritendonitis crepitans 129
  radial fracture 124
  scaphoid bone fracture 128
  shin pain 103
  small wounds 414
  torus fractures 125
  trigger finger 130
  ulnar fracture 124
  upper limb 113, 114*b*
splinters under the nail 421
spontaneous bacterial peritonitis 316
sports injuries
  eyes 431
  limbs 91
  pretibial pain 104
  shin splints 103
sprays, incapacitating 302
stable angina 196–7
stab wounds 73*b*, 392, 417–18
  abdomen 82, 84
  back 63
  chest 75
  great vessels 80
  haemothorax 75
  heart 80
  pneumothorax 75
staphylococcal toxins 266
Staphylococcus aureus 252, 360, 423
Staphylococcus saprophyticus 335
status epilepticus 244
Steatoda nobilis 418
sternal fractures 50, 79
sternoclavicular joint disruption 113
steroids *see* corticosteroids
stimulant drugs, poisoning 292
stings 419
strangulated bowel 320
Streptococcus pneumoniae 218, 220–3
Streptococcus pyogenes 361, 424
Streptococcus viridans 252
streptokinase
  contraindications 191*b*

stridor 208–9
 children 348–50
  upper airway obstruction,
   partial 2
stroke 240–2
stroke volume 4
structured communication 17
strychnine poisoning 246
ST-segment elevation myocardial
   infarction (STEMI) 187–91
 ECG changes 187–8
 reperfusion therapy 190–1
 treatment 190
subacromial bursitis 114–15
subarachnoid haemorrhage
   (SAH) 47, 238
subconjunctival haemorrhage 431
subdural haematoma 46, 379
subendocardial infarction 193
subungual collections 421
sudden infant death syndrome
   (SIDS) 371–2
sudden unexpected death in
   childhood procedures
   (SUDIC) 372
Sudeck's atrophy 130
suffering, relief of 10, 11b
suffocation 31
suicide 384
 alcohol addiction 379
 depression 383
 risk assessment 305, 384b
sulfonylureas 288
sulphur dioxide poisoning 303
sumatriptan (Imigran) 239b
sunburn 143
superficial reflexes, nerve roots
   supplying 50t
supracondylar fractures 120–1, 120f
supraglottic swelling, throat
   examination/instrumenta-
   tion contraindicated 2
supraspinatus tendinitis 114–15
supraventricular tachycardia
   (SVT) 175–7
 infants 177, 179
 irregular/broad-complex 175
surgical airway 2, 205
surgical care 454–455
surgical cricothyroidotomy 22b, 205
surgical emphysema 75, 76
surgical skills 455
sutures 414
 facial wounds 69
 skin grafts 417
swallowed foreign bodies 438
sweating
 breathing problems 3

cardiac dysrhythmias 172
chest pain 185, 186, 196
circulation problems 4
syncope 236
syndrome of inappropriate
   antidiuretic hormone
   secretion (SIADH) 261
Syntometrine 327, 331
syphilis 338
syringing an ear 436
systolic blood pressure 5

tachyarrhythmias 175
tachycardia 172
 algorithm 178f
 breathing problems 3
 electrocution 150
 myocardial infarction 195
 supraventricular 176–7
 ventricular 180–1
talar fractures 107
tampons, retained or infected
   vaginal 334
tarsometatarsal fracture and
   dislocation 109
Taser injuries 400–1
tazobactam
 biliary disease 316
 neutropenic sepsis 273
 peritonitis 317
 pneumonia 222
 variceal haemorrhage 314
team wellbeing 18
tear gas 302
technetium bone scanning
   (scintigraphy) 128
teeth
 injuries to 70–1
teicoplanin 273
temazepam 130
temporal arteritis 239
temporomandibular joint (TMJ)
   dislocation 66
tendon reflexes, nerve roots
   supplying 50t
tenecteplase 192b
tennis elbow 122
tension headache 240
tension pneumothorax 24, 75–6,
   75b, 77b, 162, 168, 201
terbutaline 215, 217, 352
terfenadine 181
terlipressin 314
terrorism
 police, release of information to
   the 401–2
testicular swelling and pain 336
testicular torsion 336

tetanus 245–6, 441
 prophylaxis
  abdominal injuries 84
  dental injuries 71
  electrocution 145
  envenoming 299
  hand injuries 133
  limb problems 89
  small wounds 415–16
  trauma patients 28
 Renshaw cell 245
tetany 260–1
tetracaine 428
Thaumetopoea processionea 419
theophylline 213, 214, 217, 289–90
thermoregulation, impaired 54
thigh, femoral shaft fracture 91–7
third-degree heart (AV) block 173
third disease 361
Thomas' splint 95b
thoracic outlet obstruction 118
thoracocentesis, needle 77b
thoracolumbar spine
 fractures 59–60
 radiography 57
thoracotomy 75
 criteria for 80
 procedures after 83b
 resuscitative 27, 81, 83b
 technique 81
 trauma patients 27
throat problems 437–41
thrombocytopenia 271
thrombolysis
 complications 191b
 contraindications 241, 241b
 lower limb arterial occlusion 110
 pulmonary embolism 229–30
 STEMI 190–1
thrombosed external pile 325
thrombus, cardiac arrest 162
thrush 334
thumb injuries 139
thyrotoxicosis 257
tibial condyle fractures 100
tibial epiphysis
 distal fracture 107
 posterior displacement of the
   lower 107
tibial shaft fractures 103
Tietze's syndrome 204
Tillaux fracture 107
tirofiban 195
tissue donation 406
tissue glue 69
toddlers' fracture (tibia) 103
toe fractures 110
toluene 294

tolvaptan 262
tongue blade test 66*b*
tongue injuries 69–70
tonsillectomy, bleeding after 441
tonsillitis 439
tooth
    extraction, bleeding after 441
    injury 69*b*, 70–1, 70*b*
torsade de pointes 181, 181*f*
torticollis 59
Torus fractures 124–5
toxic shock syndrome 334
toxins, cardiac arrest 163
tracheitis 204
tracheobronchial tree injuries 79
tracheostomy 22, 64
Trachinus draco 419
Trachinus vipera 419
traction splints 95*b*
training
    Advanced Trauma Life
        Support 20
tranexamic acid 27
tranquillisers 291
transient global amnesia (TGA) 242
transient ischaemic attack
        (TIA) 242, 242*b*
transient loss of consciousness
        (TLOC) 236–7
transient synovitis 96
transverse processes, fractures 60
trauma care 454–455
Trauma Care Checklist 445, 447*f*
trauma, major
    Advanced Trauma Life
        Support 20
    bereaved relatives 32
    chain of care 21–2
    children 31
    definitive care 29–30
    epidemiology 19–20
    pregnancy 32
    prehospital care 21
    preparation for patient
        reception 20
    primary survey and resuscitation
        phase 20–7
    scoring systems 33
    secondary survey 11, 21, 27–8
traumatic asphyxia syndrome 80
traumatic cardiac arrest
        (TCA) 167–8
    algorithm 82*f*
    reversible causes 168*b*
travel 264–9, 299
travellers' diarrhoea and
        vomiting 266–7
trench foot 427

Trethowan's sign 97
tricyclic antidepressants (TCAs)
    poisoning 166, 288–9
trigeminal autonomic
        cephalgias 240
trigger finger 130
trimethoprim 335, 336
tripod fracture of malar complex 66
tropicamide 428
troponins 184–6, 188, 191, 192*b*,
        193, 200
true posterior myocardial
        infarction 188*b*
trunk injuries 73–87
    abdomen 81–6
    assessment 73–4
    chest 73–81
    chest wall and lungs 75–81
    pelvis 86–7
Trypanosoma cruzi 252
tuberculin skin testing (TST) 225
tuberculosis 225–6, 225*f*, 252
tubular necrosis, acute 258*b*
tularaemia 425
tumbu fly 419
turpentine poisoning 298
tympanic rupture 434
typhoid fever 267
typhus fever 268

ulcerative colitis 319–20
ulipristal 332
ulnar fractures 124
ulnar nerve 122, 123*b*
ultrasonography
    abdominal injuries 85
    Achilles tendon rupture 104
    aortic aneurysm, leaking
        abdominal 317
    hip 96
    intussusception in children 363
    peritendonitis crepitans 129
    pregnancy
        ectopic 332
        trauma 32
        vaginal bleeding 331
    trauma patients 29, 32
    venous thrombosis 111
United Nations Disaster Assessment
        and Coordination team
        (UNDAC) 448
universal health coverage 443
unstable angina (UA) 185, 193, 197
upper airways 205–9
    obstruction
        allergic reactions 306
        partial 2, 208–9
        trauma 22*b*

upper arm problems 113–18
upper limb
    elbow 118–23
    forearm and wrist 123–30
    shoulder and upper arm 113–18
    support and splintage 113, 114*b*
    vascular problems 130–1
    see also hands
upper respiratory tract infections
        (URTIs) 359–60
uraemia 254, 259*b*, 271
ureteric colic 323–4
urinary tract
    infection (UTI) 324 335–6
        children 360
    stones in the 324
urine
    output
        head injuries 39
        organ perfusion 25*b*
        retention 324, 338–9
        spinal cord injuries 54
urogenital injuries 86–7
uterovaginal prolapse 334
urticaria 306
urticarial rash 362
uveitis 433

vagina
    bleeding 326, 332
        in pregnancy 330–1
    discharge 334
    examination 311*b*
    foreign bodies 334
vancomycin 62, 253, 273
vaping 232
vapours, noxious 303
variceal band ligation 315
variceal haemorrhage 314–15
vasovagal syncope 236
vasopressin 314
venous thromboembolism (VTE)
        110–11, 224
    plaster casts 90, 111
    risk factors 228*b*
ventilation
    asthma 214
    cardiac arrest 161, 164
    mechanical *see* mechanical
        ventilation
    respiratory arrest 209
ventilatory support 3
ventricular fibrillation (VF) 158,
        168, 180
    amiodarone 161, 163
    children 343*b*
    hypothermia 248
    lidocaine 163

ventricular septal defect (VSD) 196
ventricular septal rupture 196
ventricular tachycardia (VT) 158,
	180–2
verapamil 177, 287, 289
	contraindications 177
vertebra, collapsed 323
vestibular neuronitis 243
veterinary vaccine injection
	injuries 133
vibration white finger 131
Vibrio cholerae 267
Vincent's angina 441
Violence and Injury Prevention
	programme 445
violent crime 393
violent patients and relatives *see*
	aggressive patients;
	aggressive relatives
viral meningitis 356
Virtual On-Site Operations
	Coordination Centre
	(VOSOCC) 450
visual acuity, testing for 428, 429*b*
visual loss *see* blindness
vitamin B 381
vitamin C 381
vitamin K 272
vitamin poisoning 295

vitreous haemorrhage 434
Volkmann's ischaemic contracture
	112, 121
vomiting
	bleeding after 312–13
	children 362–3
	poisoning 280, 282, 285, 288, 289,
		293, 295, 296, 306
	travellers 266–7

wanderer's foot 427
warfarin 46, 231, 272
	adverse effects 272
	poisoning 288
wasp stings 419
water quality sanitation and hygiene
	(WASH) 457
waveform capnography 162
weever fish stings 419
Weil's disease 315
Well's scoring system for DVT 111,
	111*t*
Wenckebach's phenomenon 173
Wernicke–Korsakoff syndrome 383
Wernicke's encephalopathy 383
West Nile fever 269
whiplash injury 58
white cell count (WCC) 214, 227
white phosphorus burns 149

WHO Coordination Cell
	(WHOCC) 450
whole bowel irrigation 280–1, 295
winter vomiting (Noro, Norwalk)
	virus 322
witness statements 403
Wolff-Parkinson–White (WPW)
	syndrome 176, 181
World Health Organisation (WHO)
	oral rehydration solution 322
	severe acute respiratory
		syndrome 223
wounds, full thickness 70
wrist drop 244
wrist problems 123–4, 128–9, 129*f*
wry neck 59

yellow fever 267
yellow phosphorus burns 149
Yersinia pestis 269

zanamivir 225
zoonoses 264–9, 305, 425
zopiclone 394
zygomatic arch fractures 66
zygomaticofrontal suture,
	displacement 66